MODERN CLINICAL PSYCHIATRY

ARTHUR P. NOYES, M.D.

Superintendent, Norristown State Hospital,
Norristown, Pennsylvania

LAWRENCE C. KOLB, M.D.

Professor and Chairman, Department of Psychiatry, College of Physicians and Surgeons, Columbia University; Director, New York State Psychiatric Institute

FIFTH EDITION

W. B. Saunders Company

Philadelphia and London

Reprinted, November, 1958, June, 1959, June, 1960, and June, 1961

 Made in the United States of America. Press of W. B. Saunders Company. LIBRARY OF CONGRESS CATALOG CARD NUMBER: 58–7956

Preface to the Fifth Edition

It is with much satisfaction that announcement is made of the active participation of Dr. Lawrence C. Kolb, Professor of Psychiatry, Columbia University, in the preparation of the Fifth Edition of this book. It has been our purpose, so far as facts and experience seem to warrant, to maintain a dynamic and developmental orientation in the discussion of the various personality disorders that constitute the thesis of psychiatry. Acknowledgment is made of the indebtedness due to many writers who during the past five years have contributed much to the understanding and treatment of the various disturbances of personality functioning. It is hoped that the book reflects these contributions. In response to the suggestion of friends a chapter, Psychiatry and the Law, has been added.

It is a pleasure to acknowledge the great helpfulness of Mrs. Monica Mellon in the preparation of the manuscript.

Arthur P. Noyes

Contents

CHAPTER I

Psychiatry and the "Mind"

Scope of Psychiatry

Psychiatry may be defined as that branch of medicine which deals with the genesis, dynamics, manifestations and treatment of such disordered and undesirable functionings of the personality as disturb either the subjective life of the individual or his relations with other persons or with society. By genesis one refers to the source and process of origin of these disturbed functionings and malformations of personality; by dynamics is meant the motivations, techniques and measures utilized in the psychological functioning of the personality. Psychiatry is concerned not merely with the clinical manifestations and treatment of disturbances of human thinking, feeling and behavior but also with the energizing factors and influences that determine behavior. Particularly is psychiatry concerned with the morbid personality and with psychopathology, which may be defined as that branch of science that deals with the principles of abnormal behavior, or as the science of disordered functioning of the personality. Psychiatry is concerned, therefore, with the immaturities, disorganizations and disintegrations of personality. The range of personality maladjustments is broad and their nature complex, but their study and the application of measures designed to prevent, modify or correct personality disorders come within the scope of psychiatry. Viewed a little differently, psychiatry may be regarded as the science which deals with the psychopathological aspect of human biology. The latter considers man not only as a living organism but also as a thinking, feeling and striving one.

The "Mind"

It will be noted that in the definition of psychiatry there was no mention of the word "mind." There need not be, however, any objection to the use of the word provided it is employed as a collective designation for certain functional activities of the organism, particularly those of the organism as an individual personality. As a corollary to this definition of mind the reactions of parts of the organism would be designated as physiological, and mind as the integrated response of the organism to the complex physiological, psychological and sociological forces that impinge upon it. The "mind," therefore, is merely one aspect—the psychological aspect—of biological functioning of the organism and not a metaphysical entity having an existence parallel with the body. The dichotomy which is implied by mind and body does not exist in the organism. They are equivalent and inseparable expressions of life itself—the two aspects of psychosomatic existence. They are different phases of one fundamental unity of biological functioning which we separate only for convenience of discussion. It is in this sense as a biological manifestation of the organism responding and adjusting as a whole that the word mind will be used in this book. The expression of this reacting unity of function, or mind, constitutes *behavior,* which may be defined as the sum of our responses to stimuli arising from both within and without ourselves. As we shall see later, behavior is a product of both conscious and unconscious processes acting jointly. In general, behavior which is determined largely by conscious factors, is flexibly adapted to reality and modified by experience, may be spoken of as "*normal.*" Behavior, including thoughts and feelings, predominantly determined by motivations lying outside of awareness is called *neurotic.* The study of neurotic behavior has contributed much to our knowledge of human motivations and the significance of the everyday behavior of the individual.

Evolution of Mental Functions

We know that the comparative method of examination and investigation has been one of the most useful ways of inquiring into the various biological sciences. Comparative anatomy and embryology, for example, by revealing the genetic continuity of structure, have cleared up many an obscure problem in human anatomy. A comparative study of the functions which we call mental as they are manifested by the serial line of genera in their progress up the evolutionary scale will not be as illuminating as is the case in anatomy. Yet, as we watch the evolutionary ascent of the biological ladder and observe the successively larger patterns of behavior and the constantly increasing capacity for adjustment to life conditions, we may gain a broader view of the development and purpose of those directing, co-ordinating and unifying functions of the organism that collectively we call the mind. Such a survey will assist us also in realizing that the evolutionary development of the mind, like the evolutionary process in organic structures, is one of hierarchical continuity, and that a highly differentiated psyche is derived, not from an original nonpsychic element, but from a less differentiated psyche. This aspect of living beings that we know as mental was present from the first and not added somewhere in the process of evolution. It is a part of the biological evolutionary process.

What we call the mind may be looked upon as the adaptive patterns of purpose, of motivation, which have arisen as life has emerged from matter and through evolution have become progressively more highly organized. The psychic element exists therefore in every biological organization, and the higher psyche is derived from the lower. During biological evolution one observes an increasing importance of the psychological capacities of living matter and its capacities for knowing, feeling and willing. It should be remembered, however, that psychological and somatic analyses of life are merely two approaches to one and the same thing. There is a fundamental, progressive and cumulative common character extending from the properties of excitation and transmission observed in all protoplasm (properties which, it has been suggested, entitle it to the designation of psychoplasm) to the development of a complex nervous system and those functions we call mental. This evolutionary ascent is characterized by increasing differentiation, increasing specialization and increasing integration.

Levels of Mental Functions

Since the gradations from a less differentiated psyche to a highly differentiated one are made by imperceptibly progressive steps, any attempt to divide these reactions into fixed and clearly defined levels is quite arbitrary from a biological standpoint, although for descriptive emphasis it has value. Biologists and psychologists are not entirely agreed as to where such divisions should be made, but perhaps it is justifiable to speak of four levels constituting a hierarchy of mental functions: (a) the level of tropism; (b) the level of the reflex; (c) the level of instinct; and (d) the level of intelligence or reflection. Tropisms are observed most typically in the protozoa; reflex behavior is the predominant type of response in such species as the annelids; instinct reaches its greatest complexity in such insects as the bee; intelligence appears in animals having a cerebral cortex and reaches its maximum development in man with his highly complex neopallium. If space permitted, it would be interesting to discuss the phylogenic development of the nervous system as it parallels the progressively higher levels of integration and the accompanying progress in adjustment at the successive psychic levels, but the medical student, from his previous studies in biology and comparative anatomy, will easily refresh his memory.

Tropism

Tropism is a fixed type of behavior, or method of adjustment, characteristic of plants and certain primitive forms of animals in which the integrations are largely at the chemical level. Probably to be regarded as tropistic are certain highly adaptive instances of behavior seen in protozoa —activities some of which in higher animals would be described as examples of "trial and error." Jennings, for instance, relates that a paramecium, if it meets with an obstacle as it swims about, will first retreat and then advance in a different direction until finally the obstacle is avoided. In swimming, too, the paramecium usually advances in wide spirals, but if confined in a capillary tube too narrow to permit this it will swim by a rotary movement.

Reflex Adjustment

The earthworm offers a good example of the reflex level of the psyche. The stimulation of a receptor leads to a specific and constant response produced by the passage of the impulse from the receptor to a definite effector by way of determined adjustment center and conductors. While not at all on a conscious level it nevertheless shows interesting capacities for effecting adjustment. For example, it is stated that when attempting to drag a leaf into a burrow the worm will seize it by the narrow end. The vegetative life of man, regulated through the autonomic nervous system and its effectors of unstriated muscle and gland, is conducted on the level of the reflex. At this level we first find inherited networks of neuronal synaptic patterns.

Instincts

In the protozoa we find that tropism represents the mechanism of adjustment, and adjustment is secured by reflex behavior in the worm. In the insect we meet with much more elaborate behavior patterns made possible by a higher adjustment mechanism known as instinct. Behavior at this level may produce instances of exquisite adaptation. The ammophila, or solitary wasp, for example, affords an interesting example of adjustment effected by this type of behavior. As the egg-laying season approaches this insect digs a hole in the ground about 3 inches in depth; then, having found a caterpillar of a particular species, it stings the worm in one of its important ganglia, thus paralyzing but not killing the caterpillar. The wasp then proceeds to drag the defenseless worm into the burrow that has been prepared. After several caterpillars have been stored in this manner, the wasp deposits her eggs upon the helpless worms which continue to live until the eggs are hatched, when they are consumed by the young ammophila. Although this striking behavior is apparently intelligent, the fact that it is really stereotyped and unmodifiable does not become apparent until the sequence of events (chain reflexes?) is interrupted in some way. If, for example, one pushes aside from the entrance of the burrow a caterpillar awaiting storage, the wasp is unable to search for its victim, even though it be within range of sight and smell. The business of nest-making is either abandoned entirely or the procedure started afresh, beginning with the construction of a new burrow.

From what has been said, it might be inferred that reflex and instinct[1] are unallied types of behavior. Such a conclusion is unwarranted as the lower type of behavior passes into the higher by a continuous gradation. Both are innate reactions to stimuli and arise from the adjustment needs of the organism. Complex as it is, instinctive behavior, particularly in the lower forms of organisms, is an inelastic and stereotyped mechanism of

[1] The term "instinct" is unfortunately used in different ways. Here it is used to indicate a genetically inherited and relatively fixed, unlearned pattern of behavior which operates in the service of the organism. The behavior pattern is probably determined by the inherited pattern of neuronal network. In a dynamic psychiatry, however, the word is used in the sense of a hypothetical energy or drive to specific aims on the part of the individual.

adjustment with little capacity for modifiability. This fixity in the pattern of behavior is well illustrated in the case of the salmon, originally probably a fresh-water form which made a permanent migration seaward in some remote period. Each year now when the procreative impulse awakens the salmon is impelled to return to its ancestral home to bring forth its young, even though the act proves to be suicidal so far as the individual is concerned.

The concept that instinctive drives may prompt and direct our behavior is one that persons without biological training are often reluctant to accept. Not realizing that expressions of instinctive behavior may be disguised in the form of laudable activities possessing great spiritual value, they feel that such a conception is one that devaluates the motives of our behavior and therefore meet it with a resistant attitude. They fail to realize, too, that if through the process of evolution extending over millions of years nature succeeded in the lower animals in developing exquisitely adapted behavior based on those urging drives we know as instincts she would not, in her most highly evolved species, discard a plan that had served her purpose so efficiently in prehuman species and create a new and untried principle governing behavior.

Any discussion of behavior suggests a consideration of motives and doubtless leads one to ask if behavior should not be interpreted in terms of motives rather than of instincts. To such an inquiry one must reply that motives are but instinctive drives which man, because of his capacity for abstract thought, has been able to transform and thereby, in some measure, conceal.

If throughout the whole range of life the driving or initiating force is derived from instinctive urges, what, it may be asked, is the function of consciousness, or awareness of self and environment, in behavior? It is not the same thing as mind but is merely one attribute of mind—one that seems to become more prominent as the brain becomes more and more complex in the ascent of the phylogenetic scale. Its office, there is reason to believe, is largely selective and inhibitive, while to a small degree only is it creative. Similarly viewed, intelligence would be an instrument of instinct which remains the fundamental initiating condition of behavior and uses intelligence for determining how the goals of the organism can best be reached. Intelligence plays a much smaller part in determining behavior than we have been accustomed to believe. Behavior is based on a need to react, and needs do not arise out of intellectual considerations. They arise only out of instinctive and emotional drives in search of satisfaction. Intelligence is used in attaining the ends determined by these drives.

Instincts, therefore, have been considered, firstly, from an evolutionary and a physical point of view and, secondly, from a psychological standpoint. Viewed from the first standpoint they have been described as inherited patterns of action, as experience written into patterns of behavior. Psychologically, however—and in psychiatry we deal with psychological concepts—instincts are to be regarded as the innate biological urges or impulsions that drive the organism toward certain ends. They are the dynamic agents not merely for the maintenance of the individual or of the species but for creative purposes in art, philosophy and science. To return to the use of the singular number, we may speak of instinct as the constitutional factor in behavior.

Affects

Other important elements entering into the dynamics or motivation of behavior are affects and conation. While these dynamic elements must be discussed separately, their influence in determining behavior is so coordinated that they act largely as one. Affects, which may be defined as feeling-tones, are pain-pleasure accompaniments of an idea or mental representation. By stimulating or facilitating some instinctive tendency, they exercise a strongly determinative influence in giving direction both to thought associations and to overt behavior reactions. The terms affect and emotion are often used loosely and therefore as if these two aspects of mental life were the same. This is because the term *emotion* is used with many and, therefore, ambiguous meanings. Its use should probably be confined to indicate either the complex biochemical, physiological processes or functions concerned with the somatic expression of feeling, or else the patterns of behavior that express affect rather than subjectively experienced feeling phenomena to which the term affect is more applicable.

There is much to suggest that the processes, activities or patterns which we call emotion appear when there is some bar to the smooth and complete execution and satisfaction of an instinct. If there had been no interference with the satisfaction of the instinct, all the auxiliary activities stimulated by the vegetative nervous system and felt in consciousness as affect would not have taken place. When, however, there is interference with the execution of an instinctive activity, the vegetative nervous system initiates such activities of the organs under its control as will assist in carrying out the activity. If, for example, there is obstruction to an activity that would serve the instinct of self-preservation, both epinephrine and norepinephrine may be poured into the blood, as a result of which the blood pressure is raised, the heart and lungs work more rapidly, the arterioles of the skin contract—all being processes that force blood into the lungs, muscles and brain, where, during the emergency, it will be of maximum service. At the same time sugar is mobilized for the production of energy in the muscles, the coagulability of the blood is increased so that wounds are less likely to be fatal and the pupil of the eye is dilated so that the field of vision may be widened. All these changes serve to aid the instinct of self-preservation and are fused in the fields of sensation and consciousness into an affect which we speak of as fear. The subjectively experienced feeling aspect of an emotion may be regarded as an *affect.* The physiological and psychological aspects are, however, integrated and nonseparable.

Conation

Containing components from both instincts and affects, and in many ways merely a name for the urge created by these two dynamic agents, is that striving aspect or urge of the personality for expression known as *conation.* As conations we include those intention sets of the personality having motivating urges behind them. Here, too, one would include attitudes, or those responses determined with special reference to feeling states. Conation lacks the degree of consciousness which we usually associate with the idea of will or volition, since the individual may not recognize the affective-instinctive sources from which his action was prompted.

The concept that behavior is motivated by the psychobiological needs of the organism and that dynamic, striving impulses and tendencies act as prompting agents both in normal and abnormal behavior is one of the cornerstones of psychiatry. The fact that if incompatible they may give rise to neurotic reactions is the best criterion of their psychological strength and importance. Running constantly through the mental life of the individual, behavior has for its purpose the satisfaction of deep-seated, frequently unrecognized, instinctive and affective drives. If these strivings and drives, or goal-seeking impulses, find a harmonious satisfaction in socialized form, the result is a well adjusted personality. If, on the other hand, compelling impulses and tendencies find it impossible to exist harmoniously beside each other the personality may suffer such disorganization that mental disorder is said to exist. Instinctive impulses and deep-seated emotional needs may be blocked in their effort to secure satisfaction. They may therefore find substitute, often symbolic, satisfactions in forms which constitute symptoms of mental disorder. A psychiatry based on an attempt to obtain a penetrating understanding as to how these factors may have operated, often unconsciously, to produce personality disorders is known as dynamic psychiatry. In the light of such a psychiatry, the beliefs and behavior of the patient are rendered intelligible. They are studied in terms of cause and effect and reconstructed in terms of beginning and development.

Intelligence

In vertebrates the modifiable and integrative aspects of behavior are greatly increased. In them appears the cerebral cortex, developed for the purpose of providing a mechanism capable of elaborating, integrating and controlling impulses and functions more perfectly than is possible with a more elementary nervous system. In fact, evolutionary stages in development are traceable in the cerebral cortex itself, associated with a corresponding hierarchy of functions. The older part of the cortex, the archipallium, is concerned with olfactory and visceral functions, while the more recently developed portion, the neopallium, is essential for the highest psychic functions. The biological purpose of its development was that the organism might thereby avoid rigid domination by reflex and instinct and secure a more flexible adjustment.

An attempt has been made to show how psychological capacities and functional activities together with the structures which have made them possible have developed by successive steps. Like other biological processes, they have evolved from conditions of simplicity and diffusiveness to complexity, differentiation and definiteness. They have been traced through the stages of tropism, reflex and instinct—stages, we have observed, which merge imperceptibly one into the other. Similarly we find an imperceptible transition from instinct to cognitive ability or that adaptive attribute we call *intelligence*. Since, from a practical standpoint, the intelligence of an organism is fundamentally its psychological capacity for adapting to, and for making use of, its environment, it is quite arbitrary to say where in the phyletic series intelligence is acquired. In fact, intelligence probably was not superimposed on earlier instinctive processes at some definite stage of evolution but was an outgrowth of them. Those, be they species or individual human beings, that possess the greatest capacity in these respects are the most intelligent.

Consciousness

A prerequisite for that degree of adapting to, and making use of, the environment to which we apply the term "intelligence" is that mental function we know as consciousness. By this term, as already indicated, is meant a sense of awareness of self and of the environment. Its major biological purpose is to permit the organism to adapt itself to novel circumstances. How consciousness develops we do not know but it seems reasonable to assume that in common with higher functions in general it is a specialized development of lower ones. Such an assumption would be in agreement with the general proposition that if we trace back higher functions to their primary source, we find their beginnings in the general characteristics of living substance. While no conclusions as to the origin or nature of consciousness can be secured by objective observation, it is possible in an effort to trace it back to properties common to all protoplasm, to speculate that it goes back to the properties of irritability and response. When protoplasm—let us assume it to be in the form of an extremely simple organism such as a protozoan—is stimulated, a response occurs. A response, however simple, implies a change, a difference. As evolution progresses and the organism becomes more complex and as the types of stimuli and of responses multiply, one can imagine that the organism becomes gradually but dimly aware that modifications are induced, that changes occur in itself; a sense of comparison arises, until finally sensations are produced, an awareness of which constitutes the dawning of consciousness. These beginnings of perceptive processes undergo evolutionary expansion from the simple to the more complex until finally a conceptual consciousness with ideative and affective components is reached. Whether the dawning phases of consciousness arose in some such way can only be conjectured, but it seems safe to assume that its development was through an expanding process, a successive integration, which has progressed simultaneously with zoological evolution. At the psychological level is to be found the highest phase in integration in the continuity of nature. Looking back from this phase one notes how the inorganic integrates with the organic, the organic with the biological, and the biological with the psychobiological in which such attributes as consciousness exist. A consideration of the evolutionary process suggests that there is no sharp distinction between the conscious and the unconscious, and that conscious thinking represents the most highly developed and most fully integrated process of organizing and dealing with experience.

Degree of Consciousness. A phenomenon that should be mentioned in the consideration of the dynamics of behavior is that many psychobiological activities that we term mental occur without conscious awareness. It was formerly assumed that consciousness, or sense of awareness, was a prerequisite for all those expressions of the organism we refer to as mental. While many of these psychic functions are manifested only under conditions of clear awareness, observation of mental processes, particularly of those occurring in mental pathology, reveals that many highly significant psychic processes operate under widely varying degrees of awareness and even in the absence of awareness. Most students of man's mental life agree that he is greatly influenced by unrecognized psychological forces, and that much behavior originates from motives of which one is not aware in his normal waking state. Psychological motivations are undoubtedly a result usually of combinations of causes of which those which are least acceptable socially and morally possess the greatest driving force and are farthest removed from consciousness, whereas those which the individual considers the most acceptable are in the forefront of consciousness and are the manifest ones.

"The Unconscious"

In order to explain many mental phenomena the features of which are not manifest, it is necessary to hypothesize the existence of a stratum of the personality referred to as "the unconscious." It includes material which under ordinary circumstances is unable to enter the conscious part of the personality. Resistance must be overcome before the ordinarily inaccessible part of the unconscious can become conscious. These psychological activities and states are nonconscious and therefore beyond our conscious commands. They operate without awareness and are manifested in such forms as dreams, amnesias, purposeful forgetting, mistakes, split personality and other products. There is abundant evidence that unconscious motivations exercise a fundamental influence upon behavior, feelings, decisions and interpersonal relationships. In psychopathological states it is particularly apparent that unconscious psychic forces may be powerfully active in influencing personality. Motivations often spring from causes too deeply seated to be apparent and may therefore be described as having their origin in the unconscious, *i.e.*, in such a dim periphery of conscious recognition or memory that they do not come within the scope of awareness. Emotional forces of which the individual is unaware may be in conflict and act on him in such a way as to determine his behavior even though he knows nothing about them consciously. As will be discussed later, conscious and unconscious forces or motivations may pursue opposite goals. Much behavior, in fact, is a complex of conscious and unconscious motivations. It is only through active repression or through dissociation that any sharp division is introduced between the conscious and the unconscious. A great deal of our knowledge concerning motivations has been acquired by the psychoanalytic method of studying the unconscious through free-association technique. Some psychiatrists raise the question whether, instead of speaking of the unconscious, one should not emphasize unconscious mental processes.

The Preconscious

The preconscious is a term applied to mental processes which have not become conscious but possess the attribute of being admissible to consciousness. The material in the preconscious needs to pass only a slight barrier, so to speak, before entering consciousness.

BIBLIOGRAPHY

Bergson, Henri: Creative Evolution, Translated by Arthur Mitchell. New York, Henry Holt & Co., 1926.

Cannon, W. B.: Bodily Changes in Pain, Hunger, Fear and Rage. 2nd ed., New York, D. Appleton Co., 1929.

Child, C. M.: Physiological Foundations of Behavior. New York, Henry Holt & Co., 1924.

Cobb, Stanley: On the nature and locus of mind. Arch. Neurol. & Psychiat., *67*:172–177, 1952.

Gerard, R. W.: Higher levels of integration. Science, *95*:309–313, Mar. 27, 1942.

Gregg, Alan: What is psychiatry? Bull. Menninger Clin., *6*:137–146, 1942; also, Brit. M. J., *1*:550–553, Apr. 22, 1944.

Huxley, Julian: Knowledge, morality and destiny. Psychiatry, *14*:129–151, 1951.

Jennings, H. S.: The beginnings of social behavior in unicellular organisms. Science, *92*:539–546, Dec. 13, 1940.

Loeb, Jacques: Instinctive Movements, Reflexes and Tropisms. Philadelphia, J. B. Lippincott Co., 1920.

Margetts, E. L.: The concept of the unconscious in the history of medical psychology. Psychiat. Quart., *27*:115–138, 1953.

Novikoff, A. B.: The concept of integrative levels and biology. Science, *101*:209–215, Mar. 2, 1945.

Ritter, W. E.: The Unity of the Organism, or the Organismal Conception of Life. Boston, Badger, 1919.

Whitehorn, J. C.: Concerning emotion as impulsion and instinct as orientation. Am. J. Psychiat., *11*:1093, 1932.

———: Basic psychiatry in medical practice. J.A.M.A., *148*:329–334, 1952.

CHAPTER II

Development of Dynamic Psychiatry

"Now we, like all animals, carry with us vestigial traces of our past ancestry, not least in our mental processes. To develop psychologically we must understand ourselves, and it should help us to do so if we can find ways to investigate those hidden depths in our minds from which we draw our impulses." SIR WALTER LANGDON-BROWN

ALTHOUGH mention will be made in Chapter V of the development of some of our concepts concerning the causes and nature of mental disorders, and of the contributions made to that knowledge by certain psychiatrists, it may be well to refer now to the development of opinion concerning the entering of psychological forces into the formation of personality and its disorders. During the latter part of the nineteenth and the first quarter of the present century there was a rapidly increasing acceptance of the theory of a *dynamic psychiatry*—a psychiatry based on psychological influences and motivations. A chain of mental events and experiences is produced by pathogenic forces which may ultimately come to have determinative influence on behavior. Various factors and emotional experiences may, for example, lead to feelings of insecurity, these in turn to anxiety followed in a vicious circle by aggressiveness, feelings of guilt and further anxiety. According to this theory the behavior of a person, no matter how "abnormal," is considered to be the result of the driving forces and emotional needs that have entered into the structure and development of his personality as complicated and modified by counterstrivings and counterforces of other needs. Some of the driving and determining or motivational aspects of personality are conscious but more are beyond awareness. Entering, too, into the dynamic or cause-and-effect organization of the personality are the social and cultural influences to which it is exposed and the feeling-experiences growing out of interpersonal relationships.

Since throughout this book there will be repeated reference to "psychodynamics" it may be well to quote the definition of the word as adopted by the Conference on Psychiatric Education held at Cornell University in 1951. This Conference defined psychodynamics as "the systematized knowledge and theory of human behavior and its motivations." It is through the principles of psychodynamics that one obtains a penetrating understanding of human personality and behavior. Let us therefore review briefly some of the more important theories offered during the period mentioned that have contributed to our present assumptions concerning the operation of mental forces in the production of both normal and psychopathological reactions. While many others have supplemented the work of Janet, Freud and Meyer these three were largely responsible for the development of psychological medicine from a descriptive and classifying stage into one based on psychodynamic formulations with their emphasis on a dynamic interplay of emotional forces and other motivational aspects of personality.

Jean Martin Charcot

Charcot (1825–1893), by his recognition of the profound influence of ideas and by his study of hypnotism, may be looked upon as having paved the way for psychotherapy and for a psychological approach to the causes of mental disorders. His demonstration that the physical manifestations observed in hysteria are due to "ideas" has been called the most revolutionary conclusion in the history of psychiatry.

Weir Mitchell

About this time Mitchell (1829–1914) began actively to treat psychoneurotics but apparently he did not adequately recognize the influence of psychic factors or appreciate that his form of treatment was in certain respects admirably fitted to fix permanently the invalidism pattern he desired to remove. He believed the psychoneuroses were due to fatigue and treated them by rest and overfeeding. Through his forceful personality, a certain element of persuasion, and the confidence and regard in which he was held by his patients, many of them enjoyed at least a remission of their symptoms. The improvement was frequently but brief, a fact which is not surprising since we now know that the psychoneurosis is often a product unwittingly created for the sake of the gain that the illness brings; that therefore a treatment that surrounded the patient with all the accoutrements of the sickroom, made him the center of attention and increased his power and domination over his environment yielded gains which the patient was reluctant to forego. In Mitchell's day it was not adequately realized that the psychoneuroses are psychologically motivated and that a permanent cure cannot be expected until either the motives for recovery are greater than those for disease, or until the patient becomes aware of his motivations and is able through conscious reflection to solve the conflicting demands that beset him. Although Mitchell was one of the great psychotherapists of his day, he really contributed very little to our understanding of the disordered personality.

Hippolyte-Marie Bernheim

The work of Bernheim (1840–1919), professor of clinical medicine at Nancy, on hysteria, hypnosis and psychotherapy was of outstanding importance. He stripped the subject of hypnosis of much of its mystery, dispelled all ideas of special hypnotic powers and magnetic influences, and showed that patients could be susceptible to suggestion in the waking state and even to autosuggestion. He advanced the theory of a mental origin for hysteria and was probably the first to use the term "psychoneurosis" for hysteria and allied conditions. How nearly he approached our present understanding of the cause and treatment of hysteria is revealed in his expression, "The therapy of hysteria is not suggestion but de-suggestion." Bernheim apparently recognized, too, that acts might be devoid of conscious intent or even of conscious origin.

Through their work on hypnotism Bernheim and Charcot demonstrated the importance of ideas in the development of mental symptoms.

Pierre Janet

Attracted by his work on hysteria and hypnotism a brilliant group of pupils, of whom Pierre Janet and Sigmund Freud became the best known, gathered about Charcot at the Salpêtrière in Paris. As time went on these two pupils not only added to the work of Charcot but came to differ sharply from him and one from the other.

Janet (1859–1947) recognized that mental forces must be operative in producing the phenomena manifested by the psychoneuroses. Janet rested his theory of the neuroses on the lack of an adequate psychic tension on the part of the patient. By psychic tension Janet meant an integrating psychic energy which, when abundant and adequate, holds the stream of conscious activity together through its force of cohesion and thereby produces an integration of personality. If this cohesively-acting tension is deficient constitutionally, or becomes deficient through fatigue, stress or shock, the integration of the elements of consciousness becomes defective, the deficiency manifesting itself in the phenomena of the psychoneuroses. Janet introduced the term "psychasthenia"—psychic weakness. Under this term he included reactions characterized by phobias, anxiety, obsessions and compulsions—in fact practically all the mental disorders he had not already included under hysteria. If this lowering of psychic tension is general, then the manifestations are those of psychasthenia; if the lowering is localized, confined to a certain level, then the phenomena are those of hysteria. According to Janet, emotions, being of a low order in the psychic hierarchy, exhaust large quantities of energy, thus lowering tension and weakening the synthesizing forces. He laid little or no stress on intrapsychic conflict as a cause. Based on his concept of a deficiency or lowering of cohesiveness or tension, Janet formulated the idea of dissociation as a result of which certain elements of consciousness take on an independent or separate existence, manifesting themselves as alternating personalities, fugues, paralyses, anesthesias and other hysterical and dissociative phenomena. His conception of dissociation as a mental state in which there is a piece of consciousness split off from the main bulk has established a place in abnormal psychology. Janet, who became professor of psychology in the Collège de France, studied particularly the various phenomena of suggestion, phobias, automatism and compulsive acts and brought together in one systematic framework all the strange phenomena of hysteria.

In addition to the concepts of dissociation and of psychological tension, Janet introduced that of a subconscious. He recognized that factors of which the patient was not aware were important in the production and manifestations of hysteria but assumed that certain mental processes go on in the subconscious independently of (dissociated from) the main stream of consciousness. This dissociation was due, he believed, to a constitutional deficiency in the hypothetical psychological tension. The splitting was therefore largely mechanical and caused by lack of psychological tension or energy and not to repression, a concept which he did not accept. "Repression," Janet said, "is not a normal phenomenon which through clumsy handling becomes the cause of subsequent disturbance; it is itself already a morbid disturbance."

Most of Janet's formulations now seem inadequate and superficial, yet he played an important part in the discovery of some of the essential tenets of modern psychology and laid the groundwork for an explanative psychopathology. He just failed of constructing a penetrating, dynamic psychology of the neuroses. He did, however, show that ideas caused such symptoms as paralysis following emotional shock and that hypnosis could be used for tapping the patient's memory and discovering the origin of symptoms. His contributions as a pioneer in psychological medicine merit much gratitude.

Sigmund Freud

In 1885 Freud (1856–1939), attracted by the fame of Charcot, went to Paris and studied with him for a year. He was much impressed by Charcot's use of hypnosis as a method of treating hysteria. After his return to Vienna he used hypnosis as his chief method of treatment but without satisfactory success. He then became associated with Josef Breuer in the study of neuroses. Breuer was the first to discover that neurotic symptoms had "meaning," a relation to the patient's previous life. He observed, too, that when under hypnosis his patients "re-lived" previous emotional experiences. Under hypnosis their minds went back to old ideas and impulses which they had had to suppress. As these were brought into consciousness by hypnosis and the patient "talked out" his emotional difficulties he improved. In spite of the promising beginning which Freud and Breuer achieved in removing pent-up emotion by this method, the latter became dissatisfied and discontinued it, leaving Freud to carry on alone. Left to himself, Freud soon dropped hypnosis and continued the talking-out method without it. He persuaded the patient to talk freely, to say whatever came into his mind, holding back nothing because it was thought to be irrelevant or distressing. He had already noted that events causing shame or similar emotional disturbance were violently repressed and so made "unconscious" or forgotten. He soon noted that this "free association," or unconstrained expression of mental content, could be used as a means of extending the range of exploration of the patient's mind.

Basing his concepts on observations secured through explorations of the unconscious and its relations to consciousness, Freud soon departed widely from Charcot and Janet and gradually developed what was in many ways an entirely new system of psychology. To this new psychodynamic system which he first employed as a technique for treating psychoneurotic disorders, but which soon became a psychological theory and method of psychic research, and finally in some respects a speculative philosophy, Freud gave the name "psychoanalysis." Freud and some of his adherents have extended certain deductions from psychoanalysis to a degree that seems to many psychiatrists to be extreme. Many of the basic principles of psychoanalysis have now, however, been widely accepted by non-Freudians and extensively permeate psychiatric theory and practice. It is generally considered beyond dispute that his concepts have contributed more to an unlocking of the secrets of the human personality and to an understanding of the psychogenesis of mental disorders than have those of any other system of psychology. One of its basic features is its genetic approach by an attempt to explain the present by reconstructing the past and its continuing influence. To psychoanalysis, in fact, we are largely indebted for our knowledge concerning psychopathology and psychodynamics. Through its stress on the significance of childhood experiences and relationships and of the unconscious as an integral part of the mind, psychoanalysis has shown that behavior and symptoms which seem incomprehensible become significant and meaningful.

SOME PSYCHOANALYTIC CONCEPTS. The notion of unconscious mental processes is to be found already in the writings of Augustine and of Thomas Aquinas yet Freud was undoubtedly the first to apply such a concept to the problem of human motivation. Through his study of dreams, hysterical symptoms and hypnotic phenomena, Freud was able to demonstrate that mental forces and processes of which one is unaware are of great importance in the motivation of his behavior. It is perhaps not too much to say that the basis of dynamic psychiatry and psychotherapy rests on the concepts of unconscious mental processes and of methods for the study of the deeper motivational aspects of behavior.

One of the most practically useful concepts introduced by Freud is that of hypothetical divisions of the personality. These divisions, the id, the ego and the superego, each with its specific functions, will be discussed in Chapter III, Personality Development and Structure.

Another concept is that of the Oedipus complex, so named from the legend of King Oedipus, who, moved by forces over which he had no control and without knowledge of his parents' identity, slew his father and married his mother. As the developmental stages in the love or, as Freud would broadly designate it, the sexual aspects of the personality take place, the first love-objects of the child are naturally found within the family circle. Thus there arises an attitude of sexual attraction on the part of the child toward the parent of the opposite sex and one of rivalry and hostility toward the one of its own. The child enters this phase at about the third year and normally works through to a satisfactory solution by the age of five. This complex Freud regarded as the central one in the whole unconscious, as the nucleus of all human relationships. In his opinion, the way the child deals with it determines more than does anything else the individual's character and temperament as well as any neurosis he may develop.

Many psychiatrists, while acknowledging that the Oedipus relationship is of significance in personality development, doubt that such a cross-sex parental preference is universal. They conceive of love and attachment to the one parent as not being necessarily a sexual one, and of the hatred or resentment against the other as not necessarily stemming from sexual rivalry. The antagonism between father and son may be caused, not by the latter's incestuous strivings, but by his resentment of paternal authoritarian power.

Evaluation of Freud's Contributions. Freud's supreme contributions consisted of demonstrating that there are processes that go on outside awareness and of discovering techniques for bringing them into consciousness. To him, too, are we largely indebted for the emphasis on early life experiences as extremely important sources of personality disorders. The criticism may be made that his concepts of personality structure suggest the animism of prescientific psychology. If, however, his more ultraspeculative concepts and his emphasis on infantile sexuality as a source of basic conflicts be discounted, we shall find in his theories many of the most illuminating and widely accepted interpretations of personality disorders. (His theory, however, has been subject to much misapprehension partly because of our habits of thinking in terms of adult sexuality, and partly because Freud came to give the word sexuality such a singularly wide meaning that many think it has largely lost its usefulness to thought.) In justice to Freud it should be said that he distinguished sharply between "sexual" and "genital" and that in speaking of infantile sexuality he did not at all have in mind the adult sexual urge that is focussed on the genital organs. By "sexual" Freud meant merely the pleasure satisfaction that the child secures from the sense-stimuli of special zones of his body. At the stage of personality development designated by Freud as pregenital, the genitals have not yet become the dominant pleasure zone. Another factor which has doubtless produced confusion and misunderstanding among dissenters from his tenets is Freud's extensive use of metaphors and analogies.

While accepting in the main the theories which Freud has presented, many psychiatrists prefer to supplement them with other observations and theories. Many feel that Freud, in spite of the unquestioned importance of the early experiences of childhood as determinative influences, of intrapsychic conflicts and of the mutual interactions of impulses and defensive measures which ward off anxiety, did not sufficiently emphasize the compelling part played by reality and by actual experiences occurring in many phases of life throughout post-childhood years, or by feeling tones and emotional reactions representing conditioned responses. As fundamental as is the concept of unconscious motivations, the prompting basis of behavior is probably broader than Freud conceived it. We are greatly indebted, not so much to Freud himself as to his students, for a recognition of the important emotional and dynamic implications of personal relationships and interpersonal attitudes. Many psychiatrists now feel that Freud overemphasized the concept of libido, an instinctive creative impulse, and did not adequately emphasize the results of socializing forces on the personality. General psychiatry has now assimilated many psychoanalytical principles. Certain Freudian concepts, including those of exploration, have greatly broadened and deepened the study of psychiatric problems. It is probably not too much to say that the greatest advances ever made in psychotherapy are based on psychoanalytical principles. To no other person are psychiatrists so indebted as to Freud for a recognition of the fact that in mental as in physical science no event or phenomenon is to be regarded as isolated but rather as a link in a chain of inevitable sequence. One of the greatest contributions of psychoanalysis has been to show the continuity of principles governing "normal" and "abnormal" behavior alike. Psychoanalysis is gradually growing less dogmatic and undergoing modifications and changes both in theory and practice that promise to reveal even further the moving forces in personality and to make it possible to guide or redirect them more effectively. An adequate recognition of the great value of its contributions has doubtless been retarded in part because of its highly esoteric terminology.

America and Psychoanalysis

In 1909 Freud was invited by G. Stanley Hall, president of Clark University, and by Dr. James J. Putnam, a Boston neurologist, to give a series of lectures at Worcester, Massachusetts. In the same year Dr. A. A. Brill (1874–1948), a former pupil of Freud's at Vienna, translated the latter's Selected Papers on Hysteria. Soon the influence of William A. White and Smith Ely Jelliffe gave an added impulse to the acceptance of psychoanalysis in America. Through the medium of their Nervous and Mental Disease Monographs and through the Psychoanalytic Review founded by them in 1913 they made many original contributions to the theory and therapeutic principles of psychoanalysis. With his inquiring and analytical mind, always eagerly in search for underlying factors in the development of abnormal reactions, it was natural that White should adopt a Freudian orientation toward psychiatry. A facile writer and speaker, interested in the dynamic forces of the personality, White perhaps contributed more than any other American psychiatrist to a recognition of dynamic factors in the causation of mental disease. Incidentally, it may be added that White, imbued with the newer trends in psychopathology, contributed immensely to the understanding and treatment of legal problems and to a scientifically valid basis for the present-day mental hygiene movement.

Adolf Meyer

While a more comprehensive presentation of Meyer's (1866–1950) contributions to psychiatry will be made in Chapter V, The Causes and Nature of Mental Disorders, mention should be made at this point of some of their more dynamic aspects. Meyer proposed that the development of the personality, whether normal or disordered, could be explained by an approach which he termed "psychobiological." Such an approach would utilize relevant and applicable data from "all the sciences entering into the understanding of the human life-processes and life problems." By such an approach, one would consider not merely the physical organism but all the social, cultural and emotional factors and experiences that make the individual what he is. Psychobiology, therefore, is a biology of the whole personality—the whole person in the whole situation. Mental expressions of life are no less biological than physical ones. It would not be doing justice to his great influence on psychiatry were it not added that although Meyer did not wholeheartedly accept the theory or even the method of psychoanalysis he nevertheless emphasized the importance of its dynamic concepts. In fact Meyer was one of the first to introduce the concept of genetic-dynamic formulations in explaining the development of mental disorder. In his reconstruction of the patient's mental illness, Meyer did not exclude unconscious and other psychological processes to the extent suggested by many psychiatrists and did thoroughly appreciate the sensitizing or conditioning influence of environmental factors, the significance of disturbing emotional experiences, of substitutive and evasive reactions, of symbolic expressions and the patient's various modes of securing satisfaction for his complicated needs. He did, however, think of much mental disorder as a process of progressive habit formation. In his teaching Meyer condemned the method of choosing one complaint, one aspect of the patient's problem, and of examining it from the viewpoint of any one particular system of psychiatry. Meyer distinguished types of reaction on a descriptive basis but stressed that psychiatric disorders, like normal behavior, represent adaptive reactions of the individual organism and that every such reaction is an understandable result of the total psychobiological development of the individual up to the occurrence of the disordered reaction. He was among the first to formulate personality studies. Meyer stressed the continuity of the forces which produce both personality and the mental illness. He taught that one should attempt to understand all maladaptive behavior by a comprehensive study of the life history of the individual and by tracing the development of his personality and his general life adjustment. He pointed out that the individual human being is both product and victim of his own life experiences. In his approach to therapy he carefully assessed the patient's personality "assets and liabilities," emphasized the study of faulty "habit patterns" and the possibility of re-socialization. Both Meyer and Freud taught that the occurrence and nature of the psychiatric symptoms can be understood only by an apprehending and insightful study of their development and not by attributing them to a specific cause.

As the first to emphasize that psychiatry is a biological science and that its practitioners should study the actual and complete dynamic situation in which the patient finds himself, Meyer left an indelible imprint on the form and content of American psychiatry which may now be regarded as a psychobiology extended in breadth and depth by many psychoanalytic principles.

BIBLIOGRAPHY

Alexander, Franz, and Ross, Helen, Eds.: Dynamic Psychiatry. Chicago, The University of Chicago Press, 1952.

Allport, G. W.: The trend in motivational theory. Am. J. Orthopsychiat., *23:*107–119, 1953.

Bailey, Percival: Janet and Freud. Arch. Neurol. and Psychiat., *76:*76–89, 1956.

Bernheim, Hippolyte: Suggestive Therapeutics. New York, London Book Co., 1947.

Brill, A. A.: Freud's Contributions to Psychiatry. New York, W. W. Norton & Co., Inc., 1944.

Cameron, N. A.: The Psychology of Behavior Disorders. Boston, Houghton Mifflin Co., 1947.

Freud, Sigmund: Collected Papers. New York, International Psychoanalytical Press, 1924–45.

----: New Introductory Lectures on Psychoanalysis. New York, W. W. Norton & Co., Inc., 1933.

Hall, J. K., et al.: One Hundred Years of American Psychiatry. New York, Columbia University Press, 1944.

Hinkle, B. M.: The Re-Creating of the Individual, 2nd ed. New York, Dodd, Mead & Co., 1949.

Hunt, J. McV.: Personality and the Personality Disorders. New York, The Ronald Press, 1944.

Jacobi, J.: The Psychology of C. G. Jung, 5th ed. New Haven, Yale University Press, 1951.

Janet, P. M. F.: Psychological Healing. New York, The Macmillan Company, 1925.

Lief, Alfred, Ed.: The Commonsense Psychiatry of Adolf Meyer. New York, McGraw-Hill Book Co., Inc., 1948.

Meyer, Adolf: Objective psychology, or psychobiology with subordination of the medically useless contrast of mental and physical. J.A.M.A., *65:*860, 1915.

Mullahy, Patrick, Ed.: The Contributions of Harry Stack Sullivan. New York, Hermitage House, 1952.

Murphy, Gardner: Personality: A Biosocial Approach to Origins and Structure. New York, Harper & Brothers, 1947.

Obendorf, C. P.: A History of Psychoanalysis in America. New York, Grune & Stratton, 1953.

Schwartz, Leonhard: Die Neurosen und die dynamische Psychologie von Pierre Janet. Basle, Benno Schwabe & Co., 1951.

White, W. A.: Twentieth Century Psychiatry. New York, W. W. Norton & Co., Inc., 1936.

Winters, Eunice, Ed.: The Collected Papers of Adolf Meyer, Vols. I-IV. Baltimore, Johns Hopkins Press, 1950.

Zilboorg, Gregory, and Henry, G. W.: A History of Medical Psychology. New York, W. W. Norton & Co., Inc., 1941.

CHAPTER III

Personality Development and Structure

"During man's growth, mere individuality becomes personality: and the developed individual personality is not only the most complex type of organization known, and one which exhibits a far greater range of diversity among its members than any other single type of organization, but the highest product of evolution of which we have any knowledge."[1]

Personality Development

It is obvious that an organism undergoes a process of development of biological structure from the time of the fusion of the male and female germ cells until adult maturity has been reached. At any time during this biological development noxious factors may limit the growth of the organism, produce malformations or impair the functioning of an organ or of the entire living being. Each person, therefore, has an anatomical structure conforming in general to the species pattern yet unique in certain details. So, likewise, he has more or less enduring and consistent patterns of temperament, character, intelligence, beliefs, desires and adjustmental tendencies that give him an individual uniqueness. The distinctive whole formed by the integration of these relatively permanent patterns and tendencies which are distinctive of a given individual may be spoken of as *personality*, in considering which it will be helpful to apply the concepts of developmental evolution and functioning.

To a limited extent certain patterns are already laid down at birth, yet for the most part only the potentialities for the development of personality components exist at that time. Whether the successive stages of the unfolding personality proceed in a wholesome manner and in a

[1] Huxley, Julian: Knowledge, morality and destiny. Psychiatry, *14*:131, July, 1951.

normative, harmonious sequence of biopsychological and biosocial maturation through infancy, childhood, maturity and old age with subjective happiness and social adjustment, or whether there is an arrest or uneven growth of various personality components depends upon complex genetic, environmental, social and emotional factors. In personality development there is normally a maturational sequence, each stage developing as a logical sequel to the previous one—an emergent growth through distinctively different stages each of which has its particular needs and problems. If residues of an earlier stage are carried over to later ones, they may serve to produce malformations of the personality and to become a source of psychopathology. Early experiences, too, continue to exert their influence on the developing personality even though they are not available to conscious recall. The operation of the processes by which, through interactive and reactive relations with these complex factors, the development of the personality proceeds is spoken of as *dynamic; i.e.*, the processes are prompted by psychological or perhaps, better, biopsychological forces that drive and direct human nature. As will be repeatedly emphasized in succeeding pages a psychiatric diagnosis must be a genetic and dynamic formulation of the processes, largely unconscious, responsible for the personality structure and the behavior of the individual patient. The most important contributions to the understanding of personality development have come from the study of persons suffering from personality difficulties.

Genes cannot transmit acquired characteristics. Although, therefore, the biological development of the fetus may be influenced by the intrauterine environment there is no reason to believe that personality, as just defined, is largely influenced by prenatal life or even that it exists in the newborn infant. This is not to say that there is not a genetic anlage or that there are not congenital aspects of biochemistry and reactivity that may create biological predispositions to the temperamental components of personality in later life. However, while extreme abnormalities in vegetative, central nervous and endocrine systems may have a demonstrable relation to personality characteristics, there seems to be very little relation between them and persistent features of the normal personality. This is not to say that social and psychological forces, important as they are, do not act upon a biological organism and a particular set of biological dispositions. To what extent the development of personality represents an unfolding of constitutionally derived action patterns can scarcely be said but psychiatry now tends to minimize this element.

It is difficult to state just when evidences of personality formation appear. It is certain, however, that maturity of personality is attained only through successive stages of maturation. The processes of maturation and personality development involve several steps or phases which are actually never separate and distinct but may be distinguished for purposes of discussion. There is a process of repeated relinquishment and supersedure of an earlier pattern of functioning or conduct by another pattern more appropriate to the growing, developing, aging individual. Personality development is therefore an ongoing process of maturation which may be stunted, distorted or even prematurely developed. Issues at one level must be dealt with fairly conclusively before those of a higher level can be managed. Each stage of development, too, should be characterized by patterns of thinking and feeling appropriate to it.

Present concepts of the development of personality in infancy and early childhood no longer assume that the infant has no relationships with people until he has reached the age of a year or more. On the contrary, it is believed that object relationships develop from birth on, although it is obvious that early relationships must be quite different in character from those experienced later. Differences in the manner in which infants respond to people are manifested by the three-to-four months child and are probably determined by previous relationship experiences. For the first two years the personality is largely infantile and under the domination of feelings. Primitive instincts are still in control. The young child therefore demands immediate satisfaction of desires in accordance with the "pleasure-principle." Not until the development of a relatively mature personality is one able to defer pleasure, to undergo discomfort in order to reach future gains or to satisfy desires by socially approved substitute activities—to be guided by the "reality-principle." Even though the personality remains infantile for a considerable period this does not mean that it is not being molded by psychological experiences. Of all experiences and factors those that have the most determinative influence upon the growing, plastic personality are those that spring from the emotional, personal, interacting relationships between the child and members of his family. The external shaping of the personality starts with parent-child relationship. It is the relationship between mother and child that is particularly significant. It is now generally accepted that an abundant and consistent "psychological mothering" tends to create a wholesome sense of satisfaction and security that may promote a healthy emotional, social and perhaps ethical development free from irreversible anxiety and tensional states. Many consider a wholesome mother-child relationship as vital for emotional growth and personality development as are vitamins for physical growth. Essential as a foundation for future healthy personality development, the child must have a feeling that he is wanted, loved and enjoyed by his parents. He should not, however, remain childishly dependent on a mother for maintaining emotional security. With the early emotional experiences the concept of father and mother is established, and along with these experiences basic interpersonal reaction tendencies which are important in determining later personality. The earliest experiences of the child are in the family setting and his interpretation of these experiences will most likely determine his interpretation of later, even adult, experiences that contain some apparent similarity. Such a transference of an attitude from some family situation may exert a favorable or an unfavorable influence upon personality development. Hostilities or other feeling tones may be built into the personality structure through early interpersonal relations. If a young child, for example, sees the comforting and protecting mother repeatedly hurt or made to cry by a cruel father he may acquire a lasting hatred for the father and perhaps for all men who resemble him. Again, if the mother is sometimes cruel, sometimes comforting, and not consistently one thing or the other the child may be unable to discriminate and will feel baffled and anxious. Ambivalent attitudes of love and hate are created and the foundation for a mixture of basic urges may be laid. A sense of security or of insecurity of personality is largely laid down, too, through the early parent-child relationships. If this relationship is a warm and friendly one and the child feels that he is loved and cared for, a desirable security of personality free from anxiety will follow. On the other hand, if he experiences frustration, rejection, harshness and uncertainty, his personality will be characterized by anxiety and insecurity and especially by hostility and aggression. Although many of the attitudes and patterns of responses established early through interpersonal experiences with parents or other significant persons are nonconscious they become of meaningful, dynamic importance in determining the personality and in shaping the child's attitudes toward himself and the world. It should be remembered, too, that in the family each child's situation is a unique one, entirely unlike that of the other children.

Suckling, feeding, weaning and toilet training may be of much significance because they are among the first experiences which may be accompanied by special meanings and therefore influence the direction of the child's development. Special meanings with their dynamic influence will be created by the attitude with which these functions are handled by the mother. If, for example, the child is punished for urinary or bowel incontinence before physiological maturation has made him capable of recognizing or announcing his need, or before he can walk to a toilet or manipulate his clothing, anxiety may be aroused in the child and he may respond with resentment and hostility. Perhaps as a reaction to such an experience the child may soil himself as a form of aggression against the parent. Unfortunately such punitive parents continue to use similar training methods in the problems of later childhood with cumulative influence on personality formation. Also of great influence in personality development and growing largely out of the interpersonal relationships experienced by the child are direction and training of aggression and whether he learns to give constructive or destructive expression to it.

Attention has been called to the complex crosscurrents of interpersonal relationships as significant agents in affecting personality. One of the most fundamental requirements is that these relationships supply the child's emotional needs. A mental mechanism that is early established through child-parent relationship is that of *identification.* By this mechanism the child, through his love for and wish to be like the parent of the same sex, unconsciously and automatically molds himself after the fashion of this parent and reproduces his values and characteristics. This is an unconscious process and not a mere imitation. If the parent is an emotionally mature person, this mechanism may be of profound influence in the promotion of a healthy mental and emotional maturation.

While the family with its emotional attitudes and atmosphere is the first social factor that influences the individual personality, other social contacts later exert more or less influence on the direction of personality and emotional development. Among them are school and social groups with which the individual may identify himself.

During middle childhood, identification and other parent-child relations continue to influence personality development, although not always uniformly. Other mental mechanisms, motivated largely through interpersonal relations, assume an increasing role in personality development. Compensation, prompted particularly by desire for attainment of status, is one of the more important. This may act constructively, or again a feeling of inadequacy may stimulate aggressive traits. At this time cultural and social influences with their associated values and prejudices help to direct the expanding personality. Problems involving security, dependence and independence, passivity and aggression, competition, hostility and love continue to arise and may stimulate personality growth or they may block or distort natural maturation processes with resulting immaturities or deviations of personality. Generally speaking, however, healthy personality growth occurs only if emotional needs are met. From early childhood, too, sociological and cultural factors constitute a molding influence on the developing process of personality formation. There should be a continual differentiation and expansion in the individual's responses as event follows event. His selection of responses should be of those that are progressively finer and more mature.

Since it began to occur much earlier than the period of personality development now under discussion, attention might well have been previously called to the fact that early in the unfolding of the child's personality a division arose between those psychological processes which develop on a conscious level and those which evolve on an unconscious level and exert their influence on the individual's life without his knowing of their existence. While further development of the personality continues to be directed by forces from both of these levels, its pattern, whether rigid and neurotic or flexibly adaptive to changing external realities, will depend largely on the extent to which forces from these two levels pursue incompatible goals and to what extent forces from the unconscious level dominate the personality.

Important as is childhood for the development of personality, its formation does not cease with the termination of that period. With adolescence new manifestations in the continuity of personality development appear almost automatically with the biological maturation of that period. Childhood experiences and the background of family relationships continue, however, to promote or interfere with personality development. There is an intensification of drive for self-sufficiency and independence which should be accompanied by growing vocational aptitudes and interests and by a sense of personal and social responsibility. The adolescent stands midway, nevertheless, between dependence and independence and therefore may experience difficulty in meeting the new problems of the latter. Frequently his emotional reactions are an expression of his emancipatory strivings. At puberty there are developmental changes in endocrine activities which are reflected in alterations of feeling and action.

Coincident with the physiological development of sex, there should be a maturation in its emotional, dispositional and socialization aspects. This development should continue until a mature disposition to heterosexuality, one of the basic aspects of a well developed personality, is established. The intensified emotional and instinctive drives of puberty are important factors in the development of this stage of personality growth. Intellectual growth which has developed simultaneously with biological growth reaches its maturity in middle or late adolescence. With the biological process of maturation, a corresponding emotional, psychological development should take place. Late adolescence, however, is usually characterized by a self-conscious, idealistic, cynical or romantic attitude. Each developmental period carries with it varying drives and defenses against these drives. In some instances the defenses may have an unfortunate effect on later personality development.

By the time adulthood is reached, the successive stages of personality development should have been worked through to a well adjusted degree prepared to meet the responsibilities and demands of mature relationships. Later changes are normally those of further integration and consolidation but preferably without the establishment of a cramping rigidity. With the attainment of adult personality organization, the individual should be more absorbed in work or family than in self-assertion and should be reconciled to limitations through satisfaction in real achievement. If he meets adult problems with attitudes more appropriate to a less mature stage of personality development, anxiety which will require some character or neurotic device for its alleviation will be created and render him unable to utilize his assets to the full. Pathological changes may, of course, occur in the adult personality as well as arrests and deviations in the course of its development. These, the particular subject with which psychiatry is concerned, will be discussed in later pages.

What we have attempted to point out in the preceding paragraphs is the fact that personality development is a genetic-dynamic, progressive, organizing, evolutional process and that it is biologically, culturally and psychologically determined. The fusion of the male and the female germ cells determines certain hereditary potentialities and probably certain constitutional predispositions. To an important degree, however, personality is shaped by environmental and subjective experiences and the manner in which the individual organizes them. This shaping starts with one of the most important of psychological relationships—that of parent-child. Sibling and other significant interpersonal relationships as well as social and cultural factors soon add a molding influence. As later discussion will show, the extent to and manner in which emotional and instinctive needs, both conscious and unconscious, are met exercise also a profound influence upon degree and direction of personality development. This implies that there are both conscious and unconscious forces in the personality and that it has both consciously and unconsciously organized levels. Personality, therefore, is a product of many interacting factors and includes all those inner dynamic expressions of thought, striving and feeling that characterize each person as a unique individual.

The behavior of the individual, whether normal or abnormal, will reveal recurring patterns partly determined by constitution but probably much more by feeling-experiences dynamically built into the personality during childhood. The type and degree of personality development depends to no small extent on the stability of the family and on the dynamics of the relationships which exist in it. All too often emotional disturbances in the family are perpetuated from generation to generation thus becoming familial rather than hereditary in nature.

As already stated, the development of personality has been presented as a complex evolving process in which there occurs a progressive maturation in the emotional, social, intellectual and physical spheres. This maturation is affected by the interplay of various forces, particularly hereditary, somatic, cultural and interpersonal ones. In many aspects the maturational process is guided, promoted or restricted by the progress and degree of emotional development. It is exceedingly difficult in a given individual to evaluate the relative importance of constitutional factor and of subjective experience in determining personality development. Doubtless biologically innate tendencies, including intelligence, have a marked and continuing effect on personality growth but this effect is extensively modified by the individual's feeling-experiences and the influence of his culture. It must be remembered that the significance of any experience is special or peculiar for each developing personality. It is certain, however, that an understanding knowledge of the personality and its pathology must be largely based on data that go back to and include the beginning of the psychological and social career of the individual. It is usually assumed, therefore, that the unique individuality of a personality is to a considerable degree developed and directed by psychologically dynamic interactionisms as they have been consciously and unconsciously stimulated through social and cultural influences, but perhaps most of all by affective mechanisms prompted by interpersonal relations. The stage in personality growth which an individual attains depends, as already indicated, upon many things but to no small part upon the degree to which he has been deprived of such wholesome interpersonal emotional experiences as tenderness in infancy, participation with others in the activities of childhood, the sharing of experiences with peers in the juvenile period and a close relationship with a member of the opposite sex in adolescence. We have tried to emphasize that the factors involved in the formation of the personality are exceedingly complex and that its structure is dynamically organized.

The type of personality pattern the individual works out for himself in his effort to meet the stresses of life will be influenced by many things. Among them will be the nature and number of the defenses which he constructs against unacceptable strivings, against aggressive tendencies and against socially unacceptable feeling-attitudes toward persons who have occupied key positions in his life, particularly during childhood. If one develops a multiplicity of such defenses designed to reduce tension and anxiety, a constricted type of personality characterized by rigidity, narrowness and lack of spontaneity results. If these defenses become pathologically exaggerated or disorganizing, they eventuate in the neurotic or psychotic personality. One's basic personality, the kind of person he really is, continues to be the same throughout both prepsychotic and psychotic states. This remains true even though during a psychotic breakthrough it may appear to be quite at variance with the prepsychotic personality.

Psychoanalytic Concept of Personality Development

Probably all psychiatrists and psychologists think of the adult personality as having been gradually attained through an orderly developmental sequence and an inherent process of maturation. In this process one observes successive steps, each normally merging into a successive "higher" one, until a mature, adult, socialized personality is reached. There are many aspects of personality any one of which might be selected for emphasis and its gradual growth traced from infancy to maturity. This method of approach to the study of personality is advantageous since when the pathology of personality is considered it will be found that many of its disorders are best explained on the assumption of an arrest (fixation) or deviation occurring at some point in the progressive sequence in maturation of an important component or aspect of the personality.

Since the pleasure derived from the satisfaction of psychological and physiological impulses is a matter of much importance in personality functioning and the means of securing this satisfaction a good indicator of the degree of personality development, Sigmund Freud attributed a predominant place to this phase of personality to which he applied the term sexuality. The selection of this term for pleasure-seeking impulses was unfortunate since it erroneously carries the implications that have become associated with the word through its usual application to genital sexuality and pleasure. In using the term infantile sexuality, Freud never attributed to infants and children the complex pattern of adult sexuality. If the restricted, even figurative, use of the term sexuality is borne in mind, one may, following the terminology of Freud, trace what should be an orderly and step-by-step development of the psychosexual aspect of personality from its earliest expression to a mature, heterosexual, socially approved mating upon the basis of which the family is founded. His psychoanalytical concepts have constituted important contributions to an understanding of personality development.

Oral Stage. Prior to birth the infant is fed through the maternal blood stream and has never experienced the satisfying pleasure provided by the gratification of an instinctual need. With birth, however, a biological need for food arises and receives satisfaction through sucking. Not only is the discomfort from hunger relieved by this sucking but as other and more complex tensions arise the infant turns to the most available substitute as a source of security and satisfaction and therefore sucks his thumb. The mouth becomes, accordingly, the part of the body in which interests, sensations and activities are centered and through which gratification is secured. Some analysts speak of a second phase (from about eight to eighteen months of age) of the oral stage in which the pleasure of biting is added to that of sucking. It is sometimes referred to as the period in which aggression appears.

It is conceivable that the oral satisfaction secured from nursing may be the first primitive manifestation of what through many subsequent stages of development will ultimately become adult heterosexuality. At this stage, however, the pleasure-seeking is related to the mouth and contains no discernible relation to the genitals as in the adult. To speak of this oral phase as the first stage of psychosexual development is more figurative than actual but has become an accepted term in psychoanalytic terminology. Because of its pleasure-giving potentiality at this stage of psychosexual development, the mouth is spoken of as an erogeneous zone. Satisfactions thus secured from such pleasure-giving zones are called autoerotic. Too little or inconsistent "psychological mothering" is apt to promote autoerotism in the form of prolonged or excessive thumb-sucking, constipation or in early and excessive masturbation. On the other hand, consistent and healthy emotional satisfactions in the child's relationships to his parents shorten the autoerotic period of development and promote a natural sublimation of the instinctive drives—a wholesome progress in the successive stages of these aspects of personality development and differentiation. If the individual, far beyond the age when the mouth should have ceased to be a focus of satisfaction, continues to be mouth-centered, he is said to be of an oral type of personality. Although this stage of personality development is one of dependency in which the child gives nothing, it is a normal one, unless it is pathologically prolonged.

Aggression. Although the subject of aggression will be discussed later at length, it may be mentioned at this point since, in the opinion of some psychiatrists, its initial manifestation is during the oral stage of psychosexual development. Even at a very tender age the nursling is not a mere passive recipient of his mother's milk. On the contrary the milk is secured by a surprisingly vigorous activity. According to this point of view, aggression makes its first appearance in personality traits characterized by energy, application and determination and is thus of a constructive nature. Other psychiatrists stress that aggression arises relatively later in personality development and as a reaction to frustration, particularly to the frustrations which the child inevitably feels that he suffers at the hands of parents during the process of being brought up. Doubtless, therefore, there are many occasions in the child's life for developing resentments and aggressive impulses against the frustrating parent.

Anal Stage. At about the end of the first year with the termination of the nursing period the mouth begins to share its pleasure-giving role with that of the organs of elimination. Not until that age does the child's ever-widening awareness extend to and include this function. The interest in excrement and excretory functions which appears at this stage of maturation is probably but an illustration of the fact that the exercise of primary body functions is a source of pleasure. The retention and passage of feces leads to pleasurable irritation of the anal zone. The child becomes as much interested in his excretory functions as the parent is in controlling them. The mother, on the other hand, has the usual adult's feeling of revulsion for excreta, not yet at all shared by the child. Probably conscious cortical control of the rectal sphincter is not fully developed until after cortical development makes standing and walking possible. This period of interest and gratification in the processes of elimination is one of normal physiological and psychological development. If the mother, unmindful of these pleasurable elements and that toilet training is not possible until a certain stage of nervous system development has occurred, and before the child has a sign language with which to make his wants known, attempts to enforce training by severe and punitive repression of the pleasure-giving impulses, many conflictful emotional elements which will harmfully influence the developing personality may be aroused. There is much to suggest that permanent personality scars such as hostility, resentment or ambivalent attitudes to parents may be thus created. Psychoanalytically trained physicians point out also that an extremely rigid and severe toilet training combined with special pleasures secured through the child's control of excretory functions may produce a fixation in personality development which Freud designated as an anal type of personality characterized by excessive orderliness, parsimony and obstinacy. It is in a fixation at this stage of personality development that we find the roots of the adult compulsive neurosis with its uncontrollable impulse to perform certain obsessional acts and the ambivalence of personal attitudes.

PHALLIC STAGE. Attention has already been called to the theory that at about one year of age the source of pleasure shifts from the oral to the anal region. Similarly at about three years of age there appears another stage in the development of pleasurable interest with a shift of source from the anal to the genital region. This phase continues until about the seventh year. With the advent of this phase, there is a concern with the difference between sexes and the size, presence or absence of the phallic organs. There is a predominance of genital sensations and masturbation may become a source of psychosexual pleasure. The interest is not a sexual one in the adult sense of the term. The boy merely comes to realize that his penis is important and devotes narcissistic attention to his own. Some Freudians contend that the girl becomes aware that she has no penis and believes she must have had one but has lost it, with the result that she has feelings of inferiority and jealousy. The oral, anal and phallic stages of libido development are often spoken of as the pregenital stages.

Oedipus Complex. Continuous throughout the phallic stage up to the fifth or sixth year there exists, according to the conception of Freud, a period of attraction to the parent of the opposite sex accompanied by jealousy and rivalrous hostility toward the parent of the same sex. To this situation between father, mother and child Freud gave the term Oedipus complex.

Various anthropologists reject the universality of the Oedipus complex. That it is, however, a basically correct psychological feature of our own culture is generally accepted. Some suggest that the Oedipus reaction is determined by the behavior of the parents, not of the child. It is certainly frequently true that fathers are more severe with their sons and more indulgent with their daughters. That mothers frequently reverse this relationship is constantly observed by the psychiatrist. In either case the rivalry and hostility associated with the Oedipus reaction would follow quite naturally. Others regard the Oedipus period as a convenient and expressive metaphorical term for designating the phase of personality development in which the child feels and expresses hostility against one of the parents because of the frustrations experienced.

Normally this potentially pathogenic relation is resolved by the mechanisms of identification in which the boy identifies with his father and incorporates the father's goals and standards into his own pattern of behavior. Likewise the girl identifies with her mother, advances toward a healthy emotional maturation and finds gratification and security in a feminine role.

From clinical observation, it is frequently recognized that when the Oedipus complex is inadequately resolved the individual may introject some of the qualities of the parent of the opposite sex with the result that the development of "normal" relationships, including marriage, with persons of the opposite sex is precluded. Familiar examples are the adult son who lives with a widowed mother and is oblivious to the charm of women of his own age, or the young man who falls in love with a woman much older than he and who in some way resembles his mother. It may be said that a fixation occurs at the homosexual stage of personality development.

While acknowledging the universality and the jealousy aspect of the Oedipus complex, some psychiatrists ("neo-Freudians") believe it is based not on sexual rivalry but on the prolonged dependency of the human infant on its mother's care with a reaction of hostility and jealously to any competition for the affection and possession of the mother. This reaction becomes directed toward the father since he is not only the main obstacle to the possession of the mother but because he is also the more severe disciplinarian and therefore the object of fear.

Some psychoanalysts, following Freud's theories rather closely, stress these stages of psychosexual development and the importance of the Oedipus complex as the dominant factors in character development, while others emphasize the social and cultural experiences to which the individual is exposed, also his feeling-experiences growing out of interpersonal relationships.

These developmental phases of the personality—oral, anal, phallic and Oedipal—overlap and are not as sharply delimited as the previous discussion may suggest. Emotionally retarding or deviating experiences occurring during these developmental stages may leave a permanent influence upon the personality with the creation of defenses against the expression of fixated and deviated impulses. Conditions favorable for the subsequent development of a neurosis or for a disturbance of later sex life are therefore created. Rejection, dependence, overprotection, domination, frustration or situations that create hostility and resentments, singly or in various combinations, may be particularly pathogenic agents during the stages of personality development included in the periods of infantile sexuality.

Latency Period. From about the sixth year until the eleventh or twelfth year there is a relative decrease in sex interest. This is known as the latency period. While sex interests and activities do not disappear there are no such marked and significant psychosexual changes as are seen in both the preceding and following periods. The child does, however, identify more strongly than before with the parent of the same sex and begins more differentiation along masculine and feminine lines. At this time it is important that there be close association with a parent or some other satisfactory person of the same sex with whom the child may identify in establishing masculinity or femininity. This period is notably one of training in the customs and attitudes of society. There is a progressive development of the ego as a result of growth on the one hand and of education and experience on the other. It is a period during which ideals are formed. The child is exposed to more complex social pressures; also environmental opportunities play an important part in directing individual interests and capacities. In the latter part of the latency period a quest for status becomes a strong motivating force. It is, too, the period when inner control of aggressive-destructive impulses should be attained.

Genital Stage. Adolescence with its rapid physiological development of the sex organs and the maturation of sexual and reproductive capacities stimulates genital and heterosexual interests and activities. Sexuality is no longer diffused throughout the body as in the pregenital phases of personality development but becomes focalized on the genital organs. The sexual area, however, is only one aspect of the personality in which there is an inherent drive toward maturation. A psychological maturation with more mature emotional satisfactions should follow upon the biological. Reinforcement of masculine identifications should be sought by the boy and feminine identifications by the girl. Heterosexuality with its essence of love and the integration of its functioning into the purpose of mating, reproducing and the establishment of a family under conditions providing security and independence is a part of the individual's total development to maturity of personality.

Attention has been called to the successive stages of the development, as psychoanalytically conceived, of personality. As this development proceeds to successively higher phases, characteristics normal to lower, less mature levels, should be left behind. Some analysts point out, however, that certain personality elements derived primarily from pregenital levels may, if wholesomely modified, be of value in promoting social adjustment and individual success. They note, for example, that enough aggressiveness carried over from the late oral stage to aid in carrying on the struggle for existence, and also endurance and perseverance from the anal stage, may be personality assets.

The genital stage of personality development is usually regarded as the final and determinative one of personality formation. By the time this stage is fully attained a mature personality with a balanced structure of id, ego and superego should have been attained. Early adulthood is, however, with considerable individual variability, characterized by both maturity and immaturity of personality. Physical, physiological and intellectual maturity are already well established but patterns for the most efficient use of these aspects may not have been attained. In many individuals the maximum of psychological and social maturity of personality may not be reached for several years.

For the most part, those processes which have passed through successive stages of maturation and finally constitute what we call the adult personality remain relatively permanent in their dynamic patterns. This is not to say, however, that serious disturbances do not occur. To study and treat these various pathologic conditions of personality, whether developmental or acquired, is the task of psychiatry. The individual should progressively supersede or replace previously acquired patterns, relationships, ideas, feelings and conduct with new patterns appropriate to his age. To fail to do so means that he is compelled to meet life handicapped by patterns established at an earlier stage of maturation. As age advances, a relative rigidity in the structuring of the personality occurs. This decreasing spontaneity, originality and individualism and a corresponding increase in stability and inflexibility may in old age become so extreme as to result in disorganization of personality.

Personality Structure

We have discussed how that functioning organization of the whole of an individual which we call personality evolves through a developing process. It is convenient, too, to think of this organization as having parts or divisions performing specific functions—as having structure. Such a concept facilitates the idea of dynamics in the functioning of the personality. We must not, however, think of them as concrete realities or self-acting entities but as three groups of forces and functions. The concept of personality structure now generally followed is that proposed by Freud. Using a motivational approach, he postulated three psychic segments in the structure of the personality. While these structural divisions are purely hypothetical, they offer a useful classification of the systems of drives. Many of the terms used in describing their dynamic interrelationships are highly figurative.

The Id

The id is a collective name for the primitive, biological and aggressive impulses. It therefore represents the emotional and instinct-driven part of the personality. From it come such basic drives as those for food, sexual satisfaction, for aggressiveness and the gaining of immediate goals set by our loves and hates. Morality and discipline are no part of this level of personality organization. If ego functions are impaired, id impulses may erupt into consciousness in the form of fantasy or in more overt expression.

The Ego

The ego, or reality-testing self, is that part or function of the personality which establishes a relationship with the world in which we live. The ego, of course, is really a group of functions but for ease of conceptualization we employ a metaphor and speak of them collectively as if the group constituted an entity or organ located somewhere in the body. It deals with the environment through conscious perception, thought, feeling and action and is therefore the consciously controlling portion of the personality. It contains the compromising, solution-forming and defense-creating aspects of the personality. It evaluates situations and forms judgments. The ego organization, being in charge of such important functions as perception, memory, reality evaluating and testing, synthesizing of experience and of acting as intermediary between the inner and outer world, may be regarded as the integrative and executive agency of the personality. The ego develops by a gradual learning process and is determined largely by the individual's growth experience and education and by environmental influences. Its functions are to deal rationally with the requirements of reality, to adapt behavior to the environment and other reality situations and to maintain harmony between the urges of the id and the demands of the practical, outer world. In other words, it adjusts behavior so as to effect a suitable compromise between instinctual demands and the world of reality. For normal development and functioning of the personality, the ego must be able to modify both the id drives and the superego's demands for acceptable conduct without extreme sacrifice either of satisfactions of emotional and instinctive needs or of ethical ideals. In this way the ego serves as mediator and directs behavior into acceptable compromises between the blind drives of the id and the inhibitions of the superego. The guiding role of the id is that of the pleasure-principle but that of the ego is the reality-principle, *i.e.*, the demands of the external world to which practical adaptation must be made. The ego directs instinctual energy into channels which will, in the long run, bring the maximum pleasure and satisfaction. Its processes take place largely, but not entirely, at the conscious level. It constructively integrates impulses and thus secures mastery over them. If through conscious control it deals effectively with inner and outer stresses and through reason and circumspection it deals rationally with the requirements of reality and of society, the ego is said to be strong and healthy. A "strong ego" achieves an integration of the demands of the id, the superego and reality. It modifies or sublimates primitive urges into socially acceptable patterns. The individual with a "strong ego" shows flexibility in handling the various stresses of life without resorting to those defenses that lead to neurotic or psychotic symptoms or to characterological defects. If the ego is "weak" and easily controlled by unconscious factors it may undergo disintegrative processes. It may be unable to withstand the strain of continued repression with the result that mental symptoms or characterological defects appear.

The Superego

The third hypothetical segment of the personality structure is the superego or inhibiting and conscience-including component of the personality. This represents the internalized moral and social values, and is a conceptualized advisor, admonisher and threatener with both conscious and unconscious aspects. The basic process of organization of this function of the personality is quite advanced by the age of five but it continues through adolescence and probably through young adult years. During this period, figures of authority capable of punishing or rewarding become incorporated into the personality to form the distinguishable part known as the superego. It is particularly derived from identification with parents and their substitutes. The prohibitions and obligations noted in these identifications are internalized and incorporated into the unconscious psychological structure of the child. Later, the injunctions and prohibitions of other authorities and of cultural influences are absorbed into the superego, the whole acting as censor. The ascetic and moral demands of one's social group become introjected and organized into an uncompromising, unconscious, internal inhibitory law of which the superego is the personification. The superego acts as the supervisor of the ego and of inner, unconscious tendencies and therefore as the repressing part of the personality. It criticises the ego and causes pain to it whenever the latter tends to accept impulses from the repressed part of the id. It may contain irrational and even sadistic elements. It may threaten and punish and thereby seek to maintain its authority. It does this by creating anxiety and by producing guilt and remorse. If the superego is severe and inflexible, the resulting fear of it will lead to a rigid, inhibited, unhappy, anxious and often neurotic personality. A superego developed on the basis of fear and imitation is much less firm in its structure than one established through the healthier pattern of identification and introjection.

In the well adjusted person, his behavior simultaneously and successfully meets the demands of the id, the ego and the superego. On the other hand, the behavior of the neurotic, of the psychotic and of the pathological personality with serious and repetitive social maladjustment may be conceived of as resulting from a disturbance in the dynamic checks and balances of the id, the ego and the superego.

Other Personality Considerations

Psychobiological Constitution and Types

While not strictly relevant to the subject of development and structure of personality, there are other aspects of personality which are usually mentioned in a discussion of the subject.

A study of the personality from a psychophysiological approach has suggested to some biologically minded psychiatrists that there is a tendency for certain features of personality to be constructed upon a certain type of constitutional make-up. These observers point out that the dynamic process within the organism results in a psychophysiological unit that expresses itself in a specific morphological, metabolic and psychological reaction. Some suggest that certain psychological types of personalities and their particular attitudes toward life seem correlated with certain physical characteristics. Perhaps the endocrine system and the vegetative nervous system form a link between the metabolic processes on the one hand and certain personality features on the other. Some biochemists assert the belief that different personality make-ups are based on differences in brain tissue, be they at the histological or the molecular levels. While there seem to be types of psychophysical constitution that have a disposition to respond in certain ways, yet psychological types of reaction are by no means always correlated with biological constitution and no diagnostic conclusions can be drawn from such apparent correlation.

Ernst Kretschmer (1888–), professor of psychiatry at the University of Tübingen, emphasizes the morphological-physiological-psychological unity of the individual. He maintains the hypothesis that a common constitutional matrix links the phenomena of the mind not only with the functions of the brain and endocrine glands but also with the general body structure. According to Kretschmer the individual's life "style," his attitude and temperamental reaction tendencies are reflections of his physical make-up. Most American psychiatrists do not accept Kretschmer's emphasis on a somatype approach to personality with its constitutional predestination of the form of mental phenomena, even though he concedes that the content of these phenomena is conditioned by individual experience.

Kretschmer describes four types of physique into which the configuration of the body may often be observed to fall: pyknic, leptosomic, athletic and dysplastic.

PYKNIC PHYSIQUE. The person of pyknic physique is characterized by short stature, short, large neck and stocky, round figure. The contours of the body are rounded, the extremities are short and large; the hands are large and lacking in dexterity; the skin is often florid; the head and thorax are large and the face round. Persons of this type frequently accumulate superficial fat, particularly on the abdominal walls. They tend to be of the outgoing, energetic type known as extravert (page 39).

LEPTOSOMIC PHYSIQUE. The leptosomic is described as a spare, angular, narrowly built person with flattened chest. He has narrow shoulders, "from which hang lean arms with thin muscles and delicately-boned hands." The growth in height is usually normal although a few always remain short. Some leptosomes show a childish, undeveloped facial expression although many, on account of their sharp, thin faces, appear older than their actual age. Visceroptosis is not rare. Leptosomes seem predisposed to be introverts. The secondary sex characteristics are usually not pronounced. Many writers prefer the term asthenic to Kretschmer's designation of leptosomic.

ATHLETIC PHYSIQUE. The athletic type is characterized by strong development of the skeleton and muscles, particularly of the trapezii and those of the lower extremities. The bony prominences of the face are distinctly evident. The shoulders are broad, the chest wide, the pelvis narrow and the hands large. The skin is usually thick and firm. Many consider the leptosome and the athletic but extreme varieties of one group.

DYSPLASTIC PHYSIQUE. The dysplastic type of physique is characterized by aberrations. Among these physical aberrations one finds the myxedematous product of hypothyroidism, growth disorders of pituitary disturbances, infantilism and eunuchoidism. A large percentage suffer from disturbances of the endocrine glands. Some dysplastics are biological inverts, while other personality anomalies are not rare. In the opinion of some psychiatrists, the incidence of manic-depressive psychosis is higher among pyknics and schizophrenia more common among the leptosomic, the athletic and the dysplastic types. This conclusion is open to question.

"Temperament"

Formerly many psychiatrists, notably Kretschmer, spoke of "temperament," meaning thereby the predominant mood background of the personality, its reactive affectivity and tempo. It was regarded as being shaped largely by the general biochemical factors of the individual organism, particularly as they are determined by the endocrine glands, and perhaps by the thalamus. Kretschmer believes that certain types of temperament are associated with certain types of physique. This opinion is regarded as questionable. For the most part, therefore, psychiatry lays little stress on classifications of temperament. There are, however, definite types of personality which have come to occupy an important place in psychiatric concepts.

CYCLOTHYMIC PERSONALITY. Kahlbaum introduced the term "cyclothymia" to designate the predisposition of the individual to alternating moods of cheerfulness and vivacity and of mild depression; cyclothymia also indicates the tempo of the personality, *i.e.*, whether it is lively or retarded. While oscillations are not uncommon, mood and tempo continue to harmonize and the different components of the personality in their reactions and expressions function as a unit. Kretschmer characterized as "cycloid" those people who are subject to cyclic variations of mood that tends to swing between exhilaration and depression but not to pathological extremes. As might be expected, the cycloids or "cyclothymes" are predisposed to the development of manic-depressive or affective psychoses. Christopher Smart (1722–1771), the English poet who on at least one occasion developed what was undoubtedly a manic-depressive psychosis said of himself, "I have a greater compass both of mirth and melancholy than another."

HYPOMANIC PERSONALITY. The hypomanics are outgoing, cheerful enjoyers of life. They are free from internal inhibitions, many being vivacious and sprightly and showing a sustained buoyant, confident, aggressive, optimistic, perhaps exhilarated reaction. They are usually energetic, gregarious, pleasure-loving, unstable, given to fleeting enthusiasms and easily swayed by new impressions. Some are blustering, domineering, argumentative and hypercritical. Their judgment is superficial and they have a ready excuse for their failures. The hypomanic cannot subordinate himself, resents frustrations and disappointments and is usually adept at talking himself out of difficulties. The hypomanic woman is often a chatterbox.

MELANCHOLIC PERSONALITY. Those cyclothymics at the melancholic pole are often kindly, quiet, sympathetic, good-tempered people, lacking in strained eccentricity but tending to be easily depressed. They feel but little of the normal joy of life and are inclined to be lonely and solemn, to be gloomy, submissive, pessimistic and self-depreciatory. They are prone to express regrets and feelings of inadequacy and hopelessness. They are often meticulous, perfectionistic, overconscientious, preoccupied with work, feel responsibility keenly and are easily discouraged under new conditions. They are fearful of disapproval, tend to suffer in silence and perhaps to cry easily, although usually not in the presence of others. A tendency to hesitation, indecision and caution betrays an inherent feeling of insecurity. A few are irritable and paranoid. Many psychiatrists feel that the melancholic temperament of personality has developed its characteristics as a reaction formation against aggression.

SCHIZOID PERSONALITY. The schizoid (Bleuler) or schizothymic (Kretschmer) personality is marked by incongruities of the feeling-life coupled, characteristically, with a poorly socialized personality. It will often be found that the prepsychotic life of the psychotic schizophrenic was characterized by schizoid tendencies. In the schizoid personality the feeling-life lacks the resonance and responsiveness that characterize the cyclothymic. Its contrasting affective poles are sensitiveness on the one hand and dullness or coldness on the other. The sensitive schizoid feels lonely, imperfectly understood and isolated. Timid, shy, self-conscious, often self-dissatisfied, perhaps stubborn, secretive and suspicious, he is constantly wounded. In childhood he is often teased by his playmates who look upon him as "queer." In school or college he rarely takes part in rough-and-tumble games but strives for a sense of security through superiority in school work. Silent and unsociable, his love of books is often a substitute for human companionship. He chooses subjects of an abstract, perhaps philosophical, nature rather than those of a concrete, objective type. He may be imaginative and idealistic, perhaps with vague schemes for bettering humanity. Not a few schizoids of this group attempt art or poetry. Some are successful in transmuting their daydreams into cultural values. Many of these sensitive plants suffer from a sense of isolation. What their thoughts may be is often unknown even to their friends since others are rarely admitted into their confidence. Many have feelings of inferiority and of discomfort in interpersonal relations and are aloof to the opposite sex. In speaking of the sensitive schizoids Kretschmer comments that they close the shutters of their houses in order to lead a dream life. Many have a genuine love of nature, while those who have had cultural opportunities often show a rare esthetic taste, gentle manners and an uncommon avoidance of the coarse or vulgar. Frequently they are ambitious, conscientious, meticulous and perfectionistic. The overconscientiousness of the schizoid tends, however, to exert a paralyzing effect on initiative or variation, with the result that he often performs his duties in a stereotyped, almost ritualistic manner. Some schizoids are overscrupulous and by making a virtue of their repression become ascetics or prudes. To a certain number of these frail, sensitive individuals the harsh realities and frustrating experiences of life become too painful and they retreat into a world of fantasy.

Many schizoids, while retaining an imaginative attitude toward life and its experiences, lack the finer sensibilities shown by the type just described.

The most attractive members of this second group are kindly and honest but they are also emotionally dull, taciturn, unsociable and given to rites and cults. Because of a lack of spontaneity, they appear indifferent and indolent, colorless personalities. The less attractive members are often cold, reserved, callous individuals, frequently jealous of those more happily adjusted. Some shrink unhappily away into themselves and become preoccupied with unwholesome ruminations. In adolescence they are usually willful, disobedient, headstrong, moody, passively stubborn, ill-tempered, easily offended and resentful of advice, supervision or correction. Such a schizoid may be described as a "lone wolf" who prefers to get along without strong ties to other people. Often his early relationships within the family are disturbed and unsatisfying. The self-confidence which not rarely characterizes these unfeeling, distrustful individuals will be found to be of compensatory origin and to arise from a sense of insecurity which in turn stimulates defensive attitudes and reactions that tend to increase and complicate the problems of adjustment. They may have to show the world how tough they are lest they betray their shyness, diffidence and sense of insecurity. The mistrustful schizoid who expects and detects disapproval and insult may feel safer to endure in silence with self-restraint and sullenness, retaliating, as it were, in daydreams, fancying how he may punish and destroy his alleged adversaries. In less marked types the dearth of esthetic sensitiveness may be shown by a neglect of personal appearance, of home and family, or by a lack of tact and other evidences of social sensibilities and amenities. A rigid moral idealism expressed in inflexible rules of conduct and associated with a self-satisfied intolerance is not rare.

Actually but few schizoids belong to the purely sensitive or to the purely unfeeling type. In the majority of them we find characteristics from both groups. Not rarely, to our surprise, we find a sensitive and tender nature hidden beneath a cold and unresponsive exterior. Similarly one must not conclude that the schizoid type always exists in pure culture. Often it is not clearly differentiated from the cyclothymic, between which and the schizoid there is a sliding scale.

Bleuler preferred the term "syntonic" to Kretschmer's "cycloid" to describe a personality tendency opposed in characteristics to the schizoid. The syntonic person is in vital contact with his environment, is emotionally lively and responsive and his affects are versatile in expression and appropriate to the occasion. Syntonic characteristics reach their greatest development in harmoniously adjusted persons whereas schizoid elements reach their maximum development in the schizophrenic psychoses.

Psychological Types: Extraversion and Introversion

Psychobiological constitutions and personality types have been discussed from the standpoints of physique and of emotional characteristics. The personality may also be classified according to psychological type. One of the most widely followed classifications is that of a Swiss psychiatrist, C. G. Jung (1875–). This classification is based on the direction toward which the individual turns his fundamental energy-tendencies (libido[1]). Jung did not, like Freud, regard libido as a drive solely pleasure-striving and sexual in nature but extended it to include all the psychic urges of life. Depending upon the direction of this life energy and of interests, Jung spoke of *extraversion* and *introversion.* It is usually difficult to formulate the process of their development. The *extravert* is one who concerns himself with objects, persons and the realities and activities of his environment. He has a pragmatic outlook and his values and activities are governed by the objective facts of his environment. He is more interested in persons than in abstract ideas. He is characteristically energetic, aggressive, enthusiastic, friendly, emotionally responsive to his environment, sociable, self-confident and freely expresses his feelings. Often he is an adventurous spirit whose reactions tend to be immediate rather than logical. He is frequently a leader although more through comradeship and humanism than through creative thought. His emotional expression is spontaneous and natural but lacks the delicacy of feeling of the introvert. The interest and attention of the *introvert* are directed, not toward objects and persons about him, but toward himself and his subjective life, although he need not be selfish in the sense of regarding his own advantage at the expense of others. He is reserved and is unable to form the free and easy contacts of the extravert; in fact he often seems cold and aloof. Introversion should be regarded as a matter of direction of energy rather than as one of deficient facility in making social contacts although the introvert's herd instinct is usually less developed than that of the extravert. The introvert tends to be contemplative, serious, studious and sensitive. He is usually lacking in self-confidence and boldness of activity. He may become an artist or a philosopher. He has a less practical mind than does the extravert and often reacts in fantasy to failures and conflicts.

Jung concluded that to divide people into extraverts and introverts was not sufficiently discriminative since individuals were further characterized by the relative degree to which the fundamental psychological functions as thinking, feeling, sensation and intuition also determine personality type. He therefore described four subtypes of extravert: extraverted thinking, extraverted feeling, extraverted sensation and extraverted intuitive types. He described four subtypes for the introvert in the same manner.

Jung's classification has considerable usefulness, yet most people are not habitually extraverted or introverted in type of reaction. The factors governing the development of personality are too complex to permit such a simple dichotomy. Personalities tend to be distributed between extreme extraversion and extreme introversion with a majority falling in the middle

---

[1] In Freudian theory, libido is conceived of as a force working in the organism to bring about a pleasurable and satisfying state of affairs. Pleasure strivings, Freud believed, exist from the beginning of extrauterine life and are comparable to the appetite in the nutritional system. About the fourth year this pleasure striving appears to have, for a period, a relation to adult sexuality; then for a time its sexual goal is not apparent (latency period). At adolescence it again manifests itself as a maturing form of genital activity.

zone. This is not to say that each individual does not have a certain pattern of inner psychological forces which cause him to develop a characteristic personality.

BIBLIOGRAPHY

Adler, Alfred: Individual Psychology. New York, Harcourt, Brace & Co., Inc., 1924.

Brown, G. G.: Culture, society and personality: A restatement. Am. J. Psychiat., *100*:173–175, 1951.

Dollard, John: Frustration and Aggression. New Haven, Yale University Press, 1939.

English, O. S., and Finch, S. M.: Introduction to Psychiatry. New York, W. W. Norton & Co., 1954.

Frank, L. K.: Play in personality development. Am. J. Orthopsychiat., *25*:576–590, 1955.

Freud, S.: The Ego and the Id. Translated by J. Rivière. London, Hogarth Press, 1927.

———: Collected Papers. London, International Psychoanalytic Press, 1924.

Greenacre, Phyllis: Trauma, Growth and Personality. New York, W. W. Norton & Co., 1952.

Harsh, C. M., and Schrickel, H. G.: Personality, Development and Assessment. New York, The Ronald Press Company, 1950.

Healy, Wm.: Personality in Formation and Action. New York, W. W. Norton & Co., Inc., 1938.

Hendrick, Ives: Facts and Theories of Psychoanalysis. New York, Alfred A. Knopf, 1941.

Hunt, J. McV.: Personality and the Behavior Disorders. New York, The Ronald Press Co., 1944.

Hurlock, E. B.: Child Development. New York, McGraw-Hill Book Co., 1950.

Jacobi, Jolande: The Psychology of Jung, 5th ed. New Haven, Yale University Press, 1951.

Jung, C. G.: Psychological Types. New York, Harcourt, Brace & Co., Inc., 1923.

Kretschmer, E.: Physique and Character. New York, Harcourt, Brace & Co., Inc., 1926.

———: Medizinische Psychologie, 11th ed. Stuttgart, Georg Thieme Verlag, 1956.

Masserman, J. H.: Principles of Dynamic Psychiatry. Philadelphia, W. B. Saunders Co., 1946.

Murphy, Gardner: Personality: A Biosocial Approach to Origins and Structure. New York, Harper & Brothers, 1947.

Ribble, M. A.: Infantile Experience in Relation to Personality Development. Chapter 20, in Personality and the Behavior Disorders, ed. by J. McV. Hunt. New York, The Ronald Press Co., 1944.

Saul, L. J.: Emotional Maturity, The Development and Dynamics of Personality. Philadelphia, J. B. Lippincott Co., 1947.

Senn, M. J. E., Ed.: Symposium on the Healthy Personality. New York, Josiah Macy, Jr. Foundation, 1951.

Sheldon, W. H.: Constitutional Factors in Personality. Chapter 17, in Personality and the Behavior Disorders, ed. by J. McV. Hunt. New York, The Ronald Press Co., 1944.

———, and Stevens, S. S.: Varieties of Temperament. New York, Harper and Brothers, 1942.

Simpson, S. L.: Hormones and behavior pattern. Brit. M. J., *1*:839–842, 1957.

Symonds, Hedy: The emotional development of children. Lancet, *269*:814–816, 1955.

Whitehorn, J. C.: Basic psychiatry in medical practice. J.A.M.A., *148*:329–334, 1952.

CHAPTER IV

Mental Mechanisms and Their Functions

Need for Adaptive Mechanisms

During the course of its evolution every species has developed various means and mechanisms whereby it may obtain an adjustment to the life conditions it must meet. Many butterflies, for example, develop a protective coloring whereby they so simulate the appearance of the surface on which they rest as to escape detection by their enemies. Since adaptation is the very essence of life it is not strange that man as the most highly developed species has developed not only anatomical adjustments which protect him structurally or physiologically in respect to his environment but that he has evolved psychological devices that assist him in dealing with his emotional needs and stresses. These mechanisms or devices may, for example, help to meet such emotional needs as those for affection, personal security, personal significance and for defense against perturbing anxiety. By acting without conscious recognition on one's part, these mental devices effect an adjustment to inner situations and experiences that would otherwise be sorely, even intolerably, troublesome. The self-conscious personality with its intense need for a sense of security and self-esteem evokes mechanisms of a protective nature as instinctively as self-preservation prompts the avoidance of approaching physical danger. Just as the body through its physical and biochemical processes strives to maintain a physiological equilibrium, or homeostasis, so the personality through automatic and unconscious psychological processes seeks to maintain a psychological stability. The personality, by various techniques to be considered in this chapter, attempts to enhance and defend itself, to establish acceptable compromises between conflicting impulses and to allay inner tensions. By these internal mechanisms of control, unconsciously selected and automatically operating, the personality develops defenses designed to manage anxiety, aggressive impulses, hostilities, resentments and frustrations. All of us make continual use of defense mechanisms. In themselves they are not necessarily pathological. Life would be unbearable without resort to rationalization and similar psychic protections. It is not always, either, the goal of therapy to eliminate them. Since at times they may promote the individual's ability to live in peace with himself, it may in fact be a therapeutic objective to strengthen them. The type of motivating device unconsciously selected to meet emotional needs and stresses and to provide a defense against anxiety, the extent of its employment, the degree to which it distorts one's personality, dominates his behavior and disturbs his adjustment with others determines the measure of his mental health. Processes similar in kind take place therefore in both the "normal" and the "abnormal."

Conflict

Unfortunately the conscious desires of the individual, the recognition he craves or the gratification of biological impulses with which he was endowed are frequently not compatible with the conventionally sanctioned habits, attitudes, demands and values of the larger social group of which he is a member nor with the prohibiting and censoring forces of his personality. Conscious and unconscious forces pursue incompatible goals. A struggle exists between two powerful incompatible response-tendencies —between the attitudes, habits and values he has absorbed from the family, school, church and various other carriers of ethical and moral standards and traditions on the one hand and his unconscious needs and strivings on the other. The dilemma in which the individual is impelled by mutually incompatible mental forces and irreconcilable, competing impulses and personality needs is known as a *psychic conflict*. The conflict may be thought of as a clashing—an internal struggle—between different parts of the personality. According to psychoanalytical theory, many conflicts have their origin in the early struggles of infancy and childhood but through repression become inaccessible to conscious introspection. In his dynamic clashing of impulses the individual is torn between his conflictful drives, his wishes and his aversions, his loves and his hostilities, between his fears and his longings, his urges and his resistances. His satisfactions, stability and peace of mind may be seriously disturbed because of conflict between his drives and wishes on the one hand, and the codes, traditions, beliefs and loyalties which he has adopted from his social group on the other. There is, as it were, a civil war within the personality. The individual is driven simultaneously toward behavior of opposite types. The personality becomes divided against itself and a sense of *tension* or inner restlessness exists. It is the task of personality, and it is often a difficult and painful one, to establish a compromise satisfactory to its conflictful strivings. Frequently it is not successful and as a result the individual experiences *anxiety*, a condition of diffuse apprehension and of heightened and persistent inner tension. This concept of a self struggling against tendencies and strivings of which it is unaware, or only partially aware, leads to the theory of *psychodynamics*, or the study of how the mind works. The term psychodynamics is sometimes referred to as an analogue of physiology which may be defined as the study of how the body works. Later we shall see how unwholesome or extreme psychological devices or mechanisms for dealing with conflicts, frustrations and other anxiety-producing factors may lead to disorders of the personality. In other instances the energy-consuming conflicts may not lead to serious disorders of the personality but may limit and distort the fulfillment of the individual's inherent potentialities. As has been stated, many conflicts are established in childhood and there is reason to believe that much later behavior and the fabrication of many adult personality patterns rest upon conflicts established at that time and upon the psychological mechanisms with which the individual has attempted to deal with them or with the anxiety which they have created.

Types of Adaptive Mechanisms

The various adjustive techniques by which individuals strive to protect the personality, to satisfy its emotional needs, to establish and maintain harmony among its conflicting tendencies, to reduce tension and anxiety arising from unacceptable impulses that must be counteracted or restrained, or to modify reality in order to make it more tolerable and acceptable, are, it is found, of such systematized, standardized types that we call them mental mechanisms. These *mental mechanisms* do not represent isolated activities of definite psychic instrumentalities but rather are reactions of the personality designed to allay anxiety and secure substitutive satisfactions. We see the same mechanisms running through the individual's total life pattern. In these defensive mechanisms are to be discovered the dynamics through the action of which outstanding characteristics of the personality have been constructed. These intrapsychic operations, acting largely automatically and without conscious recognition of the individual, become inextricably woven into his personality pattern and will be found to be operative in a variety of mental manifestations ranging from character traits through slight deviations from the norm to profound psychotic disturbances. In the operation of these internal dynamics of the personality are revealed many of the basic principles of both normal and abnormal behavior. The mechanisms, the anxiety-relieving devices and defenses, habitually used by the "normal" person to make him emotionally more comfortable, are of relatively subtle construction and enable him to meet his personality needs without resorting to those overt and extreme measures which constitute the symptoms of the neurosis or psychosis. Unless anxiety becomes too great, the individual continues his successful and socially acceptable defenses against it. On the other hand if anxiety is too threatening, the defenses against it tend to become less efficient and less rational. As a result the defenses lead to personality and character traits that disturb personal and social realtions, or even to reactions which we designate as neurotic or psychotic.

Repression

One of the commonest of mental mechanisms developed for the purpose of dealing with the conflict, *i.e.*, with irreconcilable desires, competing strivings, with action-tendencies that constitute a threat to the image which we have of ourselves and with divided and antagonistic loyalties, is that of repression. By this mechanism desires, impulses, thoughts and strivings which would be incompatible with or disturbing to the individual's conscious self-requirements and motivations are excluded from the field of conscious awareness, being pushed down, as it were, into the unconscious. Here, through a psychological inhibition of recall, they remain inaccessible in order that they may not be recognized and give rise to unbearable anxiety. Repression acts as a defense against drives and memories that cannot be controlled by the ego. It is not produced by a deliberate and conscious effort of rejection on the part of the person in whom it operates. Rather it is an involuntary repudiation or denial, a nonconscious process acting automatically. It exercises a resisting, rejecting influence against those unacceptable feelings, strivings, memories, hostilities, aggressions, inferiorities and other mental contents, a conscious acknowledgment of which would be inconsistent with the individual's self-respect, his estimates of self, or the demands of his own conscience. By this mechanism emotion-laden experiences are pushed out of conscious memory to an area or level of hidden memories where they are no longer accessible to direct, conscious self-examination, and are permitted to emerge only in incomprehensible and perhaps incapacitating patterns of thinking and behavior—in symptoms. Experiences involving guilt, shame or the lowering of self-esteem are particularly apt to be repressed. In repression there is an elimination from consciousness of unrecognized motives and of all ideas or memories that might tend to arouse a painful anxiety. Impulses which the ego cannot handle except by repression nevertheless retain their dynamic drive and tension. They continue to lead a subterranean life beneath a conventional surface, yet they are liable to manifest their influence in traits of personality, in special interests, in some system of beliefs or code of values, or in more marked form as neurotic, psychosomatic or psychotic symptoms. Frequently repressed material may be dealt with rationally if it can be rendered accessible to the scrutiny of consciousness. It is therefore often desirable to make such recall possible. As will later be pointed out, this may be done by the technique known as free association.

The psychiatrist usually thinks of repression as a primary defense against anxiety which is prone to arise when unbearable ideas and impulses threaten to enter conscious awareness. From a little different point of view, one may think of repression as having been induced by anxiety rather than the reverse. In either case the present tendency is to think of repression as the cornerstone of dynamic psychiatry. If repression is unable to prevent anxiety then other mechanisms, such as projection or symbolization, may be called on to assist in its failing efforts. If repression breaks down the capacity for evaluating, reality may be impaired and defenses disregardful of reality may be called into action. These may, for example, permit the patient to disown an unacceptable impulse or threatening feeling of hostility by having it attributed to a source, perhaps a voice, outside himself. As we come to consider symptoms we shall find that the patterns of defense against anxiety may be of various and even of changing forms.

By forbidding the undisguised expression of instinctive strivings and socially forbidden tendencies, repression operates to maintain ethical and social conventions, thus assisting the individual in adjusting to the mores and social institutions. Unfortunately repression is not without disadvantages. Deep-seated drives and urges are not destroyed by repression but, on the contrary, although automatically restrained, they remain unchanged in quality and intensity. These drives and urges are, in fact, unmodified in any respect save that the individual is not consciously aware of the disowned strivings. Though frustrated they constantly seek satisfaction. To make sure, however, that the undesired awareness and expression of these strivings and wishes may not be permitted, the mind, automatically and without conscious deliberation, seeks to crush the strivings, wishes and thoughts and to reverse their effect by the cultivation and promotion of characteristics sharply opposed in nature. These contrasting aims and efforts, designed to reinforce repression, lead to the formation of prejudices and of pronounced character defenses known as *reaction-formations.* These will be discussed later in the chapter. The more repressions a person has, the more prejudices and biases it will be found he develops in order to prevent the arousal of his repressed desires. Similarly, intolerance of the wrongdoing of others is often indicative of the effort required to repress similar unrecognized tendencies on his own part. When complete repression is no longer possible impulses may push up and secure a disguised expression not in the form of prejudice or reaction-formation but in the form of neurotic or psychotic symptoms.

It must not be concluded from what has been said that repression is always pathological and its results undesirable. It is a mechanism which, if it operates smoothly and without undue effort, may result in a well adjusted life, but if with difficulty and with a drastic intimidation of impulses, it may easily lead to breakdown and symptom formation. In some instances repression and other mechanisms designed to deal with conflicts and unacceptable impulses may result in the formation of qualities of character that are estimable and yet, because of the sources from which those qualities have arisen, the psychological purposes and needs they fulfill and the uncompromising tenacity with which they are pursued, they must be looked upon as psychopathological products. Since, however, a tree is better known by its fruits than by its roots we need not be unduly concerned as to the genetic source and psychodynamic function which these commendable personality traits are serving. Such desirable character traits might be characterized as representing the conversion of liabilities into assets. A careful scrutiny often reveals the same psychological theme running through character, personality traits and the neurosis or psychosis. This is consistent with the principle of scientific thinking—that boundaries in nature are not fixed. One is forced to the conclusion that an unbroken line of continuity exists from normal behavior through neurotic to psychotic behavior. From the standpoint of dynamic development, many personality traits serve the same psychological purpose as do neurotic symptoms. Intolerance, submissiveness, meticulousness, extreme shyness and other traits may, like neurotic symptoms, have developed as protection against an awareness of early fear, hate or resentment long buried in the unconscious.

Repression should not be confused with *suppression*, in which a conscious effort is made to dismiss repudiated strivings and undesired memories from awareness.

COMPLEX. Because of the important part that repression plays in its origin, that mental product known as the complex[1] should now be considered. Not only may instinctive strivings and tabooed tendencies and desires be repressed, but also ideas, particularly those imbued with emotionally painful feeling-tones. A group of associated ideas which are thus invested with common affective[2] accompaniments that are highly troublesome in nature and have therefore suffered repression is known as a complex. The affects impart a dynamic element to the complex as a result of which it comes to constitute a sphere of thought and interest to which great emotional significance is attached. Such a center of emotional disturbance may exercise a strong nonconscious influence. Even though such associated ideas and their attached emotions be repressed they continue to possess the capacity for unrecognized activity with the result that the latent tension in their affectively-toned content may be touched off by some apparently insignificant remark or experience and manifest itself in various forms. A not uncommon manifestation of the complex is in the form of excessive behavior reaction or sudden emotional outburst in response to an apparently slight stimulus. A marked disproportion between stimulus and mental reaction suggests that the latter may be complex-conditioned. The disproportionate reaction shows that the external stimulus has added itself to a subconscious situation. Such emotional storms over trivial occurrences will usually be found to be linked up with something very personal and significant.

Sometimes the response arising from complexes does not consist of a sudden emotional outburst or of a more or less isolated instance of striking behavior. In some cases the complex may lead the person to see certain aspects of life in a particular way, or again it may lead him to establish some sustained idiosyncratic pattern of behavior. It may manifest itself, too, in various character traits, mannerisms, slips of speech or in forgetting to carry out some intended action. When one exhibiting the complex-determined behavior is asked what has prompted his apparently causeless acts, he will reply that they are merely matters of accident or chance. We know, however, that mental phenomena, like

[1] The psychoanalysts no longer apply the term "complex" in its original sense. They look upon it as a typical attitude connected with certain special inner needs or topics. They particularly stress the so-called "Oedipus complex" and the "castration complex." The term "complex" originated with Bleuler and Jung.

[2] It will be remembered that by *affect*, derived from the Latin word *affectus*, meaning feeling or disposition, is meant a certain feeling-tone that tends to color experience and one's outlook on life.

physical phenomena, are due to definite causes although the primary etiological agent and the sequential steps may often be unknown to us.

Resistance

This defensive mechanism produces a deep seated opposition to the bringing of repressed (unconscious) data into awareness. Through its operation, one seeks to avoid memories and insights which would arouse anxiety and be painful for him to face consciously. It is also observed in psychoanalytical therapy when the psychiatrist, through free associations, encourages the patient to bring repressed material into awareness. It was through the difficulties and obstructions encountered in free association—the blocking, embarrassment, silences and anxieties shown by the patient to which he gave the name resistance—that Freud built up his concept of repression. Resistances afford a clue to repressed material.

Denial

Denial is an intrapsychic defense mechanism by means of which consciously intolerable thoughts, wishes, facts and deeds are disowned by an unconscious denial of their existence. What is consciously intolerable is unconsciously rejected by a protective mechanism of nonawareness. Reality is regarded as nonexistent or is transformed so that it is no longer unpleasant or painful. The term *denial* used in a psychiatric sense does not include a consciously attempted endeavor to repudiate or disown, as in malingering or lying.

Sublimation

We have seen that repression is a mental mechanism designed to deal with conflicting drives and desires. If it is successful in its purpose and there are no accompanying feelings of anxiety, it facilitates a well adjusted life. Since, however, repression is in effect the overcoming of one force by another, the energy in the repressed impulse is not available for constructive, consciously directed activity. It would be highly desirable, therefore, if the energy inherent in primitive or unacceptable impulses could somehow be transformed and flow with relative freedom into the conscious mind and there direct the individual's interests and activities. The mechanism by which this energy is transformed and directed to socially useful goals is known as sublimation. Instinctive needs and unacceptable impulses find an acceptable outlet and mode of expression. Anxiety arising from the threat of these needs and impulses is channeled into patterns of social acceptability. Instead of utilizing primitive tendencies and impulses for selfish or forbidden purposes, sublimation transforms and directs them into such channels as art, literature, religion, science, or other activities that promote cultural development and a richer life both for the individual and the social group. Aggressive impulses, for example, may be sublimated through sports and games or other socially accepted channels. The energy transformation by sublimation may be compared to the transformation of the hydrodynamic energy in such falls as those at Niagara where the electric generator transforms this hydrodynamic energy into highly useful electric energy. The primitive energy of the waterfall is no longer expended in erosion or some other crude form but, refined and disguised, it serves the material and cultural needs of man.

Rarely does the individual recognize that his activity which serves the material, mental and cultural welfare of himself and his fellows derives its energy from impulses originally developed for biological and selfish ends. The scientist engaged in research on problems of importance to the health or welfare of the entire race does not consciously recognize that his researches are but the disguised and refined expression of a pronounced, innate drive of curiosity.

By repeated sublimation, impulses are gratified at progressively higher levels resulting in a constant cultural advance. For example, the child who is instinctively cruel and is destructive to his toys and unkind to animals may in youth be an enthusiastic hunter and in adult life a successful surgeon. The same impulses serve as the dynamic agent but become progressively refined and socially more serviceable. The social sublimation of aggression may result in constructive leadership of great value. Through sublimation, too, the fundamental drives of the organism are made to employ intelligence and its product, knowledge, for promoting adjustment and achievement. Successful sublimation is one of the most important mechanisms in the formation of sound character. At times, however, as we study personality disturbances we find that some outstanding personality trait which the possessor interprets as a good sublimation is but a neurotic symptom; what he thinks is an important element of his character is but the thinly disguised expression of an unsuccessfully resolved conflict. If sublimation is impossible, the personality is in constant conflict and may suffer disorganization.

Conscious Control

From what has been said, it is plain that repression is a mechanism which, when employed, operates without conscious recognition, and that sublimation, much like the electric generator to which it was compared, acts without apprehending the nature or meaning of the forces it transforms and renders available for utilization for higher purposes. The most successful adjustment to life conditions is not possible if there are tendencies or feelings of which one is not aware and which are therefore beyond the reach of control. The motives directing our behavior cannot be guided into desirable constructive channels unless their hidden sources are exposed to the light of full consciousness where we may face all the facts and direct our promptings by the mechanism of conscious control. It enables us to replace automatic adaptations and repressions by conscious and flexible adjustments. Likewise, if we can learn to recognize and understand our mechanisms of escape and defense, we may exercise a greater measure of conscious control. Conscious control requires a realistic and efficient capacity for perceiving, deciding and regulating—a strong ego.

Rationalization

Probably none of us realizes the extent to which the mental mechanisms operative in our everyday lives are defensive in nature. One of the commonest of these devices designed to maintain self-respect and prevent feelings of guilt is that of rationalization, a term introduced into psychiatric literature by Ernest Jones. It is a self-adjusting mechanism by which we first act in response to unrecognized motives, and after the action offer various supposed "reasons" for the action. We prefer to believe that our behavior is the result of thoughtful deliberation, unbiased judgment and a full awareness of all the motives prompting it. As a matter of fact, to a minor extent only, is behavior the result of such conscious intellectual considerations. To a large degree behavior is the product of motives of which we are not aware. After we have acted in response to these unrecognized motives we formulate presentable reasons which we believe determined our conduct although they are really but *ex post facto* justifications. This mechanism provides rational, intellectual explanations of behavior which has really been prompted by unrecognized motives. We think we can fully explain our conduct but are deceived by pseudo-rational explanations. Our real desires and attitudes remain concealed and disguised. At times certain of our rationalizations contain a minor element of truth which, however, is so unduly emphasized that it serves to conceal the essential prompting motive. Those motives which are acceptable are selected and considered to be the only ones. Our thinking defends our feeling. Since we believe that our behavior ought to be determined by certain motives, rationalization through its self-deception leads us to believe that it is. Frequently several motives participate in initiating behavior. In fact several motives usually combine and are operative in originating our behavior, some of them having a distinctly ethical value, other components being of a more selfish, emotional, or instinctive nature. When behavior is determined by such a coalescence of motives, it will be found that the individual selects the most acceptable from the complex group to explain his behavior. The more selfish and instinctive ones are the more dynamic, and these exercise greater influence in determining behavior yet are not the ones that are recognized in consciousness as determinative of it. The most highly sublimated motives, the ones that from an ethical standpoint are the highest, are the ones that dominate consciousness and are therefore offered as the real motives although they are of less influence in determining behavior than are those components which are unrecognized.

The student may ask if the individual is not aware that the reasons he offers for his behavior are not the actual ones and that he is therefore guilty of a falsehood. To this, one must reply that in the case of a lie one consciously knows that the reason is fictitious, whereas rationalization is so thoroughly a nonconscious mechanism that he does not recognize that motives cannot always be taken at face value. To employ rationalization in discussing his behavior does not mean that he is not honest and sincere. The self-deceptions of rationalization are usually defended with great emotional intensity since the truth they are created to conceal would be painful to the ego.

Rationalization is a mechanism that serves a useful purpose insofar as it is conducive to psychic self-protection and comfort. It leads, however, to self-deception and its conclusions are untrustworthy guides for further conduct. Its products, which are often employed deductively as premises, are so fallacious that they may readily contribute to the formation of delusions.

A not uncommon reaction closely allied to rationalization which helps to maintain self-esteem in the face of inadequacy is one of depreciation often somewhat inelegantly spoken of as the "sour grapes" mechanism. In this defensive, devaluation reaction, the individual disparages some particular goal which, inwardly at least, he would greatly like to attain but which because of some obstacle, often personal inadequacy, he cannot reach. An expression of depreciation for that for which one is unqualified is not infrequent. It is, of course, one form of response to anxiety. A bit allied as a defensive mechanism is a blasé indifference in the face of circumstances that would naturally offend self-esteem. We should remember, too, that irritability and evasion are often merely defensive techniques.

Compensation

Physiological and physical compensations are phenomena which the internist and the surgeon observe daily. If a valve of the heart is incompetent the heart muscle hypertrophies in order that additional force may be available to compensate for the impairment in circulation that would otherwise result from the valvular defect. If from disease or faulty habits of posture, a spinal scoliosis develops, a secondary curve, opposite in direction to the primary one, is produced above or below the former in order that the center of gravity may not be displaced. Such compensations represent attempts of organs to adjust to physiological defects and inadequacies. Similarly the organism as a whole, in distinction from its component organs, by compensating for its inadequacies and imperfections attempts to secure the recognition which it craves. Such compensations may easily become exaggerated and are often unwittingly betrayed by behavior. The person of small stature but with aggressive and dominating traits is an example of overcompensation familiar to all. His pompous and pretentious manner may have been unwittingly adopted in order that it may indicate a strength and authority which a diminutive size fails to suggest. His deportment may make the undersized person feel more comfortable and secure and help him forget his physical inadequacies. Prestige seems to be one of the fundamental needs of the personality. Methods of enhancing our self-feeling and of covering up deficiencies are widespread and vary from the simple "showing off" seen daily on the playground or the pretentious display observed in Peacock Alley to the formations of delusions of grandeur. It should not be forgotten, moreover, that socially acceptable degrees of compensation and even admirable personality traits may be an expression of neurotic needs. Their neurotic origin is often betrayed by the striking degree to which they are developed.

Handicaps and limitations, as factors in the production of compensatory products, may be of a widely diversified nature, in some instances being physical, in others mental. The inferiority, too, which lies at the basis of compensatory mechanisms may be either real or fancied. In persons whose reactions in relation to reality, in general, and to social stimuli, in particular, are well integrated, the existence of a physical inferiority may provoke constructive activities that result in qualities of outstanding social usefulness. Handicaps may spur one on to greater efforts, as in the case of Wordsworth's happy warrior who "turned his necessity to glorious gain." On the other hand, diseases or deformities that thwart normal instincts or ambitions or cause the individual to stand out unpleasantly from the group may fail to promote desirable qualities of the personality but may lead to wishful thinking, to unpleasant traits or even at times to a psychotic sacrifice of reality. In whatever form manifested, the products represent the results of the personality's efforts to attain a satisfying self-esteem and sense of security. All too often, unfortunately, the mechanism leads to overcompensations which, although satisfying to the individual, are fictitious so far as social values are concerned. A boy who was so tall, angular and ungainly that he had always been extremely self-conscious enlisted in the Army. (It is quite probable that without consciously realizing it he had been prompted to enlist because the military uniform and a certain glamor connected with the military life seemed to offer hope of relief from the unpleasant sense of being different, produced by his tall, ungainly figure.) Here he soon became an object of raillery because of his clumsiness in attempting to execute the various drills. After having struggled in vain for adeptness the boy was placed in the "awkward squad" where he naturally felt even more self-conscious and more painfully aware of his deficiencies. The indignity suffered by his self-esteem was too great; the need of his personality for a more satisfying recognition and for a sense of security exceeded its limited resources and he therefore constructed a fictitious substitute by developing the belief that he was a major general. He was no longer the awkward soldier unable to compete with his associates but was their commander and directed affairs of great military importance. The compensatory delusion satisfied the recruit's emotional needs but destroyed his usefulness for the realities of military life and required his hospitalization.

Feelings of inferiority are frequently not consciously recognized. With their concomitant insecurity and anxiety they may lead to reactive aggression, depreciation of others and fantasies of superiority.

Reaction-Formations

As already indicated, compensation is a dynamic determinant which, if of appropriate technique and limits, is often beneficial, serving as a spur to purpose or acting as a stimulus to the maximum development of the resources of the personality. Just as the cardiac compensation may repair a failing circulation, so a wholesome compensatory reaction may repair certain defects of the personality. Compensation contributes to that mental process by which one not merely becomes blind to undesirable characteristics of his personality but stimulates the development of traits that serve as personality or character defenses. A character trait, usually the exact opposite of that which would naturally have followed from the expression of unfettered tendencies, a trait developed to maintain the repression of these impulses and to deny and disguise personality trends that have existed under cover, is known as a *reaction-formation.* Perfectionistic and uncompromising character traits are often reaction-formations against forbidden tendencies, desires or impulses. Often such traits unwittingly reveal troublesome aspects of the personality. The defensive character of conspicuous traits and attitudes is betrayed by the very quality of their exaggeration and at times by their inappropriateness. Such overemphasized character and personality traits may be described as constituting the first line of psychological defense. They can scarcely be called pathological unless they disturb adjustment. Feelings of rejection and hostility may be disguised by scrupulous politeness or effusive expressions of gratitude. So far as conscious intention is concerned a reaction-formation is always honest and sincere. The overtly aggressive person, constantly demanding his rights and ready to fight at any provocation, may be defending himself against a deeply seated sense of insecurity. On the other hand, submissiveness may be a reaction-formation that serves to cover up unrecognized aggressive tendencies. A façade of excessive amiability may conceal intense hostility.

Many reaction-formations are developed as defenses against the anxiety stimulated by disturbing and unacceptable feelings and impulses. Hostility, with its feeling state of anger, hate and resentment may, for example, be so charged with guilt that, to prevent its overt expression and its accompanying feelings of guilt, significantly overdetermined reaction-formations may be created to act as defenses against the anxiety aroused by it and its associated feelings. Great concern for a certain person may be a disguise for unrecognized feelings of hostility, jealousy or even for wishes for his death. Beneath a façade of devotion there may lurk a concealed wish for the death of a widowed mother for whom a spinster daughter has sacrificed herself and refused an offer of marriage in order to remain with her. Such devotion may serve to appease a sense of guilt. If employed within rational limits reaction-formation may be a very desirable choice of defense against anxiety.

Mental mechanisms may supplement and reinforce one the other. Reaction-formation and sublimation, for example, may be employed simultaneously as means of dealing with an unacceptable drive.

Restitution

The mechanism of relieving the mind of a load of guilt by restitutive acts (a making up for, or reparation) is not uncommon. Restitution arising from feelings of guilt may become the main motive of life, as exemplified by the indefatigably, almost wearisomely, benevolent person.

Operating to a less extreme degree and in a less obvious manner, the restitutive reaction to unconscious guilt may play a large part in a drive toward creativeness.

Symbolization

At first men communicated with each other through the use of concrete objects but with the development of language they used words in place of objects. Gradually words were employed to represent ideas as well as objects. Similarly, objects became the symbols, or substitutes, for ideas, feelings and tendencies. Symbolization with its meaning-carrying signs is therefore a mechanism whereby one idea or object is employed to represent some other idea or object. It is characteristic of words or objects used symbolically that they thereby become significantly charged with meaning. This arises from the fact that the displacement of emotional values from the object to the symbol is the essence of symbolization. The symbol may therefore come to represent mental experience heavily laden with meaning. It is a mechanism extensively employed in psychopathology.

We have seen that conflicting drives and ideas, or groups of associated ideas, with which painful emotions are associated may be repressed because they are distressing to the conscious personality. Such repressed material is still too active, too heavily charged emotionally, not to be constantly seeking for expression. Since denied direct, conscious, and frank expression the repressed impulses and other psychic content break through and obtain expression at the conscious level in indirect, disguised form. The wish or drive, therefore, that cannot be acknowledged consciously may be dealt with or satisfied in a symbolic manner. The resemblance between the symbol and the object symbolized is generally so slight or superficial that the conscious mind would overlook it. The individual is therefore quite unaware of the meaning of the symbol he has employed; indeed, he is often unaware that he has used one at all. To his conscious mind the symbol is not a symbol; it is reality in and of itself. He therefore treats symbols as if they were real and directs his behavior in accordance with the affective value with which the symbols are invested. In both the normal and the psychotic individual, repressed material may be expressed through symbolism. It is manifested, not in forms of esthetic value, as in the case of the artist, but in forms equally symbolic although often in disguises more difficult to read. It is frequently said that symbolism is the language of the unconscious. Symbols, therefore, become the language whereby material that may not appear in conscious awareness in undisguised form finds expression. Appearing in the content of dreams, hallucinations and in obscure or apparently meaningless ideas, symbols express particularly those contents of the individual's inner life with which much feeling is connected.

The disguises under which such material may be manifested are numerous. Various affectations of dress, gait, speech or manner as observed among persons who are never regarded as suffering from mental disorder are often symbolic disguises expressing products of repression.

Dreams, which are products of thinking lacking the awareness and direction supplied by consciousness, involve various processes, one of the most frequent of which is symbolization. Although not all dreams contain symbolic material, nor do all psychiatrists agree as to the interpretation to be placed upon given dream imagery, many of the images and experiences of dreams represent such products of repression as unacknowledged motives and desires. Frequently dreams are a symbolic expression of inner tension.

In the psychoses, particularly in schizophrenia, repressed and emotionally charged material may find disguised, symbolic expression at the conscious level in the form of hallucinations, *i.e.*, in images of the visual, auditory or other sensory fields.

Displacement

Another anxiety-reducing device which also operates by a process of substitution is displacement. By this defense mechanism an emotional feeling is transferred from its actual object to a substitute. The feeling originally directed toward a certain person, object or situation is transferred and attached to another person, object or situation which becomes invested with the emotional significance originally associated with the former. In a phobia, for example, there is an unconscious transfer of fear and threat from its original hidden and internal (unconscious) source to another one which is external and apparently unrelated insofar as the patient is consciously aware. In the frequent handwashing observed in certain compulsive neuroses, affect is displaced from an earlier experience with which a feeling of moral uncleanness was associated to the idea of dirt which comes to possess the feeling value originally attached to the consciously repudiated experience. Feelings and attitudes, such as love and hate, are particularly apt to be displaced from one person to someone else who comes to be a surrogate for the first person. A feeling of hostility toward a parent may, for example, be so intense that it cannot be consciously entertained. By shifting the hatred to someone who has a resemblance to the parent the person may be protected against conscious recognition of his attitude toward the parent. In many instances symbolism is a kind of displacement. An object to which a feeling or impulse is displaced becomes a symbol of the person or object which originally stimulated the feeling or impulse. Displacement enables the individual to maintain repression of dangerous or unacceptable impulses, wishes or thoughts. The displacement of anxiety from the significant to the less significant is a common defense mechanism. Allied to displacement is the mechanism described by Freud whereby the conscious may defend itself from material in the unconscious by treating it as a joke.

Substitution

Substitution is a mechanism which may be employed to reduce tension resulting from frustration. Through it are secured alternative or substitutive gratifications comparable to those which would have been enjoyed had frustration not occurred. To yield satisfaction and reduce tension, the substitutive action must have certain similarities to the frustrated one. Many psychiatric symptoms represent substitutive and symbolic satisfactions.

Projection

This mechanism is, in many respects, a form of displacement, a means of defense which to a limited degree one may observe daily among his associates and which is seen to a psychotic degree in paranoia and in other paranoid psychoses. Acting as a defense against anxiety, projection directs outward and attributes to others one's disclaimed and objectionable character traits, attitudes, motives and desires. The mechanism enables one to remain blind to important dynamic factors in the personality, while their influence distorts his picture of the outside world. One constantly meets people who severely criticize in other persons the very same faults which are the weak points of their own character, utterly failing to recognize the fact that they themselves possess the despised traits and motives. The material projected might be said to be an echo of the projector's own unconscious. By projection, one's own aggressive designs and id impulses are attributed to others. Through it repudiated tendencies find outlet. Feelings of guilt that give rise to anxiety may be alleviated if he is able to cast the blame for shameful tendencies or wishes onto the outer world leaving himself guiltless or even victimized. He may feel less guilty, too, if he can make someone else feel guilty. As a further defense against anxiety, he may respond with hostility and aggressive behavior toward the external object which is the focus of projection. Some treat others as projections of certain of their own unconscious trends—hate, fear, etc. Many times they hold others responsible for their difficulties. Sometimes a depressive affect is produced even though the anxiety has been alleviated by a defensive projection. Such a sense of guilt may even give rise to a need for self-punishment.

It will be noted that projection is often closely associated with the mechanism of denial, already discussed. This is well illustrated by the formula stated by Freud: A, unable to tolerate the anxiety aroused by his hatred of B, unconsciously changes his attitude, "I hate B," to "B hates me." Repression and projection protect the ego from being overwhelmed or disorganized by the effects of aggression, hate or guilt.

In the discussion of the mechanism of compensation, mention was made of the fact that physical inferiorities may stimulate compensatory reactions. In some instances such handicaps may be dynamic factors in the development of other defensive reactions, including projection. Although the anatomical defect may be of wide variation, yet malformations or hypoplasia of the genital organs or disfiguring cutaneous lesions seem especially provocative of defensive reactions. Feelings of inferiority arising from defects of organs so highly prized biologically as the genitals, or so valued as a determinant of physical attractiveness as the skin, may give rise to sensitiveness, dissatisfaction, embitterment and resentment. Such emotional attitudes readily lead to misinterpretations or even cause a person thus handicapped to attach to others any weaknesses in his own personality. Sometimes a striving for supremacy and security by persons who, compared with others, are actually or in imagination at a disadvantage in life may lead to projection as a defensive means. If the ego fails or becomes disorganized other phenomena—hallucinations, ideas of reference and delusions—often become associated with projection.

DELUSIONS AND PROJECTION. Material may be projected either in the form of ideas or of perceptions. In the former case, projection may lead to the formation of delusions, particularly ones of persecution. During World War I an American soldier in order to escape from a highly dangerous situation in the front-line trenches shot himself in the foot. He was at first treated in an Army hospital in France and later transferred to the United States where the self-inflicted wound healed but slowly. The retrospective discomfort or sense of guilt created by his cowardice and dereliction was alleviated psychologically by projection. He believed that the delay in the healing of the wound was a result of neglect on the part of his physician. The soldier felt no self-reproach since it was not he but the physician who was culpable. He was, of course, quite unaware that the attempt he later made on the life of the physician was an effort to destroy qualities of which he was the actual possessor. Such a projection stimulated by a sense of guilt is at times one of the important mechanisms in the production of paranoia. By this mechanism, a patient may persuade himself that his persecutor is so unspeakably evil that he deserves death and that to inflict this, far from being a criminal act, is a laudable one.

HALLUCINATIONS AND PROJECTION. Frequently in the psychotic the disowned aspects of the personality are projected not in terms of ideation but in terms of perception. In such a case the repressed mental material or unacceptable tendencies, strivings or qualities may be externalized in the form of hallucinated voices accusing the patient of practices that represent the rejected aspects. The soldier mentioned above, in his effort to kill the physician, naturally did not destroy the sense of guilt produced by the violation of his code of mental honor, nor did his attempt to kill his physician destroy the despised defects of character. Finally their projection led to a still greater distortion of reality in the form of hallucinations. One day as he was walking along a city street he heard accusing remarks that seemed to refer to him. Glancing about he saw that the person in the direction from which the accusing voices apparently came was the driver of a passing automobile. Without warning the former soldier shot and killed the man. Thus he killed a person who, by projection, had become the representative and incarnation of his own hated but unrecognized qualities.

Ideas of Reference. The symptom known as "ideas of reference" arises through the operation of the mechanism of projection. The individual who utilizes this type of projective mechanism egocentrically believes that he is the object of special and ill-disposed attention by those about him. Casual remarks by others, for example, are understood as relating to him and interpreted as accusatory or vilifying.

Projection is a psychological expedient which by its defensive process makes the individual more comfortable. It is less disturbing for him to discover an undesirable tendency in someone else than consciously to admit that he possesses it himself. Protection against disowned impulses and wishes and the anxiety which they would stimulate is secured by their paradoxical denial and reversal. Even in the so-called normal person, the mechanism of projection may be employed for its protective function, but it readily becomes a danger to peace of mind and to the integrity of the personality. It prevents him from seeing himself as he really is and leads to excessive criticism, sarcasm, pessimism, cynicism, brooding, prejudice, intolerance and hatred. While defensive against anxiety, it is often highly provocative in producing disturbance of human relations. It is a mechanism which may set in motion a process that leads to a vicious cycle. The attitude of the projecting person toward those on whom the projection is focused frequently becomes one of suspicion or even of overt hostility. This attitude readily leads to one of mutual estrangement which in turn activates in the projector a sense of an increasingly hostile world. This feeling easily promotes misinterpretations and perhaps the formation of delusions that tend to create more problems. Thus the mechanism feeds on itself.

Identification

Perhaps it is most convenient at this time to consider a mechanism which in certain respects is the reverse of projection. By this mechanism, known as identification, we do not disown and reject certain qualities and wishes of our own personality by imputing them to others, as in projection, but attach and transfer to our own ego certain qualities or elements associated with the personality of another. It originates in the wish to be like another individual in some way and leads to the assimilation of the desired traits as stable and permanent elements of the personality. Under favorable conditions, therefore, the mechanism plays an important part in the healthy growth of the ego. Through this mechanism, the child takes over attitudes and behavior patterns from his parents or others. It contributes much to the formation of the superego. A boy, for example, may identify himself with his father and thereby mold his own personality after that of his parent. He follows the father's patterns and shares his ways. It should be remembered, however, that the mechanism is not a deliberate and conscious process. The values and attitudes that accompany and grow out of this mechanism may contribute much constructive influence to the development of personality. Identification may be wish-fulfilling in its psychological purpose. This function may, for example, be observed in the self-gratifying sense of superiority felt by the servant of a distinguished personage with whom he identifies himself, or again it may explain the self-satisfaction of the psychotic patient who believes he is Christ and who, to complete the role, wears his hair and beard in the manner in which Christ is ordinarily represented. Through this mechanism certain circumstances, including relationships with certain people, may be selected because they fit into specific personality needs. The exaggerated sympathy at times shown by one person for another (even though the second person may be charged with some serious legal offense) results from identification—from a certain unconscious sensing of a common quality of impulse shared with the second individual. Through this mechanism, some desire may be vicariously satisfied, any fulfillment or even a conscious recognition of which would not be knowingly permitted. The false confessions of crime of which one occasionally reads in the newspapers are the result of identification which is based on a desire to commit the offense which the confessor alleges he has committed.

As thus far described, identification is an individual's unconscious molding of himself after the fashion of another, or a feeling of a sort of affective oneness with a second person. It is more than the conscious modeling of a child after the pattern of a loved and admired parent. In a second type of identification, the image of one person is unconsciously identified with that of another. The more recent acquaintance becomes the surrogate of the person previously known and is invested with the same emotions with which the individual had come to surround the image of the original party. In this way are to be explained some of our apparently causeless likes and dislikes of persons whom we have unwittingly identified with someone who had once aroused similar emotions. A person representing authority may come to be identified with a tyrannical father and the surrogate be regarded with the same emotions as was the original image. This is doubtless the dynamic determinant of the activity shown by some persons who constantly struggle against societal regulations and institutions. Hostile and other negative feelings having their original source in attitudes created in early childhood may be displaced or transferred to others in later life and thereby seriously distort human relationships.

A form of identification that is limited and temporary but that enables one person to feel for and with another and to understand his experiences and feelings is that known as *empathy*. By means of this quality, the individual possesses a warm capacity for projecting himself into the situations and feelings of others.

Introjection

In many respects the first type of identification is but a particular instance of the operation of the mechanism of introjection by which the conception of another person and the sentiments and affects with which he was invested are incorporated and re-erected within the individual's own personality. It is essentially the converse of projection—an "internalization." Sometimes hostility instead of being objectively directed toward other persons may be introjected with the creation of anxiety. Such an introjection of hostility may result in melancholia. An attempt to kill the enemy created by this introjected hostility may be expressed by suicide.

Fixation

We know that from infancy to maturity there should be a progressive development, differentiation and maturation in the instinctive, emotional and other aspects of the personality. There should not only be a progressive development in the psychosexual aspects of personality but also in methods of thinking, in meeting difficult situations and the frustration of wishes, in dealing with reality and in the control and expression of emotions and instincts. Unfortunately the development of some aspect of the personality may be halted at an incomplete stage of its evolution with a resulting persistence of certain incompletely matured elements. Such a personality shows a lack of harmonious integration. Its emotional organization particularly remains at an immature level and there is a lag between biological status and emotional independence. This cessation of the process of development of the personality at a stage short of complete and uniform mature independence is known as *fixation.* Certain phases of development are not successfully passed through and left behind. Just as the child may continue his baby talk and his dependence on his mother beyond the period when these characteristics should have been outgrown, so phases of his personality development may be arrested at various stages. The arrest is not in the intellectual but in the emotional, dispositional aspect of personality maturation. There are many theories concerning the origin of fixation. According to one theory, fixation is the result of experiencing such excessive satisfactions at a given level that this level is renounced with reluctance. According to another theory, a similar effect may be produced by excessive frustration at a given level.

An analogy from somatic pathology will illustrate the mechanism of fixation. It will be remembered that before birth the blood of the fetus passes directly from the right auricle to the left auricle through the foramen ovale thus short-circuiting the pulmonary circulation the activity of which is not necessary during fetal life. Sometimes the patulous condition of the foramen ovale persists after birth with the result that the individual suffers from a congenital heart disease. This passage between the auricles is normal for a certain stage of development, but if this fetal arrangement persists beyond the period of its usefulness, its existence constitutes a serious biological handicap. In the same way, the persistence of tendencies and emotional attitudes that should have been relinquished prevents mature development and harmonious integration of the personality.

While everyone experienced in the study of personality disorders will recognize that incomplete and irregular developments in the emotional and dispositional aspects of sex occur, yet the concept may well be extended to other aspects of the personality. The individual may be so well satisfied with the arrested stage of some aspect of his personality, sexual or otherwise, it may give him so much pleasure, that its natural development ceases. A fixation in some phase of personality development will frequently produce a lag in the evolution of other personality aspects.

One of the most important problems of personality maturing is concerned with the emancipation of the child from the binding influence of the parent. This persistence of child-parent ties with a resulting arrest in growth of the child's personality development may be a result of overprotective or possessive attitudes on the part of a parent or other relationships or experiences in early childhood. All too often a dominating or indulgent mother may not permit emancipation of her son with the result that he remains overdependent upon her and an identification with the father is difficult. Under such circumstances there is apt to be a persistence of an immature type of psychosexual development. This immature development frequently leads to deviations of the sex impulse and accounts for much unhappiness in married life. Not rarely, too, it is an element in the causation of neurosis.

Regression

Attention has just been called to the fact that certain aspects of the personality may be arrested in their maturative process with the result that a full and harmonious development never occurs. By another anxiety-evading mechanism known as regression, the personality may suffer loss of some of the development already attained and revert to a lower level of integration, adjustment and expression. If the individual is unable to deal realistically and constructively with the various problems and frustrations of life including those that arise from outside himself, but particularly those that arise from his inner mental life—his conflicts, instinctual drives and emotional needs—a normal progression to successively higher levels of adjustment may be checked and he may retreat to a lower level of personality development characterized by immature patterns of thought, emotion or behavior. An infantile or juvenile approach to the world which may have been latent for many years may be awakened by some frustrating experience or situation. Regression represents the existence of a personality status or reaction which is less highly organized and more poorly adapted to the meeting of external realities or of social relationships than had once been achieved. Regression to the dependence of infancy or childhood allays the fears and insecurities which arise from the necessity that adult existence meet life situations and responsibilities in an independent fashion. While adjustive in its purpose, regression is disruptive and deteriorative. It is not a constructive, wholesome mechanism of adjustment and does not promote a desirable adaptation.

The stronger any fixations which may have been established during the course of development the more readily will frustrating and conflictive situations be evaded by regression to those fixations. Extreme forms and degrees of regression result in a serious disorganization of personality and often constitute an important element in schizophrenia. In the process of regression, the total personality, or the whole of the personality, does not regress from one developmental stage to the next lower in clearly defined stages nor as a total unit. Certain aspects of the patient's feelings, thinking and behavior may be perceived as operating at various levels within various stages concurrently. The patient may, for example, think, feel and behave partially as an adult but at the same time may manifest infantile oral needs.

Fantasy

In mental health the freely wandering thought of imagination promptly corrected by reality plays a useful part in constructive thinking. If, however, the gratifications of reality are insufficient, thinking may not be controlled by the demands of reality but may serve as a regressive or substitute satisfaction. Such musing is known as fantasy. Fantasy provides the illusion of a fulfillment of wishes that cannot be satisfied either because of the frustrations of reality or because the individual's standards of behavior forbid actual gratification of strivings and wishes. Often these strivings and wishes are of such a character that directed reflection on them would scarcely be permitted. Fantasy is a defensive or tension-relieving mechanism offering either solace and an illusionary release from unsatisfying reality or an imaginary satisfaction of wishes any actual gratification of which has been forbidden by repression. In Freud's words: "The pleasure-principle triumphs over the reality-principle." By the former he meant the unconscious processes that strive toward the immediate gaining of affective pleasure. By the latter he meant the conscious tendency of the individual in his attempt to satisfy his pleasure to consider such practical necessities as the outer world imposes and, if necessary, to postpone the satisfaction of these pleasures. Because so seductive and so satisfying in itself, fantasy replaces necessary reality thinking or effective acting and serves as a substitute for directed effort at adjustment to the actualities of life. Fantasy has much in common with dreams, differing chiefly in being more coherent and in occurring during waking hours.

Fantasy is not an isolated function but an integrated synthesis of idea, conation, feeling, interpretation and memory in which instinctive and affective elements predominate and largely direct it. By disregarding reality and providing a substitute satisfaction, it aids in resolving conflicts and in preventing the development of anxiety. In extreme cases it tends to enlist the aid of delusions and hallucinations; wishes, particularly those that remain unsatisfied and beyond full conscious awareness, are projected and come back realized. In many cases, at least, fantasy may be regarded as a defense against anxiety.

The psychotic patient may live simultaneously in two unrelated worlds—one of fantasy and one of reality. One patient in his fantasy world owned the United States Treasury and its contents; he built and controlled the hospital in which he lived but had just lost the key to it. Almost daily he would hand his physician an order for a billion dollars, at the same time begging for some tobacco and that he be given parole of the grounds. This coexistence of the consciousness of fantasy and the consciousness of reality is made possible by the mechanism of rationalization and its production of what is known as a "logic-tight compartment." Related ideas exist in each compartment undisturbed by those in the other, each group pursuing its course segregated from those which are incompatible by a barrier through which no reasoning or argument can force a passage.

"Logic-tight" and "affective-tight" compartments produced by rationalization are not confined to the psychotic but may be seen among those who are considered of sound mental health. In such cases the compartments assure an effective segregation of incompatible strivings and emotional material.

Dissociation

Another mechanism to the employment of which the organism may resort in order to secure a measure of satisfaction when the various components of the personality are not well integrated is that of dissociation. A portion of the personality that is a source of emotional distress may be eliminated by this mechanism. In dissociation, certain aspects or activities of the personality escape from control of the individual, become separated from normal consciousness and, thus segregated, function as a unitary whole. We are accustomed to look upon our perceptions, ideas, emotions, memories and wishes as all belonging to a consciousness, a personality, that cannot be divided. Ordinarily a given topic occupies one's consciousness one moment and some other the next but it is felt that there is some connection between the two topics, that both are part of awareness, that consciousness has been continuous and that one's mental life has not been divided. Occasionally, however, in a person in whom there is an active incompatibility between repressed elements in his mental life and the rest of his personality, the repressed components may escape from the forces that are repressing them, become separated from the usual consciousness, organize a personality of their own, as it were, and thus dictate behavior. This new, or *secondary personality*, has its own consciousness which has no recollection of the usual or *primary personality* and carries out acts independent of it. The consciousness possessed by this independently functioning experience was designated by Morton Prince as the co-consciousness. The disposition and character possessed by the secondary personality may be quite different from that shown by the primary personality. This contrast should naturally be expected since the secondary personality is made up of material that has been repressed, that is, has been rejected by the primary personality because it was not of a nature to be consciously entertained or satisfied.

One of the simplest forms of dissociation is that of somnambulism in which, while the usual personality is asleep, a fragment or some aspect of the personality assumes direction with the result that without the awareness of his usual personality the sleeper arises and executes some complicated act. Other examples of automatisms, or dissociations of personality in which unconscious factors temporarily gain control, act independently and dictate behavior, are automatic writing, fugues and multiple personalities. In all these dissociated states, the organization of the repressed tendencies and desires into systems has usually been aided by daydreams.

In *automatic writing* the usual consciousness may or may not be aware that an automatism is being executed, but in all others the usual or primary personality is not aware.

Sometimes the organized material that has broken away from usual consciousness to form the secondary personality may initiate activities that lead the patient far from the scenes and efforts of his ordinary life. Stengel defines such a flight or *fugue* state as consisting of "transitory abnormal behavior characterized by aimless wandering and more or less alteration of consciousness, usually, but not necessarily followed by amnesia." A desire for escape from some intolerable situation is usually the immediately precipitating factor in the production of the fugue. Frequently the prompting desire is to escape either from justice or from domestic stress. An accompanying depressive mood is common. In fugues of short duration the patient wanders aimlessly, is highly emotional and when found is agitated and confused. In long fugues he travels far, appears self-possessed and lives in every way like a normal person except that he is not where he should be. The patient may be his normal self when he emerges from his fugue, aware of his identity with full memory of his past life except for the fugue period, or he may be unaware of his identity and of his past life. Clinically most cases fall into a poorly defined psychopathic-neurotic group. Many have shown a previous tendency to lying or to hysterical features.

Occasionally more than one body of associated repressions and affective experiences may become sufficiently organized to acquire independent activity, in which case there will be more than one secondary personality each possessing a character and disposition different from the others and from the primary personality. To these independently acting personalities is given the term *multiple personalities.*

Conversion

A mental mechanism the operation of which is confined to hysteria and in fact is distinctive of that disorder is one known as conversion. Acting subconsciously, this mechanism, by a poorly understood psychophysiological process, suspends or alters some physical function and thereby creates a disability, the existence of which serves a definite and useful purpose in the life of the person in whom the mechanism operates, although this fact is not consciously recognized by him. Conversion reactions find symptomatic expression in only the voluntary muscular and special sensory organ systems. Psychogenic symptoms occurring in organ systems supplied by the vegetative nervous system are classified as *somatization reactions.* Conversion phenomena suggest that mental content, highly charged with affect and prevented from finding an outlet along normal conscious paths, is diverted to wrong paths and finds an outflow into somatic innervation. The term *conversion* was applied to the mechanism inasmuch as it was considered that through its action the affect associated with some repressed but perturbing conflict produced expression of the mental content in the guise of symptoms. The symptoms, often symbolical and in disguised form, afford the patient an emotional satisfaction even though he may not recognize that such is the case. The form of the symbolic physical symptom into which the repressed ideas or wishes are converted is frequently determined by the nature of their emotional content and the character of the invalidism which will best offer relief to the particular mental problem with which the patient is confronted. Among the physical symptoms into which the perturbing emotional problems may be converted are paralyses, tremors, aphonia, blindness and many other disorders. When a conversion reaction occurs, the psychiatrist endeavors to ascertain the nature of the emotional conflicts that gave rise to the reaction as well as the symbolic meaning and purpose of the presenting functional symptom.

In this chapter various techniques and automatic protective devices have been discussed by which the human personality attempts to repair its defects, meet the demands of life without and of instinctual drives within, attain a sense of security, reduce tension and anxiety, preserve its self-esteem and satisfy its various emotional needs. Many blind spots, many of the attitudes and beliefs, many self-defensive reaction formations, personality facades, much behavior observed in everyday life, as well as many symptoms of the neuroses and psychoses, may be explained and formulated in terms of these mental mechanisms which should be regarded as reaction patterns occurring in the setting of the person's life experience. Pragmatically they should be regarded as pathological but are nevertheless quite understandable. Although varying with each individual, many of them may constitute important dynamics in the process of personality development. The pathological defense reactions may merely produce rigid, constricted personalities too impoverished emotionally to enjoy the positive aspects of living or they may so disorganize the personality that it cannot tolerate reality.

BIBLIOGRAPHY

Berrington, W. P., Liddell, D. W., and Foulds, G. A.: A re-evaluation of the fugue. J. Ment. Sc., *102:*28–286, 1956.

Darmstadter, H. J.: The superiority attitude and rigidity of ideas. Arch. Neurol. & Psychiat., *61:*621–643, 1949.

Fisher, Charles: The psychogenesis of fugue states. Am. J. Psychotherapy, *1:*211–220, 1947.

Freud, Anna: The Ego and the Mechanisms of Defense. Translated by C. M. Baines. London, Hogarth Press, 1937.

Freud, S.: Psychopathology of Everyday Life. Translated by A. A. Brill. New York, The Macmillan Co., 1923.

Hart, Bernard: The Psychology of Insanity. New York, The Macmillan Co., 1912.

Holt, R. R.: An inductive method of analyzing defense of self-esteem. Bull. Menninger Clin., *15:*6–15, 1941.

Kant, Fritz: Investigations into the dynamics of paranoid reactions. Dis. Nerv. System, *11:*268–272, 1950.

MacKinnon, D. W.: The Structure of Personality. In Personality and the Behavior Disorders, ed. by J. McV. Hunt, pp. 3–48. New York, Ronald Press, 1944.

Meerloo, J. A. M.: Patterns of Panic. New York, International Universities Press, 1950.

Murphy, Gardner: Personality; A Biosocial Approach to Origins and Structure. New York, Harper & Brothers, 1947.

Nicole, J. E.: Psychopathology: A Survey of Modern Approaches, 3rd ed. Baltimore, Williams & Wilkins Co., 1942.

Romano, John: Adaptation, pp. 79–96. New York, Cornell University Press, 1949.

Saul, L. J.: The Development and Dynamics of Personality. Philadelphia, J. B. Lippincott Co., 1947.

Symonds, P. M.: The Dynamics of Human Adjustment. New York, D. Appleton Century Co., 1946.

Whitehorn, J. C.: The scope of motivation in psychopathology and psychotherapy. Am. J. Psychoanalysis, *14:*30–39, 1954.

CHAPTER V

The Causes and Nature of Mental Disorders

PERHAPS there is no phase of psychiatry that has given rise to so much discussion and dispute as has that concerning the causes and even the nature of mental disorders. With the emphasis in his medical education placed on biochemistry, tissue pathology and other objective and impersonal sciences it is but natural that in his approach to personality disorders the physician should seek to place these too in the same category as organic diseases and find their causes in the operation of the same sciences. He should realize, however, that patients may become ill from disturbed human relations as well as from metabolic or other physical causes. He should recognize, too, that mental disorders are not so much diseases as disturbances of persons. It is becoming increasingly emphasized, moreover, that even when anatomical or physiological disturbances in brain elements are known to exist they cannot adequately explain the behavior that accompanies them. In varying degrees this behavior will be colored by and express the primitive impulses, affective experiences and other needs and purposes of the patient's inner life. Stresses in interpersonal relations and in the sociocultural field are no less to be considered than stresses in the biophysical sphere. Behavior cannot be adequately described in the terms of an impersonal disorganization of cellular structure or physiological processes, nor do there seem to be any psychiatric symptoms—except in some cases of toxic-organic syndromes—that can be considered as correlates of brain changes, physiological, biochemical or electrical. While other branches of medicine deal with parts of the organism, psychiatry or psychobiology studies the individual as a whole, as a biological unit living in an environment that is essentially social in nature, and deals with the biopsychic life, the total integrated behavior of the human organism. It deals with data from the biological, social and psychological sciences. Forces from all these fields determine life expression which should therefore be considered from all these frames of reference.

Proven facts concerning the causes of mental disorder are regrettably limited. Since neither its process nor its product can be demonstrated either in the test-tube or under the microscope, this is not surprising. In most cases there is not yet any established evidence of abnormality of tissue function or of any underlying histopathological changes in the brain. However, as psychodynamics, the general science of motivation, is explored, theories may be formulated as to how abnormalities and disorders of personality have developed. Since many of these theories have borne the test of experience, their continued use is permissible until others more elucidating and assured have been evolved. It is important to remember that human maladjustment can be the result of a multiplicity of causes. The pattern of morbid personality reactions is likewise, therefore, the consequence of a multiplicity or synergy of causes. Therefore one should not be too restricted or naive in assigning determinative etiological factors as the cause of a given case of mental disorder. Etiology cannot be thought of in mere terms of a stimulus-response pattern. It must be remembered, too, that the organism cannot be separated from its environment.

Physiogenic versus Psychogenic

A balance of forces entering into the organization of the personality, both those that are organic and those that are psychic, is essential to mental health. If the disturbances in integration which lead to personality disorders and maladjustments are in the organic sphere, the disorders are spoken of as *physiogenic*. If the integrative disturbances arise in the field of inner psychic experiences and situations, the disorders are called *psychogenic*. In the psychogenic mental disorders, the direct effects of structural, biochemical and physiological factors are minimal or absent, while psychological and social factors are maximal. Except in those mental disorders in which there is a physiological impairment of the brain through toxic or structural changes, it is a postulate of psychiatry that human behavior is explainable and understandable in terms of various psychological experiences and needs. Even in many cases where such toxic or structural changes exist, it will often be observed that the personality with its conscious and unconscious impulses, fears and wishes is projected in the morbid symptomatology.

Emotional maladjustments, behavior disorders and those unsuccessful attempts to solve life problems which we know as mental disorders are symptoms as susceptible of scientific study as are physical disorders. Although psychological in nature, thoughts, emotions, strivings and other personality needs become no less valid scientific facts than chemical equations or tendon reflexes. Every mental disorder is an individual problem which can be formulated only after a study of the whole personality, physical, mental, emotional and social, and of the evolution of these aspects of the particular personality.

A study of the causes of mental illness is a study of the underlying forces at the bases of the individual's blind spots, attitudes, interests, moods, beliefs, behavior and code of values. Psychiatric formulations should not be permeated with dualism or with quasi-animistic concepts that tend to exaggerate the antithesis of mind and body. They should be expressed in terms of the somatic, biological, psychological and sociological factors that may affect attitude and behavior. It should be borne in mind, too, that the fundamental, dynamic laws of behavior and of personality development are the same for the normal and the abnormal. Psychopathological research has disclosed that there is a large field between "normality" and complete psychotic breakdown.

Heredity

To paraphrase a quotation from Compoyré, one may say that both normal and diseased personalities are works written in collaboration where it is hard to discover which parts really belong to each of the collaborators, to nature or to education, meaning by education the sum of the individual's environmental conditionings and life experiences. Each stage of development is determined by the co-operation of heredity and environmental forces. Since the earlier stages influence the character of the development of late stages, the hereditary and environmental factors interpenetrate more and more as development proceeds until finally this interpenetration of biological and social influences becomes so complex and complete that the hereditary and experiential factors cannot be separated. Nor is there yet adequate knowledge concerning the relationship between heredity and the psychophysiological processes of development.

Before attributing a mental disorder to heredity, the psychiatrist should remember that parents frequently transmit their own emotional difficulties to the next generation, not because of a hereditary transmission through their germ cells but because of the influence of neurotic parents after birth. In most cases of mental illness in a parent one can presuppose a prolonged period of maladjustment with difficulties and inconsistencies in personal relationships that preclude the existence of a home atmosphere conducive to healthy emotional growth and future mental health. A failure to find gratification of psychological needs in one generation may, too, be reflected in the behavior of the next with the result that difficulty of adjustment and social misbehavior may thus follow through several generations. The patient has been conditioned by his interpersonal emotional experiences with parents and siblings; his parents, in turn, had been conditioned by their experiences with *their* parents. Neurotic patterns seem to have been communicated from one generation to another rather than inherited. A negative and hostile relationship toward parent or sibling may, too, carry over and transfer negative, hostile psychopathogenetic feelings towards persons who stand in a parental or sibling role. More than formerly it is held that many instances of nervous and mental disorder once looked upon as inherited or of constitutional origin are in reality due to crippling fixations, to hostile, aggressive or other attitudes growing out of early family interpersonal relationships. The individual's conscious and unconscious defenses against these difficulties may lead to a wide variety of personality disturbances. Whatever, therefore, may be the contribution of heredity in relation to mental disorder the postnatal influences and growing-up experiences have been of importance in determining personality structure and pattern. It is well recognized that a parent accelerates or blocks the developmental processes of the child's personality.

Up to the present time, therefore, knowledge as to a hereditary or constitutional predisposition to mental disorders is incomplete and opinions must remain subject to revision. It must be said, however, that the investigations of Kallmann as to the familial occurrence of schizophrenia and manic-depressive psychosis are suggestive. He found that schizophrenia occurs much more frequently in families which include a known case of schizophrenia than it does in the general population. He found that the average expectancy in any group of persons who are not characterized by blood relationship to a schizophrenia case is 0.85 per cent but that the children of one schizophrenic parent have a probability of developing the disease which is 19 times that of the general population. Kallmann reported that the morbidity rate among the children of two schizophrenic parents is about 80 times the average expectancy, and that among uniovular twins of such parents the expectancy rate is 85.8 per cent. He does not mean that a person is "born" a manic-depressive or a schizophrenic, rather that one inherits a specific capacity for reacting to personality stresses with either a manic-depressive or a schizophrenic psychosis while others do not. He believes that health and adequate adjustment are fundamental biological properties, with hereditary potentiality as the common denominator.

Incidence of Mental Disorder

According to reports of the National Institute of Mental Health 186 persons out of every 100,000 in the general population were, in 1903, to be found in state mental hospitals, whereas by 1954 this number had increased to 340. This increase in rate of hospitalization cannot be ascribed solely, or even largely, to an upward trend in the incidence of mental disorders. Rather, it is a result of several factors. Among them is the more adequate provision of facilities for the care and treatment of the mentally ill. There has also been a considerable and fairly continuous increase in knowledge concerning the nature of mental illness on the part of the general medical profession. This has resulted in an increased number of patients formerly not recognized as mentally ill being diagnosed and committed to hospitals. There has, too, been a growing realization on the part of laymen that mental illness is a problem in which the patient requires psychiatrically oriented treatment; also there has been an increasing knowledge that the individual is susceptible of improvement and recovery if treatment is taken in time. In addition, increasing confidence has been shown in the management of hospitals for the mentally ill with a resulting increased use of their facilities.

There has been, however, a major increase during the past thirty-five years in the number of admissions of elderly persons. During that period the incidence of admissions in New York, and doubtless in other populous states, of persons suffering from cerebral arteriosclerosis has increased six-fold. This is a result of increased longevity and the resulting increase of persons in the upper age brackets.

Age

Psychoses are rare until adolescence, when their incidence rises sharply and continues to show a definite upward trend with the advance of age. This rate of increase is especially sharp at the older age levels. In Northeastern United States, over 30 per cent of first admissions to public hospitals for mental diseases are sixty or more years of age. In proportion to the population, more than five times as many persons enter hospitals for mental disorders at the age of eighty as at the age of twenty. As indicated, psychoses are uncommon among children. Those that occur at that age tend to be strongly influenced by situational and psychological tensions. Both later in the present chapter and in subsequent ones reference will be made to the importance of interpersonal experiences of early childhood in determining personality development and attitudes. The unconscious factors derived from those experiences may be important in relation to future mental disorder.

The critical constitutional turning points of adolescence, involution and senility bring not only physical changes but also new psychological problems. The rapid increase of psychoses in adolescence is due to many causes. Frequently at that time there is an incongruity between various phases of personality growth; there is the new problem of the integration of sex into the personality pattern. There are also social and employment problems and those of emancipation from parents. No other period requires so radical a reorganization of the emotional life. The involutional period brings an increase in mental disorders due in part to declining activity of the endocrine and reproductive glands and to other degenerative involutional changes but more to the frustrations, threats and other problems which the patient then meets. It has been suggested that the age at which a person develops mental disorder is an index of his frustration or conflict tolerance. After the age of sixty there is a distinct increase of emotional disorders, an apparent contributing factor to which is insecurity. The increase in mental disorder at the senium is largely due to the degenerative processes that may occur in the higher cortical neurons in old age, yet in some instances it is due to the fact that the changes in psychological situations which arise at that time cannot be met successfully. Sometimes, for example, the fact that an individual has to be supported by children, or by children-in-law, or by others who have developed a feeling of resentment may be productive of psychosomatic or neurotic symptoms on his part. Since one-half of the population in United States lives past the age of sixty-five, the incidence of senile and arteriosclerotic mental disease is high. Omitting diseases of the senium the occurrence of mental disorder reaches a peak in the forties and then drops sharply.

Marital Status

Statistics show that mental disorder is more common among the single than among the married. While this may be due in part to the more stable and regular mode of life led by the married person with the accompanying sense of domestic responsibility, this is probably only a minor reason for the better mental health among married persons. It should be remembered that the marital association is one of the most important of all human associations. It provides not merely for the satisfaction of sexual urges but for various important securities the absence or loss of which may be very disturbing to the personality. The feeling that one is desired as a marital partner, that one is appreciated and is the subject of interest and affection contributes greatly to a sense of security. The security from loneliness, the emotional satisfactions of parenthood and frequently in women the added sense of economic security, add wholesome satisfactions. With marriage the individual may be compelled to adjust to a very different type of environment and to personal relationships quite foreign to those in which he was reared. The development of mental disorder before marriage naturally decreases greatly the prospects of subsequent marriage; many whose affective and other personality limitations are so great that they are predisposed to mental disorders are never sought as partners because of their obvious maladjustment.

Statistics show that there is a marked preponderance of mental disorder per unit of population among divorced persons. There are several reasons for the more frequent occurrence of mental disorders among this group. In many cases maladjustments representing early stages of mental disorder led to domestic discord and divorce before the personality disturbances were sufficiently developed to be recognized as constituting mental disease, or were so serious as to require commitment. On the whole divorced persons represent a group suffering from conflicts so unusual both in number and intensity that the high incidence of mental illness is not surprising. The same deep-seated mechanisms tend to lead to marital maladjustment and to the psychosis or neurosis. It should be remembered, too, that marriage is a relation that demands a most highly sustained adaptation. The unmarried woman may have been unable to achieve the adult toughness necessary to stand the give and take of adjustment to marriage and parenthood. Perhaps she may have been unprepared for this adjustment because her parents before her had not been healthy models for identification as mates and parents. A mental illness may be precipitated by factors concerned with sexual function, such as concern over adjustment to motherhood, pregnancy or abortion.

A person the psychosexual aspects of whose personality never reached a mature, heterosexual level but remained, even though unconsciously so, with a basic sex interest in persons of the same sex, may be unable to establish an abiding harmonious partnership with one of the opposite sex. Usually there will be no physiological interference in the exercise of sex functions natural to his or her sex but the emotional, dispositional tendency of sex expression is directed to one of the same sex. The attempt to meet this conflict between emotionally determined and biologically determined impulses may be made by projection or other psychopathological mechanisms that eventuate in mental disorder.

Pregnancy

Mental disorder may be associated with pregnancy or the postpartum period. There are, however, no mental disorders specific to either of these periods. Latent or repressed psychological material may under the stress of maintaining physiological homeostasis and of the emotionally significant situation prove too great for the patient's ego resources with the result that psychopathological reactions occur. What her pregnancy, perhaps unconsciously, means to the mother psychologically may be of significance, also the birth of her child. Doubtless, sometimes, it reanimates the patient's old attitudes toward her own mother. Sometimes the patient expresses delusions indicating hostility for either the husband or child, thus reflecting a conflict about married life or motherhood. Rejection of the child may be expressed by a delusion that it is dead, by abusive treatment of it, or by fear that something will happen to it.

About 50 per cent of the mental illnesses associated with pregnancy or the postpartum period are schizophrenia, about 25 per cent are manic depressive and 20 per cent are psychoneurotic reactions. These disorders occur with the same frequency in the postpartum setting as they do in any other setting.

Alcohol

The role of alcohol in the production of mental disease contains many complex elements, and while in some respects our ideas are becoming clarified there are still many unknown and variable factors. That there is a direct relation between the amount of alcohol drunk in a community and the incidence of psychoses classified statistically in the alcoholic group is certain, as shown by experience in the United States during the past third of a century. In 1920, immediately following the enactment of the prohibition amendment, the number of first admissions of alcoholic psychoses to New York State hospitals for mental diseases per 100,000 of general population fell to 1.2. This rate gradually increased to 7.1 in 1941, decreased until 1945, and has again continued to rise since World War II. During three years (1919 to 1921) of relatively successful observance of the prohibition amendment to the constitution there were 720 first admissions with alcoholic psychoses to all hospitals for mental disease in New York State. The total of such first admissions increased to 2,013 in 1929 to 1931 and reached 3,132 in 1939 to 1941, since which time there has been no appreciable change per unit of population. The more carefully the history of a patient suffering from a chronic form of mental disorder is studied the more frequently it will be found that any associated alcoholism is either a symptom of the psychosis or another method of dealing with the same personality problems which contributed to the mental disorder rather than an essential cause of it. The role of avitaminosis in producing a psychosis in the chronic alcoholic must be borne in mind.

Infections

Of all infections syphilis still plays the most active part in causing mental disease. The most common psychosis resulting from such infection is that associated with syphilitic meningoencephalitis (general paresis) which accounts for about 2 per cent of all first admissions to public mental hospitals. During the past twenty-five years there has been a constant decrease in the relative prevalence of syphilis with a resulting decrease in general paresis. Also, the treatment for general paresis is now begun much more promptly and carried out much more efficiently.

Drugs

Certain chemicals and drugs may give rise to acute brain syndromes, not infrequently in the nature of a delirium of brief duration, although occasionally a delirioid state of such an origin may continue for several weeks. The most frequent agents producing mental symptoms are bromides, barbituric acid derivatives, sulfa drugs, morphine, cocaine, marihuana, thiocyanates and lead.

Endocrine Disturbances

Abnormal functionings of the endocrine glands will undoubtedly influence personality. Such disorders, for example, may lead to changes in general efficiency of bodily functions with resulting feelings of frustration or insecurity. The quality of autonomic functioning will also influence the pattern of personality. Occasionally neuroendocrinal dystrophies produce biological defects that cause the individual to stand out from the rest of the group in physical appearance. This dissimilarity may contribute to a self-consciousness which favors the development of defensive and compensatory mechanisms that may distort the personality and render adjustment more difficult. The question, however, whether minor or major mental symptoms have any endocrine pathology to which they can be related is highly debatable.

Physical Defects

Physical anomalies or disturbances not caused by endocrine dysfunction, yet ones that occasionally provoke resentment and other undesirable psychological reactions, particularly of a compensatory, aggressive or other defensive nature, are genital deformities, clubbed feet, scoliosis, kyphosis and congenital defects of vision and hearing. Cleft palate, also, tends to create a sense of inability to meet social situations and to lead to feelings of inferiority and insecurity. Adolescence is the period when physical defects are most apt to evoke unwholesome psychological reactions. It must be said, however, that the personalities of individuals having physical defects are not always affected by such handicaps.

Vitamin Deficiencies

Certain vitamin deficiencies are known to produce encephalopathic syndromes resulting from metabolic or organic disturbances in the cerebrum. Pellagra and Wernicke's syndrome are among the most clearly recognized of the deficiency reactions. Brain syndromes rather than disorders of psychogenic origin usually occupy the foreground in personality disturbances associated with these deficiencies, although trends that have been developed for dealing with anxiety-producing situations and persons may be revealed.

Disease of the Brain

It was formerly assumed that every mental disease was a cerebral disease and that a psychosis without disease of the brain did not exist, also that specific brain lesions were accompanied by special mental symptoms. While in some instances of mental disorder an associated disease of the brain is known to exist, in most instances there is not, so far as our present knowledge goes, any cerebral pathology. Even when mental symptoms accompany disease of the brain, they cannot be explained by considering the location of the brain pathology alone.

Mental symptoms arising from disease of the brain are dependent to a large extent on whether the brain disease is of an acute or chronic nature, and if chronic whether the involvement is diffuse or circumscribed. The resulting symptom pattern tends therefore to fall into one of three types: (a) an acute organic syndrome; (b) a chronic syndrome due to a diffuse lesion; and (c) a chronic syndrome due to a localized lesion. The *acute* organic reaction is the result of temporary, reversible, diffuse impairment of brain tissue function and is characterized by a disturbance of consciousness, difficulty of apperception, somnolence, coma and cloudy and delirious states. The disturbance of the sensorium may release hallucinations and poorly organized transient delusions. *Chronic* organic brain syndromes result from relatively permanent, usually irreversible, diffuse impairment of cerebral tissue function. The chronic brain syndrome may vary in degree of progress but usually some disturbance of memory, judgment, orientation, comprehension and affect persists permanently. Frequently the organic syndrome is colored by the patient's individual personality with its particular conscious and unconscious impulses, fears and wishes. It should therefore be remembered that structural changes in the brain may release symptoms of a neurotic or "functional" nature.

Trauma

Trauma of the head with lesions ranging from a diffuse but minute separation of neuron structure through edema and hemorrhage to destruction of brain tissue with subsequent scar formation may be followed by varying defects of mentation. The clinical picture is usually at first that of an acute organic syndrome. If the impairment of brain function is persistent the clinical picture becomes that of the chronic organic brain syndrome with a permanent impairment of mental function. Trauma of any part of the body may be reacted to, usually after a latent period, by a traumatic neurosis. The possibility that some advantage or compensation may accrue to the patient as a result of the trauma often conduces to the development of a traumatic neurosis.

Sex Distribution

More men than women are admitted to hospitals for mental disorders, the ratio among first admissions being six men to five women; however, because of the greater longevity of women, the number of them in public mental hospitals exceeds that of men. General paresis, alcoholic psychoses, traumatic psychoses, psychoses with epilepsy and psychoses with cerebral arteriosclerosis are more frequent in men. Manic-depressive psychoses, involutional melancholia, paranoia and psychoses with somatic disease are more frequent in women. Schizophrenia appears to be a little more frequent in women.

Overwork

Overwork was formerly ascribed an important place in the etiology of mental disorders. It is now generally held, however, that so far as unusual application to work constitutes exhausting effort it is a symptom of mental disorder rather than a cause. The compulsive neurotic may work excessively hard, his job serving as a means of reducing anxiety and of support. Work may be the only outlet for an otherwise creative person. It may also in some instances serve as a neurotic outlet for aggression. It may give strong ego support through success or prestige to a person besieged with feelings of inferiority. For the withdrawn person, work may be his chief means of contacting others in a nonthreatening manner. Again the close interpersonal contact required in certain occupations may be threatening to schizoid persons. Finally, satisfying work is important for mental health. It brings such healthy gratifications as creative expression, companionship and a feeling of accomplishment. The mental disorder, as recognized by the patient's family, may have been preceded by unaccustomed effort but if a complete knowledge of the motivating forces is available, we should discover that the unusual assiduity represented an attempted flight from conflicts and problems for which satisfactory and successful solution had not been reached. It should undoubtedly be conceded that fatigue may at times weaken the controlling strength of the ego. Probably the factors in modern life productive of nervous and mental disorder lie less in overwork, in the speed and stress of work, distraction of noise and the like than in dissatisfaction, insecurity, distasteful work and lack of incentive. There is no evidence showing that mental effort in the absence of emotional stress and tension can produce either neurotic or psychotic reactions. There is no justification for the pessimistic suggestion frequently made that the pace of modern life conduces to mental breakdown.

Environment

More patients per unit of population are admitted to public hospitals from urban than from rural communities due in part to the greater incidence of mental disorder in cities and in part to the fact that admissions vary inversely with the remoteness of the community from an institution for mental diseases. Alcoholic psychoses, general paresis, psychoses due to drugs, manic-depressive psychoses, paranoia and psychoneuroses are more frequent in urban areas. Senile psychoses, psychoses with cerebral arteriosclerosis, involutional melancholia and psychoses with mental deficiency occur with relatively greater frequency in rural regions. Schizophrenia occurs with about equal frequency in urban and rural regions.

While the subject of environment is usually presented in much the manner just described, yet this is by far too limited a consideration of it from a psychiatric aspect. The environment in which an individual—the patient—lives is really a close interaction situation. Life is a series of processes of participation in a social setting, a total environment-person situation which the individual has helped to create. It is important to remember, also, that the significance of the environment, of the social constellation, is not what it appears objectively to others but how it is felt and lived subjectively by the patient. In making a distinction between person and environment we cannot consider that the environment has an independent existence. There is a functional relationship between the two. It is not likely that any so-called functional mental disorder can be said to have developed entirely independently of environmental influences. The content of the neurosis or psychosis, too, will vary with the emotional experiences and repressions of the developing personality, and these, in turn, will vary with the given culture and with the given family group.

Physical Illnesses

Acute physical illnesses with an associated toxic state frequently lead to an acute brain syndrome with an accompanying delirioid state but are rarely directly responsible for neuroses or the so-called functional psychoses. Chronic illness, however, with its handicaps, frustrations and unhealthy methods of attempting to surmount them is a severe neurosis-producing stress. The patient with an organic illness is confronted with two types of problems for which he must mobilize a variety of defenses and mechanisms of adaptation: (a) problems, largely conscious, related to the realities of the pain, inability to make a living and handicaps imposed on his family and (b) problems arising from emotional needs and from the activation of hitherto repressed, unconscious conflicts. There will be noted, however, a relationship between the psychological symptoms released by the ego-weakening effect of the illness and the premorbid personality of the patient.

Constitution

From the standpoint of psychiatry, constitution may be looked upon as the hereditary and developmental psycho-physical formula of the individual's organization, as the sum and synthesis of inherent conative, affective and temperamental qualities. It is therefore the sum total of physical, physiological and psychological attributes of a person as determined largely by heredity and only secondarily modified by developmental and environmental influences. Representing as it does the reactive potentialities of the individual, constitution is important in determining modes of behavior that are considered basic to the personality. Constitutional factors and predispositions must, however, be regarded as highly complex and as yet poorly understood. We do not yet know to what extent characteristics are gene-carried, but the tendency is to minimize the degree. It is difficult to discriminate between the effects of heredity and those resulting from family influences, because of the fact that the same relatives through whom hereditary characteristics might be traced are also the ones whose personality characteristics permeated the offspring's social environment in childhood and doubtless greatly influenced his developing personality. We must consider not only constitutional predispositions but also emotional states, interpersonal relationships and personal experiences in family life. The largely unchangeable groundwork of the personality is therefore probably determined by the influence of the intimate personal environment, particularly of childhood, upon a given hereditary substratum. As life progresses, behavior becomes an increasingly complex resultant of constitutional, genetic and experiential factors. As yet, however, our knowledge as to constitutional and genetic determinants and as to physiological mechanisms concerned in personality functioning is incomplete.

Psychogenic Causes

Mental disorder is not a disturbance in the function of a single organ, like the brain, but the maladapted and disordered psychobiological functioning of a social organism. Impersonal disturbances of tissue cannot alone explain disturbances in belief, mood and behavior. In most forms of mental disorder there is apparently no functional imperfection in the nerve tissue of the brain; rather does the mental disturbance represent the reaction of an individual personality to his special life situation including his interpersonal and emotional experiences. Much mental disorder and many maladaptations cannot be ascribed to physical pathology and can be understood only in terms of life-long dynamic interactions between the individual and all the forces, internal and external, which have impinged upon him. Such disturbances are described as psychogenic, *i.e.*, they are life-experienced or "mental." They are usually associated with emotional needs, guilt-producing situations, conflicts and disturbing interpersonal relations and other antecedent psychological determinants. The mental and emotional factors, the meaningful situations, are numerous.

In the psychogenic mental disorders we deal with concepts of genetics and of dynamics. Genetics refers to anxiety-producing sources, the factors involved in the origin of the anxiety. Dynamics refers to the pathogenic mental forces which have been evoked as defenses against the anxiety. While genetic factors tend to represent certain general themes, they are uniquely individual in each case. Generally speaking, the emotional and unconscious aspects of personality with their unrecognized motivations are the ones which are of significance in mental disorders and other disturbances of personality. No mental illness, psychoneurotic, psychotic or psychosomatic, can be understood without taking into account the unconscious dynamic mechanisms designed to deal with anxiety.

Interpersonal Relationships

The earliest and some of the most dynamic stresses, which perhaps can later be met only by psychopathological techniques, so disturbing to the happiness and efficiency of the individual or so disrupting to his social adjustment as to be regarded as mental disorder, arise from repetitive, early interpersonal attitudes and stresses within the family. This is not surprising since human relations involve problems of pain, pleasure, love, hate, guilt, jealousy, envy, security and status. Frequent among such themes are desires for protection and security, the demand for the satisfaction of deep inner needs and for relief from situations which fail to meet them. Likewise are strivings and impulses so strong that the individual can neither repress nor accept them without anxiety or emotional disturbance. It should be remembered that many interpersonal attitudes and their resulting influence on behavior are unconsciously determined but continue nevertheless to exercise a continuing and dynamic influence on the developing personality.

Of all interpersonal relationships of childhood, the attitude of the mother is frequently the most determinative of the future mental health of the individual. A strangling, perhaps guilt-ridden, overprotection on her part may prevent the development of a mature, independent personality by the child. Again the maternal relationship may fail to give him the warmth, security and support necessary for the emotional and social growth of his personality. For example, instead of providing a healthful emotional climate of affection, acceptance and approval, the mother may to varying degrees reject or overprotect the child with consequent misshaping of his developing personality. Such attitudes, which exist particularly among mothers who have been damaged emotionally by their own life experiences, are usually unconscious ones. Other attitudes, often covert or ambivalent, which may also be manifested by psychologically important persons are hostility, aggression, dominance, sadism and dependence. Out of such relationships emotions frequently arise which are culturally so unacceptable that they are repressed and give rise to conflict and anxiety. Ambitendent attitudes *i.e.*, confusions of hostile and affectionate impulses, which had their origin in some childhood intrafamily relationship, may continue to influence the personality pattern throughout later life and constitute, often unconsciously, a conflictful problem which cannot be met except by psychopathological methods.

Psychiatry now places much emphasis on the fact that adult behavior is apparently determined to a considerable degree by events which took place in the preverbal age period or through later unliquidated childhood situations. The *anlage* of many neuroses and of many other personality difficulties and characteristics is found in emotionally traumatic experiences of early childhood. Early tension-laden relationships with parents seem to be particularly apt to become pathogenetic. Interpersonal situations in later life may awaken previous feelings and unresolved difficulties and lead to the re-enactment of problems generated in prior relationships. Difficulties in these relationships may therefore be both expressions and sources of personality disturbances. Not only may aggression and hostility arise out of family relationships but many other emotional reactions such as feelings of insecurity, rejection, guilt, dependency, overprotection and jealousy be acquired in response to repetitive, early interpersonal experiences. They may have great influence upon the child's personality and the course of its development with the result that later mental disorder may be the working out of a pattern of childhood origin. Clinical experience certainly seems to show that many anxieties, and therefore the self-defensive reactions habitually used to minimize them, arise out of early interpersonal relationships and attitudes. While the emotional reactions and inner experiences growing out of early disturbing relationships rarely lead to psychotic reactions during childhood, yet in them is frequently to be found the genesis of neurotic and behavior disorders occurring at that age. The personality pattern laid down through such experiences may, however, in later years prove inadequate for the stresses and problems confronted with the result that a neurotic or psychotic reaction occurs.

In the previous paragraphs much emphasis was placed on the stress of interpersonal situations as important genetic factors in the creation of life-problems, in the formation of symptoms and in the production of various degrees of personality disorders. When we come to consider psychosomatic symptoms we shall find that physical complaints and symptoms may also arise from interpersonal issues as well as from toxic, metabolic or other organic causes. Deep seated, cumulative resentment and hostility, conscious or unconscious, while held under apparent control, may in some persons find expression in tensions, instability, cynicism, or even in more extreme cases in neurosis or psychosis. In other persons these same factors may be expressed in somatic symptoms.

Aggression

In recent years there has been emphasis on aggression as a participating factor in the psychogenic production of personality disturbances. Aggression may be defined as a goal-directed self-assertion with an associated implication of attack, often of hostile, destructive intent. There are two contradictory theories of aggression. The first, stemming largely from the later writings of Freud, holds that aggression is a primary, instinctual drive (more accurately a component manifestation of Freud's death instinct). According to this view, each individual requires a certain amount of gratification of this destructive impulse which if not attained in one way will be achieved in some other.

The second theory may be characterized as the "reactive" theory in contrast to the more speculative "death-instinct" theory. According to the "reactive" theory aggressive behavior is provoked through emotion aroused by thwarting, frustrating experiences. If an individual's habitual modes of action lead smoothly to accustomed gratifications, little or no impulse to aggression will be generated, but if obstacles arise in the habitual paths to established goals, there will be correspondingly strong instigation to ever-pressing aggressive behavior. The sequence, then, is frustration-anger-aggression, the latter aiming to remove the source of frustration and thereby clear the path to the desired goal. Presumably the formation of the aggressive personality pattern is frequently established by reason of the fact that frustrating forces are applied too early, too harshly or too intensively in the family with the result that an unconscious aggressive and hostile attitude may be developed. Such unconscious hostile impulses stimulate anxiety which gives rise to neurotic guilt, depression, displaced hostility and other psychopathological clinical expressions. The fact that the child is dependent on the very persons, the parents, who are the chief frustrating agents further psychologically complicates the situation.

Other Factors

At times failure results in the attempt to discover interpersonal and experiential factors that may have contributed to the patient's mental disorder. This does not exclude their existence but merely means that their presence or nature can be ascertained with difficulty only. It must be remembered, too, that in their bearing on mental disorders it is not what the facts of an experience were that is significant but what the experience meant to the person and how much anxiety it created. A situation or experience which in itself seems insignificant may mobilize unconscious material which is highly significant. Emotional experiences involving a frustration of hopes, wishes and instinctive drives, as well as those that beget fear, humiliation, loss of prestige, resentment and guilt may stimulate anxiety and constitute too great a problem for the individual to meet without resorting to defensive or evasive psychopathological methods.

The creation in early life of feeling patterns of fear, guilt, resentment, hostility, insecurity or inadequacy, even though the feelings were never consciously verbalized, tends to favor the later development of personality maladjustment. The emotional problem of the child may grow into the mental disorder of the adult. Unhealthy reactions are prolific in their propagation. A chain of dynamic sequence may be established. The result of one faulty method of reaction may become the cause of another. In this way the burdens of adjustment are increased and the measures for meeting them rendered less efficient. A sense of insecurity, for example, cannot be complacently accepted. As a result one may become aggressive in order to construct a spurious feeling of assurance. Aggressiveness leads to hostility, the hostile act often leads to guilt which creates further insecurity. Again a sense of insecurity may tend to separate a person from his social group. This isolation, in turn, contributes to the development of pathological fantasy; from this it is not a far step to the projection, in the form of hallucinations, of wishes which cannot be fulfilled in reality. In searching for the causes and development of mental disorders, as well as of other behavior, it is necessary to connect a series of experiences into a meaningful pattern. It will usually be found that a constellation of factors has led to a mental disorder.

Social Factors and Cultural Mores

In approaching the relation of culture to mental disorder, it must be remembered that cultural factors are important ones in determining personality. Cultural demands upon the individual are highly coercive and many of his inner pressures are the reflections of these requirements. The mental disorder from which a person suffers is a highly individual problem, yet social pressures and attitudes are important factors in producing personality disturbances. Cultural anthropologists and those psychiatrists who have worked among peoples of different cultural institutions agree that cultural factors influence the etiology and psychopathology of mental disorders. Frequently the individual's disorder cannot be understood without a scrutiny of the psychic difficulties presented to individuals by the prevailing cultural mode of life. The fact that man, unlike other organisms, is a socially patterned and constituted one is doubtless the most important factor in producing neurotic and psychotic forms of reaction. More and more have such reactions come to be regarded as issues of conflicting attitudes and tendencies learned from and reinforced by the cultural environment. The demands of the social environment, its excessive competitiveness, its sex repressions and its contradictory codes bring individual frustrations and dilemmas and engender psychic conflicts. Social factors and standards help to shape the adaptive efforts of each individual and, operating with biological and psychological ones, are partly responsible for the formation of personalities that eventually succumb to neuroses and psychoses. Social factors, too, often participate in the constellation of forces usually spoken of as "precipitating causes." The conscious content of the disordered mind, the symbols it uses and the form of its delusions are determined by the prevailing ideology and social attitudes and practices of the environment. From one point of view the mentally disordered person is one who has not been able to make the exacting grade required by the culture in which he lives. The neurotic or psychotic reaction, therefore, would represent the failure of the individual to cope with the stresses of adjustment to society.

Finally, the psychiatrist should bear in mind the significance of the patient's immediate social situation. He should, for example, consider the impact of this situation on the development of the patient's illness in terms of the familial, vocational, economic and cultural pressures upon him.

Mental Conflict

One of the most important psychogenic factors in the production of mental disorder is the problem of reconciling discordant desires and conflicting psychological needs and of dealing with incompatible response-tendencies. Conflicts may be of the greatest variety but tend to be between the ideals of the individual, his socially conditioned disposition to comply with the customs and standards of society on the one hand, and socially unacceptable impulses, motives, wishes and strivings on the other. Frequently the conflict is between instinctual drives on the one hand, and socialized and religious values on the other. Instinctual urges may be beyond the capacity of the ego to handle at the time. Unrecognized motivations, repressed hostilities and resentments, aggressive tendencies, disturbing memories, sensitive scars and other results of unresolved childhood anxieties may continue to persist beneath conscious awareness.

Particularly important are persistent emotional conflicts that arose during earlier stages of personality development. The conflicting and discordant components of personality, the many people that make up a person, engender anxious tensions for the relief of which the individual may employ various neurotic or psychotic devices. Conflicts at a deep level may appear on the surface in the form of far removed symptoms. For example, an unwillingness to accept a feeling of hostility toward a parent may cause the patient to focus his attention upon a local manifestation, such as a difficulty in swallowing. Sometimes an apparently insignificant experience may set off a chain reaction of deeper emotional conflict within the individual with conflicts spreading from one situation to another. Some situation, specific to the individual, may be so highly charged with symbolic content that it may touch off a major psychotic explosion. Whatever the cause of the inner disharmony the mind has not been at peace with itself. Caught in a tangle of attitudes the unification of the personality has been disturbed. Unless opposing impulses are blended, the individual is constantly prompted by contradictory drives and disconcerted by the tensions of his emotional dilemmas. Faced with highly charged emotional issues he is unable to attain a working harmony in his personality. Since our most important conflicts take place on levels which our conscious self-perceptions cannot reach, we cannot apply reason, reality and common sense to their solution. If the internal conflict is great, there is relatively little resistance to external stress with the result that an immediate environmental difficulty may appear to have been the basic cause of the mental disorder, whereas in reality it was only the releasing agent.

The personality, if confronted by conflict and by the fact that the repression of forbidden wishes and of instinctual tendencies is in danger of giving way, tends to develop *anxiety*, a persistent fear arising from threatening factors deep in the mental life accompanied by a vague but disquieting, anticipatory feeling of prospective harm or disaster. In the sources of this anxiety, whether it be overt or hidden, are to be found many of the causes of mental disorder, while the personality devices designed to serve as defenses against anxiety constitute the symptoms of the neuroses, of many of the psychoses and even of personality traits, particularly those known as reaction formations.

Far more than formerly it is now believed that not only are internal (instinctual) dangers the source of anxiety but also attitudes growing out of troublesome interpersonal relationships. While the greater part of one's satisfactions arise from his emotional relationships with others so, also, do a large part of his dissatisfactions. Many of the self-defensive reactions which one habitually utilizes for minimizing his anxieties are developed for the purpose of decreasing anxiety that has arisen out of interpersonal relationships and attitudes. Anxiety, guilt and depression may develop as a breakdown of defenses against hostile and aggressive impulses is threatened.

The ways of dealing with anxiety may be various and range from those which have social value to those which disorganize the personality.

Which of the various defenses are used depends largely on the personality structure of the individual. Both behavior which is socially useful and constructive and character traits which are desirable may be the products of neurotic drives unconsciously directed to the prevention or relief of anxiety. The degree of anxiety from which an individual suffers, its manner of expression and the types of defense which he utilizes against it largely constitute the difference between mental health and mental sickness and the various shades between.

A frequent source of anxiety is an unsuccessful attempt to secure the satisfaction of a basic emotional need. Much behavior may therefore be explained on the basis of attempt to secure some degree of satisfaction of such a need. Not a few personality and character and even psychotic traits arise from the anxiety caused by the frustration of a basic need for being loved, accepted and belonging.

The methods of dealing with anxiety may so disturb personality functioning that social adjustment is destroyed and the individual must be removed from his usual environment and placed in the controlled and protected one of the hospital for mental diseases. The more the individual is threatened and the less effectively his conflict is tolerated, the more he is driven to defend himself. Among the less malignant devices for minimizing anxiety are the phobic, conversion and compulsive reactions—neuroses which do not seriously disorganize the personality. Devices which may serve a similar purpose but may so disorganize the personality and produce such a serious break with reality that the patient is called psychotic are the paranoid and the schizophrenic reactions. In the former the patient attributes hostile or aggressive motives to others and thus by blaming another he relieves his own guilt and anxiety for possessing such attitudes. Again, the defense against anxiety may be through a schizophrenic delusional and hallucinatory preoccupation that disorganizes the personality and disregards reality.

Role of Organic Factors

There is as yet no proof as to whether underlying physiological disturbances exist in all cases of mental disorder or whether some types arise in their absence. In certain types, such as general paralysis, organic factors clearly exist and explain the signs of dementia that are found in that disease. The impairment of memory, of apperception and of other higher mental expressions occurring as general paralysis progresses may be looked upon as resulting from the disturbances in the physiology of cortical neurons. Probably most psychiatrists would agree that the individual patient's disturbances of mood and behavior, frequently more conspicuous in the early stages of the disease than is any accompanying dementia, are determined by the patient's particular psychological problems and stresses and by the patterns of reaction that have long characterized his personality. As the higher organic integrating mechanisms suffer destructive physical changes there appear personality maladjustments, psychotic in type and with characteristics determined by personality and psychogenic factors. The organic factors may be the pathogenetic agent that so disturbs the integration of the personality that the psychosis follows, but the psychological factors, the problems and needs of the personality, are the pathoplastic agents that determine the picture of the mental disorder. There is an increasing effort to discover physiological or biochemical changes in the nervous system that may be operative in the production of mental disorder. Some psychiatrists believe that all such major forms of mental disorder as schizophrenia, manic-depressive psychosis and paranoid states are produced through undetermined physical or chemical changes which, although not irreversibly destructive like those in general paralysis, are sufficiently disturbing as to impair the functions of the central integrating mechanisms of the organism and thereby permit the psychotic personality reactions. The fields of structural, and particularly of physicochemical, alterations in the central nervous system have not yet been fully explored. It is known that certain cortical strata are unusually sensitive to toxins or injuries. This is especially true of the third layer the cells of which have a particular need for oxygen with the result that they are easily affected when the blood or oxygen supply is impaired. Those attempts, however, to find changes of ganglion cells characteristic of certain diseases or injuries has been successful in only rare cases. This is not to say that time may not bring a greater correlation of psychological dynamics with the functioning of the central nervous system. Human behavior, however, cannot be reduced to a matter of disturbed chemistry. For the most part, American psychiatrists do not look upon mental disorder as a form of dissolution of psychic activity that is *always* conditioned by an organic process.

Of much interest is the fact, discovered in recent years, that certain substances, notably LSD (lysergic acid diethylamide) and mescalin produce artificial psychoses. In such experimental psychoses a small amount of a drug or poison introduced into the human organism changes the biological pattern of personality in such a way that everything becomes distorted. It would appear that a change occurs in some metabolic processes in the brain which causes a shift in the normal spectrum of perception, intensifying some reactions and dimming others, thus producing a twisted conceptual world. Such experimental psychoses suggest that in certain psychoses there may be abnormal, noxious metabolic products formed in the endocrine glands which affect the brain function in a way similar to that of LSD.

Mental Disorders: Some Comments on Causes and Nature

To a large degree, the causes of mental illness, the factors that eventuate in the psychically or emotionally sick personality, are presumably the familiar difficulties of human existence. The so-called abnormal is but an exaggerated or unbalanced expression of the normal. For the present, therefore, it seems most fruitful to look upon most mental disorders not as the result or expression of some "disease" but as a mode of behavior or of living that is the logical, although socially maladjusted, outcome of the particular individual's original endowment, of the molding influence of the home, of traumatic experiences that modified personality development, of the stresses and problems springing perhaps from deep within his emotional and instinctive life, of his inability to meet these strains, of the type of self-defensive reactions habitually utilized for minimizing anxiety, and of any bodily ailments that may impair the integrity or efficiency of his biological organism. Mental disorders should therefore be regarded as patterns of human reaction set in motion by stress. The tendency to look on those who manifest nervous or mental symptoms as being different in their organization from the so-called normal is therefore erroneous.

Just as mechanical objects, if subjected to stress beyond the limits of their elasticity, suffer distortion, so the personality, if subjected to anxiety-producing stresses beyond the limits of its capacity for adaptation, may suffer disorganization in both overt and symbolic behavior. Doubtless everyone, however healthy his adaptation appears to be, has particular psychological spheres which are vulnerable to stress. If his experiences touch these areas and the degree of their anxiety-producing nature exceeds his ability to deal with their stresses by healthy, adaptive methods, he will be compelled to deal with them by neurotic or psychotic ones. Through repeated or cumulative stress the individual's "normal" defenses no longer suffice and his capacity for adjustment becomes exhausted, so to speak. Stress alone, however, should not be considered as the precipitating factor in mental disorder. It must be a particular stress for a particular person and perhaps at a particular time.

Since all behavior is but a reaction to personality and life factors, it is not always easy to define exactly any criterion of mental illness. An unbroken line of continuity exists from "normal" behavior through neurotic to psychotic behavior. In the mental field as elsewhere we find that no boundary in nature is fixed. Perhaps the criterion is largely the degree to which behavior becomes undesirably substitutive and symbolic, and the extent to which one deals with problems in a neurotic manner rather than by rational decision. As Meyer has stressed, however, the form and coloring of mental illness is as wide as life itself.

Like more narrowly biological phenomena, such as fever, inflammation and other morbid processes, mental disorders are defensive, protective and reparative in purpose; but, as they deal with the affective and psychosocial aspects of the organism, the adjustive ends they serve are those of personal situations. The neurosis or the psychosis represents either the individual's attempt to effect an adjustment to the interplay of psychological, social and physiological forces impinging upon him or his failure in that effort. Again the symptoms may represent an attempt of the individual to hide the truth from himself, to retreat from difficult situations, to deal with anxiety, or to shut out the stresses of life, but with the result that he employs substitutive methods of adjustment that lead him away from reality which he may even sacrifice in order to attain the objective that offers him emotional comfort, maintains his self-respect or provides satisfaction in the easiest way. His comforts and compensations, however, are highly egoistic and are often disserviceable or even objectionable to the social group.

A longitudinal study of the patient's behavior pattern will often reveal the neurosis or psychosis to be the culminate but logical result of the basic mental habits and personality trends of the individual, an accentuation and distortion of the reaction patterns which he has long employed to meet the stresses of life. The same complex forces that determined the prepsychotic personality play also an important part in determining the clinical picture of the psychosis. The mental disorder reveals more sharply both the attitudes which have been subtly developing for years in response to anxiety-producing situations and to deep-seated psychological needs and the manner in which the personality has attempted to meet its stresses. The formative factors may be detected in the early patterns and responsive tendencies characteristic of the individual personality. An urge for self-assertion, for example, may have been an attitude or personality trend found useful in dealing with certain anxiety-producing situations or persons. So long as such an attitude or trend remains adequately effective in its purpose, the individual maintains a satisfactory personal adjustment. Should, however, such a personality attitude not continue to provide the needed relief from his anxiety, the individual may resort to an exaggerated or unbalanced manifestation of self-assertion in the form of a manic attack. Various personality traits may have represented compromises with unconscious conflicts and unconscious purposes. Through such compensatory compromises the individual may have achieved a certain mastery over them although never free from their influence. Finally, under some unusual stress, the compromise may fail and the neurotic or psychotic symptoms appear.

When one discovers the significance of the patient's life pattern his personality disorder comes to have a logical place in the evolution of that particular pattern. Personality trends and characteristics and neurotic or psychotic symptoms are often allied efforts toward the same goal. Any absence of continuity between the individual's prepsychotic personality and psychic characteristics and those existing after the development of the mental disorder is only apparent. There is a definite correlation between the kind of person an individual is in health and the type of disorder he develops if he becomes mentally ill. In psychopathology, too, we are able to see in isolated and exaggerated form many dynamic mechanisms that are easily overlooked in normal behavior and personality development. The mental disease often represents the result of a progressive development of the prepsychotic characteristics to a degree that constitutes a caricature of the previous personality or leads to disintegration and breaking up. The embryology of the psychosis may be studied in the habitual reaction patterns employed by the patient in his prepsychotic life. The psychological process may lead from a long standing character disorder into the early stage of an acute psychosis. The person who cannot modify his ways of thinking, feeling and behaving as his life advances may find that an adjustment is possible only through a psychosis. The same psychological theme or conflict runs through personality, character traits and psychosis. In all we discover certain attitudes—"sets" of the organism to respond in a given manner.

Sir Russell Brain, the English neuropsychiatrist, in an apt selection of characters from Shakespeare, points out certain well-recognized types of personality and the form of mental disease in which they are prone to culminate. On the one hand, he says, is Cassius with his lean and hungry look and his propensity for thinking too much. In him is typified a form of personality calculated to develop a malignant, paranoid type of psychosis. On the other hand, is the fat, jovial Falstaff, in whom a psychosis, if it occurred, would probably be of a benign, affective type. It will thus be seen that mental disease is not a partial expression but one that goes to the very depths of the personality.

Conceptions of Mental Disorder: Psychiatric Theories

Just as there has been remarkable development in our knowledge of physical diseases during the present century, so clinical, psychological and neuropathological researches during that period have clarified our ideas concerning the causes and nature of mental disorder and educed theories which seem to offer rational explanations for observed mental phenomena.

CONTRIBUTIONS OF KRAEPELIN. Prior to the work of Emil Kraepelin (1856–1929), a German psychiatrist, psychiatric attention was directed largely to the mental symptom which was in itself generally regarded as constituting the mental disease. Kraepelin gave psychiatry the first comprehensive descriptions of what he believed to be mental disease entities. Assuming that mental disorders are definite disease entities analogous to physical diseases and therefore defined by etiology, symptomatology, course and outcome, he stressed clinical observation and searched for an organic background for mental diseases. If brain histopathology failed to reveal structural changes considered to be responsible for the "disease," he sought for metabolic and constitutional etiological factors. Since it was frequently impossible to make a diagnosis by the microscope or test tube he attempted to make a diagnosis by the general pathological evolution of symptoms and the outcome of the illness. Kraepelin's classification of mental diseases was therefore based on description, symptoms and outcome rather than on an understanding of the nature of the diseases or of their psychological dynamics. While Kraepelin brought clarity in what had been a chaos of psychiatric thought and helped to introduce scientific methods of investigation, yet it was his belief that mental disease is the result of an attack upon the individual by an impersonal something rather than the logical outcome of unique psychodynamic experiences the story of which should be reconstructed in order to understand the patient's personality reactions.

To Kraepelin, abnormal behavior was a sign of brain disease. Symptoms did not have a psychological significance. The theory of unconscious mental activities and attitudes was not accepted. In view of the assumption of a mind-body dualism with parallel activities of the two there was no stress on interpersonal relationships as the source of emotional experiences that may be pathogenic. He had, in fact, little or no appreciation of the patient's inner life. Although Kraepelin, with his emphasis on description and symptomatology, contributed very little to an understanding of the nature of mental disorders and nothing to their psychological dynamics, he gave a great impetus to their study and scientific investigation. Psychological medicine has given a much clearer perception of mental disorder than did the medical science of Kraepelin's day. For that reason, there is sometimes a tendency to belittle his contributions to psychiatry. His name, however, deserves to stand among the great ones of psychiatry. Kraepelin observed with discernment and systematized the results of his observation—a stage through which a science must pass. He was the first to establish the homogeneity of various forms of mental disease. Even though it is unsatisfactory today, his classification of mental disorders was clinically useful and facilitated an orderly approach to their study.

CONTRIBUTIONS OF ADOLF MEYER. Psychiatry is immensely indebted to Adolf Meyer (1866–1950), professor of psychiatry at Johns Hopkins University from 1910 to 1941 and founder of a system of psychiatric concepts which he designated psychobiology.[1] In introducing the term, Meyer sought to eliminate the contrast between physical and mental, as well as theories about mind-body relationship. He stressed the concept that psychiatry is a part of human biology and that mental expressions of life are no less biological than physical ones, that psychic aspects of life cannot be considered apart from the biological. Psychobiology emphasizes the importance of the patient as a person and yet as a natural, biological creature whose total life history as well as his physical and mental capacities must be studied in order to understand his behavior and his problems. Meyer urged that the psychiatrist study the activity and behavior of the patient as the interaction of an individual organism with its life situations. He regarded each individual as a human organism, as a natural biological phenomenon, a physical-chemical-social-psychological interacting unit, and that therefore the etiologic bases of mental disorder may be multiple. While his approach to personality functioning was that of biology it was that of a broadly conceived humanized biology. He insisted on the consideration of all pertinent data concerning the life of the patient as a biological and social organism. He believed, therefore, that not only should the organic, including constitutional and structural, aspects of the individual be studied but also the sociological, cultural, experiential and psychological components. To Meyer, all life is a biological reaction and he held that the individual is a living, behaving being in action and that his particular genetic heritage, intellectual endowment, social environment, cultural influences and personal experiences mold him in a unique manner. He therefore regarded mental illness as a psychobiological response to the special, complex life situation in which the individual is placed.

Meyer introduced the term "reaction type" as a designation for the

---

[1] The word "psychobiology" was first used in 1886 by Hippolyte-Marie Bernheim. professor of clinical medicine, University of Nancy, but was introduced in United States by Meyer in 1915. "Psychobiology studies not only the person as a whole, as a unit, but also the whole of man" (Meyer).

clinically recognizable patterns of behavior which characterize the major forms of personality disorder, previously assumed to be disease entities. These patterns or "reactions," he urged, should be regarded as meaningful forms of behavior understandable in terms of personality development and life situation. He was perhaps the first psychiatrist to see the individual in terms of his own life history.

Probably we are indebted more to Meyer than to anyone else for the concept that mental disorder is not "a standard disease picture" but the behavior of an individual who is unable to maintain his adjustment to pressures and threats, to emotional and instinctual needs and to the demands of reality. He taught that one must consider the whole setting and uniqueness of circumstances in which the mental disorder occurred and that the disorder should be looked upon as a reaction or mode of behavior which constitutes a faulty adaptation dynamically understandable in terms of the individual's life history. Meyer often characterized his approach to psychiatry as "common sense," *i.e.*, the emphasis should be on the facts that could be observed.

The naturalistic, biological approach to a study of the personality, including its psychological aspects, as proposed by Meyer was more comprehensive and meaningful than any previous one. He was the first to stress what is now the trend of modern psychiatric thinking, *i.e.*, emphasis on the whole organism, the total personality, the psycho-socio-somatic unit. He did not, however, adequately recognize the importance of the unconscious and its dynamic role. Probably, too, more than Meyer realized are the causes of contemporary difficulties to be found in early interpersonal emotional experiences. Enriched, as it now has been, by many psychoanalytical concepts, psychobiology perhaps represents the point of view most widely accepted by American psychiatry which postulates that important among the facts for consideration are the concrete genetic-dynamic data gained from a study of the life of the individual as he has developed in his specific social and interpersonal situation.

CONTRIBUTIONS OF MASSERMAN. Since man is a biological organism, his behavior may well be considered from the standpoint of biological dynamics, *i.e.*, from that of biological response to an acute or continuing situation. From his experiments with animals and the production of neurotic behavior in them, Masserman of Chicago developed a concept which he has termed biodynamics, the principles of which he applies to psychiatry. The four main principles of biodynamics are as follows: (a) That all motivation, or nearly all, derives from the biological needs of the organism; (b) that every organism adapts itself to its environment in terms of its own life-experiences; (c) that the organism reacts to frustration from its own environment either by a change of technique or a change of goal; and (d) that when two strongly motivated methods of adaptation are mutually incompatible an impasse results and the organism develops what we call a neurosis.

Masserman's concept of biodynamics appears superficially to be a much less comprehensive one than that of Meyer's psychobiology, but it is nevertheless a thought-stimulating, biologically-based theory the principles of which offer a common denominator for the behavior—including neurotic—both of higher organisms (men) and of lower ones (cats in Masserman's experiments). Many psychiatrists are of the opinion that Masserman applies to too great a degree his observations of behavior of animals to a theory of human behavior.

Contributions of Freud. It is no disparagement to Kraepelin, to Meyer or to the many others who have contributed much to our knowledge of mental disorders to state that our greatest indebtedness for an understanding of personality disturbances is to Sigmund Freud who was born in Freiberg, Moravia, in 1856, and died in London in 1939. His influence upon psychiatry was revolutionary. After a period in the neuroanatomical laboratory, Freud decided to become a neurologist and therefore, wishing to prepare himself for the treatment of hysteria and allied conditions, he studied under Charcot at the Salpêtrière in Paris and under Bernheim at Nancy. As he continued his study of hysteria, he noted that experiences which caused shame or similar emotional disturbance were forced out of awareness and were not accessible to the usual process of memory. Continued observation convinced Freud that this material which had been forced out of awareness could still influence behavior. This area of the mind beyond or beneath conscious awareness and into which material was repressed Freud designated "the unconscious." He soon perceived that if, by free thought association and by dream interpretation—devices which will be discussed in Chapter XXXVI—he probed into the unconscious, he discovered the cause of conscious symptoms. He discovered, also, that the unconscious is a great reservoir of early established wishes, desires and drives of a sort not permitted expression by the personal and social ideal. This material, he concluded, had been forced from the conscious state into the unconscious by a process or mechanism he designated as "repression." A second use of the term "unconscious" is as a collective term for those phases of psychological activity which cannot be consciously observed. These activities, taking place without conscious recognition and serving such psychological purposes as reduction of tension and anxiety, have been discussed under mental mechanisms.

While some psychologists dislike the use of such a metaphorical word as "the unconscious" for those impulses, desires and emotional responses which are inaccesible to our introspective observation, such a hypothesis is required for the explanation of many mental phenomena. This concept has been one of the greatest contributions to psychiatry. Many, too, do not accept Freud's concept of infantile sexuality with its uncompleted differentiation and the influence of its persistent hangovers on personality. His emphasis upon personality as a process developing step-by-step has, however, given a clearer understanding of personality manifestations. Freud's demonstration of the importance of inner conflict with its dynamically opposed impulses has also contributed greatly to our knowledge of the genesis of neurotic and psychotic reactions. Although some would interpret Freud as referring to the generalized systems of drives, the id, the ego and the superego, as if they were entities, yet the use of such terms for certain dynamic parts or functions of the personality has simplified our thinking concerning the personality. Freud's emphasis upon a determinism of psychic processes has led to a greater clarity of our thinking. We are largely indebted to Freud for a recognition of the dynamic importance of experiences in early life and the importance of parental attitudes and influences on the growing child. His psychological theory revolves around the problem of the development of infantile drives into adult personality. He contended that psychopathology resulted from a failure of a smooth, scheduled progress through the successive stages of infantile sexuality development described in Chapter II. Through his establishment of a dynamic psychology of behavior, Freud greatly broadened and deepened our psychiatric concepts and our understanding of human motivations and the causes and nature of personality disorders. While Freud emphasized the id as the primary source of motivation in psychodynamics, later psychoanalytical writers, notably Karen Horney (1885–1952), have included factors of social origin and social significance.

CONTRIBUTIONS OF OTHERS. Various psychiatrists have formulated other theories as to the formation of personality and as to the causes and nature of its disturbances which are considered as mental disorders. While their theories have not, in full, stood the test of clinical experience and have largely given place to those of Freud or Meyer, or to eclectic concepts selected from these two, yet the student should have some acquaintance with them.

Adler. Alfred Adler (1870–1937), a Viennese psychiatrist, was an early student and associate of Freud but later came to dissent from Freud's emphasis on infantile sexuality and believed that the child's resistance to domination and his drive to self-assertion, domination and superiority, were more important than the sexual drive in the development and structuring of the personality. Adler's psychological formula would be as follows: Because of a sense of inferiority—organic, intellectual, social or the result of past experiences—a will to power is stimulated, resulting in compensatory reactions directed to goals of superiority. Adler included these various compensatory activities under the term "masculine protest." He adopted this term on the assumption that the exaggerated "will to power," with its drive to prestige, superiority and achievement, implied a struggle for power which might be compared to what he believed was the reaction of women to their feminine status. He observed that in European culture women were usually regarded as inferior, a status to which he believed they reacted by a so-called masculine protest, that is, by trying to act like men. This "will to power" need not have its origin in a patent organ defect but in whatever feeling of inferiority, be it organic, sexual, economic or social, may lead to feelings of inadequacy. Adler gave his psychological movement the name "individual psychology," to indicate that each individual has his own special goals and a unique manner of attempting to achieve them. These methods, which mark the individual off from others, largely determine the structure of his personality. The various psychological processes by which he seeks to deny his inferiority and maintain the fiction of achievement constitute the symptoms of the neurosis. Adler's emphasis on power and prestige motivations, on cultural determinants of neurosis, and therapy as a re-education have been absorbed to a greater extent than is conceded by adherents of other "schools."

Jung. C. G. Jung (1875–), a Swiss psychiatrist, became closely associated with Freud during the early days of the latter's development of psychoanalytical theory and became a leader in the movement. In 1911 he broke with Freud over the all-importance of infantile and childhood levels or stages of sexuality development and the effect upon personality of their fixations.

Like Freud, Jung assumed the existence of an unconscious but he did not conceive of it as containing the same type of material or as acting in the same way in the production of psychopathology. Jung presented the belief that the unconscious is made up of material derived from two sources. These he called the personal unconscious and the collective, or racial, unconscious. He proposed that in the more superficial and accessible level, the one nearer consciousness and known as the *personal unconscious,* are the personal urges and thoughts developed in the history of the individual, forgotten impressions and incidents concerned with one's actual life, the instinctive activities and reactions to environmental experiences which have disappeared from consciousness. To the deeper layer of the unconscious Jung gave the name *racial or collective unconscious.* The contents of this are not related to any personal experience but consist of instinctive impulses and primitive fears, feelings, trends and thoughts not connected with personal, but with racial experience and thought. The form of feeling and thinking was once universal and general and is known to us as archaic. In the collective unconscious are feelings and desires, according to Jung, which belong to a mode of thinking and acting which has undergone racial repression and belongs to phases of past human cultural epochs. To this psychological movement Jung gave the name *analytic psychology.*

While Freud attributed the nonorganic mental disorders to unresolved, unconscious conflicts, Jung explains them on the assumption that the individual is overwhelmed by the contents of the collective unconscious, that the psychic organization is broken down by its phylogenetic determinants, with the result that its impulses and feelings sweep the individual along regardless of his conscious will or reason. In such disorders as the compulsion neuroses, the individual, according to Jung, is not overwhelmed by the uncontrolled impulses of the collective unconscious, but the individual's self-imposed rituals and compulsive ceremonials serve as defenses and protections against the domination by the collective unconscious, which Jung regards as more important than the personal unconscious.

Jung not only developed his hypothesis of a racial or collective and of a personal unconscious but contributed many other concepts some of which have received wide acceptance. Among them was the word association test for investigating hidden regions of personality. This laid the foundation for the psychology of free association. It will be discussed in Chapter XXXVI. Jung was among the first to emphasize the nature of the child's interpersonal relationships and to point out that neurotic difficulties of parents are decisive influences in the difficulties of children. Working with Bleuler, Jung applied psychoanalytical concepts to the psychoses and was the first psychiatrist to suggest a psychological approach to the study of dementia praecox (1907). He presented a penetrating, analytical description of personality types and developed the extravert-introvert concept. He studied artistic creations, mythological themes and religion and their relation to dreams, fantasies and the neuroses. He greatly stressed symbolism and religion. His critics comment upon the extent to which he combined psychological, philosophical, mystical and metaphysical elements.

The theories of Freud, Adler and Jung as to the causes of mental disorder have been presented, but it should be added that the Freudian psychoanalytical school has constantly gained recognition while other groups have lost in acceptance.

Janet. Pierre Janet (1895–1947), a French psychiatrist, laid important groundwork for a psychopathological consideration of the nature of mental disorders but this will be considered in Chapter XXXVI.

Finally, it must be said that no one theory does justice to all the problems presented by psychiatry. A conception as to the causes and the nature of disorders of the personality must be holistic and take into consideration a wide variety of factors which have acted and, directly or indirectly, are continuing to act, dynamically upon the personality. Among them are constitutionally genetic, somatic, social and cultural factors and that great group of psychological ones uncovered by psychoanalysis. Among the latter are the warpings and stuntings of personality that occur during the developmental phases of childhood, the attitudes created through family and other interpersonal relationships, the perceptions of self, the place of sexuality, aggression, hostility and emotional needs, the phenomenology of conflict, anxiety and guilt and the role of mental mechanisms and their functional operation in the service of forces and counterforces. Stated with extreme brevity, and therefore inadequately, it may be said that both abnormal and "normal" behavior are the products of a complex constellation of biological and psychological forces, the latter being to variable proportions conscious, preconscious and unconscious.

Although disruptive to the individual's personal happiness and efficiency or disturbing to his social adjustment, it follows from what has been said that mental illness is the expression of a way of living. Even though it is in certain respects somewhat extreme, there is much truth in H. S. Sullivan's (1892–1949) statement that the phenomenon of mental illness may be regarded as a type of participation in the social process rather than as an entity residing within a person.

BIBLIOGRAPHY

Adler, Alfred: The Practice and Theory of Individual Psychology. New York, Harcourt, Brace and Co., 1929.

Ansbacher, H. L., and Ansbacher, R. R.: The Individual Psychology of Alfred Adler. New York, Basic Books, 1956.

Bleuler, M.: Endokrinologische Psychiatrie. Stuttgart, Georg Thieme, 1955.

Braceland, F. J.: Kraepelin, his system and his influence. Am. J. Psychiat., *113:*871–876, 1957.

Brill, A. A.: Freud's Contribution to Psychiatry. New York, W. W. Norton & Co., 1944.

Cameron, N. A.: The Psychology of Behavior Disorders. Boston, Houghton Mifflin Company, 1947.

———, and M. A.: Behavior Pathology. Boston, Houghton Mifflin Company, 1951.

Clark, R. A.: Jung and Freud. Am. J. Psychotherapy, *9:*605–611, 1955.

Dunham, H. W.: Some persistent problems in the epidemiology of mental disorders. Am. J. Psychiat., *109:*567–575, 1953.

Farnsworth, D. L.: Mental Health in Colleges and Universities. Cambridge, Harvard University Press, 1957.

Foundeur, Marvin, *et al:* Postpartum mental illness. Arch. Neurol. & Psychiat., 77*:* 503–512, 1957.

Freud, S.: Collected Papers (4 Vols.). New York, The International Psychoanalytic Press, 1924.

Hare, E. H.: The ecology of mental disease. J. Ment. Sc., *98:*579–594, 1952.

Himwich, H. E.: Thought processes as related to brain metabolism in certain abnormal states. J. Nerv. & Ment. Dis., *114:*450–458, 1951.

Hoch, P. H., and Zubin, Joseph, Eds.: Current Problems in Psychiatric Diagnosis. New York, Grune & Stratton, 1953.

Hooker, D., and Hare, C. C., Eds.: Genetics and the Inheritance of Integrated Neurological and Psychiatric Patterns. Assoc. for Research in Nervous and Mental Diseases, Vol. 33. Baltimore, Williams and Wilkins Co., 1954.

Jung, C. G.: Psychological Types. New York, Harcourt, Brace and Co., 1923.

———: Contributions to Analytical Psychology. New York, Harcourt, Brace and Co., 1928.

Kallmann, F. J.: The genetics of human behavior. Am. J. Psychiat., *113:*496–501, 1956.

———: Heredity in Health and Mental Disorder. New York, W. W. Norton & Co., 1953.

———: Genetic Aspects of Psychoses. Chapter 19, in Biology of Mental Health and Disease. New York, Paul B. Hoeber, Inc., 1952.

Kretschmer, E.: Textbook of Medical Psychology. Translated by E. B. Strauss. New York, Oxford University Press, 1949.

Lemkau, P. V.: Prevention of psychiatric illnesses. J.A.M.A., *162:*854–857, 1956.

Lief, Alfred: The Commonsense Psychiatry of Dr. Adolf Meyer. New York, McGraw-Hill Book Co., 1948.

Malzberg, Benjamin: A statistical analysis of patients in the New York civil state hospitals, April 1, 1947. Psychiatric Quart., *22:*495–515, 1948.

———: Rates of discharge and rates of mortality among first admissions to the New York civil state hospitals. Mental Hygiene, *36:*104–120, 1952.

Marmor, Judd, and Pumpian-Mindlin, E.: Toward an integrated concept of mental disorder. J. Nerv. & Ment. Dis., *111:*19–29, 1950.

Masserman, J. H.: Principles of Dynamic Psychiatry. Philadelphia, W. B. Saunders Co., 1946.

Meyer, Adolf: Scope and teaching of psychobiology. J. A. Am. M. Coll., *10:*93, 1935.

———: Objective psychology, or psychobiology with subordination of the medically useless concept of mental and physical. J.A.M.A., *65:*860, 1915.

———: The "complaint" as the center of genetic-dynamic and nosological teaching in psychiatry. New England J. Med., *199:*360, 1928.

———: The Psychobiological Point of View. In The Problem of Mental Disorders by Bentley, N., and Cowdrey, E. New York, McGraw-Hill Book Co., 1934.

Muncie, Wendell: Psychobiology and Psychiatry, 2nd ed. St. Louis, C. V. Mosby Co., 1948.
Ostwald, P. F., and Regan, P. F., III: Psychiatric disorders associated with childbirth. J. Nerv. & Ment. Dis., *125:*153–165, 1957.
Overholser, Winfred: The meaning of Freud for our time. Internat. Record Med., *164:*249–257, 1951.
Report of Milbank Memorial Fund Conference: Biology of Mental Health and Disease. New York, Paul B. Hoeber, Inc., 1952.
Sprague, G. S.: Etiology of mental disease, a changing concept. Am. J. Psychiat., *100:*785, 1944.
Sullivan, H. S.: Conceptions of Modern Psychiatry. Washington, William Alanson White Psychiatric Foundation, 1946.
Whitehorn, J. C.: The scope of motivation in psychopathology and psychotherapy. Am. J. Psychoanalysis, *14:*30–39, 1954.
———: Stress and emotional health. Am. J. Psychiat., *112:*773–781, 1956.

CHAPTER VI

Symptoms of Mental Disorder

Symptoms as Psychobiological Reactions

The symptoms of mental disorder were formerly thought of as disturbances of different mental faculties. We now know that the mind is not made up of an aggregation of isolable and more or less distinct, independent functions or faculties, such as memory, will, association, etc. These are simply convenient names for groups of mental processes that appear to have some feature in common but are in no sense unitary capacities. They are but different aspects of one homogeneous process. Mind is an integral function of the organism and cannot be split up into components. We must therefore not think of it as a sort of machine, different parts of which sense, perceive, imagine, remember, associate, reason about, desire, choose, etc. We recognize that the metabolism of an organism is an integrated process, yet to describe it one must consider one aspect at a time. Similarly, behavior is a function of the entire personality, yet in discussing what we speak of as mental disorder, it is convenient to look upon the different symptoms as disturbances of distinguishable phases of the mind. We must remember, however, that such a division into disturbances of emotion, association, memory, etc., is artificial.

Origin and Function of Symptoms

Some symptoms, such as impairment of memory in senile dementia, or confusion in a toxic state, are the results of physiological disturbances of neuron activity involved in the process of thinking. Neurotic symptoms, however, in contrast to organic and toxic ones, are manifestations of psychological processes of which the patient is but relatively little, if at all, aware. Symptoms, then, are not abnormal functionings of unitary faculties but are really psychobiological reactions or expressions of the total organism at the mental level and should be approached in terms of biological and dynamic concepts. This is particularly true of symptoms which do not arise from disturbed physiology of cortical neurons but arise through the influence of psychological factors. In the latter, the symptoms are the results of many forces, some from without but more of them from within the patient. Such symptoms indicate particularly his problems and the way he is struggling to meet them. His symptoms may indicate his inability to deal with such problems as instinctive drives, with a difficult relationship to parents, wife or children, with a feeling of guilt or insecurity or with disturbing residuals from past experiences. Symptoms, therefore, even though they be weird and bizarre and therefore baffling to our understanding, have a cause and meaning. To discover the meaning of those unusual personality manifestations that we call symptoms and the functions they are performing in the life history of the patient, we must ascertain the needs and meaningful factors or situations that led to their production. We should remember that the pathological psychiatric formations that we call symptoms represent the patient's attempt, in the face of great difficulties, to maintain his existence in the best possible way. Symptoms, too, may not only be an expression of a mental illness but also an attempt of the patient to fight the illness. Regression, for example, with its withdrawal to an earlier developmental level, may not only be a symptom of mental illness but also an attempt to deal on that level with tasks consonant with his reduced ability to deal with them.

The method of approach to mental disorder is to correlate the symptoms with the whole life history of the patient and with the forces which have played a part in molding his personality. The psychiatrist attempts not only to interpret symptoms in their relationship to past experiences but also in terms of the known dynamics of behavior. Clearness of thinking is promoted, too, by efforts to explain psychiatric symptoms in terms of methods of adjustment observed in everyday life or of methods allied to them. Through his symptoms and their motivational sources and adaptive functions, we hope to read the riddle of the patient's inner life, to see the personality back of the symptom.

The study of a psychiatric symptom requires, if possible, a knowledge of the history of that symptom within the patient himself. The major contributions to this history are not so much a knowledge of the events of the patient's childhood and adult years but in what way these events and experiences were understood by him unconsciously. The patient is therefore not considered from the standpoint of his symptom alone without regard to the context of his total situation and history. In studying mental symptoms, it is important to remember that their manifestations are specific and intimate life-revealing signs and that they have but little meaning apart from the setting in which they have developed. All symptoms have a fundamental connection of some sort with the life of the individual. Frequently they are expressions of, and a defense against, troublesome repressions and their resulting anxiety. Much mental material that cannot be expressed in frank, conscious form may be neurotically expressed in the imagery of the symptom. Again, the symptoms may represent the tension-reducing devices or other defenses to which the patient must cling. If the individual's former choice of defense against anxiety (repression, reaction-formation, symbolization and others) proves inadequate, his next resort is symptom formation. Symptoms may therefore appear as defenses decompensate or disintegrate. Delusions, hallucinations, compulsions and other symptoms must accordingly be traced back to their source just as a physical pain is traced back to its source in order that the factors that produced it may be understood and removed. As we consider them in the following pages we shall discover disabling compromises with threatening situations and harsh reality; again we shall see the results of various protective and safety devices adopted in order to serve the needs and aims of the personality. At times we shall find that symptoms represent the means employed by the patient in dealing with disowned and terrifying tendencies within him. We shall also note that many symptoms are produced through the operation of the mental mechanisms described in the previous chapter. Anxiety-laden situations will be found to evoke psychological defenses which we label as symptoms. Unfortunately many symptoms while representing efforts of the personality to satisfy its fundamental needs do so with results that disturb inner harmony or prevent social acceptance. They represent failures to deal adequately with frustrations, insecurities and undesirable impulses.

It will be found that any explanation of symptoms often requires the assumption that material beyond conscious awareness may possess psychodynamic or motivating qualities and to varying degrees may dominate the conscious personality; also that many symptoms express the patient's feelings and problems in a symbolic rather than a direct way and have a meaning of much greater significance than their manifest appearance. In order to understand the symptoms of mental disorder, we must understand the forces that have gone into their formation, and seek to ascertain what the patient is reacting to and expressing in them. It is therefore necessary to have the same understanding of fundamental psychodynamic processes and mechanisms as is required of physiological and biological principles in the case of physical disease. To the psychiatrist the patient's behavior and reactions are what symptoms are to the general medical practitioner. He goes behind the particular deed and tries to ascertain the motive for it since he realizes that a reaction itself is not important unless it is judged in the light of the underlying purpose and motivation. It will be found, too, that in the symptoms of mental illness the dynamic relationships that frequently occur in normal behavior occur in isolated and exaggerated form. An individual may use a variety of means (symptoms) to achieve the same goal. It will therefore be noted that similar genetic and dynamic factors may lead to symptom formation in psychological, in somatic, or in behavior and social fields. Also, the same or nearly identical conduct or emotional response exhibited by different persons may be the result of different life experiences or the expressions of very different affective reactions, and the patient may be greatly plagued and distressed by his symptoms.

Disorders of Perception

Illusions

It will be remembered that the various end-organs or receptors are so constructed as to analyze the environmental energy and select certain kinds which are transformed in the receptor and give rise to a nervous impulse. On arrival in the appropriate area in the brain, this impulse produces a visual, auditory or other sensory image, the interpretation and meaning of which will depend upon one's previous experiences and interpretations. One of the ways by which the mental life of the individual may express emotional or striving elements that touch it with peculiarly keen significance is through a perceptual misinterpretation of such sensory images. The elements which are particularly likely to lead to misinterpretations of these images are deeply intense affective states, ardent wishes or strongly urgent drives and impulses. Repressed elements are especially apt to be highly dynamic and produce misinterpretations that reflect some affect or express some wish or drive. A patient with a deep feeling of guilt, for example, may interpret the rustling of leaves as reproaching voices. Such a perceptual misinterpretation is known as an *illusion.* The illusion has the same psychological function as a hallucination but less reality distortion is involved. The nature of illusions is especially likely to be determined by the prevailing trend of the patient's emotional state and needs. Strained expectation or fear predisposes to illusional interpretations. In mental health, but particularly in mental disorder, the emotional life imbues and tends to influence perceptual experience according to the needs of the personality. In confused, toxic states, caused either by ingested poisons or by infection, perceptions, especially visual ones, may be misinterpreted because the sensory stimuli and impressions are not sharply defined. Such illusions usually possess less psychological significance than do those occurring in fully clear consciousness.

Hallucinations

In an illusion an image symbol of a real object is formed but for psychological reasons it is misinterpreted. In a still larger number of cases a more serious falsification of perceptions occurs consisting of the formation of image symbols when there is no impulse created by the stimulation of a receptor. Such a mental image projected outward as a perception in the absence of an external stimulus is known as an *hallucination.* The word was introduced by Esquirol (1772–1840), a pupil of Philippe Pinel (1745–1826). He defined it in accordance with its present meaning as a perception without object and clearly differentiated it from illusion.

Although lacking a basis of reality, hallucinations constitute an actual part of the patient's mental life. They should not be looked upon as spontaneous perceptions but as the outcome of a long series of morbid mental processes intimately linked up with the total personality, as mental products which, arising from within and therefore not related to any external stimulus, come to possess the peculiar vividness which is usually associated with impressions derived from the external world. The content of the hallucinations usually suggests their dynamic significance. They may be regarded as representing a breaking through of preconscious or unconscious material into consciousness in the form of sensory images in response to psychological situations and needs. Anxiety often plays an important part in their genesis. These hallucinated images which the patient accepts as reality represent the projection onto the outer world of such psychological needs and situations as wish-fulfillment, enhancement of self-esteem, criticism, censure, a sense of guilt, self-punishment, the satisfaction of repressed and rejected impulses or the desire for a more satisfying reality. The dreams of normal persons are prototypes of the mental patient's hallucinations. Sometimes in case of internal conflict there is hallucinatory expression of the internal debate, some of the hallucinations expressing approbation or commendation while others, representing the other side of the issue, express insults and antagonism. It will be seen, therefore, that hallucinations are never symptomatic of a given morbid condition.

The way in which escape from a harsh and unsatisfying reality may be secured through hallucinatory perceptual experiences is illustrated in that of a woman whose natural biological tendencies had been frustrated and who, because of personality inadequacies, had found economic and social adjustments too great a burden. One day as she was sitting on the bank of the Potomac River, preoccupied with her problems and dreaming of some means of satisfactory escape from them, she heard the voice of a former lover who had ceased his attentions as her personality limitations had become more apparent. In this thwarted and distressing state of affairs she received from the old admirer a message pointing the way to an enchanting fulfillment of her fondest hopes. Although she could not see him, the patient heard the lover direct her to jump into the water, from which he promised to rescue her and row her to Norfolk whence they would sail to Egypt there to occupy a beautiful castle. So convinced by the vividness of the message that reality was ignored the woman threw herself into the water where she would have perished except for some chance passers. A correct appreciation of her experience would have been too painful and disillusioning so she continued to believe in the reality of these autogenous perceptions.

In mental health we ignore as devoid of interest the majority of perceptions produced by casual stimuli from our environment, but the content of perceptions in hallucinations is so intimately subjective that in their acute phases, at least, they cannot be ignored and therefore not only absorb the attention but require that reality be made to harmonize with them. As a result, the functional capacity of the ego for testing of any reality that does not harmonize with the hallucinations is usually suspended.

In so-called "anticipatory" illusions and hallucinations, a person in a tense emotional state, say of fear, intently expects to see or hear the object which has excited the emotion. The result is that the perception, momentarily expected in vivid clearness, appears, but in a projected, hallucinatory or illusional form.

Sometimes various gradations between normal representation and hallucinations may occur, with the result that the patient is uncertain as to whether his mental experience has been of a perceptual (unreal) nature or whether it has been merely a thought.

Hallucinations may occur in diseases associated with toxic or organic states. Although in these cases there is perhaps an irritation of the association centers connected with the special sense hallucinated, the nature of the material hallucinated is doubtless influenced by the psychological experiences of the patient.

Psychological material may be projected in the image symbols of any of the senses although the images are characteristically of that sense best fitted to symbolize the particular material seeking expression. Feelings of guilt, for example, may best be expressed in spoken language, so the patient hears accusing voices. Such accusing voices represent the projection of the critical voice of the superego. Fear of some aspect of the personality may well be symbolized by the sight of terrifying objects, so the patient sees frightful animals. One patient with an experience which he looked upon as one of moral contamination complained of a constant odor of carbolic acid. To him this chemical had always represented a purifying agent and its hallucination was well adapted to symbolize his desire for a feeling of moral purification.

Hallucinations are more marked during the early and acute stages of a psychotic reaction. This is to be expected, since it is the period when repression is failing and the solution of the conflict is proving unsuccessful. Hallucinations with clearness of consciousness are of much more serious prognostic import than those occurring with clouding of consciousness. Hallucinations occur less frequently when the patient is occupied with reality than when attention slackens or he begins to daydream. They are often associated with delusions to which they add a support or corroboration. At times they seem to be the concrete symbolic expression of delusional ideas.

1. Hallucinations of Hearing. As already indicated, hallucinations of hearing are the most frequent form of perceptual disturbance. Sometimes the hallucinations are in the form of various noises but most often in words arranged in more or less complete sentences. Usually these sentences are remarks concerning the patient or addressed to him. The patient may converse or quarrel with the "voices." He may locate them as coming from any part of the body or from a distance. Sometimes the remarks are of a pleasant nature but usually they are unpleasant, derogatory, obscene or in the nature of accusations. These unpleasant remarks represent the projection of disowned personality aspects and desires which may not be allowed in consciousness in undisguised form. Hallucinations conveying a command are often convincing and compelling. They may therefore lead to direct and dangerous action. Considerations of reality are of little weight in comparison to their influence.

2. Hallucinations of Sight. These are not rare but are much less

frequent than auditory hallucinations. They occur most typically in the deliria of acute infectious diseases or of toxic psychoses. In each of these states the visual hallucinations are apt to be accompanied by some clouding of consciousness. In general, visual hallucinations are confined to acute, reversible organic brain disorders. Visual hallucinations more frequently excite fear in the patient than do auditory ones since they produce a greater distortion of reality. One of the most frequent forms of mental disorder accompanied by visual images is delirium tremens in which the images tend to be of a terrifying nature.

3. Olfactory Hallucinations. Hallucinations of smell are not uncommon in schizophrenic states. Olfactory hallucinations are usually of an unpleasant or even of a strongly objectionable character. Their repulsive nature is not surprising since they are particularly apt to represent feelings of guilt.

4. Hallucinations of Taste. True gustatory hallucinations are uncommon but at times are associated with hallucinations of smell. Illusions of taste are much more frequent.

5. Tactile Hallucinations. Hallucinations of touch occur principally in toxic states, such as delirium tremens, and in cocaine addiction.

6. Sexual Hallucinations. Hallucinated sexual sensations are not of rare occurrence in schizophrenia and are often associated with grotesque delusions concerning bodily organs.

Disorders of Thinking

The joining of ideas one to another by imagining, conceiving, inferring and by other processes, and the formation of new ideas by these processes constitute a function we know as thinking. This may be looked upon as a form of internal or implicit behavior. Thought is the most highly organized of psychobiological integrations. In considering this function from the standpoint of psychiatry, attention should be directed to: (*a*) the production of thought; (*b*) the progression of thought; and (*c*) the content of thought. It should be remembered, too, that thought takes place on several levels ranging from that on a fully conscious level, dealing perhaps with highly abstract topics, to that on a primitive, emotional level.

Disorders in Form of Thought

As just indicated, the psychiatrist looks upon thinking as a form of behavior, which implies the existence of stimulus and response, the latter serving some psychologic purpose. In mental health the stimuli for thought come from various sources, including unconscious and affective ones, but thinking is corrected by reason and logic. Such thought is known as *rational or realistic thought.* It appears to be directed by and to take place in conscious awareness. In daydreaming, thinking is not fully guided by realistic considerations but to a considerable extent by egocentric wishes and instinctual needs. In mental disorder, and particularly in schizophrenia, thinking may be directed even more by unconscious factors and become of the type first designated by Bleuler as *autistic* and later as dereistic. In dereistic, in contrast to realistic, thinking complexes, drives and other affective and conative thought motivations are given free rein and operate without conscious regard for reality. As a result associations of ideas are no longer logical but assume the nature of "free" associations.

Disorders in Progression of Thought

The rate and manner of associative activity cannot, of course, be learned except through the patient's stream of talk. It is a matter of familiar observation that as one's thoughts are expressed in language there is a pertinent association or linkage of each idea with the one that has preceded, that one's thinking moves in a logical progression toward a more or less definite end. This progression of thought is often known as the *stream of thought* or stream of talk. Normally there is a logical and coherent sequence of related ideas passing uninterruptedly and without digression from an initial to a goal idea.

FLIGHT OF IDEAS. In certain mental disorders there occurs a disturbance in the progression of thought characterized by an increased associative activity, a rapid digression from one idea to another. Ideas follow in quick succession but do not progress toward the goal idea which is therefore never reached. This disturbance of the stream of thought in which the thinking processes appear to run too quickly and in which no idea is completed is known as flight of ideas. Flight of ideas is associated with an accelerated inner tempo; also with a distractability as a result of which the patient is unable to sustain his attention and hold it directed toward a goal idea. Observation will usually disclose an associated relation between the thought and a prompting stimulus springing from either an external or an internal source. Not rarely a word similar in sound, but not at all so in significance, calls up the new thought. This is known as *clang association* and may lead to a jejune type of pun or a senseless rhyme.

One patient with a rapid flow of thought, when asked if he were sad, replied, "Yes, you have to be quiet to be sad. Everything having to do with 's' is quiet—on the q.t.—sit, sob, sigh, sin, sorrow, surcease, sought, sand, sweet mother's love and salvation. This is my first case—I am kind of a bum lawyer or liar—too damned honest to be a lawyer, so had to be a liar."

RETARDATION. As already seen, the flow of thought in flight of ideas is abnormally rapid. In retardation, on the other hand, the initiation and movement of thought are slow. Often the patient will state that his thoughts come slowly or that he has difficulty in thinking. It will be noted that he speaks slowly and usually in a low tone. Retardation is most frequently observed in the depressive phases of the affective psychoses but may be noted in schizophrenia.

PERSEVERATION. By perseveration is meant an abnormally persistent repetition or continuance in expression of an idea. This clinging to a thought may be observed at times in aphasia and in catatonia.

CIRCUMSTANTIALITY. Another disturbance in the flow of thought is that known as circumstantiality. In this disturbance the patient finally reaches his ideational objective, but only after many unnecessary and trivial details have led him into tiresome digressions. Circumstantiality occurs largely among persons who do not form sharply defined concepts or are unable to distinguish essentials from nonessentials. In mental disorder, therefore, it is frequently observed among the feebleminded, epileptics and in cases of moderately advanced senile mental disorder.

INCOHERENCE. Sometimes the progression of thinking is so disorderly that one idea runs into another without logical consecution, and speech is not bound by any law. The result is a disorganization of syntactical structure with a lapse into disjointed phrases or even into parts of sentences and known as incoherence. One schizophrenic patient, when asked how long she had been in the hospital, answered, "Oh, three weeks—since different statements are made—because it is hot—Mr. Smith is a cheap guy—French—how goes about it?" In incoherence there is a tendency for ideas to arise from a confusion of complexes, *viz.*, repressed material highly charged affectively. As might be expected, incoherence occurs particularly in schizophrenia, a disease in which the thinking is characteristically dominated by complexes. Much of the thinking of the schizophrenic is described as "scattered," which simply means that the thinking is a little less disorderly than in incoherence.

BLOCKING. Another disturbance in the flow of thought is that known as blocking. In this disorder, sometimes known as thought deprivation or thought obstruction, both expression and progression of thought suddenly cease. To a degree it may be considered as having a prototype in the sudden inhibition of the train of thought sometimes occurring when one is overcome by some strong affect, such as anger or terror. After a time, the apparent obstruction seems to be removed and the flow of thought is resumed. This interruption of the progression of thought is probably caused by the activity of a dominant complex with its associated unpleasant affect. At first the blocking may be caused by some definite thought, or rather by the disagreeable affect attached to it, but it quickly becomes general so that nothing more is initiated. Blocking seems to be confined to schizophrenia.

Disorders of Content of Thought

TRENDS AND OVERDETERMINED IDEAS. There is a tendency for the associative evolution of ideas, and therefore for thought content, to be determined more by affective factors than by logical reasoning. Ideas having the strongest feeling tones tend to dominate. It is because of this fact that thought content may exhibit a *trend*, *viz.*, a propensity to center around a special topic. In case an idea comes to have an extreme feeling-tone connected with it, it is spoken of as an *overdetermined or overvalued idea.* The importance or value and the meaning attached to an idea are directly proportional to the inner need for such a belief. When an overvalued idea exists, it blinds the individual to all else so that only those observations and memories are selected which suit its purpose or confirm it. Anything which conflicts with it is denied admission into consciousness. The whole personality, including its thinking and feeling aspects, is absorbed by the idea and placed at its disposal, so to speak, with the result that the overvalued idea becomes one of the most important determinants of behavior. Trends and overdetermined ideas, like delusions, to be discussed presently, serve to satisfy some pressing inner need of the personality, such as a sense of security, defense or self-esteem.

DELUSIONS. We are all prone to develop comforting and other psychologically useful fictions to afford support and security to the personality. Always, apparently, mankind has developed or adopted elaborate beliefs in an effort to satisfy inner needs. The construction of reassuring delusive beliefs as protection against anxiety and insecurity has been universally characteristic. This has been the unrecognized purpose in our fairy tales, in the folk stories of powerful persons and in our father-image myths, beliefs and creeds. Sometimes the demand for the satisfaction of special inner needs of the personality may be so insistent that the claims of reality are disregarded and delusional ideas appear. Actuality is transformed to make it compatible with the emotional needs of the personality. The delusion is usually defined as a false belief. As we consider delusions and their meaning, value and purpose, we shall see, however, that such a definition is fallaciously inadequate. It is often said that to be considered delusional a false belief must be one that a person of similar education and experience would consider improbable or impossible and is not corrected in response to reason or logic. Even this definition is inadequate since it ignores any consideration of the important principle that the incorrect understanding and use of facts and evidence are in response to definite purposes and needs of the personality and that the prevailing factors that control delusional thinking are affective rather than ideative or cognitive.

How inner needs may produce misinterpretations, denial and misuse of facts in a way to be considered delusional is illustrated in the following: During World War I a woman was notified by the War Department that her husband had been killed on a certain date and buried at a certain place in France. Several months later she visited the Department and expressed the conviction that her husband was alive and that the body of her supposed husband was actually that of no person known to her. The military authorities presented evidence that no error had been made but the widow remained unconvinced and demanded that the body of her alleged husband be returned to America and examined. This was done and the identification number and the location of wounds were found to correspond with the records of the War Department. Still the woman remained unconvinced. Finally the reason for the delusion appeared. Among the officer's papers collected after his death and forwarded to the widow were affectionate letters from another woman. The patient had protected herself from the painful realization that she was not first in the affections of her husband by developing the belief that the man who had been killed and whose papers had been forwarded to her was someone other than her husband. We thus see that situations containing highly affective factors are accompanied by a lowering of the critical faculty and of the threshold of beliefs. Attempts through factual disproof to convince the patient that his beliefs are delusional are therefore rarely successful. The patient's experiences are assimilated and the picture of the external world supplied by his thinking is falsified according to his nonadjusted affective and instinctive demands. He acts as if his delusional system constituted reality—as to him it does.

As already indicated, the thinking which we characterize as delusional is quite similar in kind, although different in degree, to that in which we all indulge. Our beliefs tend to be subjectively colored and doubtless all of us resort to certain fictions of security. Employment of wishful thinking by "normal" persons in their struggle for a realization of their hopes, and of rationalization or projection for defensive purposes, serves the same psychological ends as do the delusions of the psychotic and imperceptibly merges into them. Prejudices, likewise, often arise from intrapsychic conflict and serve as defensive measures.

From what has been said, it will be seen that delusions are attempts to deal with the special problems and stresses of one's particular life situation. In many cases fantasy is called upon to supply what real life has denied, but, as Macfie Campbell expressed it, "The fantasies are not woven into a structure which is compatible with a normal social adaptation." Delusions, therefore, require an individual approach. Their trend is determined by the prepsychotic personality problems and needs of the patient; their content will be found to reveal significant aspects of the patient's personal problems. The sources of these problems may often be found in thwarted trends and drives, frustrated hopes, feelings of inferiority, biological inadequacies, rejected qualities, teasing desires, gnawing feelings of guilt and other situations which require a defense against anxiety. A deep-seated need for consolation, for example, may be met by self-flattering delusions. Often the problem-solving value of the delusion and its relation to the situation by which it was produced are psychologically plain. Many times, however, the function of the delusion is far from obvious and its interpretation must remain a matter of speculation. This does not mean that the delusion is without significance or purpose. It possesses a definite adjustment value but its source and purpose are concealed by its symbolically disguised content.

Systematized Delusions. On careful scrutiny and analysis the apparently complex ideas in the delusion can be reduced to a simple theme which has been elaborated. When this central theme is extensively developed and conclusions are so logically deduced from the premises assumed that a coherent and connected organization of ideas is established the patient's delusions are said to be systematized.

Since the psychological purposes and needs for the satisfaction of which delusions are created fall into certain general classifications, and as well defined mental mechanisms are employed in their creation, we find that for convenience of description delusions may be classified in accordance with certain type-similarities.

Delusions of Grandeur. Expansive delusions, or delusions of grandeur, arise from feelings of inadequacy, insecurity, or inferiority, any conscious recognition of which is prevented by the exaggerated ideative and affective components of the delusion. The content of grandiose delusions frequently suggests the nature of previous frustrations or insecurities. The patient who insists that he is God has by the aid of his delusion escaped from the troubles of reality which were too great a threat to his emotional security. If his distress was one of guilt, he has achieved perfection; if it was one of intolerable inferiority, he has achieved distinction; if it was one of fear, he has gained security and safety. The symbolic meaning of grandiose delusions is not greatly complicated and is fairly easily analyzed.

Delusions of Self-Accusation. Delusions of self-accusation are believed to arise because the repression of unacceptable trends and desires weakens and the superego becomes increasingly critical. In such a case repression is not destroyed but the threat, as it were, that consciously forbidden tendencies might be permitted expression creates in the patient a vague feeling of guilt. This sense of guilt is then rationalized in consciousness into ideas of remorse and self-accusation. Feelings of guilt may be appeased through self-punishment.

Delusions of Persecution. Ideas of persecution are among the most frequent forms of delusions, occurring especially in chronic psychotic disorders. The threat of unworthy desires and of troublesome and disowned aspects of the personality is projected as hostility from the environment. Sensitive dissatisfactions with self, arising from unadjusted elements in the personality, may be projected as a dissatisfaction, and therefore as hostility felt toward one by others. The formation of delusions of persecution is facilitated by the mechanism of projection which easily leads to misjudgments of reality. The hostile and aggressive motives which the patient attributes to others reflect his own inclinations. High aspirations without qualities necessary for satisfying success accompanied by an inability to accept defeat may lead to brooding, distrust, suspicion, misinterpretations, resentment and ideas of persecution, coupled perhaps with aggressiveness. Delusions of persecution permit a shifting of responsibility and otherwise serve to relieve a guilt anxiety. As a further measure for averting blows to self-esteem, the patient with ideas of persecution may develop compensatory reactions in the form of an exaggerated self-assurance. It will often be found that persons who develop delusions of persecution have, since childhood, been critical, resentful, suspicious and unhappy. Not a few of them have been lonely, brooding and insecure, and have lacked friends with whom they could share confidences. Ready to criticise others, they have been unable to tolerate criticism themselves.

It is not uncommon to find delusions of grandeur and of persecution associated. This is not surprising since they serve much the same purposes, one tending to supplement the other. By his delusions of grandeur, the patient psychopathologically enhances his self-esteem and magnifies his ego, while in the delusions of persecution he repudiates and rejects by attaching to others those aspects and tendencies which self-respect would disavow. The two types collaborate to relieve anxiety.

Ideas of Reference. Through ideas of reference, remarks or actions on the part of other persons, although in no way referring to the patient, are interpreted by him as being significantly related to himself and often as expressing accusation or depreciation. In paranoid states, ideas of reference represent a projection of the patient's own self-criticism onto the external world. In depression, feelings of guilt may stimulate ideas of reference and these, in turn, contribute to loosely organized paranoid delusions.

Depressive Delusions. Depressive delusions frequently represent the ideational expression of rationalization of an affective depression. If repression weakens, material, such as wishes, memories or ideas, which is of such a nature that it would cause emotional pain if admitted to consciousness, is apt to give rise to depression. Depressive delusions often represent the rationalization of a sense of depression that has had its source in unconscious hostile tendencies felt toward persons against whom such feelings and tendencies should not be directed.

Depressive delusions are most frequently expressed in ideas concerning guilt, disease or poverty. Ideas of guilt and of loss of self-esteem may arise when the repression of unconsciously desired but consciously repudiated tendencies is weakened. The patient in his attempt to rationalize the vague feeling of wickedness rising into consciousness formulates ideas of self-accusation based on criticisms by the superego. Unconscious hostile tendencies may be projected outward giving rise to fear of punishment. Any psychological factor which makes the patient feel that he stands out in an undesirable or unacceptable way from the rest of his social group may lead to delusions of guilt and therefore of depression.

Ideas of disease seem occasionally to have their origin in disturbances of cenesthetic sensations springing from the viscera which through the vegetative nervous system and endocrine glands are influenced by emotional states. Attempts to rationalize these cenesthetic sensations may lead to delusions concerning disease.

Ideas of poverty are often the ideational representation of a subjective sense of loss of social value. Such ideas of poverty may accompany delusions of guilt, the idea of unworthiness being displaced to the most generally recognized symbol of value—money. Appearing at times with depressive delusions are nihilistic ideas expressing the patient's belief that he has no brain, that he has no feeling, that he is dead, or that other sections of reality no longer exist. Such nihilistic ideas probably have their origin in vague feelings of emotional change and in a subjective feeling of unreality and of changed personality. This subjective sense of absence and of change is rationalized into ideas of annihilation.

In passivity feelings or ideas of control the patient may express the delusional belief that he is controlled or that people read his mind. Such feelings probably represent the denial of an impulse to yield to threatening internal needs or demands which, however, are disowned through the mechanism of projection.

Hypochondria. Although containing important affective elements of a depressive nature, the symptom, hypochondria, with its exaggerated concern over physical health, may perhaps best be considered as a disturbance of ideational content. In hypochondria the patient's attention is abnormally concentrated on his own body; he is depressed and his thoughts are obsessively preoccupied with some bodily organ which he is convinced is incurably diseased although no pathological process can be demonstrated. A changed feeling of self may be present. Probably hypochondria should be basically regarded as an organ neurosis, in which tensions generated through psychological factors produce disturbances of organs innervated by the autonomic nervous system. Anxiety is displaced from unconscious mental sources to organs which thereby become the center of affective distress and preoccupation. The organ which is the focus of bodily complaint is usually one particularly subject to physiological expressions of anxiety or to the muscular tension of the anxious state. Hypochondria is more frequently manifested by persons who have shown a previous tendency to solicit desired affection or to evade the responsibilities of life through illness. In its milder forms hypochondria may have its origin in a sense of insecurity which is rationalized as a threat to physical health. Because of the changing psychological outlook on life, as well as the regressive physiological processes and the failing psychobiological security at that time of life, the involutional period may be marked by hypochondria. If hypochondriasis is consistent with the mood, it tends to disappear as the mood goes. If it is symbolic or inconsistent with the mood, as in schizophrenia, it indicates a serious disorder.

Obsessions. Thoughts that persistently thrust themselves into consciousness against the conscious desire of the patient are known as obsessions. Obsessions persist in the conscious mind so tenaciously that they cannot be dispelled by conscious processes and are uninfluenced by logic or reasoning. The obsessive thought is strongly charged with emotion, is unwanted and usually plagues the individual almost constantly. He cannot understand why he is obsessed with the thought. Obsessive ruminations are of various content. Not rarely the constant preoccupation is concerning some metaphysical question. The patient, for example, may be compelled to keep asking himself why he was born. The explanation of obsessive thought is to be found in the activity of the unconscious and of repression. As a defensive device a guilty anxiety is displaced to an innocuous idea and the anxiety thereby decreased. The obsessive thought that is consciously distasteful may be related to what is unconsciously desired. Obsessive thoughts are closely related to compulsive acts in which after a distressing resistance to its performance the patient feels impelled to perform some act which because of its elaborate and repetitive nature often seems almost ritualistic.

Phobias. Allied to obsessive thoughts are phobias or fears, doubts and indecisions. Like the obsessive idea a phobia thrusts itself persistently into consciousness. Since morbid anxiety always accompanies a phobia, the patient is constantly depressed. Among common phobias are fears of dirt, of bacteria, of cancer or of crowds. In general one may say that the patient's anxiety becomes detached from a specific idea, object or situation in his daily life and is displaced to some symbolic idea or situation in the form of a specific neurotic fear. The fear that he feels in the presence of a certain object or experience is really the displaced fear of some anxiety-producing component within his own personality. The patient is not, of course, aware of the psychological source or significance of his fear, and while he may acknowledge that his fear is irrational he is quite unable to regulate his life except as dictated by his phobia. He constantly attempts to control his anxiety by avoiding the object or situation to which the anxiety has been displaced.

Finally, before concluding the discussion on ideational content, the student should be reminded that the thinking and behavior of the psychotic are just as "rational" as those of the personality usually and pragmatically called normal, but are called irrational because we are ignorant of all the experiences and conditioned responses, and more especially the conflicts and anxieties requiring defense. In connection with the subject of ideational content, it should be remembered that the conscious thought content concerning any topic may be self-defensive and therefore directly opposite to that which deeper aspects of the personality would dictate.

Disturbances of Consciousness

Perhaps from a descriptive standpoint the word "clear-mindedness" or "awareness" best indicates what we designate as consciousness. The sensorium is clear, *i.e.*, the functioning of the special senses is intact and the apprehension of external stimuli presented to them is unimpaired. The individual is able to apprehend his environment as to place, time, person and general setting, to understand questions and to reflect upon them.

Confusion

Confusion is a disturbance of consciousness characterized by impairment of the sensorium, by difficulty of grasp, and by bewilderment, perplexity, disorientation, disturbance of associative functions and poverty of ideas. The face of the confused patient presents a distressed, puzzled, and at times a surprised expression. Confusion is confined largely to conditions in which there is a diffuse impairment of brain tissue function, especially impairment associated with toxic, infectious or traumatic agents, although it occurs also in dissociative reactions and epileptic dream states. Most psychiatrists believe that the term *confusion* should not be loosely applied to those subjects, such as retarded depressive or perplexed schizophrenic patients, whose replies are not prompt or pertinent. Many believe that true confusion is found only in toxic-organic reactions. Certainly clouding of the sensorium is the basic feature in the toxic-organic states.

Clouding of Consciousness

Clouding of consciousness is a disturbance in which clear-mindedness is not complete, usually because there are physical or chemical disturbances producing functional impairment of the associative apparatus of the cerebrum. The threshold of consciousness is high and perceptions are not produced by those sensory stimuli which ordinarily result in clear perceptions. The capacity to think clearly and with customary rapidity, to perceive, respond to and remember current stimuli is impaired. To make the patient understand a question, it may be necessary to shake him, to shout the question and perhaps to repeat this procedure several times before he apprehends sufficiently to reply. Attention wanders and the patient's apprehension of his environment is incomplete and inaccurate. The symptom is frequent in general hospitals where it is often seen in patients suffering from infectious diseases. Clouding of consciousness may also occur in psychogenic disturbances, such as dissociative reactions. In this the clouding and the subsequent amnesia for events of the clouded period may serve the purpose of excluding from awareness material which deep-seated wishes would shut out. Clouding of consciousness may be of various degrees, ranging from mental hebetude to somnolence, stupor or coma.

Stupor

Stupor occurs both in the toxic-organic and in the psychogenic groups of mental disorders but the similarity of disturbance of mental processes in the two groups is more apparent than real. Stupor may occur in such a diversity of physical and mental conditions as toxic states, organic brain disease, intense apathy, profound depression, blocking, in epilepsy and in dissociative reaction to overpowering fear. In neither toxic-organic nor psychogenic stupor does the patient move. In toxic-organic stupor conscious thought processes are suspended; in catatonic stupor there is intense preoccupation of thought which is often dereistic in nature. There is a loss of reality sense but no real suspension of consciousness. A sudden change from stupor to activity, often impulsive or excessive, occurs in psychogenic stupor only.

Delirium[1]

Although involving much more than a disturbance of consciousness, mention should be made of the symptom-complex known as delirium. This syndrome, ordinarily acute both in development and course, consists of clouding of consciousness, bewilderment, restlessness, confusion, disorientation, incoherent or dreamlike thinking, illusions and hallucinations and not rarely apprehension or fear. Its occurrence is usually associated with infections with fever, toxic states, metabolic disturbances (uremia, pellagra, pernicious anemia), cardiac decompensation or head trauma. Some persons develop delirium more readily than do others. Perhaps in some cases this tendency is caused either by an inherently greater vulnerability of the brain to toxins or by a less resistant blood-cerebrospinal

[1] The clinical picture of delirium is well depicted in Shakespeare's description of Falstaff's death:

"For after I saw him fumble with the sheets, and play with flowers, and smile upon his fingers' ends, I knew there was but one way; for his nose was sharp as a pen, and a' babbled of green fields." King Henry V, Act II, Scene iii.

fluid barrier. On the other hand, the susceptibility may depend upon the integration and stability of the personality. Electroencephalographic changes are usually found in delirium. Generally, the greater the reduction in the level of awareness, the greater the shift toward slower frequency ranges. The changes are reversible to the extent to which the clinical delirium is reversible.

Delirium is usually more marked at night and at times may be limited to it, the patient being seemingly normal mentally during the day. The most frequent prodromal symptoms are drowsiness, restless sleep, difficulty in grasp and impaired attention. In very mild cases the patient may merely appear mentally dull and sluggish and not keenly aware of just what is happening about him. He may show a little "wandering" but become clear when addressed. Attention is impaired and there is a reduction in capacity for abstract thinking. The patient will usually have difficulty in performing tests requiring concentration and sustained attention, *e.g.*, the serial subtraction of 7's from 100. As the delirium becomes more marked the patient seems dazed, baffled and bewildered and fails to recognize members of his family.

Important symptoms are fluctuations in grasp, orientation and consciousness. Shifting degrees of awareness and of orientation should always suggest the possibility of delirium. Moments of rationality often alternate with ones of irrationality. If the clouding of consciousness has been marked, the patient, after recovery, has no recollection of what occurred during the delirium. Frequently the memory is "patchy," varying with the fluctuations of consciousness that occurred during the delirious episode. Other variations in the clinical picture often coexist and are also suggestive. Comparative calmness, for example, may exist for a period to be suddenly followed by restlessness or impulsive activity. The patient's mood may shift rapidly or be characterized by doubt, perplexity, irritability, apprehension, fear and even panic. Frightening dreams and fantasies may occur, and both illusions and hallucinations occur, the former being more frequent. Visual hallucinations are more frequent than auditory and at first are often in the form of shadowy figures. The content of thought and of hallucinations is more dependent upon the patient's personality problems and tendencies and his previous life experience than upon the nature of the underlying physical process responsible for the delirium. Frequently the patient shows motor disturbance, manifested in mild cases by tremulousness in writing but in more severe cases by picking, grasping and groping. Activity may vary from mild restlessness to intense and uncontrollable overactivity.

Delirium rarely continues for more than a month and in infectious diseases may be of only fleeting duration. Later delirious episodes tend to resemble any previous ones both in content and course. Following his recovery, the patient often describes his hallucinations and other delirioid experiences as having been dreamlike in nature. Although the delirium syndrome occurs frequently in infectious diseases and in their febrile period, it is by no means confined to such association. Toxic-delirioid reactions occur in old age in a wide variety of physical illnesses.

Postoperative psychoses which are more frequent in elderly patients than in younger ones usually resemble those of toxic-exhaustive and infective states and therefore present delirioid features. Puerperal psychoses, even those that are fundamentally affective or schizophrenic in nature, often show delirioid characteristics in their onset. The delirioid reaction may, too, follow the abuse of bromides and other drugs. It may occur as well in cardiac or other disorders involving nutritional or circulatory support of the brain.

Dream State

Presenting a somewhat similar but more exaggerated symptom-complex is the disturbance known as dream state, or twilight state, as it is sometimes known. Such a state does not, like delirium, arise from toxic-organic conditions, but is of affective or other psychogenic origin. Consciousness is usually disturbed, in some cases being so clouded or confused that the patient is not aware of his real surroundings. Visual and auditory hallucinations occur in response to which the patient may perform complex acts, such as running away or committing acts of violence. These dream states may last from several minutes to a few days. When normal consciousness is regained, the patient may report that during the twilight state he felt as if he were dreaming and will have little or no recollection of events that occurred during its existence. Such dream states occur for the most part in dissociative reactions and in epilepsy. In dissociative reactions they represent escapes from unpleasant reality or the gratification of frustrated wishes. In epileptic dream states the behavior is motivated by more deeply unconscious factors.

Organic Disturbances of Consciousness

In connection with impairment of consciousness resulting from physiological disturbances of the cortex, it should be remembered that sensitivity to deficiency in supply of oxygen is peculiarly great in the cerebral cortex which suffers irreversible damage in five to eight minutes of complete oxygen deprivation. Insufficient oxygenation for cerebral needs may result from cerebral anemia, caused either by diminished blood supply or by conditions in which oxygen saturation of the blood is insufficient for cerebral needs or by enzymatic disturbances.

Disorders of Apperception

Involving much more than a disturbance of consciousness are the disturbances of that complex function known as apperception, by which through active, attentive thought one analyzes, synthesizes, integrates, evaluates and absorbs experience. W. M. Wundt (1832–1920) defined it as "the single process by means of which any psychic content is brought to clear conception." By it new ideas are formulated and related to ones already familiar with the result that one is able to understand or "grasp" new situations, events and experiences. In disturbances of apperception, the patient has difficulty in understanding questions and unaccustomed situations and experiences. Disorders of apperception occur in psychogenic diseases involving intense preoccupation and other disturbances of attention, also in toxic and organic states. Faulty capacity for apperception exists, of course, in mental deficiency.

Disorders of Orientation

The process by which one apprehends his environment and locates himself mentally in relation to it is known as orientation. If he knows his position in reference to time, appreciates his situation both as to space and circumstances and understands his relationship to other individuals, he is said to be oriented. If he does not recognize and locate himself in respect to any one of these matters he is said to be disoriented in the particular sphere of which he has an inadequate grasp.

Disorientation may occur in any mental disorder in which there is extensive impairment of the patient's memory, of the extent or accuracy of his perceptions or of his attention. Disturbances of orientation may therefore exist in toxic-organic diseases and in psychogenic disorders. Their occurrence is more frequent in toxic disturbances or in organic destruction of the neurons when the functions of the physiological mechanisms essential for memory, perception and attention are impaired. Less frequently, disorientation is caused by acute conflicts, intense affective factors, distractibility or lack of interest or attention.

Disturbances of Affectivity

By affectivity is meant the feeling-life or emotional feeling-tone of a person. The strong, temporary variations, modulations and expressions of this self-feeling are known as *affects.* Although the term emotion is often used loosely as if synonymous with affect[2] it connotes rather the physiological correlate that accompanies or expresses affect. By *mood* is meant a sustained, constant, affective state of considerable duration. Affectivity penetrates and colors the whole psychic life determining the general attitude, whether of rejection or of acceptance, in relation to any experience, promoting any tendency in harmony with it and inhibiting any impulse not in agreement. It therefore contains an inherent dynamic component that serves to influence both thought content and conative activity. Affective factors may interfere with associative tendencies and prevent one from becoming aware of certain strivings or other consciously unacceptable aspects of his mental life. There seems reason to believe that profound disturbances of affectivity may even produce disturbances of consciousness, as in the perplexed, bewildered states of deep depression.

[2] The question of a possible relation of the hypothalamus to affect has often been raised. There is apparently no basis for the suggestion that the hypothalamus governs or even mediates affective experiences themselves, yet body functions which are controlled by the hypothalamus are subject to psychogenic stimulation.

In fact, as patients are observed while they are suffering from mental disorders and their feelings are largely determined by unconscious factors, it becomes evident that affective factors influence not only all other psychic functions but often physiological ones as well.

The role of affects for psychopathology was well summarized by Bleuler: "Just as those abnormalities which we call psychopathies are practically nothing but thymopathies (disturbances of affects) so affective influences play such a dominant role in psychopathology in general that practically everything else is merely incidental. Only the feeblemindednesses, the confusions and most delirious states are predominantly disturbances of intellect. But even these are colored by affective mechanisms, and often in both their practical and theoretical significance are determined by affective factors."[3]

Psychiatric literature strongly stresses the importance of psychogenic factors in the production of mental disorder. Although not clearly so denoted, such dynamic etiological factors are really affective in nature. It is not ideas themselves which are the important factors in determining the patient's mental content or his forms of behavior but the affects that are attached to his ideas. One thinks, therefore, according to the nature and intensity of his moods.

To evaluate fully the significance of affect or feeling-tone in mental disorders, its consideration must not be confined to that of pathological variations, since, directly and indirectly, it exercises profound influence upon the thought and behavior of every individual. Not only is the thought content composed largely of affectively valued ideas but judgment is constantly distorted and rendered unreliable by those ideas that are overvalued for emotional reasons. Associations are to a large degree directed by affective factors which facilitate those associations that tend to magnify the ego or aid in attaining some objective, while affects inhibit those associations which are unpleasant or opposed to some psychological need. The alteration of mental content by affective influences is sometimes spoken of as catathymia. If the tension of his emotional need or conflict exceeds the individual's capacity for evaluating reality, for appreciating its significance and remaining in contact with it, his experiences may be interpreted in accordance with affective needs and become hallucinatory or delusional.

By the mechanism of identification, an affect may extend or irradiate from the subject to which it was originally attached to one associated with or suggested by it. If, for example, a child came to hate a person who chanced to have some particularly striking physical characteristic, then the child might always thereafter dislike persons who had a similar physical characteristic. In psychopathological states there is this constant tendency for the transfer of affects from material beyond conscious recognition to conscious thought content. In the psychoses, affective states of great intensity are often determined by unrecognized but highly dynamic factors. All affects possess conative elements; for this reason there is a delicate responsiveness of associations and behavior to affect.

---

[3] Naturgeschichte der Seele, Zweite Auflage, S. 185. Julius Springer, 1932.

Pleasurable Affects

A moderately pleasurable affect is known as *euphoria.* The euphoric patient is of an optimistic mental "set," is imbued with a subjectively pleasant feeling of well-being and is confident and assured in attitude. Euphoria is most frequently noted in hypomanic states and in certain organic disorders such as general paresis, multiple sclerosis and in some cases of frontal lobe tumor. In *elation* an air of enjoyment and of self-confidence radiates from the patient. His circumstances may be such that unhappiness should be produced yet everything that would normally produce that feeling is lightly brushed aside. It imparts a false sense of reality. Elation is often a labile type of emotion and readily shifts to irritability.

In *exaltation* there is an intense elation accompanied by an attitude of grandeur. A less frequent affective disorder is *ecstasy*. In this the mood is one of a peculiar, entrancing, peaceful rapture and tranquil sense of power. A religious feeling is an essential part of the state. The patient identifies himself with an immense cosmic power. He feels detached from outside things and on a new plane of existence, accompanied often by a feeling of having been reborn. That is attained beyond which there is nothing better. After having emerged from the experience, the patient retains a vivid recollection of it. Dynamically, ecstasy probably represents the achievement of the maximum of wish-fulfillment. Sometimes ecstasy occurs in persons who have had a strong sense of guilt. It has been observed in dissociative, epileptic, schizophrenic and affective reactions.

Depression

Depression is an affective feeling-tone of sadness probably arising from various psychopathological sources to be mentioned later. It is probably the commonest type of complaint in psychiatric patients. Depression may vary from a mild downheartedness or feeling of indifference to a despair beyond hope. In the milder depressive syndrome, the patient is quiet, restrained, inhibited, unhappy, pessimistic, self-depreciative and has a feeling of lassitude, inadequacy, discouragement and hopelessness. He is unable to make decisions and experiences difficulty with customarily easy mental activities. He is overconcerned with personal problems. Some depressed persons are petulant, querulous and distrustful. In somewhat deeper depression there is a constant unpleasant tension; every experience is accompanied by mental pain; the patient is impenetrably absorbed with a few topics and these are of a melancholy nature. Conversation may be painfully difficult. He is dejected and hopeless in attitude and manner. The patient's dispirited affective attitude is projected toward his environment which reflects his dolesome outlook. He feels rejected and unloved. He may be so preoccupied with depressive ruminations that attention, concentration and memory are impaired. Some patients are anxious, perplexed, complain of a feeling of unreality or of inability to think. Bodily complaints such as headache, tightness in the head, fatigue, loss of appetite and constipation are common and occur in more than half of all cases of depression. Insomnia, especially that caused by awaking early, is the rule. Since mental content is greatly influenced by affective states ideas of reference are frequent. Delusions are common and are prone to express ideas of guilt, unworthiness and self-accusation. Suicidal thoughts are frequently entertained. Events and peccadilloes long past come to receive an interpretation determined by the present mood. Initiative is lost and replies to questions are delayed and often monosyllabic. The facial expression is one of dejection, perplexity, hopelessness and perhaps of fear; the lower eyelids droop and the skin on the forehead may be furrowed, the corners of the mouth sag and the eyes are often directed downward. In agitated depression there are deep furrows between the eyebrows. Antagonist groups of muscles show slight imbalance, the flexors and adductors being moderately contracted with the result that the neck, trunk and extremities present the so-called "flexion" attitude of depression. All movements are executed slowly and with apparent difficulty. Depression is often accompanied by poor appetite, loss of weight, coated tongue, foul breath and constipated bowels. Brain metabolism apparently remains normal in depressive states.

Depressions, in respect to their source, may be classified as reactive and autonomous. *Reactive depressions* are those that arise in reaction to obvious external causes that might naturally produce sadness, such as bereavement, business difficulties or other adversity. They are not usually of protracted duration and are more responsive to the immediate environment than are the endogenous depressions. Retardation is more unusual in reactive states. *Autonomous depressions* are of endogenous rather than of situational or experiential origin. They arise from unrecognized affective factors within, the nature of which is beyond the patient's capacity for understanding. Not rarely such a source is the anxiety associated with a sense of guilt stemming from irrational and unconscious sources. The guilt-producing anxiety giving rise to autonomous depression is one of the most important of psychological forces. It may, for example, have its origin in the threat of conflicts arising from instinctual wishes and drives. Again, depression may have its roots in unconscious guilt arising from interpersonal issues, perhaps from unconscious ambivalence and hostility with resentful and aggressive impulses directed toward persons who are the objects of an undesired obligation (a mother whose dependency prevents her daughter's desired marriage) or toward persons on whom one is dependent for security. The hostile impulses originally directed against other persons become directed against one's own self. Depression may arise not only as an affective repercussion to such a psychologically unhealthy method of dealing with aggressive impulses but it may also become directed toward the individual's self with a resulting affective reaction of depression. Feelings of remorse and guilt are more common in endogenous depressions than in the reactive ones. In depressions of a simple, retarded, type, the anxiety may arise largely from past events, whereas in the aggitated depressions common in elderly patients the anxiety may be relative to future security.

Tension, fear, anxiety, panic, suspicion, hate, petulance, perplexity and irritability, in addition to their ideational implications, contain so much feeling that they are sometimes spoken of as "impure" affects.

Tension

In tension, the patient has a continuing feeling of tautness both emotionally and in his muscles. He senses a restlessness, dissatisfaction, dread and discomforting expectancy. He presents a strained, tense expression of the facies, his fingers are tremulous and he manifests an abrupt haste in movement. The patient may experience difficulty in concentration and complains of tightness or other unpleasant sensations in the head. Tension may arise when a person is torn between contradictory desires and strivings, by a struggle for security and by various other situations. Its origin may be from either conscious or unconscious sources. It is accompanied by, or more accurately, is a component of, anxiety.

Anxiety

Much of psychological theory rests upon the concept of anxiety. It will therefore be discussed at some length. By anxiety is meant a condition of heightened, and often disruptive inner tension accompanied by a vague but often most disquieting feeling of uneasiness and apprehension.

Anxiety and fear have much in common, both being responses to and signals of danger. The physiological reactions in the two conditions are similar, if not identical, and the individual's emotional tone is much the same. There are, however, certain very fundamental differences. Fear is a response to an actual, present, external danger. Fear does not persist since the external danger that gave rise to it is soon eliminated either through conquest or escape. Anxiety, with its persistent feeling of dread, apprehension and impending disaster, is a response to threats from repressed dangerous impulses deep within the personality or to repressed feelings striving for consciousness, a warning of danger from the pressure of unacceptable internal attitudes. It differs from fear in not being referable to specific objects or events. The patient is ignorant of its source.

Most psychiatrists in using the word "anxiety" without a qualifying adjective mean neurotic anxiety arising from self-inaccessible sources as just described. Some speak of "normal" anxiety meaning thereby that there is an actual danger which is realistically appraised and that the degree of anxiety is not out of proportion to the threat. Such an anxiety does not have to be managed by forcing it out of awareness by such mechanisms as repression or dissociation or by using neurotic defenses.

Anxiety, with its threatening feelings from within, occupies a most important place in the dynamics of human behavior. As one of its most frequent roles, anxiety may serve as a painful warning signal that disturbing, unwanted impulses are approaching awareness. Anxiety is one of the most distressing and intolerable of mental states with the result that adjustmental defenses designed to avoid, disguise or relieve it become exceedingly important determinants of behavior. As previously stated, much anxiety has its source in repressed impulses the emergence of which become particularly threatening if repression weakens. It may also arise from frustrations, dissatisfactions, insecurity, and more frequently than usually realized, either directly or indirectly from hostility or other interpersonal issues. In the process of their personality development, all people evolve certain adaptations or personality trends which are habitually employed in dealing with such anxiety-producing situations. Naturally the effectiveness of these means of dealing with anxiety-producing problems varies greatly. Some of these unconsciously developed devices not only serve as successful habitual responses to conflict and anxiety but become the foundations of character traits of great social value. In other cases these personality defenses against excessive and irrational anxiety become such exaggerated and unbalanced automatic defense mechanisms that they constitute reactions which we designate as neurotic or psychotic. In his symptoms, the patient both expresses and wards off his anxiety. Many personality and behavior characteristics as well as blind spots and most neurotic and psychogenic psychotic reactions are therefore dynamically explainable on the concept of anxiety and of defenses against it. Anxiety is an individual matter and can be understood only through a study of the experiences and personality of the individual in whom it exists. Perhaps one should speak of "anxieties" rather than "anxiety" as a single entity. It has been said that the degree of anxiety from which a person suffers, its various modes of expression and the varying types of defenses which people utilize against it constitute a means of differential diagnosis between healthy and mentally sick people.

Anxiety is often displaced from its original, but unrecognized, source to some other situation which appears to the patient to afford reasonable grounds for apprehension, to be the excitant of his diffuse, unformulated uneasiness and painful apprehension. Sometimes the anxiety is not attached to any ideational content but is felt as a morbid fear without apparent source. Anxiety which is directly felt and expressed in this manner is known as *free-floating* anxiety. Again anxiety may be *covert.* In this hidden form there is no obvious tension and painful apprehension with their physical manifestations. The various personality traits of the individual together with the mental mechanisms which he has developed to conceal or displace his anxiety may serve sufficiently well as defenses to prevent its overt expression. It may still, however, be the fundamental basis for the development of serious personality deviations or disorders. Anxiety is the presenting symptom in the so-called anxiety neuroses and may often be openly manifest in other neuroses. Anxiety, therefore, together with the various defensive mechanisms, such as repression, regression, conversion and displacement, developed to avoid it, constitute important factors in the psychopathology of abnormal personalities, psychoneuroses, psychoses and psychosomatic disease.

Anxiety occupies a position of great importance in psychoanalytical theory according to which it results from the threat either of uncontrollable id forces or of self-destructive superego forces. According to this theory, anxiety is of significance in two roles: It serves not only as a signal or indicator of conflict but also as a reinforcing agent for repression, reaction-formation and projection. In fact the various mental mechanisms and devices that serve a defensive purpose exercise that function through their ability to reduce the strength of anxiety. Through its effect upon the autonomic system, anxiety is particularly apt to disturb physiological functions and to find expression in psychophysiological symptoms. In acute forms, it may, through stimulation of the autonomic system, produce generalized visceral tension and therefore spasm of the cardiac and pyloric portions of the stomach, intestinal spasms, hyperchlorhydria, diarrhea or constipation, palpitation, tachycardia, extrasystoles, vasomotor flushing and respiratory distress. It may be accompanied by fainting, weakness, nausea and tremor. Hands and face may perspire; the patient may assume tense posture, show excessive vigilance, fidgety movements of hands or feet, the voice may be uneven or strained and pupils be widely dilated. When anxiety is severe and overflows in this way into the muscular system, with its production of gross motor restlessness, the reaction of the patient is spoken of as "agitation."

Panic

Marked affective elements enter, too, into panic, one of the best definitions of which is that of Diethelm: "Panic is not merely a high degree of fear, but a fear based on prolonged tension, with a sudden climax which is characterized by fear, extreme insecurity, suspiciousness and a tendency to projection and disorganization."[4] Misinterpretations are followed by projections that may assume the form of hallucinations having a threatening and accusatory content, also in the form of delusions of persecution. The situations giving rise to panic are ones in which some long-standing insecurity of the personality has created tension and become particularly threatening. Homosexual and occasional disowned heterosexual tendencies are the most frequent factors. Because of the underlying sense of insecurity, the patient may react with self-assertion, aggressiveness, may rush about or, in other cases, exhibit dilated pupils and the other usual sympathicotonic manifestations of great fear yet remain immobile because he does not dare move. There is often difficulty in thinking and at times a sense and appearance of bewilderment. The reaction usually contains both affective and schizophrenic features, the latter often including considerable temporary disorganization of the personality. Suicide is not uncommon in panic states.

Inadequate Affect

Emotional dulling or detachment in the form of indifference or *apathy* is a frequent form of affective disturbance and is characterized by an inadequate sensitiveness to those experiences that normally give emotional pleasure or pain. The facies shows an emptiness of expression. Patients suffering from this affective impoverishment show a lack of drive and interest in those matters that have previously appealed to them. There is an indifference to esthetic and other finer sentiments. Such qualities as gratitude, sympathy, hope, anticipation, grief, regret, pride or shame no longer form part of the patient's subjective experience. This absence of emotional responsiveness may cause the patient to appear out of touch with reality. Apathy may be regarded as a protective, defensive reaction, perhaps against painful perceptions.

---

[4] Diethelm, Oskar: Panic. Arch. Neurol. & Psychiat., *28*:1153, November, 1932.

Inappropriateness of Affect

Disharmony of affect is a common emotional disturbance particularly noted in schizophrenia. In this disease it is a logical result of the disorganization of personality and the conflict between dominant complexes.

Ambivalence

Recognizing that each feature of the personality has a double aspect, each having a counterpart closely connected with it, Bleuler introduced into psychiatric thought the concept of ambivalence. In affective ambivalence, contradictory feeling attitudes may exist toward the same object. Both of these conflicting attitudes are faces on the same coin; while only one may be visible, the other is nevertheless present. One of the two components of ambivalence remains repressed but may nevertheless give rise to anxiety and feelings of guilt. A common form of ambivalent polarity is a subtle combination of love and hate. A person caring for an invalid member of his family may, for example, have mixed feelings. One feeling may be that of love, of wanting to be helpful, but another, of which he is not conscious, may be that of annoyance and hostility. Affection is linked with a sentiment of rejection. In the confusion of hostile and affectional impulses there may be an intensification of conscious love in order to repress the fundamental hatred. An expression of hostility toward one to whom a person should be indebted, a parent for example, is not consciously tolerable. The hostility, therefore, necessarily remains unconscious lest it give rise to anxiety. The ambivalent attitudes of hostility and love are accordingly developed. Not rarely when ambivalence of feelings exists the repressed component of the dual affective attitude will be projected. The repressed hatred existing in the ambivalent feelings felt toward another person may be projected and therefore experienced as hatred directed toward one's self by the other party.

Depersonalization

Depersonalization, a pervasive and distressing feeling of estrangement, known sometimes as the depersonalization syndrome, may be defined as an affective disorder in which feelings of unreality, a loss of conviction of one's own identity and of a sense of identification with and control over one's own body are the principal symptoms. The term was introduced by Dugas in 1898. The unreality symptoms are of two kinds: a feeling of changed personality, and a feeling that the outside world is unreal. The patient feels that he is no longer himself, but he does not feel that he has become someone else. The condition is therefore not one of so-called transformation of personality. Experience loses emotional meaning and may be colored by a frightening sense of strangeness and unreality. The onset may be acute, following a severe emotional shock, or it may be of gradual onset following prolonged physical or emotional stress. It is more frequent in personalities of an intelligent, sensitive, affectionate, introverted and imaginative type. The patient may say his feelings are "frozen," that his thoughts are strange; his thoughts and acts seem to be carried on mechanically as if he were a machine or automaton. People and objects appear unreal, far away, and lacking in normal color and vividness. The patient may say he feels as if he were going about in a trance or dream. He appears perplexed and bewildered because of the strangeness of unreality feelings. He has difficulty in concentrating and may complain that his brain is "dead" or has "stopped working."

Depersonalization is probably not a specific disorder but occurs in various neurotic and psychotic states such as depressions, hypochondria, obsessional states, hysteria and in some early schizophrenias. Apparently it may occur in some normal persons after exhaustion or shock. It is more common at puberty and in women. The reaction may be regarded psychopathologically as a form of withdrawal from reality, as a means of escape from an intolerable situation by an insecure and self-observing personality. The syndrome is not influenced by drugs but a remission follows a course of electroshock treatments.

Disorders of Motor Aspects of Behavior

Conation

The disorders to be considered under this heading are those formerly described as disturbances of volition, a hypothetical faculty assumed to be in the nature of a deliberative will. The disorders are those in the action sphere of the personality. While the isolation of any aspect of the mind is purely artificial, yet the disturbances to be considered here lie in the field which the psychologists designate as conation, action tendency, or impulse toward action. This term includes an implication of affect and desire as well as the concept of what was formerly included under will. Conversely, all affects have conative elements and impulses. Conation is really the intention-set or striving aspect of the personality. It represents the purposive activity of the personality but lacks the degree of consciousness that has usually been associated with the idea of will or volition. It is not a special faculty—there are no isolable "faculties"—but is the whole personality in action. Running through all behavior and expressions of the personality we find the correlating forces of affect and conation.

Attitude. Certain other terms dealing with the action sphere of the personality may be briefly mentioned. By attitude is meant a continuing predisposition to react with a characteristic feeling or manner. Attitudes are determined largely by one's feeling state and may be consciously or unconsciously acquired. They may become ingrained in the character structure of the personality and influence personality functioning. A bitter feeling, for example, may affect memory, judgment and reasoning.

Disposition. By disposition is meant the sum of one's tendencies or inclinations as determined by the affective and conative components of his personality.

Aggression. Aggression may be defined as a deep-seated drive or pattern of the personality to react in a definitely forceful way. The term carries a certain implication not only of will to power but of hostility and attack, although these tendencies need not be overtly expressed. The manner in which aggressive tendencies develop is a matter of controversy. In the opinion of some psychiatrists aggression is an inborn, instinctive urge which develops spontaneously. Others believe that aggression arises as a response to the frustration of needs and impulses. Since frustration and deprivation are inevitable accompaniments of living, aggression arises as a natural sequence. The ideas, wishes and fantasies representing aggression become intolerable to the superego and must therefore be transformed or otherwise eliminated. This may be accomplished by varying methods of defense. One of the commonest means is by repression. This removes hostile intentions or death wishes from consciousness without affecting their existence in the unconscious. To prevent their re-emergence from repression contrasting, positive, loving tendencies are overemphasized in the conscious mind. Reactive trends of excessive gentleness, oversolicitude and anxiety concerning the loved person are therefore developed. Again aggressive and destructive impulses may be projected outward and ascribed to persons in the external world. Ideas of reference and paranoid beliefs may therefore arise. If the aggression is internalized and directed toward the subject himself it will lead to depression. For this reason we may find depression and paranoid delusions in the same person. If aggressive impulses are sublimated they may serve to promote progressive and constructive forms of adaptation. Aggressive impulses may also find a healthy outlet in the form of sports. Not only because aggression is in itself so fundamental and pervading but because the individual, not daring to face its negative aspects in the form of hate and hostility, may develop a greatly disturbing reaction in the shape of anxiety, aggression becomes a highly dynamic factor in determining personality trends and patterns of behavior.

AMBIVALENCE. Mention has already been made of ambivalence of affects. There may also be ambivalence of desires. One may therefore be impelled by contrary or ambivalently mixed drives. He may, at the same time, desire both one thing and another quite incompatible with it.

Disturbance of Activity

INCREASED ACTIVITY. Disturbances of activity may conveniently be classified as those of overactivity (typically seen in mania), underactivity (depression) and dysactivity (schizoid and paranoic). An increase in pressure of occupation is known as increased psychomotor activity. Such activity is purposeful but no objective is attained as the goal of the activity is constantly changing. The patient is very busy but his activities are not productive. A new activity is undertaken before there has been opportunity to complete the task already begun. This celerity is often shared by all conative aspects of the individual so that the stream of thought is characterized by a flight of ideas.

DECREASED ACTIVITY. A distinct slowing up of conative expression occurs in decreased psychomotor activity, or psychomotor retardation. Typically there is a prolonged delay before initiating the intended activity, and once begun it is executed slowly and as if with painful effort. In extreme cases the patient is mute and motionless and does not spontaneously undertake any activity. As in increased psychomotor activity the other conative aspects of behavior may participate in the disturbance with the result that a retardation of the stream of thought is often associated.

REPETITIOUS ACTIVITIES. In certain mental diseases, especially in schizophrenia, it may be found that when an activity has been initiated there is a tendency to repeat it in the same manner for an indefinite period. This persistent and constant repetition of certain activities is known as *stereotypy*, and may be of position, movement of body or of speech. A constantly maintained immobility of position is known as *catalepsy*. A cataleptic form of immobility frequently seen in schizophrenia and probably to be regarded as the expression of a high degree of suggestibility is *cerea flexibilitas*, or waxy flexibility. This is so called from the fact that the joints of the patient's extremities may be flexed or extended with a waxlike rigidity, continuing to retain the position imposed as do the limbs of a jointed doll. The extremities may thus be placed and maintained in an uncomfortable position for a much longer period than would be permitted by a normal person. Stereotyped movements, known as *mannerisms*, are common in schizophrenia. These may be in the form of grimaces, repeated gestures, peculiarities of gait or of numerous other types. Sometimes a complicated series of movements may be repeated and constitute a fairly definite ritual. Sometimes the same rather meaningless word, phrase or sentence may be repeated. Such a reiteration in which no coherent thought is expressed is known as *verbigeration*. Stereotypies have a definite psychological meaning, the symbolic significance in each case being peculiar to the individual and determined by his complexes or other affective experiences. After a time their repetition may become a matter of habit in which case the original affective value is largely lost.

AUTOMATIC OBEDIENCE. A phenomenological but not psychological counterpart of negativism is observed in *command automatism*, in which suggestions or requests from without are compulsively or automatically followed. Automatic obedience may also assume the form of repeating words or phrases uttered in the presence of the patient (echolalia), or it may be exhibited by the imitation of movements noted in others (echopraxia). The different forms of automatic obedience with their extreme suggestibility probably represent a tendency to dissociation.

NEGATIVISM. Negativism is a psychological defense reaction characterized by opposition and resistance to what is suggested. It may be manifested by behavior which is the opposite of what would ordinarily be called for in a given situation. It is frequently expressed in such forms as mutism, refusal of food, noncompliance with requests and resistiveness to effort to care for the patient.

COMPULSIONS. A morbid and often an irresistible urge to perform an apparently unreasonable act repetitiously is known as a compulsion. The obligatory act may be of a simple nature such as touching an object twice, walking on cracks or it may be complex and constitute more or less of a ritual. A compulsion may be regarded as the result of an obsession, as an obsession in action. Such acts are so closely linked with obsession that the combination is often referred to as the compulsive-obsessive syndrome. They are not meaningless acts but through the operation of the mechanisms of displacement, substitution and symbolism serve as defenses against anxiety. A common form of compulsion is that of handwashing. Frequently the basic force behind this is guilt over masturbation, the repetitious act serving through the mechanisms of displacement and symbolism as an anxiety-relieving measure. Many people whom no one thinks of as suffering from mental disease have various obsessive-compulsive habits which serve as defense reactions for keeping anxiety, feelings of guilt and unacceptable instinctual drives at a minimum. Among such habits or personality traits is a tendency to exaggerate the importance of carefulness and of details and to stress cleanliness and orderliness. Various perfectionistic strivings and a rigid adherence to routine are obvious. Persons who possess such traits are often spoken of as having a compulsive personality.

AVERSION. Adolf Meyer applied the term aversion to the unbending and uncompromising attitude of some depressed patients to an unacceptable and unconquerable situation. It does not represent a mere passive unwillingness to accept a situation but an aggressive, self-assertive reaction characterized by resentment, hatred, sullen unco-operativeness, rejection and at times by stuporous or paranoid reactions.

Disorders of Attention

The conscious, selective reaction by which the organism examines the external world for useful data is known as attention. Successful examination requires a certain degree of vigilance and a certain length of tenacity. Attention is greatly influenced by conation, affect and associations. Feeling and attitudes influence attention not only directly but indirectly through their effect upon associations. Fatigue, toxic states and organic lesions strongly modify both vigility and tenacity and so influence attention. Toxic and organic factors, by interfering also with associations, tend to lower attention. Similarly a poverty of associations is largely responsible for defects of attention in the mentally deficient. Even a normal person who has few associations connected with an object submitted for examination will, in the absence of strongly affective factors, exhibit but little attention. The inability to hold the attention a sufficient length of time to render adequate examination possible is known as *distractibility*. In this disorder every fleeting stimulus or an abnormal lability of affect redirects the attention which is lacking in normal tenacity. Profound depression, on the contrary, may cause too great *tenacity* of attention. No stimulus or experience can divert the attention to an idea or object not related to the patient's depressive mental content or not in harmony with it. Emotional disorganization as seen in the apathetic schizophrenia may greatly diminish the degree of attention.

Disorders of Memory

The function by which data acquired and presented to consciousness through the observations of attention are stored, later to be summoned and again presented to consciousness, is known as memory. For the purpose of description, it may be considered as consisting of three processes: The reception and *registration* of a mental impression; the *retention* or preservation of the previously acquired impression; the reproduction or *recalling* of the impression. One must not conclude that memory is a special and more or less isolated function or faculty. It is but one aspect of that highly integrated part of the behavior of the organism known as mental. It is adjustive in its purpose and tends to promote adaptation with the minimum of effort by virtue of its role in assisting the individual to profit by his experience. Largely as a result of the investigation of abnormal psychology, it is known that memory is influenced by affect, the tendency being to modify it in the interests of the emotional needs of the individual.

The disorders of memory are three: Abnormally pronounced memory or *hypermnesia;* loss of memory or *amnesia;* falsification of memory or *paramnesia.*

Hypermnesia

Hypermnesia is occasionally seen in mild manic states and in paranoia. This excessive mnemonic capacity is largely limited to specific periods or to specific events and experiences connected with which are particularly strong affects. Impressions arising from emotionally colored events are registered with more than the usual intensity with the result that the patient has a vivid recollection of details.

Amnesia

Amnesia may be produced either by organic or by psychogenic factors. In *organic amnesia* physiological disturbances of neurons through chemical alterations, trauma or degenerative changes interfere with associative processes. Organic loss of memory is caused both by impairment of registration and of retention, more especially of the latter. In *psychogenic amnesia* recall, for psychologic reasons, is inhibited. Strictly speaking, forgetting in psychogenic amnesia is not a passive loss of memory trace. The absence of memory is an active defense against experiences which have proved unbearably painful or anxiety-producing. The memory of an actual event is repressed and kept repressed because consciousness finds it too painful to face. Psychogenic amnesia may not only provide escape from the memory of intolerable experiences but may serve as a device for escape from the consequences of an act. If anxiety is very severe, a dissociative reaction may occur with a resulting fugue or flight automatism in which the patient experiences a loss of memory both as to his past experiences and as to his identity. By this escape the patient's symptoms supply him, without awareness on his part, with a seeming solution for his difficulties. They also serve to cushion his anxiety in his disturbed situation.

Another and more frequent form of psychogenic amnesia is that for intended action. This is a result of conflict of wishes. We forget to perform some task or keep some appointment because the proposed act conflicts, perhaps unconsciously, with some wish or interest.

The differential diagnosis between organic and psychogenic amnesia is important. To differentiate between these two forms the psychiatrist must determine the nature of the cause. Often this is obvious but if not readily apparent a careful history should be secured and a searching examination of the nervous system be made before concluding that the amnesia is of psychogenic origin. Such an origin should not be accepted unless a psychological need for its occurrence is discovered. If there has been no disturbance of consciousness and no impairment of intellectual functions, the amnesia is probably psychogenic in origin. A selective amnesia in which inconvenient events or topics are forgotten is of psychogenic origin. A sudden and complete recovery of memory is not rare in case of psychogenic amnesia but does not occur if the amnesia has been caused by organic factors. Any recovery of memory that has been lost through organic causes takes place gradually and is often incomplete. A fragmentary type of amnesia with a scattered loss of memory for unrelated details of experience, as noted in general paralysis or senile dementia, is of organic origin. Amnesias for circumscribed periods of time may be either psychogenic or organic in nature. A generalized failure of memory for both recent and remote events denotes an organic degenerative disease of the brain. A patchy amnesia with a memory for isolated events in a period of confusion is frequent in delirium. An organic amnesia may be followed or widely overlapped by a psychogenic failure of recall, especially in head injuries.

ANTEROGRADE AMNESIA. An anterograde amnesia is one that progresses coincidently with the passage of time and the stream of experience. It extends forward to cover a period following the apparent regaining of environmental contact. Anterograde amnesia is sometimes observed in boxers who have received a severe blow on the head. The pugilist is hit but continues boxing in an apparently normal manner. Retrospectively, however, he reports a gap in his memory extending forward from the time of the injury and covering the period to the end of the fight or even beyond.

RETROGRADE AMNESIA. In retrograde amnesia there is a loss of memory extending back over a period prior to the time when the onset occurred. In cases of trauma to the head there may be a retrograde amnesia reaching back over a variable period prior to the injury with its accompanying loss of consciousness. It may also follow many other forms of organic interference with cerebral function, such as suicidal attempts by hanging or gassing, or following epileptic convulsions. It is often seen after treatment by electric shock. Recovery from retrograde amnesia is chronological, those memories nearest the injury being the last to return. The amnesia in Korsakoff's psychosis is both retrograde and anterograde. Retrograde amnesia may also be of psychogenic origin and has been known to stretch back over a prolonged period. In psychogenic retrograde amnesia, an experience has been registered but is not recalled except through an association of ideas. As it is recalled in this manner, the recall is accompanied by an emotional response appropriate to the forgotten material.

Paramnesia

Paramnesia, or falsification of memory, as well as distortions of memory, also serves as protection against intolerable anxiety. In the form known as confabulation the patient fills the gaps in his memory by fabrications which are without any basis of fact although when relating them he accepts them as actual occurrences. These fictions change from moment to moment and may often be suggested and directed by the person to whom they are related. Paramnesia is observed occasionally in the senile psychoses but particularly in Korsakoff's syndrome.

RETROSPECTIVE FALSIFICATION. Of different psychological significance are the retrospective falsifications, or illusions of memory, created in response to affective needs. We all tend to embroider the truth in accordance with these needs or unconsciously to select those memories that suit our interests. Two persons who have intense but different emotional attitudes relative to a certain event or experience will relate quite different accounts of the circumstances. Both persons may be honest but each will remember details in harmony with his emotional needs and forget those not consistent with his affects. In paranoid psychoses one meets with exaggerations of this tendency. Here one finds that the patient misinterprets an actual event, appends imaginary details to it or even relates experiences that have little or no basis of fact. Such falsifications of memory serve the purpose of supplying supporting evidence for the patient's delusions, which, too, are products of affective needs. Defensive distortions of recall may serve to avert threats to or enhance self-esteem.

"Déjà Vu." Mention should be made of the illusion of memory known as déjà vu. In this phenomenon there is a feeling of familiarity on observing something—a new scene, for example—of which there has, in fact, been no previous observation, or as having previously lived through a current experience. It arises when the present situation has an associative link with some past experience or occurrence for which the patient is amnesic. Various explanations have been offered for the phenomenon but it seems to occur when the forgotten experience has been the center of pyschological conflict and consequent repression. It may occur in normal people, especially in young people who are given to daydreaming. In the phenomenon of *jamais vu* there is a false feeling of unfamiliarity with situations that have actually been experienced. These phenomena may occur in schizophrenia, psychoneuroses, epilepsy and in states of fatigue or intoxication.

Functions of Psychogenic Memory Disturbances

It is apparent from what has been said that memory loss, in the absence of structural or toxic changes in the higher cortical neurons, is a selective process and not a matter of chance. It plays an important part in promoting the comfort and self-esteem of the individual.

Largely through the observations of Freud and of Brill it has become realized that slips of tongue and pen, such as use of a wrong word, of one opposite to that consciously intended, the loss or destruction of objects consciously valued, little forgettings, and various erroneous acts of everyday life that are ordinarily regarded as merely "accidental," are determined by unconscious motives. Since these apparently unmotivated errors resemble symptoms in their relation to repression they are often spoken of as "symptomatic acts."

Dementia

In any structural disturbance or degeneration of the higher cortical neurons, such as by prolonged intoxication or malnutrition, there results a reduction of mental stock, a permanent, irreversible loss of intellectual efficiency known as dementia. If of but slight degree the impoverishment may be manifested by defective self-criticism, by impairment in capacity for fine discriminations, in decisions involving delicate moral issues and in ability to employ abstract ideas. As dementia progresses there is an increasing poverty of initiative, a restriction of interests and a blunting of concern; impressions are taken in and assimilated slowly, with difficulty and often inexactly. There is therefore a failure to profit from experience. Aptitude and learning capacity are reduced. It becomes increasingly difficult or even impossible for the patient to understand and follow conversation. Questions are not answered or only after several repetitions. Memory is defective and disorientation and confusion may exist. There is a poverty of the imagination necessary for productive thinking. The content of consciousness is reduced in both number and variety of associations with the result that new ones are formed with difficulty, imperfectly or even not at all. The individual's capacity for integrating his past experience with his present is reduced and judgment becomes defective. Emotions are unstable or inadequate. Care must be taken not to mistake for dementia the temporary inhibition of interest caused by preoccupation, or the dulling of consciousness caused by external or internal toxins. One must not mistake the acquired dementia of organic lesions for the innate oligophrenia of the feeble-minded.

The causes of dementia may be grouped as follows:

1. Atrophic changes of the brain resulting in senile dementia.
2. Vascular disorders of the brain including arteriosclerotic dementia and hypertensive encephalopathy.
3. Inflammatory disorders of the brain, particularly syphilis and epidemic encephalitis.
4. Degenerative diseases of the brain; notably Alzheimer's disease, Pick's disease and Huntington's chorea.

5. Deficiency diseases, including Korsakoff's psychosis, Wernicke's encephalopathy, pellagra and pernicious anemia or vitamin B_{12} deficiency.
6. Neoplasms.
7. Trauma.

BIBLIOGRAPHY

Basowitz, Harold, Presky, Harold, Korchin, S. J., and Grinker, R. R.: Anxiety and Stress; An Interdisciplinary Study of a Life Situation. New York, Blakiston Division, McGraw-Hill Book Co., 1955.
Brosin, H. W.: Panic states and their treatment. Am. J. Psychiat., *100:*54, 1943.
Campbell, C. M.: Delusion and Belief. Cambridge, Harvard University Press, 1926.
———: Hallucinations: their nature and significance. Am. J. Psychiat., *9:*607, 1930.
Diethelm, Oskar: Aversion and negativism. Arch. Neurol. & Psychiat., *37:*805, 1937.
Dugas, L.: Sur la dépersonalisation. J. de psychol. norm. et path., *33:*276, 1933.
Freud, Anna: Notes on aggression. Bull. Menninger Clin., *13:* No. 5, 1949.
Freud, S.: The Problem of Anxiety. New York, W. W. Norton & Co., Inc., 1936.
———: Psychopathology of Everyday Life. New York, The Macmillan Co., 1919.
Good, Rankine: Depression. Brit. J. M. Psychol., *20:*344, 1946.
Grinker, R. R.: Psychosomatic approach to anxiety. Am. J. Psychiat., *113:*443–447, 1956.
Hoch, P. H., and Zubin, Joseph: Anxiety. New York, Grune & Stratton, 1950.
Jones, Ernest: The psychopathology of anxiety. Brit. J. M. Psychol., *9:*17, 1929.
Karpman, Benjamin: Aggression. Am. J. Orthopsychiat., *20:*694–718, 1950.
Kennedy, Alexander, and Neville, Joseph: Sudden loss of memory. Brit. M. J., *5042:* 428–433, 1957.
Kretschmer, E.: Der sensitive Beziehungswahn. Berlin, Julius Springer, 1927.
———: Textbook of Medical Psychology. Translated by E. B. Straus. New York, Oxford Univ. Press, 1934.
Lennox, W. G.: Amnesia, real and feigned. Am. J. Psychiat., *99:*732–743, 1943.
Lewis, A. J.: Melancholia: A historical review. J. Ment. Sc., *80:*1, 1934.
———: Depression. J. Ment. Sc., *90:*256–265, 1944.
Lhermitte, Jean: Visual hallucinations of the self. Brit. M. J., *1:*431–434, 1951.
Oberndorf, C. P.: The role of anxiety in depersonalization. Internat. J. Psycho-Analysis, *31:*1–5, Parts 1 and 2, 1950.
Oliven, J. F.: The suicidal risk. New England J. Med., *245:*488–494, 1951.
Parfitt, D. N., and Gall, C. M. C.: Psychogenic amnesia; the refusal to remember. J. Ment. Sc., *90:*511–527, 1944.
Prince, Morton: The Dissociation of a Personality. New York, Longmans, Green, 1906.
———: Miss Beauchamp—the theory of the psychogeneses of multiple personality. J. Abnorm. Psychol., *15:*82–135, 1920.
Rado, S.: Psychodynamics of depression from the etiologic point of view. Psychosom. Med., *13:*51–55, 1951.
Romano, J., and Engel, G. L.: Physiologic and psychologic considerations of delirium. M. Clin. North America, *28:*629–638, 1944.
Sapirstein, J. L.: On the phenomena of depersonalization. J. Nerv. & Ment. Dis., *110:* 236–251, 1949.
Siegal, L. J.: Amnesia—Its integrative analysis in psychopathological orientation. Arch. Neurol. & Psychiat., *66:*700–707, 1951.
Wilson, D. C.: Dynamics and psychopathology of depression. J.A.M.A., *158:*151–153, 1955.
Winnick, H.: On the structure of the depersonalization-neurosis. Brit. J. M. Psychol., *21:*268–277, 1949.

CHAPTER VII

Examination of the Patient

Purpose of Examination

The purpose of the psychiatric examination is to discover the origin and evolution of such personality disorders as may be interfering with the happiness, satisfactions, efficiency or social adjustment of the patient. One seeks, therefore, to secure a biographical-historical perspective of the personality, a clear, psychological picture of the living person as a specific human being with his individual problems. It will be found that there is a logical continuity in any personality manifestations, whether the manifestations be those that are called normal[1] or those that are called abnormal. The fundamental, dynamic laws of behavior and of personality development are the same for both. By securing the maximum knowledge possible concerning the personality of the patient, the forces that have determined it, and the problems of living which he has found anxiety-laden, we should be able to understand the function of the illness and the meaning of the symptoms. All phenomena of behavior, including those of mental disorders, are natural events and should therefore be studied like any other object of natural-history investigation. This requires that an attempt to reconstruct the patient's behavior, to unravel the story of his neurosis or psychosis in the light of the fullest information possible concerning physical, chemical, anatomical, physiological, pathological, social, psychological and educational factors and influences. It will be seen, therefore, that the mental examination should be a clinical study of personality and should aim at a comprehensive appraisal of the patient. Such a study must be made by a genetic and dynamic rather than by a cross-sectional method. Only by a genetic-dynamic investigation with its emphasis on developmental sequence can one ascertain how the individual came to express himself in his particular form of behavior—

[1] Normality is, of course, a vague concept since everyone projects his own ideal of perfection into it.

that of the neurosis, psychosis or behavior disorder. The psychiatrist does not, therefore, seek to make a "diagnosis" in terms of some disease entity, but after an analysis of the concrete circumstances of the individual life and of the complicated forces that have entered into the organization of the personality he will reformulate the patient's particular difficulties and behavior and reconstruct his inner life history. This formulation will include statements as to the significant personal relationships during various periods of the patient's life, with special emphasis on the patterns laid down during childhood. The formulation should include experiences that have been important in the development and persistence of personality traits, types of conflict present, the development and role of defense mechanisms and the methods of dealing with anxiety. The formulation of the patient's clinical picture is therefore in the form of probable facts and not in diagnostic labels. These facts must be orderly and intelligible. In his examination the psychiatrist tries to discover the logical dynamic progression of psychological and other factors, the links in the chain that finally led to the psychopathology manifested by the patient. The formulation will include a discussion of the processes responsible for the behavior of the individual patient, will trace the complicated but significant sequences of cause and effect, will through their dynamic relationship reconstruct past and present events and to a considerable degree predict future ones.

Adequate assessment of the patient's mental state requires that the physician should not be content with discovering, describing and classifying the manifestations of pathological mental reactions, but that he should understand the meaning and significance of the psychopathological behavior and determine its motivation. He will investigate the lifelong conditioning factors which have determined and molded the patient's behavior and personality. Symptoms should be looked upon as surface phenomena and one should attempt to determine the needs, feelings and motivations manifested in them. As already indicated, this will require a detailed study of the personality and its evolution, as well as a careful investigation of any somatic factors. The physician integrates and coordinates the data secured from the biological, psychological, social and other fields of inquiry, and in the light of all the information thus obtained he attempts to formulate his conception of the patient's personality disorder by analyzing and reconstructing in their flow of dynamic relationship the psychopathological factors that have been operating in its production. The psychiatrist seeks to organize these data into an understandable pattern or personality constellation which he will find, with few variations, constantly repeats itself in the life of the patient. A study of the personality will reveal certain themes or recurrent life issues or conflicts running through the individual's life history—topics or problems to which he may at times respond in the patterns known as mental illness. It will be found that a dynamic thread of continuity runs through both the prepsychotic personality organization and the psychotic personality. An examination of the patient's history will show that the same anxiety-relieving mechanisms, the same psychological themes, which are revealed in the psychosis have been active in determining his personality type and character traits long before the psychosis appeared, going back usually, in fact, to early life. In most persons the reaction formations in the form of character traits which result from the dynamic action of these themes are adequate to meet their emotional and personality needs. These traits form the first line of defense, so to speak. Unfortunately, if they prove inadequate the personality falls back, as it were, to the second line of defense, the neurosis or psychosis.

The significant data to be analyzed and reconstructed are obtained from two sources, from the examination of the patient and the anamnesis as given by others. It is usually well to obtain a history from more than one relative or friend. This is desirable not only because the history as given by the first informant may be supplemented, but because emotional factors such as feelings of shame or guilt may lead an informant to conceal certain facts or overemphasize others. Usually the most satisfactory history can be secured at the first interview. With the lapse of time the informant tends to omit incidents which he did not consider significant, and, if he be a near relative of the patient, he is prone to conceal important data, perhaps because of regret for previous attitudes toward the patient, because of fear that the patient may resent the disclosure of the information or because in his eagerness for the patient's recovery he is inclined to gloss over facts which he believes the physician may consider ominous. Often the informants lack the objective, detached attitude which will permit them to recall or state correctly the intra-family attitudes and relationships under which the patient was raised.

Psychiatric History

Since, in his study of the patient the psychiatrist seeks to understand the present in terms of the past, the psychiatric history is of much importance. In securing it one attempts to ascertain what environmental, social, emotional and other psychological influences and experiences influenced the patient's personality development. The behavior of the individual, whether normal or abnormal, will reveal recurring patterns, perhaps partly determined by constitution, but more by life experiences built into the personality. The psychiatric history will therefore be not merely a history of the patient's symptoms but a searching biography, a psychobiological life chart. It will begin with the family history which will not only help to indicate the patient's probable constitutional assets and liabilities but should reveal the existence of any disturbing interpersonal relations (such as parental dissension or maternal overprotection), or any unwholesome personality features in members of the household or of other important formative factors that may have existed in the intimate milieu of the family. It is important, too, to know what have been the attitudes of relatives toward the patient. In reviewing the history, the psychiatrist will consider the patient in terms of the interaction of his needs with his interpersonal environment. The relationships and experiences of the patient with the key people in his family are of particular significance. One will seek to ascertain if the patient-child relationship was one of symbiosis or of parasitism. It will be found that the prevailing emotional trend in the family and the personality patterns of the parents were of far-reaching importance in molding the child's personality. The goals, values and defense reactions of the parents have great influence on the child's developing personality. In the experiences of childhood and the feelings that went with them, even though they were never consciously verbalized, are frequently to be found the historical roots, the genetic sources of anxiety, depression and apprehension, of feelings of guilt and shame or of attitudes so defensive that they suggest the world is looked upon as filled with hostile people. One seeks to ascertain not only what influences acted upon the developing child but also what significant experiences may have occurred during the successive stages of his personality formation and the effect they had on subsequent behavior. In this connection it should be remembered that not only is the significance of any experience in childhood, but also that of the experiences, situations and relationships of adult life, determined by what they have meant to the patient. Some of the molding pressures of dynamic psychological forces will be discovered in the history, while the more subtly acting ones will be revealed only after careful study of the patient himself. As the history is secured one will note the manner in which the patient has reacted to the demands that life in its various aspects has made upon him. The psychiatrist will seek to ascertain the motivational dynamics that have shaped the patient's personality, to learn what has been his goal in life, the factors that determined it, and the manner in which he has striven to reach it. The history should show how the patient dealt with his handicaps and personality difficulties and what has been his attitude toward life and its problems. An attempt is made to discover the significant aspects of his personality and the ways in which he has revealed them. The psychiatrist will try to ascertain what have been the attitudes and special modes of reactions to experiences throughout the patient's life. It may be well to search for anecdotes and reactions in various situations that reveal his behavior pattern under conditions of stress. Such information may suggest the types of defenses which he has employed against anxiety. Through a detailed study of his life history it will be found that the present condition of the patient is but the cumulative end result of a long and gradual evolution in the course of which similar but milder types of reaction and of personality pattern have been apparent. On scrutinizing the various life data of the patient, the psychiatrist will often discover a meaningful connection among them. He will find that the life history of the individual reveals the trajectory of a dynamic process. The neurosis or psychosis is continuous with and a logical sequence of the patient's previous life. As we take a psychiatric history we observe the patient's life unfold as a sort of evolutionary process. The mental illness can therefore be understood only through a study of the patient's entire life history of which the present illness is but an episode.

Guide for Securing History

It is preferable at all times to interview the patient, when he is accompanied, prior to discussion of his illness with the family member or friend. Furthermore, the patient should be advised of the psychiatrist's wish to discuss his illness with the accompanying person. By this means the relationship with the patient is benefited. He is provided the dignity of responsibility of presenting his history prior to that of others who he may feel are motivated to distort his story. To be interviewed first may, too, allay a suspicion which sometimes exists that the physician is an enemy or is submissive to the wishes of a hostile family. The accompanying family member or friend should be seen on all occasions, and if additional information is provided that the patient has failed to present he may again be interviewed to determine his conception of the unreported events or factors. The discrepancies between the report of the patient and any other informant should be carefully noted.

The relative usually brings with him certain fears, misapprehensions and feelings of guilt concerning the patient's illness. His attitude, too, may vary from acceptance and understanding to intolerance. He may be protective, demanding, condemnatory or unrealistic. Often the relative, in an attempt to be helpful, may unwittingly contribute to the patient's illness.

In his interview with the patient the psychiatrist must scrupulously manifest respect for the patient, seek to maintain the latter's self-esteem and allow him considerable initiative in relating his history.

It is important that the initial interview be conducted under circumstances that allow for an unheard contact with the patient. This makes for fairness and also leads to further investigation as the patient often speaks more freely at this time than subsequently. The ease of a patient and his capacities for communication depend to a considerable extent on the manner of the physician's approach. The psychiatrist must be frank, courteous, show that he is genuinely interested in the patient, and by the implicit elements of his character be able to command the patient's respect. Rarely does the patient talk revealingly unless the psychiatrist shows signs of interest and understanding. The patient must be made to feel that he is being taken seriously, is being treated with dignity and as an equal with due consideration for his opinions and statements.

In order that the optimum rapport and maximum information may be secured, the examiner must be flexible and the interviewing situation be characterized by spontaneity. A spontaneous unveiling of the patient's account of himself will usually expose more informative material than the patient realizes. The physician, whether visited in his office or seen in an institution, is a stranger to the patient and often is representative to him of a new and perhaps what is regarded as a hostile environment. It is therefore too much to expect that the patient will confide extensively his feelings in the first interview. The psychiatrist will gradually seek to gain the confidence of the patient so that he will not hesitate to mention life experiences and desires which are so private that he has not referred to them to his intimates. The patient usually feels that he is understood and his point of view appreciated if the physician permits him to tell his own story with only an occasional tactful, courteous and guiding question. Judicious questioning of a patient with an emotional disturbance in such a way that psychopathological mental content will become manifest is a fine art. If the psychiatrist manifests a genuine interest and understanding the patient will rarely hesitate and will often be eager to make known any problem.

A physician who has placed his patient on the defensive has usually blundered in his technique and has perhaps greatly impaired his future usefulness as a counselor. This does not mean that a sense of delicacy should prevent a search sufficient to describe what is going on behind the scenes but, that having gained the confidence and co-operation of the patient, the questions should be put with discretion and with respect for the patient's feelings and intelligence. Care should be taken not to frame questions in such a way that they will be interpreted as accusations. Skillful questioning should enable the psychiatrist, without arousing undue anxiety, to touch upon the most intimate aspects of the patient's life and open up subjects for exploration that might otherwise remain untouched. Oftentimes the patient is not able to respond affirmatively to certain topics suggested by the questioning. However, the fact that the psychiatrist has intimated through his questioning his acquaintanceship with and availability for discussion of such problems is of utmost importance. The patient has been made aware that he has available to him a person to whom he may reveal himself at an appropriate time.

The psychiatrist will never permit himself to become involved in an argument with a patient. The beginner is apt to think that the principal object of the examination is to ascertain the existence of abnormal ideas and to forget the significance of the social circumstances under which symptoms became apparent. He is often more interested in gross disturbances of behavior or in delusional material with the result that he overlooks deviations in affect and mood, not to mention those of the sensorium. To become a successful psychiatrist, it is necessary to acquire a penetrating insight into personality dynamics although he must remember that the patient is more than a bundle of psychological mechanisms. He must also possess the clinical sensitivity and subconscious summation of knowledge and experience that we know as intuition.

The patient is initially often eager to discuss his symptoms, complaints and present illness. While it is the custom in many hospitals and clinics to record these data at a later stage in the formal documentation of the patient's history it will be found most satisfactory to allow the patient and the relatives to discuss these matters spontaneously and initially. To insist on a presentation of material relative to the patient's family and his life history is often regarded by patient and the family informant as irrelevant and irritating.

While the diagnostic interviews with the patient and his relatives and friends are to be conducted in a flexible manner, the recording of the data for analysis or future reference is best done in accordance with a definite schema. Such a schema is followed in describing the psychiatric examination and the information to be considered or arranged is detailed under the various headings. In examining a patient the error is often made of following such a schematic history with its various subdivisions in an obsessive manner, drilling the patient for information on each point. Such an effort is bound to be unrewarding as patients are usually too anxious initially to provide pertinent material and therefore will respond to a routine staccato type of questioning only by withdrawal or irritation.

Reason for Consultation or for Commitment

With the widespread extension of psychiatric services into the areas of private practice, outpatient clinics, courts of law, welfare agencies, schools and the general hospital, as well as the private and state institutions, a patient with a psychiatric disorder presents himself for examination under a variety of circumstances. The patient may come personally for examination, be referred by a physician to a private office or clinic or by a social agency or school. In other instances he may be required by a decree of court or by certification to be examined or admitted to a hospital. Under all these circumstances a brief statement of the manner and circumstances that led to examination or treatment should be obtained. This should include a record of the referring physician or agency and the reason for requesting the examination if this is offered or is available. In the private office or clinic the patient often comes alone and the account of his illness, as he sees it, and of his life history, is available only through him. This may also be the circumstance when a patient is committed to a hospital. However, if the patient is accompanied by a relative or some close friend, this person, or others with an intimate knowledge of the patient, may be able to impart knowledge of significant import in regard to the illness and the patient's life experiences beyond that immediately available from the patient. The accompanying family member or friend may thus verify or elaborate the information provided by the patient.

The Problem

A clear statement of the complaints and problems of the patient should be obtained from the patient. If possible it is best to record statements made by the patient in verbatim form.

Present Illness

A detailed account of the development of the present illness as it appears in the conscious awareness of the patient should be obtained. This account should not only include the patient's statements in regard to acute or insidious changes in character, interest, mood and attitude toward others, as well as modifications in his dress, personal habits and physical health, but it should also provide a careful description of the social circumstances in which the symptoms evolved. The psychiatrist should attempt to ascertain what relationships with others may have been significant. He should seek to learn what has taken place in the lives of these persons and in their contacts with the patient which may have had effect upon his emotional and psychological state. The psychiatrist should ascertain whether there have been deaths, separations, conflicts or losses suffered by the patient in relation to his parents and other members of his immediate family, or to relatives or friends who are not initially identified. The interweaving of these data and the patient's emotional responses to changes in his relations with others as chronologically related to the development of his symptoms often provides major clues as to the psychodynamic factors influencing the illness and its prognosis. Oftentimes such information is not immediately available and may become evident only by following a number of contacts with the patient.

In such instances, the psychiatrist should seek to ascertain what changes were first noticed in the patient's behavior and how they developed and progressed. He should secure information concerning changes in emotion and mood and when undesirable emotional and other personality attitudes were first overtly expressed and determine whether patient has appeared increasingly tense and anxious or displayed obsessive or compulsive symptoms. Details as to changes in work efficiency, degree of activity, conduct, attention, speech, memory are important as indicators of illness. Inquiry should be made as to whether the patient grasps questions and new situations as quickly as formerly and whether his judgment is impaired. Specific instances are necessary: Has he mentioned peculiar experiences? Has the patient said or done anything that suggests that he has heard imaginary voices or has had other sensory deceptions? Has he had expansive or depressive ideas, ideas of sin, unworthiness, persecution, jealousy, infidelity? Have suicidal or homicidal tendencies existed? What have been the patient's recent food habits? Has any change occurred in sexual activity or interest?

As the informant looks back over the life history of the patient what, in view of present knowledge, can be noted, the significance of which was not originally appreciated?

Information supplied by the history must not be of too general a nature. Concrete data are desired. Sometimes a direct quotation from the informant's description of certain significant productions or behavior of the patient will more vividly express the desired idea than the more formal account by the historian. A comprehensive account of the personality evolution is frequently the key to the interpretation of behavior otherwise obscure. It will frequently be found that the patient's neurotic or psychotic behavior is but an exaggerated or caricatured expression of his normal personality trends which were developed as a means of dealing with anxiety-producing persons or situations. In many instances it will be discovered that the psychosis is a dynamic scheme in evolving the purposes of the personality. Only by knowing the setting, needs and trends of the personality and the patient's defenses and compromises can his mental disorder be understood. Frequently, therefore, the present situation can be understood only in terms of the past.

Hereditary, Developmental and Home Factors Including Influences and Experiences during Childhood Personality Formation

Inquiry should be made concerning the history of mental illness, alcoholism, delinquency, emotional instability, eccentricity or suicide in direct or collateral family lines and if the patient is of illegitimate birth. Pathological factors attending mother's labor and birth of patient should be recorded. Other important factors to be noted are: only, favorite or unwanted child; congenital handicaps or early illnesses; rate of development (physical, mental and emotional); data concerning feeding and weaning; age at which toilet training began, and tolerant or punitive methods employed in training; excessive demands for obedience and manners; reared in parental, foster or institutional home; was home a broken one; exposed to parental dissension; was discipline overstrict or cruel; were parents authoritative and dominating or were they weak; were parents oversolicitous or neglectful; rejected or overindulged; were maternal anxieties obvious and excessive; what did this particular child mean to the mother; preference for parent; dependently attached to a parent; if so, to which; affectionally secure or impoverished; characteristic type of interpersonal relationship existing in family; was emotional climate of family one of warmth, friendship and understanding, or the opposite; did childhood provide satisfying emotional relationships; reaction to birth of younger siblings; treatment of and by siblings; stepparent; economic conditions of parents; cultural status of family; family emphasis on religion; family attitude toward sex; prolonged exposure to disharmonies or to poorly adjusted persons; how and to what extent was the patient punished; anxiety-producing experiences. Did the home give the patient affection, companionship and security? Any events or factors that may have modified childhood development. It should be remembered that the emotional attitudes and personal interactions in the family as felt by the child are extremely important factors in the formation and development of his personality. As fully as possible psychological data relevant to emotional development should be secured.

Childhood and Adolescent Characteristics

Was the patient passive or self-assertive; what was his response to frustration; given to daydreaming; withdrawn, timid, shy; did he feel secure; passively dependent on mother; what was patient's attitude toward respective members of his family; did he feel he was different from other children; selfish; conceited; was there sibling rivalry; cruel, stubborn, rebellious, resentful; jealous, disobedient; defiant; moody; irritable; oversensitive; overtly aggressive, submissive; type of games preferred; play fantasies; reaction to success or failure; range and use of interests; extent of group participation; character of identifications; inclined to be "sissy" or "tom-boy"; disposition; method of gaining own ends; nicknames; neurotic traits, such as thumb-sucking, night terrors, convulsions, fears, stammering, tantrums, persistent enuresis, peculiar habits, finicky or fussy as to food; lying, stealing and other delinquencies. Problems in emancipation from parents; adolescent interests and aspirations; progress in self-sufficiency.

School History

Age of entering; failure in grade promotion; age at leaving; grade completed; attitude toward school; truancy or other school maladjustments; nature of subjects in which any special interest was shown. Comment on nature of relations with teachers. Note if problems arose with instructors having common characteristics.

Occupational History

Nature of different occupations, position held, wages received, reasons for changing, periods of idleness and reason for same; regressing, stationary or progressing in efficiency and in responsibilities; attitude toward work, satisfaction from work; anything in present position that is especially difficult, threatening or failing to provide satisfaction; habits of saving or spending money; were life-aims achieved. Relations to those in authority and to peers; ability to assume authority and accept envy of former peers.

Medical History

A record should be made of all illnesses and injuries—duration, severity and sequelae; inquire particularly concerning syphilis, epidemic encephalitis and convulsions; previous attacks of mental disease, their symptoms, duration and outcome. A record should also be made of chronic illnesses in parents and siblings and the patient's attitudes and reactions toward the ill family members and others concerned with their care.

Alcohol and other toxins; exact amount and nature of alcohol drunk, duration of habit, reaction to alcohol; previous ill effects of its use. Use of narcotics, hypnotics or patent medicines; occupational poisoning (lead, arsenic, mercury).

Chronic somatic disease; physical handicaps and psychological devices employed in meeting them.

Psychosexual History

Reaction of mother to sexual curiosity and experimentation of early childhood; strong, persistent, dependent attachment to parent of opposite sex; menstruation, preparedness for and reaction to; guilt concerning adolescent masturbation; persistence of "crushes"; impulses primarily heterosexual or homosexual; attitude toward sex (frankness, prudishness); overt homosexuality; impotence; feelings of guilt concerning any extramarital relations or illegitimate pregnancies; changes in sex habits.

Marital History

Circumstances of marriage; characteristics of mate; degree of affection; are interests divergent; mother-in-law; general marital adjustment; attitudes of each toward sex relations and degree of sex satisfaction; if divorced, for what reasons; induced abortions; contraceptive measures;

concern aroused by their use; unwanted children; sterility; ages and characteristics of children; family problems, conflicts and dissensions.

Social Adaptability

Personal adjustment with various members of own family, with occupational associates and superiors; readiness in making friends; number of friends, their age, sex, social level and character; social attitudes and characteristics (friendly, socially warm, shy, suspicious, socially hostile, jealous, fearful, critical of others, bashful or at ease in presence of strangers); attitude toward authority; number of arrests and nature of charges; history of wandering or hoboing. Have relations with others been satisfying to himself and them? If not, why not? Has his inner feeling for others seemed to have been one of hatred or of liking? Has the patient enjoyed a degree of affection and respect from others that provided emotional security and self-assurance? Since interpersonal relationships with their positive and negative feelings may be of much significance inquiry should be made concerning any special attitudes toward parents, siblings, spouse or others closely associated with patient. Has filial devotion to either parent been extreme? The relationships of the patient with important figures in the family and social orbit may be of great significance and information concerning them should be sought not only from an informant but from the patient himself.

General Activity and Interests

Degree of initiative, of activity, fluctuation of activity, industrious, indolent; hobbies; interest in religion; interest in sports; any intense and poorly balanced devotion to special activities in work or recreation; range of interests; use of leisure; preoccupied, alert, talkative, taciturn. What have been the patient's dominant interests and activities? What satisfactions and dissatisfactions are experienced from work and environment?

Personality Traits and Characteristics

Given to emotional fluctuations; cheerful, light-hearted, optimistic; gloomy, pessimistic, worrisome, daring or timid; overconfident or cautious; self-reliant or dependent; does patient seek support, reassurance and approval from others; demonstrative or stolid; out-going or shut-in; frank and open or reserved and reticent; bashful or at ease in presence of strangers; talkative, taciturn; aggressive or submissive; has aggression been constructively or destructively expressed; generous or stingy; honest or deceitful; suspicious, given to misinterpretations, easily offended; prone to feel slighted, resentful, hostile, cynical, inclined to blame others, argumentative, stubborn, envious, cruel; self-conscious, self-blaming, meticulous, perfectionistic, excessively orderly, overconscientious, overscrupulous; boastful, overbearing, resentful, arrogant; calm or irritable; preoccupied with bodily complaints. Rigid or adaptable in opinion and habits; characterized by special prejudices; accept or shrink from responsibility; feelings of inadequacy; given to daydreaming; attitude toward authority; sense of humor; characteristic ways of handling stresses, failures and frustrations; tendency to evade reality (by what methods). Sets of reactions and patterns of behavior with which the patient responds to new situations. What tension-relieving devices does he habitually use? It is also helpful to ascertain the persons toward whom the patient manifests any of the special personality characteristics described.

Information concerning the patient's personality organization will be secured by ascertaining the type of interpersonal relationships which he has tended to develop, *e.g.*, those marked by a predominance of hostility or of affection, of aggression or of submission, of projection or of incorporation, of independence or of dependence. What type of emotional disturbance has the patient most characteristically manifested when defenses have broken down, *e.g.*, anxiety, depression, elation, rage, etc?

Expression of patient's attitude toward himself, his body, and an indication of his ideals, goals, aspirations and the sources of his chief identifications, if obtainable, should be inserted. In addition, a statement as to his superego function with a note as after whom he has modeled his conscience. Also, any past indication of the manner in which he placates feelings of guilt, whether, for example, by penitence, mourning, physical suffering, deprivation or bribery.

Emotionally Disturbing Experiences

Respects in which life has not been psychologically satisfying; was need for affection in childhood adequately met; frustration of hopes and wishes; wounds of pride, vanity and self-esteem; love and sex experiences of emotional significance; experiences producing pent-up emotional tension; domestic, economic or social stress; have family or environmental entanglements been anxiety-producing? The patient should be encouraged to express freely his associations with significant life events and his feelings about them.

Either at this point or in account of parental relations the age of the patient at the time of death of a parent or other significant person should be noted. Furthermore the patient's response to this loss in terms of sadness, depression, guilt, anxiety, or failure to respond emotionally, as well as the duration of the emotional response and its effect on his various activities should be determined. The psychiatrist should be extremely cautious not to attribute an episode of mental illness to any single dramatic event as the sole cause.

Psychiatric Examination

An examination must include a thorough physical and neurological examination together with all indicated laboratory examinations. These investigations, which must be sufficient to discover all structural, functional, somatic and metabolic factors, need not be discussed in a textbook of psychiatry. It should be borne in mind that psychotic patients may utter no word of complaint although suffering from serious organic disease. Not rarely, too, a lack of cooperation or an active resistance makes a desirably complete physical examination impossible.

From what has been said it will be seen that the approach to a study of the personality disorder should be a dynamic and analytic-synthetic one. By this is meant that the disturbance is a logical outcome of the constitutional, somatogenic, psychogenic and social influences to which the personality has been subjected; that its disorganization or various distortions result from an orderly working out of cause-and-effect relationships. Based on this assumption, the life history of the individual is analyzed in an effort to discover the factors which have contributed to the disturbance of his personality; then by synthesis the psychiatrist reconstructs the chain of psychological sequences through which the personality disorder of the patient has been produced. He seeks to discover the relation between the patient's past and his present. By this method, an endeavor is made to follow back the trail from the particular symptoms presented by the patient to their origin, often in deep-seated ideas, feelings and wishes; in hostilities, aggressions, inferiorities, anxieties and guilt. One purpose of the examination is to ascertain the patient's biologically, socially and psychologically determined needs. These needs may be both conscious and unconscious. The latter may frequently be learned through projective tests, dream analysis and other analytical and projective means to be mentioned later. The psychiatrist aims to see behind superficial appearances into the deeper needs, impulses and hidden motivations of the patient's personality and to discover how defensive and adaptive mechanisms have been utilized. The constitutional, physiological, psychological and other psychobiological facts are assembled, organized and formulated into a unified and comprehensive picture of the disordered personality. The psychiatrist seeks also to ascertain what personality resources and limitations the patient has.

As the patient is observed and the examination proceeds, the psychiatrist may note various characteristics in the symptomatology that suggest into which of two general types of reaction the disturbance in his mental life falls—the organic or the psychogenic. In the organic (or more inclusively, toxic-organic) type of personality reaction, there is a temporary or permanent, reversible or irreversible disturbance in the physiological functions of cortical neurons. The *toxic-organic syndrome* tends to assume one of two forms. In case of irreversible changes in the neuron with resulting permanent loss of function, the more salient symptoms are those of deprivation, such as seen in general paresis and in senile and other organic dementias, an impairment of apperception, memory, retention and judgment. The second type of toxic-organic reaction is one of confusional states, due most frequently, but not exclusively, to toxic interference with function, and characterized clinically by difficulty of grasp and clouding of consciousness. Not so rarely one finds the two types—deprivation phenomena and confusional states—associated.

In *psychogenic mental disorders* the essential character of the causal factors and processes is mental as opposed to structural, chemical or physiological, *i.e.*, neurological. These mental factors are responsible for a particular sequence of mental and behavior phenomena that can be understood in psychological terms only. Many times, too, these phenomena can be controlled or modified by psychological influences. In the more serious of these disorders we often deal with maladjusted behavior invested with irrational emotions.

General Appearance, Manner and Attitude

One will observe how the patient enters the room and how he shakes hands. He will note the patient's facies and the various psychomotor tensions through which emotions are expressed. The initial interview affords opportunity to note any obvious physiological signs of anxiety, such as moist hands, mopping of perspiration from the forehead, restlessness, tense posture, strained voice, wide pupils or guarded vigilance. Note should be made of any peculiarities in the patient's physical appearance including observation of any features suggestive of the opposite sex. Attention should be paid to his dress, gait, posture, gesture or voice as well as the care of his person and clothing. Dress often reveals much concerning personality. Note should also be made as to whether the patient is accessible, frank, evasive, self-defensive, suspicious, ingratiating, superior, disdainful, irritable, or otherwise characterized in manner and bearing and in his attitude toward the examiner and the environment. Is he assertive and aggressive or is he meekly submissive? Is he superior and condescending in speech and manner or is he self-depreciatory? Is he critical, sarcastic and verbally abusive? Is he irritable and irascible? Is he opinionated or indecisive? Is he arrogant or obsequious? The patient's general reaction to examination may be significant. Does he welcome, tolerate or refuse the interview? It will be remembered that surface attitudes are often compensatory or otherwise protective. Aggressiveness or a rugged and rough surface attitude, for example, may be a chronic defense against internal anxiety. While many of the data under this heading may be noted and recorded at the beginning of the interview they may frequently be modified or enlarged at its conclusion.

After having noted such general observations as those indicated, the psychiatrist examines the patient in respect to the following part-functions of the personality:

Consciousness

Under this heading one notes the sensorium, or functional state of the special senses, especially as it is related to the condition of consciousness which may be clear or clouded to varying degrees. Deeper states of impairment are bewilderment, confusion, stupor and unconsciousness. If necessary the patient is questioned to determine his orientation as to time, place and person. It is a matter of great importance to determine whether symptoms are presented in a setting of mental clearness or one of clouding.

Apperception

By this somewhat technical term is meant the capacity for recognizing, explaining and interpreting the new through one's previous knowledge; by apperception one recognizes the new by the old. Through it the patient formulates new ideas and relates them to familiar ideas and experiences so that he understands or "grasps" new situations, events and experiences. The capacities for comprehension and reflection must be comparatively intact. If apperception is impaired the patient loses some of his capacity for using his usual supply of knowledge. It is permanently impaired in dementia and temporarily impaired or suspended in toxic states. The state of the patient's apperception can be roughly tested by his ability to read and understand ordinary newspaper contents. His acuity in grasping the significance of his immediate situation should be noted. The patient's capacity for abstract thinking can be tested by his ability to comprehend the application of proverbs to human affairs.

Affectivity and Mood

By this, the character tone of the patient's feeling-life is referred to. The psychiatrist will note the type of affect, its intensity, depth and duration. The prevailing mood is often suggested by the patient's facial expression, muscular tensions and bodily attitude. One usually inquires, too, of the patient as to his emotional state. The question should not be of a leading or inappropriate type. One, for example, would not of course impair the confidence of an obviously depressed patient by asking him if he were happy. Frequently, the inquiry, "How are your spirits?" will evoke the desired description. Discreet questions designed to bring out the patient's estimate of self may not only elicit a reply suggesting his mood but one containing other significant information. When the patient has indicated his mood, he may be asked the reason for his feelings although the reply frequently represents the rationalization of factors not consciously recognized. In addition to the important observations as to the intensity of affect, its appropriateness, modulation, responsiveness and oscillation, such states as euphoria, elation, exhilaration, exaltation, ecstacy, depression, gloomy irritability and apathy or incongruity are noted. The patient who is euphoric or exhilarated will often be optimistic, self-assured, friendly and buoyant. The depressed patient is usually quiet and restrained, often dejected and hopeless in attitude and manner. Affective states readily influence attention, concentration, memory functions and thinking processes. Somewhat more complex states marked by disturbed affective components are fear, panic, hypochondriasis, apprehensiveness, worry, despair, chronic dissatisfaction, irritability, suspiciousness, anger, hate and silliness.

Conation and Expressive Aspects of Behavior

In this phase of the examination, observation is made of the patient's general activity with special reference to the urges, drives, tendencies and habit formations that determine this activity. The examiner notes both the spontaneous and the reactive behavior of the patient. Does he act in a reality-adjusted way? The physician should note whether the patient is ready for effort or whether he avoids it; whether he is overactive and energetic or whether he is slow and retarded and perhaps unable to initiate action. Is he restless, agitated, impulsive or assaultive? What, if any, activities does he spontaneously initiate? Distinction should be made between pressure of occupation with its eager output of energy and a mere undirected restlessness. Other disturbances of activity are inability to initiate action, reduction of activity, stupor, negativism, stereotypy, catalepsy, mannerisms, tics, posturing, grimacing, silliness, automatic obedience (flexibilitas cerea, echopraxia), playfulness, impulsiveness, combativeness and destructive tendencies. The apparent stupors designated under this caption do not include those caused by an extreme clouding of consciousness. Among these apparent stupors are those associated with deep depression, those resulting from negativism or resistance and those resulting from resentment. Note should be made of any compulsive acts or ceremonials. Any evidence of a compulsive personality as shown by scrupulosity or by excessive emphasis on orderliness or cleanliness should be described.

Considerable information can often be obtained by having the patient write a simple sentence from dictation. The handwriting may show tremors, as in the paretic. In the same disease, too, various elisions are common. The manic frequently writes in bold characters, underscoring many words or adding spontaneous productions. Negativism, retardation or pressure of activity may be demonstrated by the manner in which the patient approaches the task. Note should be made as to the patient's degree of alertness, as to whether or not he is mute, as to whether spoon feeding or tube feeding is necessary, as to the presence of queer postures or of the sustained immobility of catalepsy. If the patient is depressed, a careful effort should be made to ascertain any possible inclinations toward suicide. Inquiry should be made as to whether the patient considers life worth living. If his response is in the negative, he may then be asked more specifically as to whether he has considered doing anything about it and what thoughts and plans he has constructed. Note should be made concerning sex attitudes or habits observed, including flirtatiousness, hypereroticism, anaphrodisia, exhibitionism, homosexuality and overt or covert masturbation.

Disturbances of attention, in the form of distractibility, preoccupation, excessive tenacity of attention and absence of attention, should be included in this topic.

Associations and Thought Processes

In this field of examination the examiner observes not the content of thought but the tempo of associations and the characteristics of thought processes. Note should be made of any unusual rapidity of associations as in flight of ideas, also of any slowness in associations as in retardation. Disorders in the logical progression of thought will be shown by the patient's associations as he talks. The examiner should therefore note such disturbances as circumstantiality, incoherence, blocking or irrelevance.

Record should be made of any distortions of thought processes such as neologisms, word salad, perseveration, echolalia or condensation.

Thought Content and Mental Trend

In the investigation of this important field an error is often made by confining it to a search for delusions. The patient's dreams, the content of his fantasies, his ambitions, fears and identifications may also afford glimpses into his preoccupations and personal problems. The psychiatrist will note also the extent to which the patient misinterprets facts and reality in his unrecognized effort to meet his emotional and personality needs. The psychiatrist should be on the watch for a trend or general theme that runs through, correlates and tends to determine beliefs and conduct. Some patients are eager to express any beliefs that center around such a trend while others are evasive or suspicious. In patients who are otherwise accessible but who are reluctant to divulge such content of thought as they fear will be considered disordered, much depends on the experience of the physician and the rapport he establishes with the patient. Sometimes outlines for psychiatric examinations contain a list of fixed questions designed to bring out the commoner types of delusions if they exist. The patient soon discovers their stereotyped, uncorrelated nature and their lack of spontaneity, so may quickly become resentful and assume a defensive attitude. The wisdom of their use is therefore questionable. Usually while giving the story of his life and of his recent experiences, the patient will have divulged the fact if he has resorted to delusional beliefs in his efforts to deal with personality problems and difficult situations. If, up to this point, the patient has made no references to material which suggests that it may be delusional, its existence and an intimation of its nature may sometimes be secured by asking him if he has recently had any unusual, strange or troublesome experiences. If it is suspected that he has resorted to projection as a protective device, the patient may be asked if people have been spreading lies about him or if ill-disposed people have attempted to harm him. Since efforts to solve given personality needs are often met not only by projection and delusions of persecution but also by the mechanism of compensation, inquiry may be made as to self-flattering beliefs designed to magnify the patient's estimate of self. If the patient's mood is one of depression he may be asked if he has done anything that is wrong or if he has sinned more than other people. Escape from intolerable reality may be provided by delusional consolations. A spontaneous development of the patient's mental content should be encouraged and the narration be interrupted with a minimum of guiding questions. Such questions as are asked should be carefully individualized, be pertinent to and in logical relation to content that has already been expressed. The construction of the questions designed to search for delusional material must be determined largely by the intelligence and by the educational and social status of the patient. As the interview proceeds the patient's capacity for discriminating between reality and subjective mental experience is learned and the physician guides his questions accordingly.

Psychopathological mental content includes special preoccupations, overvalued ideas, disproportionate emphasis on certain topics, depressive ideas with expression of self-depreciation or of sin and self-accusation, hypochondriacal ideas, ideas of disease or of poverty, ideas of unreality with feelings of strangeness and unnaturalness in one's self or the environment, nihilistic ideas with denial of the existence of things, misinterpretations and ideas of reference, ideas and feelings of influence, beliefs that one is being persecuted, feelings of jealousy and accusations of infidelity and expansive and grandiose beliefs with ideas of wealth, power, etc. The psychiatrist notes whether delusions are transitory or persistent. As has been indicated, significant material is often revealed by the content of the patient's fantasies which, however, he may divulge only after tactful questioning. By asking the patient if he is troubled by the recurrence of the same thought, the existence of obsessions may be ascertained. Whether or not there is an impoverishment of thought must also be noted.

As the patient reveals his conscious ideational content, the examiner seeks, by the type of delusion, to ascertain what is being symbolically told him, also the relationship of its specific content to the patient's emotional needs as well as why at this particular time he has had to have the protection and support of his delusion. It will frequently be observed that the conscious content of the delusion is the converse of the true meaning. Statements made by the patient are often clues to the psychological realities they conceal. Motives ascribed to others, too, may represent the patient's own wishes and urges. Grandiose delusions often give a clue to previous frustrations.

If the patient is requested to write an account of his life he will frequently disclose a trend or express material of psychopathological significance. Mental content previously undiscovered is at times revealed in letters or other writings.

Perception

In deeply toxic and in organic states, consciousness may be so seriously disturbed that the mental processes necessary to complete perception are impossible with the result that imperception exists. In suspected mental disorder, particularly in delirioid or in strongly affective states, the examiner should scrutinize the accounts of the patient's perceptual experiences and his observed reactions to them in order to discover any indications that they are illusionary in nature. Illusional misinterpretations which are not of psychopathological origin are usually, in the face of reasonable evidence, recognized by the individual as erroneous. If, however, the illusions have arisen from a deep-seated anxiety or other personality basis, they are not amenable to reason. The ease with which the occurrence of hallucinations is ascertained varies greatly. One looks first for auditory hallucinations, the method of inquiring for which will depend upon many factors, particularly upon the apparent integrity of the patient's personality and the extent to which he recognizes that hallucinations are mentally pathological. If the patient's evaluation of reality is considerably disturbed, he may be frankly asked if he hears voices. The subject may often be approached somewhat more indirectly by asking him if he has observed that he has been called derogatory names or if unpleasant remarks have been directed to him. Frequently some remark of the patient affords a lead which if pursued will indicate as to whether or not hallucinations exist. It often happens that the patient will describe hallucinatory experiences if he is asked if he has had any "imaginations." The same inquiry may occasionally reveal delusions when the patient has some realization that his mental content is abnormal. This is not surprising since the unitary reaction of the individual frequently uses both perception and mental content for the same purpose. Indeed, ideational and hallucinatory content are so intimately reciprocal and complementary that in a guide for mental examination they might properly be considered under the same heading. In Chapter VI attention was called to the fact that both hallucinations and delusions represent an inner falsification of the outside world in accordance with the needs and wishes of the personality. The psychiatrist seeks, therefore, to determine what function the patient's hallucinations are serving in his total psychological experience. When the patient denies hallucinations, a suspicion that they exist may sometimes be confirmed by the nurse who may observe him in listening attitudes or responding to his hallucinations. Since, in disguised and projected form, the hallucinations express mental material that intimately pertains to his personality needs and problems, the patient is usually much preoccupied during his hallucinatory experience. In toxic states, the patient's behavior may suggest reactions to visual hallucinations; in other instances an inquiry if he has had any visions may furnish information. For diagnostic purposes, it is a matter of great importance to determine as to whether or not hallucinations, irrespective of the type of sense expression, occur in a setting of clear consciousness. If consciousness is not clear, it is probable that toxic or organic pathology exists.

Memory

If, as is frequently desirable, the patient is asked, as part of the general mental examination, to give a chronological account of his life, by his success in giving dates of entering and leaving school, the places and dates of employment and the names of employers, a reasonably correct estimate of his remote memory can be determined. Special attention should be paid as to whether the stated activities and dates are properly correlated. The patient's memory concerning events of somewhat less personal interest may be tested by asking him concerning local or national events known to have occurred during the patient's life and concerning which any person in the community would ordinarily have knowledge. Frequently, particularly if there is a history of head trauma, of delirium, of epilepsy or of fugues or other dissociative reaction, one should ascertain if there is a hiatus of memory for a circumscribed period of time.

Recent memory can easily be tested by asking the patient when he came to the hospital, from what place, by whom he was accompanied, or concerning other events in the immediate past.

If the patient shows impaired memory for recent events note should be made of any tendency to fill the gaps of memory with pseudoreminiscences (confabulation). Sometimes alleged activities and incidents can be suggested. In paranoid psychoses, especially, it should be determined if the accounts of any incidents are elaborated with details, really fictitious but believed by the patient to be facts. In more exaggerated cases, the entire account of alleged incidents may be a retrospective falsification of memory.

Retention and recall ability may be tested by giving a series of four or five nonconsecutive numbers and asking the patient to repeat them in the same or in reverse order. Another frequent test is to give him a street address or the names of a few objects with instructions that they be remembered. After a given period, *e.g.*, five minutes or an hour, the patient is asked to repeat what he was enjoined to remember.

Fund of Information

This will be indicated by the patient's replies to questions concerning current events, matters of common knowledge and retention of knowledge acquired in school. The character of the questions will depend upon the opportunities the patient has had for acquiring information.

Judgment

By judgment is meant the ability to compare facts or ideas, to understand their relations and to draw correct conclusions from them. The correctness of the patient's estimates and interpretations of external objective matters and the degree to which he recognizes the interrelation of significant factors and incidents are indexes of the quality of his judgment. Judgment is integrated in all personality functions but is particularly influenced by the patient's general grasp and by emotional factors. It might readily be extended to include the patient's estimate of his mental disorder, but his subjective judgment in this respect is so important that under the designation "insight" it is considered as a special field for examination. If objective judgment is impaired, one seeks to ascertain if the defect is caused by a toxic disturbance of the sensorium, by degenerative or inflammatory involvement of higher cortical centers, or if it is distorted by emotional influences and confined to matters conflicting with delusional trends and affective needs. In estimating the patient's judgment, an attempt is made to learn if the patient's business affairs are conducted with prudence and if his family obligations are met.

Insight

By insight one refers to the extent to which the patient is aware that he is ill, that he recognizes the nature of his illness and understands the special dynamic factors that have been operative in its production. It refers to the patient's ability to observe and understand himself—the extent of his self-knowledge. One seeks to learn the patient's estimate of the manner and extent to which personality difficulties are interfering with his social adjustment and the successful performance of his usual duties. An endeavor is made to ascertain if the patient recognizes his adaptive limitations. The patient is asked the reasons for the psychiatric consultation. If he is in a hospital, inquiry should be made as to the cause for his admission, whether he wished to come, his need of treatment, if he considers himself to be suffering from a mental illness or has so suffered in the past. Frequently it is well to ask him if he has noticed any change in himself or in his outlook on life or if there has been any change in his feelings, interest, memory or thinking. One seeks to learn if the patient desires to be helped and to ascertain what attempts he has made to adjust himself to the situation. Many patients state that they are or have been "nervous" or have suffered from a "nervous breakdown," and yet have no actual realization that they have suffered from a mental disorder. Not a few patients, on recovering, have what might be described as a verbal insight but are quite lacking in any psychological insight, *i.e.*, an appreciation of the presumed motives and the genesis of their symptoms. They are unable to reflect retrospectively on their feelings and experiences and understand how the past interferes with present functioning. They may readily admit that they have suffered from mental disorder yet have little realization as to what their symptoms have been, none as to the significance of their experiences, and no recognition of the factors which were operative in the production of their mental disorder. Absence of an understanding insight is not surprising since there is usually great resistance to the uncovering of dynamic tendencies that have been operating beyond the sphere of awareness. The patient is not emotionally prepared to face clearly and appreciate fully the existence of conflicts or the nature of the symptoms to which his symptoms constitute a defense. He is blind to their meaning since he needs his blindness. The patient must, too, avoid realizing that he has adopted delusional beliefs or otherwise disregarded reality in order to attain his ends. An inquiry of the patient if he has had any imaginations will often reveal whether or not he realizes he has entertained delusional ideas or had hallucinatory experiences. In hospitalized patients, significant information can often be secured by asking the patient why he has been detained so long in the institution. The extent to which the patient recognizes any continuing disabilities may at times be learned by inquiring as to what he expects to do when he leaves treatment. It is often well to ask the patient what the various psychopathological phenomena discovered mean to him and why he did this or that, not that he can or will give the real explanation, but that his rationalizations may at times betray significant factors or psychological areas that require defenses. At its best, insight is usually a mixture of self-knowledge and of rationalization. The goal of psychotherapy, frequently not attained, is that the patient gain such insight into and understanding of the unconscious roots of his problems, their genetics and dynamics, that changes in the dynamic structure of his personality will be promoted. Insight alone, however, does not cure; it must be applied.

Personality Maturity

As the psychiatrist continues his study of the patient's personality through successive interviews he makes an evaluation of the latter's emotional and personality maturity. He will note whether the patient's interpersonal and other attitudes are appropriate to a stage of personality development consistent with his chronological age. The degree of maturity of personality may be suggested by the perspective in which he sees his life and work. The psychiatrist will observe the patient's pattern of securing satisfaction, also the roles which he unconsciously demands from others. As a confidential rapport is established, the psychiatrist will study the patient's psychosexual development since, through the intimate and pervasive role which it plays in life, it becomes an important and sensitive indication of personality development. The evaluation of the maturity of the patient is important in assessing his capacity for various types of therapeutic endeavor.

While the levels of emotional maturity have been described previously, they are noted again in the following schematic manner. Infantile attitude is evident when the patient expects from others infinite service and tolerance and responds with petulance when his desires are not immediately gratified. Childish emotional maturity is signified in those in whom the psychiatrist finds a limited degree of responsibility with the expectation that when required his parents or those upon whom he is dependent will assume his care or excuse his defects. Such individuals also demand a complete trust in another as the basis of any acceptable relationship. The early adolescent stage is epitomized in youths concerned with the problem of independence from parents and by their tendency to admire and be devoted to extrafamilial figures. They may be much interested in social organizations and mystic rivalry. Here then is consciousness and awareness of sex. In the late adolescent stage, adult level emotional drive is for self-advancement, to growth and learning.

Those with infantile and childish emotional fixations in their relationship to the physician have expectations that the physician must be and do all for them by some magical means, or entirely through the physician's own efforts. The patient does not commit himself to participation in the treatment. A more adult development allows the patient the capacity to work with the psychiatrist and to learn to use his own assets and make full use of his resources. It is important to recognize that the individual's emotional development may not have advanced equally in all respects or in all relationships. An individual may function at different levels of maturity in relation to members of one or the other sex, to those in authority, or in group activities.

Psychometry

Although intelligence[2] is but one of many functions of a total personality, it is often desirable to determine whether or not a patient is feeble-

[2] Kanner excellently epitomizes the prevailing concept of intelligence as "the capacity to think, solve problems and analyze situations in life." He re-emphasizes that intelligence, like emotion and conation, is not a separate area or compartment of mental functioning, but merely one aspect of an integrated function of the organism.

minded, and if defective the degree of intelligence. Facilities should, therefore, be available for psychometric examinations. Since the conclusions reached by such examination are of little value unless it is performed by a trained, experienced individual no details as to the application and interpretation of psychometric tests will be given. A brief discussion of their nature will be found in Chapter XXII.

From such tests, not only is the subject's native intellectual ability determined but also the level of his functioning in different areas. Frequently the psychotic patient is unable to make use in an effective manner of the intelligence he basically possesses. In such a patient, therefore, the physician should not usually expect to ascertain accurately by psychometric tests his normal level of intellectual development. Not rarely, however, it is desirable to know how much intelligence the patient can now use, also any peculiarities and inconsistencies of intelligence now existing. In spite of the fact that in many psychotic states the patient is unable to demonstrate the intelligence he possesses, considerable interesting and frequently valuable information may be secured by a psychometric examination.

It should not be forgotten that high scores in psychometric tests are not incompatible with serious mental disorder; in fact, patients suffering from paranoia frequently have a high intelligence quotient. On the other hand some mental disorders are accompanied by an impairment of the original capacity for mental functioning, the deterioration being particularly manifested by difficulties in forming new associations, in making correct associations, in retaining recent memories and in fixing attention. Certain functions may become impaired more rapidly than others with the result that there may be a wide variation or "scattering" in the extent of the loss when one compares mental functioning in one area as against that in others. The use of the intelligence test extends far beyond that of simply stating the intelligence quotient of the individual. Modern tests are devised to examine a wide range of functions and mental deterioration as inferred from the variabilities exposed in the capacities of the patient to perform in the various subjects. A brief description of the most commonly employed tests of intelligence follows. The personality tests will be shown as well. These examinations may be supplemented by a variety of other test devices for special functions that are available for application under appropriate circumstances by the clinical psychologist. Where particular aspects of the personality deserve study, consultation with the clinical psychologist may provide advice as to methods of examination that are not described here.

The development of these tests all derive from the original work of the French psychologist, Alfred Binet (1857–1911), and Simon, a psychiatrist, in 1905. Since the series of modifications of the original psychometric test are described in Chapter XXII, entitled Mental Deficiency, as well as certain schedules to examine development, the only test described here is that most frequently employed in the examination of the adult and adolescent.

Wechsler-Bellevue Intelligence Scale for Adolescents and Adults (WAIS)

In contrast to the earlier tests of intelligence which were largely verbal, the intelligence scale constructed by David Wechsler performs its measurements on suitable verbal and performance material in such a fashion that the age of the subject is taken into consideration. This scale is an individually administered point scale which consists of eleven subtests applicable to ages 10 to 60 and over. The *verbal scale* consists of six subtests which examine general information, general comprehension, digit span, arithmetic, similarities and vocabulary. The *performance scale* includes picture arrangement, picture completion, block design, object assembly and digit symbol. In the verbal subtests, the responses to verbal stimuli are given orally by the patient. The performance scale includes certain subtests in which manipulation by the patient is important and others in which this element operates minimally. In scoring, items of each subtest are scored separately and the sum of these items yields a raw or unweighted score for particular subtests. These scores are then weighted in accordance with the average of the individual's own age group. The test is an advance over earlier examinations since it is standardized and the item selection is arranged by actual examination of individuals in the age ranges described. It provides simultaneously an examination of the verbal and performance testing which was lacking in previous tests of intelligence. The use of the numerous subtests provides an opportunity of differentiating an individual, of studying the "scatter" pattern of individuals with various types of personality disorder. From an examination of the scatter patterns, certain diagnostic impressions are obtained although experience has shown that much overlapping exists between the various groups. A similar type of test has been developed by Wechsler for children.

Personality Tests or Assessments

Although a knowledge of the individual's intellectual endowment often gives the psychiatrist useful information concerning the patient, it tells practically nothing about his personality characteristics or the underlying dynamics of his behavior. Much thought has therefore been given to the development of probing techniques whereby one may investigate factors existing in the deeper levels of the personality and uncover unconscious needs and aspects which have been important in determining its structure and the individual's behavior. Such methods are known as *projective tests* since in them the subject interprets ambiguous stimulus situations according to his own unconscious dispositions, *i.e.*, he reads into his perceptions and fantasied creations covert personality tendencies and processes. He projects out, onto the external world, the pattern of his own psychological life. The subject's performance patterns and responses being projections of himself reveal the personality structure and its underlying dynamics. The tests can also tell much concerning the patient's assets and liabilities. The projective tests have done much to close the gap between psychoanalysis and general psychology.

Rorschach Personality Assessment

This "test," devised in 1921 by Hermann Rorschach, a Swiss psychiatrist, furnishes much information concerning the patient's native intellectual endowment but is particularly valuable as a means of detecting fundamental personality characteristics. It indicates tendencies within the patient that may come to overt expression once the effectiveness of his defenses is diminished. In its application, the patient is shown ten cards on each of which is a complex standard "inkblot" picture with two symmetrical halves. Five of the ten cards are dark gray but with many different shadings; two are in dark gray and red; three are multicolored. The inkblots show a great variety of form, shading and color, so chosen that they may have suggestive value for the responsor. In the test procedure, the patient is asked to state what he sees in the relatively formless blot, what it looks like, what it makes him think of, or suggests to him. By creating meaningful forms out of the apparently meaningless material he unknowingly reveals fundamental traits and dominant trends in his personality. What the patient perceives becomes an expression of himself. In telling how the inkblots look to him, he tells the examiner about his own attitudes, feelings, conflicts and significant aspects of his personality. In the apparently meaningless inkblot the free-running fantasy of the patient discovers and reveals content that symbolizes significant and emotionally charged elements and problems of the personality. Authority figures and attitudes toward them, identifications, suppressed cravings, the quantum of aggression, conception of life role, sexual identification, the psychosexual level and specific anxiety-arousing factors and stresses are among the contents disclosed. From this material, the psychologist may determine the underlying conflicts against which the patient's symptoms have been constructed as a means of defense. He not only acquires an idea of the subject's defense mechanisms and against what impulses they are operating but also of the rigidity, flexibility and potentiality of his personality as a whole. By this projective technique, the examiner obtains a psychological portrait of the personality and may discover pointers to underlying psychopathology. The patient's responses are scored and evaluated by means of an elaborate system in which perceptions of and associations to the blots have been correlated empirically and logically with certain personality traits. The test gives indications as to how the patient operates, *i.e.*, anxiously, depressively, obsessionally, and so on. The Rorschach test cannot explain how the personality happened to develop as it did but it does reveal the underlying structure which makes the patient's behavior understandable. It should yield information concerning "basic personality configurations," intellectual aspects and emotional aspects of the personality. The interpretation of the test is a task that requires skill and should therefore not be undertaken by an untrained person. It affords much insight into the personality structure although its critics say it is difficult to tell where the test results leave off and the personality of the examiner begins. The Rorschach test is sometimes used in psychotherapy. Its value there is its shortening of the therapist's task of elucidating the patient's personality components and reaction tendencies.

Thematic Apperception Test

Another projective test is the Murray Thematic Apperception Test which was devised by Professor Henry A. Murray of Harvard University on the theory that the need is father to the fantasy and on the well recognized observation that pictures are significantly provocative in stimulating projective expression of content aspects of the personality. An analysis of the content will reveal the areas around which the patient's major problems revolve. In this test the patient is shown, one at a time, twenty pictures of persons in various, rather ambiguous, but dramatic situations. From his imagination, the patient makes up a story about each picture, telling how the depicted scene came about, the relation of the individuals in it, what has happened to them, how they feel about it and what the outcome will be. The patient usually identifies himself with a character and projects an image of himself and of the significant people in his life. He imagines situations and motives that represent projections of his own predispositions, impulses, feelings, thoughts, frustrations, conflicts and situations. The fantasies evoked reflect inner feelings and states, latent and repressed material and covert layers of the personality. The test yields information about the patient's attitudes and opinions in respect to his parents, death, violence, sex and the like. The stories he tells furnish clues as to his level of intelligence, the range and type of his interests and his unconscious directional tensions. To some degree, at least, the patient's stories represent a projection and expression of his own present or past personality. Not all the elements and incidents are significant personal references so care must be experienced in selecting those that are relevant. The stories, like dreams, may be used as points of departure for free associations.

Bender-Gestalt Test

This is a drawing test consisting of nine geometric designs chosen by Lauretta Bender from patterns first devised by Wertheimer in his study on perception. The nine patterns are presented to the patient one at a time and he is asked to copy what he sees. A frequent modification in the administration of this test is, after a short interval, to ask the patient to recall as many patterns as he can. The organization of the drawings, the page placement, the distortions and elaborations in the form of the individual drawings, any relative differences in pattern size, and other miscellaneous factors are used by an experienced interpreter to make inferences about personality functioning. Because of its dependence on visual-motor functions, the test is often helpful in detecting organic pathology. Although it was conceived of by Bender as a "maturational" test, many workers have in recent years found it more useful as a general projective technique and assign certain symbolic meanings to individual patterns.

Drawing-a-Human-Figure Test

One of the more recent but now widely used projective techniques for personality analysis is the Drawing-a-Human-Figure Test. The theory upon which this test rests is the assumption that the body or the self because of its intimate relation to the individual serves as a natural vehicle for the expression of his needs, interests and conflicts when projected by him into his drawing of a "person." In the application of the test the patient is first merely asked to "draw a person." The examiner may then ask certain questions about the drawing in order to secure associations to the drawing. The patient's concept of body image with its peculiar significance to himself is therefore elicited. This self-projection arising necessarily out of personal experience manifests itself in the attention and emphasis in certain parts of the body or in the difficulty in handling them in the drawing. Correlations of clinical observations with analyses of material secured by this technique appear to substantiate it as a legitimate testing device. It is now used to supplement other projective techniques.

Rotter Sentence Completion Test

This test consists of giving the subject an incomplete sentence and of allowing him to complete it after his own fancy. It explores various life areas and attitudes of the patient about himself and toward others. Among the areas tapped are fears, worries, aspirations, regrets, etc.

Minnesota Multiphasic Personality Inventory (MMPI)

This test is a questionnaire of 550 items designed to provide scores on all the more important phases of personality and personality adaptation. As such, it ranges across the areas of investigation explored in the psychiatric interview. The patient is given a box containing the questions printed on separate cards. He is asked to separate these cards into one of three categories, "true," "false," or "cannot say." The questions are distributed into some 26 different categories. From this usage, nine clinical scales have been developed. These are: hypochondriasis, depression, hysteria, psychopathic deviate, masculinity-femininity, paranoiac, psychasthenic, schizophrenic, manic. This questionnaire has the special feature of additional validating scales which identify the test-taking attitude of the individual and provide an index of the degree to which the subject has been guarded or evasive, overly frank and self-critical; a "lie scale," and finally, a set of items infrequently answered in the score directions by the standardization group and thus indicative of gross eccentricity, carelessness in response, or deliberate simulation.

Other studies, empirical in nature, have provided additional scales for social introversion, academic achievement, social satisfaction and social tolerance. When used, a careful study of the item analysis in conjunction with the patterning scales may yield many unexpected insights concerning the individual.

Clinical Usage of Psychological Tests

While the various techniques of personality diagnosis are of considerable assistance in determining if the basic personality pattern is one of dependence, submissiveness, self-depreciation, ingratiation, arrogance, grandiosity, resentment, aggression or other type, it must be recognized that the tests alone are not diagnostic procedures nor do they form the basis for a formulation of the personality structure and its psychogenesis. The information secured through psychiatric examination, in addition to that yielded by the projective tests, should, among other disclosures, enable the psychiatrist to acquire a diagnostic understanding of the patient's attitudes and relationships to others. As the data from the psychiatric history, the psychiatric examination and the projective tests are assembled and surveyed one may discover that a meaningful pattern of the personality of the patient has been reconstructed and that its parts and features fall into place like pieces in a jig-saw puzzle. It is well to recognize that the information derived from initial interviews is seldom adequate to answer all the questions in regard to personality organization. Areas in which information is lacking and where a satisfactory account may not be found for certain aspects of the personality should be noted. Here the psychological test may give information not initially available through the psychiatric history or psychiatric interview. Alone the psychological test is not an adequate diagnostic tool.

Examination of the Inaccessible Patient

The student often feels at a loss how to secure significant clinical data when confronted with a patient who is unable or unwilling to speak or otherwise co-operate in the mental examination. The beginner may not realize that the various stuporous states are characterized by more or less well-defined features possessing much of differential value clinically, or that the patient who fails to utter any word, as well as the one who declines to discuss certain subjects, unwittingly reveals much of psychological significance. The inaccessible states existing when the patient is first seen by the psychiatrist are usually rather acute manifestations and yield data of much value both in themselves and when considered in connection with subsequent symptoms observed at a later stage in the evolution of the mental disorder.

Since the clinical reactions of the inaccessible patient are in certain respects less well defined than in the co-operative patient, their detection and interpretation require a systematic method of study. The following plan of examination may serve as a guide to a study of personality expressions in the inaccessible patient:

General Reaction, Movement and Posture. After having described the patient's reactions in accordance with the plan noted in the paragraph entitled General Appearance, Manner and Attitude the following may be noted: Nature and degree of response to greeting. Will the patient shake hands with examiner? Is there any spontaneous speech? Are questions at times followed by replies? Is there apparent effort to reply by vocalization or by whispers, lip movements or by movements of head? Are replies confined to impersonal questions? Are there special topics that the patient refuses to discuss? If he will not speak will the patient write when offered pencil and paper?

Does the patient appear suspicious, on his guard, preoccupied, inattentive, evasive? Is patient ever observed talking to himself? If so, what is the accompanying emotional state?

Are bodily positions assumed voluntarily or passively? Are they natural, affected, comfortable or constrained? Describe any sustained, unnatural postures. Does the patient resist change of posture? Are muscles found to be relaxed or tense as extremities are passively moved? Are responses to suggested or passively attempted movements characterized by negativistic resistance or by movements in opposite direction? What does the patient do when placed in an uncomfortable position? Any spontaneous activity and its amount and rate should be noted.

Does the patient obey commands? Are reactions influenced by distraction or command? Are movements of defense evoked by painful stimuli?

What are the patient's habits as to eating and dressing? If food has been refused, is it subsequently eaten if left near patient? Is spoon-feeding or tube-feeding necessary? Attention to excretory needs.

Are the various characteristics of attitude, speech and behavior constant or do they vary from time to time? If variable, by what do they seem to be influenced?

Facial Expression and Emotional Responsiveness. Should the patient's facial expression be described as alert, apathetic, vacant, placid, solid, scowling, sullen, surly, morose, discontented, angry or apprehensive? Does his face express aversion, hatred, bewilderment, perplexity or distress? Is there any play of facial expression? Are there tears, smiles or other signs of emotion? On what occasions do they appear? Does the patient appear worried, anxious, fearful? Is grimacing noted? Describe any mannerisms observed.

Is the gaze fixed? Are furtive glances observed?

Is feeling manifested when the patient's family is mentioned? Is it shown when certain topics or certain experiences are mentioned? If so, what are they?

What reaction is shown to visits of the family? Describe any striking reaction to visits from particular members of the family or to those from certain other individuals.

Examination under Narcosis

If because of mutism, amnesia, or difficulty in establishing rapport one is not successful in securing significant mental material from the patient, an increase in accessibility can often be effected by narcosis technique. Various forms of barbiturates may be used for the induction of narcosis but one of the slowly acting forms, such as Sodium Amytal, is most frequently employed in this type of uncovering technique. A freshly prepared 10 per cent solution of Sodium Amytal is injected intravenously at the rate of approximately 1 ml. per minute. The injection is continued until the patient becomes drowsy but care must be exercised that he does not become stuporous. Usually after the patient has received 3 to 6 grains he will begin to respond to questions. In this lowered state of consciousness, midway between being awake and being asleep, inhibitory processes are released, rapport is produced and suppressed and conflict material is brought into consciousness. With his psychological resistance thus temporarily reduced, drugs may also be used on the patient who is accessible in order to bring repressed material to consciousness and to find underlying conflicts. The occasion can also be used for psychotherapeutic purposes. Since overdoses of Sodium Amytal produce a fall of blood pressure and respiratory depression, it is wise to have ephedrine sulfate and picrotoxin available.

While accessibility is not increased in patients with organic brain damage and toxic states, the narcosis technique, as shown by Weinstein, may be utilized diagnostically if the patient's attitude toward and recognition of illness and hospitalization is examined. Patients with brain damage explicitly deny their illness, become disoriented for place and misidentify the examiners. Those without brain damage fail to respond in this manner.

Diagnostic Formulation

A biographical picture of the person as obtained through a psychiatric history, together with a formal mental examination made as indicated, will serve as a guide in the search for signs and symptoms of personality disturbance and usually enable the examiner to determine the character of the patient's reaction-patterns. For medicolegal purposes, this is often all that is necessary but the physician, in order that he may intelligently attempt to redirect the personality functions, desires to know what the life problems are which have led to a disorganizing and asocialized method of meeting them. Diagnosis, therefore, should be a case analysis, a dynamic formulation in which is reconstructed the complex, impelling interplay of psychological forces which have served to disturb personality. While in most cases these psychological forces seem to be sufficient to account for the disturbed personality functionings, yet it must be remembered that disturbed brain functions may also alter personality performance. The psychiatrist therefore carefully considers and evaluates all the constitutional, neurological, physiological, social, psychogenic and other factors which the life history of the patient and the physical, laboratory and mental examinations may reveal. The object should be to obtain, not a static cross section of the psychosis or neurosis, but a dynamic, longitudinal section of the functioning of the personality. The aim should be both at analysis of the present situation and a reconstruction of the personality development from childhood on. It will be seen, therefore, that the examination as a whole should not be centered so much on the search for symptoms as for the factors and forces that have been operative in the psychological chain of events of which the neurosis or psychosis is one incident. It will usually be found that the psychic needs of the patient have long been finding expression in his dominant life-pattern which he has worked out for himself in his effort to prevent anxiety and meet the stress of life. Finally, in constructing a diagnostic formulation, an effort is made to co-ordinate and correlate the various symptoms and behavior manifestations and to articulate them one with the other with the result that a comprehensive, consistent, meaningful, natural-history picture of the personality is obtained, a dynamic formulation that avoids speculative assumption and makes sensible the patient's life history. It should become apparent that the patient's pattern of behavior represents a biological approach to his total life situation. As a corollary, it follows that the human being is so complex that every human reaction is always a consequence of a combination of factors.

As the previous discussion in this chapter is considered, it will perhaps be readily observed that a comprehensive psychiatric diagnosis is analogous to the diagnosis which the internist aims to construct in order that his treatment may be rationally directed. As a result of his various studies of the patient's organs and their functions, the internist makes an etiological, anatomical and physiological diagnosis. Through the techniques of his specialty, the psychiatrist makes a comprehensive study of his patient's personality and formulates a genetic, a dynamic and a clinical diagnosis. In his efforts to reach a *genetic diagnosis,* he searches both for any constitutional factors which may have precluded the construction of a strong and wholesomely functioning personality and for emotionally significant and anxiety-producing experiences which made successful personality functioning difficult or impossible without resorting either to reparative or to morbid measures to facilitate its functioning. These inherent limitations to personality development, its arrests in the maturational process and the emotionally disturbing impulses and events which have been experienced particularly in early life establish the primary source or determinant of the mental illness or, in other words, constitute a genetic diagnosis.

Through a study of the mechanisms and techniques which the individual has unconsciously employed to manage anxiety and enhance self-esteem, the discovery is made as to how psychological forces have operated to produce personality characteristics and how those pathological functionings of personality called symptoms have been formed; *i.e.*, a *dynamic diagnosis* that traces the psychopathological processes and their effects is formulated.

Finally, the general pattern of reaction which has resulted from the operation of genetic and dynamic factors is noted and classified in accordance with accepted clinical nomenclature. The *clinical diagnosis* conveys to the psychiatrist useful connotations concerning the reaction syndrome, the probable course and prognosis of the disorder and often the methods of treatment that will probably prove most beneficial.

The formulation of the case may be schematized in the following way:

1. Summary of patient's problems
   a. Behavioral disturbances including character traits and interpersonal attitudes.
   b. Psychological disturbances including conceptual, perceptual activities, thought awareness, attention, etc.
   c. Emotional disturbances.
   d. Physiological (somatic) disturbances.
2. Salient features of genetic, constitutional, familial and environmental influences as revealed by the history and the various medical, neurological and psychological examinations.

3. Psychodynamic explanation. Here an attempt should be made to reconstruct the origin of the various problems of the patient in terms of the interplay of the genetic and constitutional background of the individual and the impact upon the growing organism and the influences of the family life and other environmental contacts upon his emotional and psychological development. It will not be possible to provide a complete explanation of the intricate processes of the individual's life. However, where gaps are noted or explanations may not be made, a statement to this effect should be included for further reference.
4. Diagnostic classification. Utilize here the classification of psychiatric disorders as provided by the American Psychiatric Association.
5. Therapeutic formulation. Provide a concise statement as to the form of treatment considered most effective, its availability and its source, the need for indicated adjunctive therapies such as vocational, occupational or recreational therapies, and the role to be played by the social worker in treatment. The desirability of inpatient or outpatient treatment, the need for certification, and the appointment of a guardian if the individual is considered incompetent to manage his personal or financial affairs should be stated.
6. Transference relationship. The expected repetitive attitudes of the patient toward the physician should be indicated if this can be ascertained from the developmental history of the patient. If psychotherapy is recommended, an additional statement should be provided in regard to the expected countertransference responses of the treating psychiatrist toward the patient.
7. Prognostic evaluation. A statement should be made in regard to the expected modification of the patient's problems as a result of the therapy suggested above.

Classification of Mental Disorders

Before concluding this chapter, a word may be said concerning classification of mental disorders. Following the practice of other branches of medicine in which pathological entities are ordinarily demonstrable, psychiatry, usually basing its attempt either on similarity of descriptive facts or on prognosis, formerly endeavored to classify personality disturbances as if these, too, were distinct entities. Unfortunately, in such an attempt one may easily err in mistaking reaction-sets for disease entities. From a descriptive standpoint, the problem is simplified if mental disorders are divided into groups based on clinical and behavioral differences. It is more important, however, to think of a diagnostic understanding in terms of the patient's intrapsychic processes and how they reflect themselves in the patient's behavior and interpersonal relationships. It is well to avoid thinking in categories or disease entities and seek only to present a factual digest of the origins and types of reaction. While classifications are necessary for statistical and other purposes there has perhaps at times been too great a disposition in psychiatry to consider that its objective was attained when a classificatory diagnosis had been made. The principal value of classification is not in the categorizing of a disease entity but in quickly eliminating those considerations which will be least useful in understanding the patient and in directing attention to those which are likely to be relevant. Except in organic disorders, a classificatory diagnosis is less important than a psychodynamic study of the personality. The psychiatrist should be interested in process, not in labels. He should remember that a particular pattern of behavior may stem from widely varying psychological causes, also that a diagnosis on a purely descriptive level without regard to the patient's thought content and inner life is really no diagnosis at all. Even in such disorders as general paresis, where undoubted organic pathology exists, a study of the earlier functioning of of the personality will clear up many points that cannot be explained by neurohistology. It will frequently be found, for example, that organic brain disease has permitted the release of impulses that were formerly inhibited and repressed. It is not even advisable to think of "neuroses" and "psychoses" in rigid terms since there is no strict separation between them. So far as possible, the diagnosis should be in terms of the patient's problems, their sources and the methods by which he has attempted to deal with them and the anxiety they have aroused.

These remarks on classification have been introduced to emphasize the facts that many mental disorders, instead of being disease entities, are really methods adopted by the personality in its attempt to meet its problems and that it is not as important to fit the symptoms into a classificatory scheme as to understand the sick person in terms of his life experience, his motivations and goals and the obstacles he has met in his attempts to secure satisfaction for his basic needs. "In Nature there are no diseases, there are only sick persons."

Although, as just indicated, the psychiatrist should, through his study of the patient, formulate the many data he has secured into a meaningful psychobiological biography of the patient, yet for purposes of statistical study and for summarized identification of similarities discovered in the study of large numbers of patients, it is necessary to have classifications of the more important clinical features which persons with personality disorders manifest. If disturbed bodily processes have a common relation to certain types of disordered functionings of the personality these common factors, too, should be included in the clinical classification. In order, therefore, that there may be an established language reference it is necessary to have a generally accepted nomenclature and a standardized basis for the preparation of statistical data. Prior to 1917 there had been little effort to formulate an organized system according to which these data should be recorded. In that year the Committee on Statistics of the American Psychiatric Association (then the American Medico-Psychological Association) formulated, and the Association officially adopted, a classification which could be used both as a basis for preparing standard statistical data and for providing uniformity in nomenclature. The National Committee for Mental Hygiene and the American Psychiatric

Association then collaborated in securing the adoption of this classification and statistical system by publishing an informative pamphlet entitled, "Statistical Manual for the Use of Hospitals for Mental Disease."

Gradually, in spite of occasional changes, it became recognized that there were certain deficiencies in this system. Beginning in 1948 the Committee on Nomenclature and Statistics of the American Psychiatric Association began extensive studies in an effort to prepare a nomenclature system that indicated more clearly recognized pathogenetic and clinical facts. In 1952 the results of these studies were included in the Fourth Edition of the Standard Nomenclature of Diseases and Operations in a section entitled Diseases of the Psychobiological Unit. This classificatory system as prepared by its Committee was adopted by the American Psychiatric Association as its official system of classification and published by it under the title "Diagnostic and Statistical Manual of Mental Disorders." The previous classification was doubtless not sufficiently comprehensive and flexible, was limited too closely to mental disorders observed in hospitalized patients and did not make sufficient provision for the various personality disorders or for transient reactions to special stress. In general outline, the new classification will be followed in this book in its discussion of the various manifestations of mental and personality disorders. It will be noted that in several instances the presentation of material is not in such detail of classification as is set forth in the official nomenclature. It is believed, however, that this abridgement will not prevent the student from acquiring a perspective of mental, behavior and personality disorders sufficiently comprehensive to prepare him for their more detailed study, if desired.

It will be observed that the general categories recognized by the official classification are quite simple and correspond to recognized principles of organic or mental pathology. Approached from this frame of reference, psychiatric disorders fall into the three groups designated by the Manual: (1) Disorders caused by or associated with impairment of brain tissue function. The clinical picture resulting from this deterioration of function will vary according to whether the impairment is acute or chronic. (2) The second large group of disorders is that without clearly defined physical cause or structural change in the brain, but of psychogenic origin. This group is, of course, a large one since it includes the psychoneuroses, a major part of the psychotic reactions, the psychosomatic disorders and the personality disorders. (3) This group comprises the mental deficiencies. Strictly speaking it includes only those in which the mental defect is of familial origin, has existed since birth and is without demonstrated brain disease or known prenatal cause. The mental deficiencies which are secondary to or the result of chronic brain disease produced by birth trauma, Mongolian or other irreversible impairment of brain function leading to a developmental defect of mentation are for statistical purposes classified among chronic brain disorders.

The following is the classification of psychiatric disorders officially adopted by the American Psychiatric Association.

I. Disorders Caused by or Associated with Impairment of Brain Tissue Function

1. ACUTE BRAIN DISORDERS

Disorders Due to or Associated with Infection

Acute brain syndrome associated with intracranial infection.
Acute brain syndrome associated with systemic infection.

Disorders Due to or Associated with Intoxication

Acute brain syndrome, drug or poison intoxication.
Acute brain syndrome, alcohol intoxication.
- Acute hallucinosis
- Delirium tremens

Disorders Due to or Associated with Trauma

Acute brain syndrome associated with trauma.

Disorders Due to or Associated with Circulatory Disturbance

Acute brain syndrome associated with circulatory disturbance.

Disorders Due to or Associated with Disturbance of Innervation or of Psychic Control

Acute brain syndrome associated with convulsive disorder.

Disorders Due to or Associated with Disturbance of Metabolism, Growth or Nutrition

Acute brain syndrome with metabolic disturbance.

Disorders Due to or Associated with New Growth

Acute brain syndrome associated with intracranial neoplasm.

Disorders Due to Unknown or Uncertain Cause

Acute brain syndrome with disease of unknown or uncertain cause.

Disorders Due to Unknown or Uncertain Cause with the Functional Reaction Alone Manifest

Acute brain syndrome of unknown cause.

2. CHRONIC BRAIN DISORDERS

Disorders Due to Prenatal (Constitutional) Influence

Chronic brain syndrome associated with congenital cranial anomaly.
Chronic brain syndrome associated with congenital spastic paraplegia.
Chronic brain syndrome associated with Mongolism.
Chronic brain syndrome due to prenatal maternal infectious diseases.

Disorders Due to or Associated with Infection

Chronic brain syndrome associated with central nervous system syphilis.
- Meningoencephalitic
- Meningovascular
- Other central nervous sytem syphilis

Chronic brain syndrome associated with intracranial infection other than syphilis.

Disorders Associated with Intoxication

Chronic brain syndrome associated with intoxication.
- Chronic brain syndrome, drug or poison intoxication
- Chronic brain syndrome, alcohol intoxication

Disorders Associated with Trauma

Chronic brain syndrome associated with birth trauma.
Chronic brain syndrome associated with brain trauma.
- Chronic brain syndrome, brain trauma, gross force
- Chronic brain syndrome following brain operation
- Chronic brain syndrome following electrical brain trauma
- Chronic brain syndrome following irradiational brain trauma

Disorders Associated with Circulatory Disturbances

Chronic brain syndrome associated with cerebral arteriosclerosis.
Chronic brain syndrome associated with circulatory disturbance other than cerebral arteriosclerosis.

Disorders Associated with Disturbances of Innervation or of Psychic Control

Chronic brain syndrome associated with convulsive disorder.

Disorders Associated with Disturbance of Metabolism, Growth or Nutrition

Chronic brain syndrome associated with senile brain disease.
Chronic brain syndrome associated with other disturbance of metabolism, growth or nutrition (includes presenile, glandular, pellagra, familial amaurosis).

Disorders Associated with New Growth

Chronic brain syndrome associated with intracranial neoplasm.

Disorders Associated with Unknown or Uncertain Cause

Chronic brain syndrome associated with diseases of unknown or uncertain cause (includes multiple sclerosis, Huntington's chorea, Pick's disease and other diseases of a familial or hereditary nature).

II. Mental Deficiency

Disorders Due to Unknown or Uncertain Cause with the Functional Reaction Alone Manifest

Chronic brain syndrome of unknown cause.

Disorders Due to Unknown or Uncertain Cause with the Functional Reaction Alone Manifest; Hereditary and Familial Diseases of This Nature

Mental deficiency (familial or hereditary)
- Mild
- Moderate
- Severe

Disorders Due to Undetermined Cause

Mental deficiency, idiopathic
- Mild
- Moderate
- Severe

III. Disorders of Psychogenic Origin or Without Clearly Defined Clinical Cause or Structural Change in the Brain

1. PSYCHOTIC DISORDERS

Disorders Due to Disturbances of Metabolism, Growth, Nutrition or Endocrine Function

Involutional psychotic reaction

Disorders of Psychogenic Origin or Without Clearly Defined Tangible Cause or Structural Change

- Affective reactions
  - Manic depressive reaction, manic type
  - Manic depressive reaction, depressive type
  - Manic depressive reaction, other
  - Psychotic depressive reaction
- Schizophrenic reactions
  - Schizophrenic reaction, simple type
  - Schizophrenic reaction, hebephrenic type
  - Schizophrenic reaction, catatonic type
  - Schizophrenic reaction, paranoid type
  - Schizophrenic reaction, acute undifferentiated type
  - Schizophrenic reaction, chronic undifferentiated type
  - Schizophrenic reaction, schizo-affective type
  - Schizophrenic reaction, childhood type
  - Schizophrenic reaction, residual type
- Paranoid reactions
  - Paranoia
  - Paranoid state
- Psychotic reaction without clearly defined structural change, other than above

2. PSYCHOPHYSIOLOGIC AUTONOMIC AND VISCERAL DISORDERS

Disorders Due to Disturbance of Innervation or of Psychic Control

- Psychophysiologic skin reaction.
- Psychophysiologic musculoskeletal reaction.
- Psychophysiologic respiratory reaction.
- Psychophysiologic cardiovascular reaction.
- Psychophysiologic hemic and lymphatic reaction.
- Psychophysiologic gastrointestinal reaction.
- Psychophysiologic genitourinary reaction.
- Psychophysiologic endocrine reaction.

Psychophysiologic nervous system reaction.
Psychophysiologic reaction of organs of special sense.

3. PSYCHONEUROTIC DISORDERS

Disorders of Psychogenic Origin or Without Clearly Defined Tangible Cause or Structural Change

Psychoneurotic reactions
- Anxiety Reaction
- Dissociative reaction
- Conversion reaction
- Phobic reaction
- Obsessive compulsive reaction
- Depressive reaction
- Psychoneurotic reaction, other

4. PERSONALITY DISORDERS

Disorders of Psychogenic Origin or Without Clearly Defined Tangible Cause or Structural Change

Personality pattern disturbance
- Inadequate personality
- Schizoid personality
- Cyclothymic personality
- Paranoid personality

Personality trait disturbance
- Emotionally unstable personality
- Passive-aggressive personality
- Compulsive personality
- Personality trait disturbance, other

Sociopathic personality disturbance
- Antisocial reaction
- Dyssocial reaction
- Sexual deviation

Addiction
- Alcoholism
- Drug addiction

Special symptom reactions
- Learning disturbance
- Speech disturbance
- Enuresis
- Somnambulism
- Other

5. TRANSIENT SITUATIONAL PERSONALITY DISORDERS

Transient Situational Personality Disturbance

Gross stress reaction
Adult situational reaction

Adjustment reaction of infancy
Adjustment reaction of childhood
Habit disturbance
Conduct disturbance
Neurotic traits
Adjustment reaction of adolescence
Adjustment reaction of late life

BIBLIOGRAPHY

American Psychiatric Association: Diagnostic and Statistical Manual of Mental Disorders. Washington, American Psychiatric Association, 1952.

Beck, S. J.: Rorschach's Test: III. Advances in Interpretation. New York, Grune & Stratton, 1952.

Brown, Fred: Contribution of the psychologist to problems of psychiatric diagnosis and therapy. Psychiatric Quart. Supplement, *26:*8–21, 1952.

Diethelm, Oskar: The evaluation of a psychiatric examination. Am. J. Psychiat., *105:* 606–611, 1949.

Dunbar, E. F.: Psychosomatic history and techniques of examination. Am. J. Psychiat., *95:*1277–1305, 1939.

Gill, M., Newman, R., and Redlich, F. C.: The initial interview in psychiatric practice. New York, International Universities Press, 1954, Chapter 7.

Hart, W. L., Ebaugh, F. G., and Morgan, D. W.: The Amytal interview. Am. J. M. Sc., *210:*125, 1945.

Hathaway, S. R., and McKinley, J. C.: A multiphasic personality schedule (Minnesota): Construction of the schedule. J. Psychol., *10:*249, 1940.

Haun, Paul: A rational approach to psychiatric nosology. Psychiatric Quart., *23:*308–316, 1948.

Henderson, W. J., Coffer, R. H., Jr., and Cross, T. N.: The Initial Interview. Arch. Neurol. & Psychiat., *71:*24–30, 1954.

Hoch, P. H., and Zubin, Joseph: Relation of Psychological Tests to Psychiatry. New York, Grune & Stratton, Inc., 1951.

Holsopple, J. Q., and Miale, F. R.: Sentence Completion: A Projective Method for the Study of Personality. Springfield, Chas. C Thomas, 1954.

Klopfer, B., and Kelley, D. M.: The Rorschach Technique. New York, World Book Co., 1942.

Menninger, K. A.: A Manual for Psychiatric Case Study. New York, Grune & Stratton, Inc., 1951.

———: A Guide to Psychiatric Books, 2nd ed. New York, Grune & Stratton, Inc., 1956.

Meyer, Adolf: The aims and meaning of psychiatric diagnosis. Am. J. Insan., *74:*163–168, 1917.

———: The "complaint" as the center of genetic-dynamic and nosological teaching in psychiatry. New England J. Med., *199:*360–370, 1928.
(The two foregoing articles may be found in Volume III, the Collected Papers of Adolf Meyer, Eunice E. Winters, editor. Baltimore, The Johns Hopkins Press, 1951.)

Murray, H. A.: Explorations in Personality. New York, Oxford University Press, 1938.

———: Uses of the thematic apperception test. Am. J. Psychiat., *107:*577–581, 1951.

Rohde, A. R.: The Sentence Completion Test: Its Diagnostic and Clinical Application to Mental Disorders. New York, The Ronald Press Co., 1957.

Rorschach, Hermann: Psychodiagnostics, 2nd ed. Translated by Paul Lemkau and Bernard Kronenberg. New York, Grune & Stratton, 1942.

Rosenzweig, S.: Available methods for studying personality. J. Psychol., *28:*345–368, 1948.

Saul, L. J.: The psychoanalytic interview. Psychoanalyt. Quart., *26:*76–90, 1957.

Sullivan, H. S.: The psychiatric interview. Psychiatry, *14:*361, 1951, and *15:*127, 1952.

Weider, A., and Wechsler, D.: Contributions toward Medical Psychology II. New York, Ronald Press Co., 1953.
Weinstein, F. A., and Malitz, S.: Changes in symbolic expression with Amytal sodium. Am. J. Psychiat., *111*:198–206, 1954.
Whitehorn, J. C.: Guide to interviewing and clinical personality study. Arch. Neurol. & Psychiat., *52*:197–216, 1944.
Zubin, Joseph: Objective evaluation of personality tests. Am. J. Psychiat., *107*:569–576, 1951.

CHAPTER VIII

Disorders Caused by or Associated with Impairment of Brain Tissue Function

THE SYMPTOMS in this large group of disorders are caused by some agent or process which has impaired, usually diffusely, the functions of brain tissue with the result that there is a deficit in the capacity for intellectual functioning. If the brain lesion with the accompanying symptomatic syndrome is reversible, the brain disorder is classified as *acute*, regardless of the etiology, onset or duration of the mental illness. If the brain lesion with the accompanying organic syndrome is relatively permanent and more or less irreversible symptoms of loss of brain function persist, the brain disorder is classified as *chronic*. In both the acute and chronic forms the symptoms constitute what is often spoken of as the *organic syndrome*. The symptoms present vary greatly in degree in accordance with the degree to which brain function is impaired. In this syndrome are noted some or all of the following symptoms: confusion, impairment of orientation, memory, apperception, knowledge, judgment and other "intellectual" functions, and usually instability and shallowness of affect. The confusion tends to be more marked in the acute syndrome. Various psychotic, neurotic or behavior reactions may be associated with the organic syndrome. These are released by the organic brain disorder but their characteristics are determined by the patient's essential personality pattern, his immediate environmental situation, current emotional conflicts and the setting of interpersonal relations. A brain disorder which at its beginning appeared to be acute and reversible may later show that it has produced permanent damage and a resulting chronic syndrome.

Acute Brain Disorders Due to or Associated with Infection

The syndrome accompanying these disorders is more frequently produced by infections and toxic states. The basic disturbance is of the sensorium, *i.e.*, the functions of the special senses are impaired and the apprehension of the external stimuli presented to them is faulty. The clinical syndrome of delirium is largely limited to these temporary disturbances of brain function.

Acute Brain Syndrome Associated with Intracranial Infection

In their early stages many intracranial infections are accompanied by mental symptoms typical of an acute organic syndrome. Sometimes the damage to brain tissue is temporary and reversible. Not rarely, however, the impairment of brain function becomes permanent with a resulting chronic organic syndrome.

1. Mental Disturbances with Meningococcal (Epidemic) Meningitis. Probably the most important form of meningitis encountered by the psychiatrist is epidemic cerebrospinal meningitis. Actually the meningitis is but part of a septicemia caused by infection by meningococci. Delirium with confusion, muttering, rambling talk, disorientation and restlessness usually occurs early in the course of the infection but the acuteness of the mental symptoms varies as the disease is fulminating, acute, subacute or chronic in type. At first the delirium may be nocturnal or exist only when the patient is undisturbed. In the acute cases the patient is usually restless or even noisy and violent. In unfavorable cases, a terminal coma develops, appearing very early in the fulminating forms. In the subacute case, drowsiness, confusion and mild delirium occur. Recovery may be complete or there may be special sense deprivations accompanied, perhaps, by various types of motor paralyses and a varying degree of mental defect. The resulting mental change may consist merely of moroseness, inability to concentrate, impairment of memory and irritability, or, especially when the disease occurs in infants, there may be a serious arrest of intelligence.

The diagnosis is established by the existence of the above signs of diffuse cerebral dysfunction in conjunction with the presence of signs of meningeal irritation, including a stiff neck, Kernig and Brudzinski signs, and with the presence often of a purpuric rash, hyperesthesia and hyperalgesia. Spinal puncture shows a purulent fluid under increased pressure with a predominance of leukocytes. On Gram staining, the meningococcus may be cultured or tentatively identified as a diplococcus. The sugar and alkaloids of the cerebrospinal fluid are decreased.

Parenteral administration of sodium sulfadiazine, the agent of choice, should be initiated with an initial dosage of 0.05 to 0.1 gm. per kilogram of body weight (approximately 3.5 to 6.0 gm.). The agent should be given intravenously as a 0.5 per cent solution, preferably in 6M sodium lactate solution. Lactate sustains an alkaline urine and prevents the precipitation of the drug in the renal tubules. If 5 gm. of the drug is dissolved in 1000 ml. 6M sodium lactate, the proper concentration of the agent is provided. Subsequent doses of sodium sulfadiazine may be given in 500 ml. of 6M sodium lactate. A concentration of 10 to 12 mg. of sodium sulfadiazine per 100 ml. of blood is desirable. Concentrations above this level are to be avoided. If the drug is given by mouth, the patient should also receive 15 gm. of sodium bicarbonate daily, in divided doses. This should be continued for two to five days after complete clinical recovery. It is not necessary to consider intrathecal therapy.

Penicillin has been used but the results are less satisfactory than with the sulfonamides unless large doses in the neighborhood of 1,000,000 units are given every two hours intramuscularly.

2. Mental Disturbances with Tuberculous Meningitis. In both children and adults the onset of tuberculous meningitis is usually insidious. The previously active child begins to tire easily, appears weary, is irritable, peevish and disinclined to talk or play. Sleep is often restless and disturbed by mild delirium. As the intracranial pressure increases difficulty of grasp, clouding of consciousness and confusion begin to appear and headache increases. For a time the patient, if roused, may for a short period be fairly well in touch with his environment although he usually resents any disturbance. Some adults exhibit an agitated confusion. As the lethargy increases the patient is no longer capable of recognizing friends and sinks into coma.

A diagnosis of tuberculous meningitis is made in the presence of signs of diffuse cerebral dysfunction as described above, with clinical evidence of meningitis indicated by a stiff neck, Kernig and/or Brudzinski responses, hyperreflexia, patella and ankle clonus and Babinski reflexes. Later such signs may disappear with deepening coma. Cerebrospinal fluid is usually clear, with slight increase in pressure. A thin coagulum will develop if the fluid is allowed to stand. Tubercle bacilli may be found in the coagulum. The cells in the fluid are increased to 25 or more per cubic millimeter. Protein is elevated while glucose content is diminished.

Current treatment with streptomycin and isoniazid has been most gratifying. Intrathecal medication is unnecessary. With adults, streptomycin in the dosage of 2 gm. may be given intramuscularly in two divided doses in conjunction with 8 to 10 mg. per kilogram of body weight of isoniazid by mouth. This regimen should be continued for periods of six months or more after obvious clearing of the infection. The isoniazid may be decreased by 5 mg. per kilogram as improvement ensues. The clearing of the infection is indicated by the rise in the glucose content of the cerebrospinal fluid. Para-aminosalicylic acid may be given as well. In children 1 gm. of streptomycin is given intramuscularly with isoniazid 10 mg. per kilogram daily in divided doses. When the cerebrospinal glucose has increased, the same dose of streptomycin is given twice weekly for one or two months followed by sulfone (Promizole) by mouth for several years (0.25 to 8 gm.).

Close observation is required in order to detect signs of intoxication with isoniazid and streptomycin. The symptomatology of toxicity with isoniazid is described in the next chapter. Deafness and other disturbances have been observed with streptomycin. It has been shown that the prognosis for survival is related to the time of initiation of therapy and the severity of the illness. The state of consciousness, the degree of abnormality detected in the electroencephalogram and the increase in cerebrospinal fluid protein with decrease in glucose provide indicators of the latter.

3. MENTAL DISTURBANCES WITH ACUTE CHOREA (SYDENHAM'S). Sydenham's chorea is now regarded as an infectious encephalitis involving both the cortex and basal ganglia. It is thought that it results from the same factors which produce rheumatic fever or from similar factors. It is probably a rheumatic encephalitis and represents an exudative stage of cerebral involvement similar to the exudative changes which may be observed in the joints and heart. It seems certain that a streptococcus is involved in the process. The involuntary, jerky movements, the muscular inco-ordination and the grimaces are important symptoms of the disease but only its mental aspects will be considered here.

Symptoms. In addition to an easy mental fatigability, many psychic symptoms may be associated with chorea. One of the most constant of these is an emotional instability. The choreic child becomes preoccupied, sensitive, irritable, restless, quarrelsome and resentful of correction. Insomnia, night terrors and sleepwalking may occur. Heedlessness, impairment of attention and of concentration are frequent, also an apparent inability to remember. The majority of these children are tearful, cry at the slightest provocation, are peevish and fretful. Many show a lack of concern for ordinary duties and obligations. Occasionally there may be considerable depression. The facies is sometimes described as wistful in expression. Selfishness and disbedience are common, and many feel that the somewhat frequent association of behavior disorders and delinquency with the disease is more than a coincidence. Sometimes the behavior disturbances are not unlike those following encephalitis or trauma of the head. Delirious episodes may occur. Unfortunately the family may fail to appreciate the seriousness and significance of the disease, and therefore scold and punish the child for the emotional and other rather trying behavior characteristics. Such ill-advised treatment tends to aggravate the emotional behavior and reactions. At best the disease often leads to undesirable defense reactions. Chorea sometimes occurs for the first time or recurs in young women, associated with their first pregnancy.

Diagnosis. A history of rheumatism or of repeated attacks of tonsillitis and the presence of heart disease or of high fever may be helpful in establishing the diagnosis. It must be differentiated from hysteria, from tics, athetoid movements and from a restless, general hyperactivity. Sydenham's chorea usually continues for two or three months and occasionally for longer periods. Relapses are not uncommon. The disease occurs much more frequently in girls than in boys. There is much to suggest that a postinfectious encephalopathy may exist following chorea and that it is accompanied by permanent personality changes in the form of hyperkinetic or neurotic symptoms and peculiarities of character or temperament.

Treatment. One of the most essential requirements of treatment is physical and mental rest. The earlier the child is put to bed the shorter, usually, will be the course of the disease. The disturbing presence of other persons should not be permitted. Treatment in a hospital away from disturbing home influences is often wise. Sodium salicylate and aspirin have long been used. In children over thirteen, fever therapy induced by means of the air conditioned, thermostatically controlled hypertherm has been recommended by some as a means of shortening the course of the illness. The patient may be given daily treatments for two hours with temperatures from 104° to 105°F. Usually eight to ten treatments are given. Some pediatricians advise against fever therapy if cardiac damage exists. Such sedatives as bromides, chloral or Sodium Amytal may be required if restlessness is marked. Since the chorea is merely a symptom of the rheumatic infection the treatment of the latter must be continued until all criteria indicating its arrest are satisfied.

4. Mental Disturbances with Epidemic Encephalitis. An infectious disease of the brain which appeared in Roumania in 1915 but was first described and identified in 1917 by Constantin von Economo of Vienna spread to America in 1919 and subsequently attracted much attention both because of its devastating epidemiological features and its remarkable symptomatological polymorphism. Economo termed the disease lethargic encephalitis but as it was not always characterized by lethargy it has become generally known as *epidemic* or *Type A encephalitis.* No cases of the acute form have been reported since 1925 but the disease continues to have clinical interest since chronic forms are still seen. It seems to be clearly established that the etiological agent was a filtrable virus although its mode of transmission is not known. The most common pathological lesion existing in this form was characterized by a cuffing or infiltration of the perivascular spaces in the brain with lymphocytes. While this may have existed in the cortex, hypothalamus or even peripheral nerves, by far the most frequent site was the basal ganglia. Ganglion cells degenerated and many disappeared. In the chronic cases, which are the only ones now being seen by pathologists, the chief findings are loss of and degeneration of neurons, especially in the substantia nigra, which may be grossly pigmented, as well as a gliosis. The virus probably remained active in the nervous tissue for years, much in the manner of the Treponema pallidum in neurosyphilis.

Since the acute form of this type of encephalitis is not now seen little description of it will be given. Not even excepting syphilis is there a disease involving the central and peripheral nervous system capable of such polymorphic manifestations. Following the general symptoms of any infectious disease there appeared the evidences of an invasion of the nervous system in which any one of its functions might be disturbed. The acute forms tended to fall into two ambitendent types: the hypersomnic-ophthalmoplegic and the irritative hyperkinetic. In the first or negative type, the most conspicuous symptoms were drowsiness with gradations to lethargy, stupor and coma, slowness of intellectual function, paralytic phenomena of cortical origin, aphasia, agraphia; astereognosis and loss of limb sense caused by paralytic lesions in the parietal cortex; ptosis, strabismus and other disturbances of the ocular apparatus as well as other paralytic phenomena indicative of localization in the brain stem. The lethargy and other sleep disturbances were often the most striking symptoms of the acute form. The patient might remain in a deep sleep for days or weeks. If aroused he promptly fell asleep again. In the irritative, hyperkinetic or positive type there was restlessness, irritability, excitability, insomnia, jacksonian or generalized convulsive seizures and other irritative phenomena. Hyperkinetic phenomena resulting from involvement of the basal nuclei occurred in he acute form of the disease and were of a great variety. Among them were tremors, myoclonias, and athetoid and choreiform movements.

Following the great epidemic mentioned, many patients who had survived the acute phase continued to show symptoms that at first were ascribed to residual lesions. Gradually, however, it became apparent that these symptoms were not stationary and that a continued, chronic activity persisted. Other patients who had supposedly recovered began, after intervals of months or years free from symptoms, to develop parkinsonism or other evidence of a continuing process. Also during the years since the epidemic many persons with a history of some previous infection, perhaps diagnosed as influenza but with no associated acute encephalitic symptoms, developed chronic encephalitis. Others with no history of previous infection insidiously developed an encephalitis that was chronically progressive from the onset.

The symptoms of a chronic encephalitis of the von Economo type are varied and depend upon the areas in which the progressive inflammatory-degenerative changes take place, although the extrapyramidal basal motor nuclei are the most frequent sites. The most common syndrome is the parkinsonian (cf. Chapter XXI). Tremors, tics, myotonias, and athetoid and choreiform movements are frequently observed. In addition to these dyskinesias and hyperkinesias, there may be paroxysmal symptoms such as disturbances in rate or rhythm of respiration, also gasping or yawning. One of the most frequent paroxysmal phenomena is oculogyric crisis in which the eyes are spasmodically turned upwards owing to the periodic activity of certain neural mechanisms. Narcolepsy and epileptic attacks may occur. Excessive flow of saliva, seborrhea and obesity are not uncommon.

The psychic manifestations of the acute phase of epidemic encephalitis presented the general characteristics of an acute organic type of mental reaction of toxic-infectious origin, *viz.*, clouding of the sensorium, impairment of capacity for apprehension, for elaborating impressions and for activizing memories. Most patients showed delirium, although in a considerable number the delirium was easily overlooked because of the more obvious stupor, some degree of which occurred in the acute stage of nearly all cases. In a rather large proportion of cases emotional alterations continued after the acute phases and often constituted the only evidence of a lack of recovery. Among such mood alterations were irritability, explosive reactions, stubbornness and apathy.

Intellectual defects did not usually follow the disease except when the infection occurred at a very early age—usually four years or younger.

Behavior Disorders. In children the chronic stage of epidemic encephalitis was often associated with serious alterations in character and behavior, the severity of which bore no relation to that of the acute stage. In some cases, in fact, it was difficult to obtain any clear history of an acute attack. The restless overactivity, emotional irritability and impulsiveness of the early period were followed in a certain number or cases by lying, stealing, running away, cruelty, gross sexual offenses and other behavior comparable in many outward manifestations to that exhibited by the psychopathic child. The troublesome behavior disorders shown by the encephalitic child were of every variety and usually in a setting of constant hyperactivity. The behavior or the adequacy of the social adjustment showed no correlation with the neurological signs. The child's personality, too, might be completely changed yet his intellectual functions not be affected.

There seems to be reason for believing that psychogenic factors may have played a certain role in the production of these behavior disorders. Not infrequently, for example, the laity looked upon "sleeping sickness" as something mysterious and was therefore prone to suspect that its victim might somehow be peculiar. Such children soon became aware of this attitude. If, too, the victim suffered from strabismus, tremor, narcoleptic attacks, or from parkinsonism with its absence of expressive movements of the face, its rigidity of posture and gait and its slowness of speech, other children often called him "crazy," "dumb," or with taunting nicknames made him the laughingstock of his associates. Under these circumstances the child's feelings of inferiority and insecurity led to all sorts of undesirable defense reactions to his handicaps. During convalescence, in some instances, the child was overprotected, its training neglected and faulty, and regressive tendencies were permitted or encouraged.

Diagnosis. As already stated, acute cases of Type A encephalitis are no longer seen in the United States. A considerable number of patients, however, who exhibit the sequelae of the disease are still seen. The most common manifestations are tremor, rigidity and slowness of voluntary movements, which combine to form a neurological picture resembling in some ways the hepatolenticular degeneration of Wilson and, in others, paralysis agitans. Chronic epidemic encephalitis does not, of course, show the corneal pigmentation (Kayser-Fleischer rings), a mixed static and intention tremor, and the evidence of liver disease seen in Wilson's disease.

In degenerative parkinsonism one does not see the bizarre postures and gaits, the muscular spasms such as oculogyric crises, the coarse tremors or the behavioral peculiarities frequently seen among the sequelae of epidemic encephalitis.

While acute forms of von Economo's disease are no longer seen, one should perhaps remember that there are other forms of neurotropic virus infections that may cause such mental and neurological symptoms as drowsiness, confusion, stupor or coma, and other focal symptoms such as convulsions, hemiplegia, aphasia, ataxia, cranial nerve palsies, tremor, chorea, athetosis and rigidity. Among such forms of encephalitis are St. Louis encephalitis, equine encephalitis, and the occasional cases of encephalitis associated with mumps, measles, infectious mononucleosis and vaccination against cowpox. Residual psychiatric effects of infection with both eastern and western types of equine encephalomyelitis have been reported in the United States and Canada, also residuals following Japanese B encephalitis contracted by U. S. military personnel in Japan and Korea since 1950.

Prognosis. From 10 to 50 per cent of patients died during the acute phase of epidemic encephalitis, usually from respiratory paralysis. Of the survivors roughly 75 per cent, within a period varying from a few weeks to six years, developed signs of a continuing infection manifested by neurological, endocrine or metabolic disturbances or by behavior, mood or other personality disorder.

Treatment. Atropine, stramonium and scopolamine have long been used for postencephalitic parkinsonism. Artane (trihexyphenidyl), which is similar to atropine in chemical composition, may also be used. The initial dose should be 1 mg. the first day gradually increased, according to response, to 6 mg. to 10 mg. daily. Rabellon is also helpful. These drugs are more effective in relieving rigidity and associated asthenia than tremor. Benzedrine sulfate, administered orally two or three times a day, in doses of 25 mg. is useful in reducing oculogyric crises and for asthenia.

Acute Brain Syndrome Associated with Systemic Infection

In the case of the mental disturbances resulting from or associated with the infectious diseases that have thus far been mentioned, the infecting organism is located in the brain or its coverings. In many instances, however, mental disturbance may be associated with infections in which the infecting agent does not invade the central nervous system. Such temporary disturbances may result from many severe infections, such as typhoid fever or pneumonia, and appear especially during the febrile period and most frequently in the form of delirium. The syndrome of delirium has already been discussed in Chapter VI.

1. Deliria. Depending on their temporal relation to the febrile stage of the infection the deliria with infectious diseases are known as *initial delirium, febrile delirium* and *postfebrile delirium.*

Prefebrile Delirium. Initial or prefebrile delirium is a delirium that rather infrequently develops during the incubation or prodromal period of infectious diseases before there has been any rise in temperature. The cause of the delirium can naturally not be ascertained until symptoms diagnostic of the infection appear. Such deliria may be marked and often imply a serious prognosis.

Febrile Delirium. The delirium occurring during the febrile period of an infection is often spoken of as febrile delirium. The intensity of the symptoms is dependent less upon the height of the fever than upon the integration of the personality and the importance of psychogenic factors. The form of this, as of other delirioid reactions, is determined largely by individual personality factors. In milder degrees there may be merely restlessness, sensitiveness to light or noise, and disturbing dreams. In the more severe cases there will be hallucinations, confusion which may become extreme, indistinct muttering, stupor, twitching, carphologia, coma and death.

Postfebrile Delirium. Postfebrile delirium may be merely the continuation of a previous delirium into the postfebrile period of an infectious disease or it may be a delirium making its first appearance after the temperature has returned to normal. Consciousness is clouded to a variable degree, sometimes even to the point of stupor. In cases showing great prostration after the fall of the fever of infection, the symptoms may be of an extreme severity constituting what H. Weber in 1866 described as *collapse delirium.* In this there is clouding of consciousness or a stuporous state, sometimes marked confusion and great motor excitement that appear to be motivated by fear and may increase even to violence and destructiveness. The stream of talk may be an incoherent flight of ideas. Emaciation and exhaustion progress rapidly and a typhoid state, followed by stupor and coma, may develop. Death occurs in a few days in most of these malignant types of delirium although a few patients recover after a prolonged sleep.

2. Postinfectious Mental Disorders. These disorders differ somewhat from the postfebrile deliria just described. Delirium is not usually a conspicuous symptom, consisting, when it occurs, of a mild confusion and fleeting hallucinations. Rather more typical of the postinfectious mental disorders are states of easy exhaustion, reduced attention, restless irritability, difficulty in thinking, suspiciousness, anxious depression and hypochondriacal ideas. The patient is frequently easily frightened, oversensitive to light and noise, morose, complaining and preoccupied with his physical sense of weakness and debility. A state of physical exhaustion and prostration exists and is doubtless an important factor in the development of the disorder. If there has been a prolonged subvitaminosis there may be a retrospective falsification of memory suggesting Korsakoff's syndrome, which may be complete even to the existence of a polyneuritis. On rare occasions some degree of mental enfeeblement follows. Although the outstanding symptoms in the postinfectious disorders may be mental, yet their cessation depends upon the recovery of the patient's physical health.

3. Mental Disturbances with Trichiniasis. Trichiniasis is scarcely comparable to the infections which have just been discussed, yet mention may be made of the fact that occasionally mental disturbances occur in this disease if the young nematodes invade the cerebrum. The symptoms are those of the toxic-organic syndrome—confusion, cloudiness, disorientation, delirium, hebetude and, at times, confabulation. Occasionally signs of focal neurological disturbances are noted.

4. Acute Viral Hepatitis. With the increased recognition of acute viral hepatitis in recent years, the occasional association of mental dis-

turbances with this infection has been observed. In some instances this is a coincidence, as has been noted in public mental hospitals in which mild epidemics of infectious hepatitis have occurred. Occasionally, however, the infection releases a psychotic disturbance in poorly integrated personalities.

TREATMENT OF DELIRIUM. The treatment of delirium is primarily the treatment of the infection, toxic state or other disturbing factor that led to the reaction. This does not mean, however, that the delirium itself should not be actively treated. Occasionally a beginning delirium may be aborted by reducing environmental stimulation, an icecap to the head, the reassurance of the nurse, the administration of chlorpromazine or a hypnotic, such as paraldehyde. Precautions should be taken to prevent accidental injury or suicide. Unless carefully supervised, the delirious patient, usually disoriented and in some cases in intense fear, may unknowingly wander into danger or may attempt to escape imaginary enemies by suicide. Measures which tend to support his contact with his environment will lessen his fearfulness and anxiety. Such measures are the presence of close family members or familiar articles from his home in the room, a quiet environment with continuous light in the room day and night. Changes of environment or of physicians or nurses are apt to be disturbing. Greatly preferable to mechanical restraint are continuous baths or cold wet packs. The patient should receive an abundance of nourishment which should include a liberal amount of proteins and of carbohydrates. Chlorpromazine given by mouth or by intramuscular injection in doses of 25–50 mg. is often effective. Nicotinamide or multivitamin preparations are usually advisable. Sodium chloride or other salts and glucose, administered orally or intravenously, should be given liberally if needed to restore normal acid-base equilibrium. Caffeine may be advisable as a cardiac stimulant. The administration of sedatives should if possible be limited to the night. From 10 to 15 cc. of paraldehyde may be given in ice water, tea or wine. Bromides and the barbiturates should be avoided. Chloral hydrate (7½ to 15 grains) may be used. After the patient's recovery, the physician may be able to give considerable retrospective interpretation of delusional and hallucinatory experiences.

BIBLIOGRAPHY

Adams, R. D., and Weinstein, Louis: Clinical and pathological aspects of encephalitis. New England J. Med., *239:*865–876, 1948.

Bender, Loretta: Organic Brain Conditions Producing Behavior Disturbances. In Modern Trends in Child Psychiatry, by Lewis, N. D. C., and Pacella, B. L. New York, International Universities Press, 1945.

Bond, E. D., and Appel, K. E.: The Treatment of Behavior Disorders Following Encephalitis. New York, Commonwealth Fund, Division of Publications, 1931.

Debre, R.: Prognosis of tuberculous meningitis. Am. Rev. Tuberc., *67:*168–180, 1952.

Des Antels, E. J., and Pfuetze, K. H.: Chemotherapy of miliary and meningeal tuberculosis in the adult. Am. Rev. Tuberc., *68:*912, 1953.

Doty, E. J.: The diagnosis and treatment of delirious reactions. M. Clin. North America, *32:*647, 1948.

Ebaugh, F. G.: Neuropsychiatric aspects of chorea in children. J.A.M.A., *87:*1083, 1925.

Kinsman, J. M., and D'Alanze, C. A.: Meningococcemia: A description of the clinical picture and a comparison of the efficacy of sulfadiazine and penicillin in thirty cases. Ann. Int. Med., *24*:607–617, 1946.

Krauss, S.: Postchoreic personality and neurosis. J. Ment. Sc., *92*:75–95, 1946.

Larber, J.: The results of treatment of 549 cases of tuberculous meningitis. Am. Rev. Tuberc., *69*:13–25, 1954.

Mulder, D. W., Parrott, M., and Thaler, M.: Sequelae of western equine encephalitis. Neurol., *1*:318–327, 1951.

Neal, J. B.: Encephalitis: A Clinical Study. New York, Grune & Stratton, 1942.

Von Economo, Constantin: Encephalitis Lethargica, Its Sequelae and Treatment, Translated by K. O. Newman. New York, Oxford University Press, 1931.

CHAPTER IX

Brain Syndromes Resulting from Drug or Poison Intoxication

1. Lead

Of the various metallic poisons, lead is the one with which mental symptoms are most frequently associated. Both the source of intoxication with lead and the clinical picture differ considerably in adults and children. With adults the inhalations of toxic lead compounds is the major means of intoxication, while in infants poisoning occurs through the eating or chewing of lead containing paint often picked up in flakes peeling from woodwork or painted surfaces. The habit of "pica" in children is frequently associated with mental deficiency but it occurs also in children of good intellectual endowment who show some emotional disturbance. In adults the history of exposure in industry or building to paint spraying, burning of lead in salvage operations, the oxygas cutting of red lead, of painted steel and the dismantling of older structures, as well as vocational employment in bronze, solder or type metal or in the modern industrial practices of enameling and glass manufacture should suggest the possibility of exposure to poisonous lead-containing vapors.

Mental symptoms associated with lead poisoning tend to be of two types: (*a*) acute delirious episodes; (*b*) progressive mental deterioration. The delirious type may occur either in acute or chronic poisoning. It is of sudden onset characterized by confusion, insomnia, restlessness, tremors, fear, outbursts of violence, visual hallucinations, and delusions which are frequently persecutory in content. Convulsions may occur and be accompanied by a delirium in which the patient experiences terrifying visual hallucinations. In the chronic form, apathy or depression, speech defect, forgetfulness and at times confabulations suggesting the Korsakoff syndrome are frequently observed. The progressive mental deterioration may suggest general paresis. Occasionally the clinical picture is one of neurasthenia; the patient is irritable, depressed and complains of weakness, fatigability and dizziness. In association with the mental disturbances there is usually a history of colic, constipation and vomiting. The former is frequently more severe in adults than in children. In adults black deposits may be seen around the gum margins of pyorrheic teeth. This is seldom visible in children. There is usually an associated hypochromic anemia with basophilic stippling. In children there may be a mild renal glycosuria. Coproporphyrinuria commonly accompanies intoxication with lead. Roentgenograms will demonstrate dense radio-opaque bands going into the shafts of long bones in children. The spinal fluid protein content is increased to levels between 15 and 200 mg. per cent.

The chronic encephalopathy of children is characterized more by failure of cerebral maturation demonstrating itself in defects in attention, judgment, self-control and visual learning. Such children may be verbally facile but find it difficult to learn the techniques of reading, writing and arithmetic. In both adults and children, a characteristic peripheral neuritis is frequently seen. The most used muscle groups are affected rather than those supplied by individual nerves. Thus the extensors of the wrist are weak in adults and the dorsiflexors of the feet in children. All tendon reflexes are lost, sensation remains intact.

Treatment with calcium disodium versenate(ethylenediaminetetraacetic acid, EDTA), a chelating agent, which has the capacity of forming stable water soluble complexes with metals, is now recommended. It may be given intravenously and by mouth, 1 gm. to 15 kilograms of body weight per day. One-half the twenty-four-hour dose can be administered at intervals of twelve hours in 250 to 300 ml. of 5 to 10 per cent glucose solution. A test dose of 10 per cent of this amount is recommended. Treatment should be continued three to four days, followed by an interval of three days, and a total of three or four courses should be given. Investigation is now under way to determine if oral versene may be used in chronic cases to remove lead stored in the skeleton. This preparation is dangerous if lead is being ingested. Neurosurgical decompression of the skull may be required in patients with evidence of medullary compression. In addition to the specific therapy described above, patients with lead encephalopathy will require the general measures used in the care of the acute or acutely delirious states. Those with neuropathy should receive orthopedic protection of the weakened muscles and ligaments. In chronic lead poison alcohol is to be avoided; a high calcium diet supplemented by vitamin B_1 is indicated.

2. *Mercury*

Among the mental symptoms manifested by patients suffering from chronic mercury poisoning are irritability, timidity, discouragement, loss of self-confidence, fear and occasionally outbursts of extreme anger. Less frequent are apathy, drowsiness and impairment of memory. Chronic mercury poisoning results from the inhalation of volatile mercury for long periods of time. The hazardous trades are those concerned with the production of mercury and its derivatives, the manufacture of scientific apparatus, preparation of hatters' fur and felt hat making, the extraction of gold from silver by amalgamation and the application of antifouling plastic paint to the hulls of ships. There is usually a moderately fine but later coarse jerking tremor of the orbit, lips, tongue, fingers, limbs. Sometimes contractions of the limbs occur. The tremor is often intentional and subsides during rest. Weakness of both flexor and extensor muscles of the hand and forearm has been reported. No specific therapy is available for chronic mercury poisoning although dimercaprol (BAL) has been used in those with acute poisoning. Recovery results following withdrawal from exposure.

3. *Manganese*

Workers in manganese may suffer from permanently disabling mental and neurological symptoms. Among the principal neurological symptoms are those of extrapyramidal involvement including the basal ganglia. Gait and speech disturbances usually exist, also tremors of tongue and of the extremities and muscular weakness. About 20 per cent of cases show mental symptoms including restlessness, elation and uncontrollable laughter or crying. There is no specific therapy available for manganese poisoning.

4. *Carbon Disulfide*

The extensive use of carbon disulfide in the manufacture of rayon has resulted in the production of toxic psychoses through its destructive effect upon the lipid content of neural tissue. Among the most commonly observed early symptoms are insomnia, bad dreams, fatigue, impotence, listlessness and loss of memory. Neurologically there may be symptoms referable to almost any part of the central and peripheral nervous system. Among them are tenderness of nerve trunks and areas of hyperesthesia followed by loss of touch and pain sensation. Irritative signs of motor nerves include fibrillary twitching and spasmodic contraction of nerves. Among motor signs are early fatigue, weakness and flaccid paralysis. Basal ganglia symptoms may include parkinsonism, thalamic syndrome and choreo-athetosis. Diminution and loss of corneal and pupillary reflexes are common.

5. *Carbon Monoxide*

The gas which most frequently produces mental disturbances is carbon monoxide. The deleterious effects of this substance, which is either inhaled intentionally or by accident from the exhaust fumes of automobiles or, more infrequently, by inhalation of illuminating gas through defective combustion of coal in stoves, are caused by anoxemia of the brain. Carbon monoxide combines with hemoglobin to form carboxyhemoglobin, a stable compound which prevents the blood from absorbing oxygen. In those patients who die after several days the central nervous system shows ischemic changes of the nerve cells as well as areas of softening particularly in the cerebral cortex and the basal ganglia. Serious mental sequelae of carbon monoxide poisoning are infrequent in relation to the number of acute intoxications.

Mental symptoms following acute poisoning occur only in cases in which the intoxication has been extreme and unconsciousness complete. Of persons developing mental symptoms about two-thirds pass directly from the comatose condition into states of confusion and delirium. In the remainder there exists a clear period of a week or more between emergence from the coma and the appearance of mental symptoms among which are apathy, lack of initiative, and indifference to duties and responsibilities. Some patients continue to show confusion, bewilderment and impairment of memory with Korsakoff-like confabulations. Amnesia lasting from six to nine months may occur. In extreme cases, the patient sinks to the level of vegetative existence with incontinence, unresponsiveness and inability to carry on any voluntary activity. Occasionally a patient suffers from auditory aphasia. At times neurological complications may occur, owing usually to degenerative changes in the putamen or globus pallidus. Frequently, therefore, there is a modified parkinsonism with stiffness of extremities caused by muscular hypertonia. Most patients with mental sequelae of carbon monoxide poisoning begin to improve within a few weeks after exposure and completely recover within two years. Those who have not recovered within that period of time remain in a state of mild or severe mental enfeeblement.

Attention has been called to the immediate and to the delayed forms of mental sequelae arising from acute carbon monoxide anoxemia. Persons repeatedly subjected to moderate or minimal toxic amounts of the gas for periods ranging from several months to many years may develop mental and nervous symptoms. Among these manifestations are emotional instability, depression, agitation, anxiety, impairment of grasp and of memory, and at times confusion. Other symptoms are headache, vertigo, neuromuscular pains, digestive disturbances, dyspnea and palpitation.

6. Bromides

If administered in toxic amounts several salts of bromide may produce acute brain syndromes. A decade or more ago, with the development of methods of determining the bromide content of blood, it was found that mental disturbances resulting from bromides were more frequent than had been realized. In some psychiatric clinics 4 per cent of all admissions have been found to be suffering from bromide psychoses. The condition is now seen less frequently. About 50 per cent of cases arise through the prescribing of bromides by physicians, the prescription being repeatedly refilled. All too frequently additional amounts of the drug are further given in an effort to rid the patient of symptoms already caused by the bromides. Many toxic states arise through self-medication, principally by the use of proprietary preparations containing bromides. The normal bromide content of the blood serum varies from 0.33 to 1.73 mg. per 100 ml. Intoxication symptoms may be expected if the bromide content exceeds 150 mg. per 100 ml. of blood serum although there is a wide variation in susceptibility to the drug. The mechanism of bromide poisoning is through the replacement of the chloride with bromide. Elderly or arteriosclerotic patients have a poor tolerance and may develop toxic symptoms even though the blood content be relatively low. Bromides are excreted slowly and a mental disturbance may develop within two or three weeks after one begins to use amounts as small as 45 to 60 grains a day. Malnutrition, dehydration and arteriosclerosis render the patient more susceptible to the effects of bromides. Their use is at times associated with alcoholism.

In mild intoxication there may be a feeling of tiredness or weakness, irritability, broken sleep, slowness of mental grasp, inability to concentrate, faulty memory, drowsiness, impaired attention and perhaps even confusion. Physically one notes a dry skin, coated tongue, digestive disorders, impotence or menstrual disturbances, ataxic gait, tremors of tongue and fingers, and hyperactive, sluggish or absent deep reflexes. Dehydration is common. Protein elevation in the spinal fluid is frequent. Acne, considered an ordinary sign of bromidism, is often absent. In more severe intoxication the clinical picture is one of delirium with fever, confusion, clouding of consciousness, varying degrees of drowsiness or stupor, disorientation, difficulty in grasp, misidentification, motor restlessness even to the point of extreme excitement, fear, and memory loss accompanied by confabulations. Speech is thick, muttering, hesitant and slurred and the face mask-like and expressionless. The mood is often one of fear or depression. In bromide as in other toxic psychoses there may be a loss of the usual forces of repression with a resulting appearance of hallucinations. The ideational content of the delirium may be colored by individual psychogenic factors. Paranoid ideas are common. Occasionally a schizophrenic-like syndrome is observed. Bromide delirium may continue for ten days to two months. Remissions and exacerbations with sudden changes in the mental state are not uncommon.

The treatment consists of stopping the drug, the forcing of liquids and the administration of 2 to 4 gm. of sodium chloride every four hours unless gastric irritation forbids such large doses. Most patients can take a total of 4 to 6 gm. a day in divided doses if it is given in enteric-coated tablets. Recent investigations seem to show that bromides are excreted more rapidly by the administration of ammonium chloride than by sodium chloride. Ammonium chloride not only furnishes a chloride for displacing bromide but acts also as a diuretic. Cathartics are usually necessary for the obstinate constipation that often exists. Paraldehyde may be advisable at night.

The following clinical report of an acute reversible brain syndrome associated with bromidism illustrates not only the type of mental disorder associated with toxic states but also the sensorial and other disturbances often seen in delirium:

C. M., aged 38, was transferred to a mental hospital on October 22 from C. Hospital to which he had been admitted five days previously. His history prior to the present illness was without particular significance although apparently he was of a somewhat immature, unstable personality. His wife commented, "He could not sit for five minutes. He had to have the last word in everything. He felt that he was never to blame for any difficulty. He lost his temper easily." For several years he had drunk moderately but was never intoxicated. In September the patient became tense and greatly concerned because, after a brief and stormy marriage, his daughter had left her husband. About October 1 he began to drink more alcohol. Between October 9 and October 13 he consumed four "large bottles" of a proprietary drug product containing a large quantity of bromides. So far as known he took no alcohol during that period. On October 13 he appeared confused, showed a slurring of speech and an unsteadiness of gait. Soon, in addition to these symptoms he stated that he would shoot his son-in-law, also other members of his family. On October 17 he was admitted to the general hospital. There he was seen by a consulting psychiatrist who suggested that the patient's blood bromide content be determined. This was found to be 600 mg. per cent. The patient was confused, refused to stay in bed, showed poor motor co-ordination and one night locked himself in a closet. He thought he had a gun in bed with him. He made such irrelevant remarks as, "I know who shot him. I was behind the curtain." He told his wife that the patient in an adjoining bed had "killed the little girl on B Street," located near his home. No such incident had occurred. On October 21 he became much more confused, was completely disoriented and his speech quite incoherent. He heard gun shots in his room, said there were dead bodies there and that his wife was sleeping in the hospital with other patients. He attempted to jump from a window and it was necessary to place him in restraint pending his transfer to a mental hospital.

On arrival at the mental hospital he was found to be heavily sedated with paraldehyde. After emerging from the effects of this he was restless and constantly responded to both auditory and visual hallucinations. When asked where he was he replied that he was at "Mom's and Pop's place." Upon being asked why he was in bed he answered, "It seems to be a precaution to be parked here to smooch." He pointed to the bedcovers and said, "That's my wife there." He felt about the covers and remarked, "See that stone. It makes me G-d mad." He turned and shouted over his shoulder, "Well, come on, you might as well take it off. Sure going to get hell over that. What do you think of buying that place out"? By October 26 the patient was more co-operative but still disorganized and restless. A physician introduced himself to the patient who then said, "Yes, I heard about Hugh Pendleton. I better sleep pretty good tonight. He's got his offices at DeKalb and Jacoby Streets. Do you know it's him"? On October 29 he knew where he was, but gave the date as October 5 and had no recollection of having been in the C. Hospital. He stated that he had been depressed over his daughter's troubles and had taken triple bromides. For several following days there were periods during which he was noisy and restless and his verbal productions were incoherent and irrelevant. By November 9 his sensorium was fully clear and his apperception was intact. When asked about his experiences he replied, "I must have caused considerable uproar at home with my antics. They thought I was drunk. I insisted I was not. I took it upon myself to take that bromide medicine for my nerves. My wife tells me I was in C. Hospital for four days. It's a blank wall. It seems I only really started remembering things from last Saturday when my family saw me. My folks were telling me about some of the stuff that I did. I sure feel like an ass."

On November 10 the patient's blood bromide content had been reduced to 75 mg. per cent. His convalescence continued without interruption and on November 20 he was discharged as recovered.

7. *Cortisone and ACTH*

These drugs may produce a wide variety of mental disturbances resulting, apparently, from their direct effect upon the central nervous system although the precise pathogenetic mechanisms are not yet determined. The total energy exchange of the brain as measured by cerebral metabolic rate does not seem to be altered by ACTH or by cortisone, yet these hormones disturb enzymatic reactions by altering the electrolyte and water patterns of the body. In general, the mental reactions do not exhibit the type of confusion, disorientation and sensorial disturbance characteristic of toxic psychoses. Nearly all patients receiving the drug show an increased joviality and optimism. Among the common disturbances are affective ones varying from depression to hypomania, also from apathy to panic, and even inappropriateness of affect. Feelings of depersonalization, or a sense of detachment or strangeness in awareness of one's body image, may occur. Disturbances of speech are frequent and may vary from mutism to flight of ideas. Illusions and hallucinations may occur, as also do delusions of depressive, grandiose or persecutory types. A wide variety of motor disturbances may appear including immobility, pressure of activity and regressiveness. In general the type of mental disturbance produced by the drug seems to be determined by the basic pattern or structure of the patient's personality. Complete spontaneous recovery occurs upon discontinuance of the drug. In prolonged cases, lucid intervals of gradually increasing frequency and duration may occur until a normal state is fully established.

8. *Isoniazid*

With the increasing use of this drug for the treatment of tuberculosis a number of cases of mental disturbance have been observed associated with its administration. The clinical picture is that of an acute, toxic, confusional disorientation for time, place, person and situation, restlessness and auditory or visual hallucinations. It is usually preceded by muscular twitching, hyperreflexias, difficulty in micturition, constipation and sometimes convulsions. Occasionally this toxic state is followed by signs of an organic cerebral impairment of the Korsakoff type. It has been stated that the toxic mental symptoms are related to the plasma level of the drug and that the majority of psychotic reactions occur in patients receiving more than 8 mg. of isoniazid per kilogram of body weight daily. Pyridoxine in large doses may prevent the appearance of isoniazid neuritis. Once established, this agent is not effective in reversing symptoms.

9. *Sympathomimetic Amines (Benzedrine, Dexedrine and Desoxyn)*

Chronic poisoning with the sympathomimetic amines, amphetamine, (Benzedrine), methamphetamine (Desoxyephedrine or Desoxyn), may be brought about by the continuing use of these agents. All have cortical excitant action in addition to their sympathomimetic action. They produce a feeling of well being and exhilaration which may lead to a persistent craving. The stimulation produced by the drug is followed by fatigue and depression. As tolerance is acquired increasingly larger doses are necessary to produce the desired stimulation. Their abuse occurs commonly in the case of alcoholics and barbiturate addicts. They are popular among thrill-seeking adolescents and inmates of penal institutions. These drugs are almost always taken as tablets. Amphetamine inhalers no longer constitute a problem since they are not available. Some users have taken individual doses as high as 250 mg. of amphetamine and a total daily intake of 1 to 1½ grams. The symptomatology produced by the drugs is similar to that of intoxication with cocaine. Tension, apprehension, jerky and tremulous movements are noted in conjunction with tachycardia, hypertension, mydriasis, insomnia and anorexia. A hallucinatory psychosis and paranoid delusions may occur in certain individuals. Treatment should include the use of sedation and abrupt withdrawal of the drug with the institution of a program of psychotherapy to correct the underlying personality defect requiring habitual use of the drugs.

10. Sulfonamides ("Sulfa" drugs)

The administration of sulfa drugs may at times cause headache, dizziness, confusion, bewilderment, inability to concentrate and hallucinosis.

11. Thiocyanates

The continuing use of thiocyanates in the treatment of hypertensive disease with the occurrence of toxic mental symptoms must be kept in mind. Levels of blood thiocyanate that exceed 15 mg. per 100 ml. are likely to produce toxic reactions. It has been shown that thiocyanates are converted to cyanide in the body and this cellular poison probably leads to depression of utilization of oxygen by inhibition of cytochrome oxidase. The consequent oxygen lack in the cerebral cortex leads to the production of the delirious reactions as well as to other symptoms such as convulsions, ataxia, aphasia and paraplegia. The usual toxic mental symptoms are incoherent muttering, slurring of speech, confusion, disorientation, auditory and visual hallucinations, restlessness, agitation, resistance, ideas of persecution and convulsions. Several deaths have been reported. In addition to withholding the thiocyanate, a trial with methylene blue or sodium thiosulfate is probably worthwhile. It has been suggested that hydroxycobalamine (Vitamin B_{12}) may serve as a potent antidote. The following case illustrates a thiocyanate intoxication:

A fifty-nine-year-old housewife, admitted as an emergency case, complained of "pain all over." She claimed she was paralyzed, yet tossed restlessly about on the ambulance cot. She was confused and unable to give a coherent story. Her daughter said the illness started with a severe dizzy spell that had occurred two months earlier. Her home physician had found that her blood pressure was "over 300," and had prescribed some red tablets. She had continued to take the medicine until she came to the hospital although at no time had a blood test been made. Three weeks prior to admission general weakness, tremor of the hands, somnolence, tinnitus and blurring of vision had developed. These symptoms had become progressively more severe in the meantime.

On physical examination the patient complained volubly of unbearable tenderness in all her muscles. Her systolic blood pressure was 150 mm. Hg. and the diastolic 80 mm. There was narrowing and sclerosis of the retinal arterioles. No neurological deficit was detected although the weakness she described was confirmed.

The concentration of thiocyanate in the blood was 17.6 mg. per 100 ml. and a diagnosis of thiocyanate psychosis was made. On mental examination she was depressed, withdrawn, negativistic and distractible. Delusional, self-derogatory thinking was disclosed by her statements that other patients regarded her as a germ carrier and that her physicians thought she was a nuisance and wanted to "fumigate" her. Hallucinations were not evident. She spoke haltingly and cried easily. She was disoriented as to time but not as to place or person. She was unable to repeat more than five digits forward and none backward. Simple multiplication was impossible and she was unable to subtract serial sevens. Her memory was severely impaired for both recent and past events.

Further studies disclosed a blood urea concentration of 60 mg. per 100 ml. and a normal urine except for albuminuria, grade 1. She had a mild anemia the hemoglobin measuring 10.3 gm. per 100 ml. and the erythrocyte count being 3,000,000 per cubic millimeter. A blood smear revealed no specific abnormalities. A roentgenogram of the thorax, an electrocardiogram and an excretory urogram likewise did not disclose any abnormality. A provocative test with histamine did not give any evidence of pheochromocytoma, a possibility suggested by the history that her blood pressure on one occasion had exceeded "300."

With a high intake of fluid, the signs of toxic delirium subsided rapidly. The concentration of blood thiocyanate decreased to 8.7 mg. per 100 ml. by the eleventh day in the hospital and there was only mild residual tenderness in the calves of her legs. When she was dismissed on the twentieth day her blood pressure was 150/90 and she was free of symptoms.

12. *Other Drugs*

Several other drugs may occasionally produce delirium, particularly belladonna, chloral hydrate and paraldehyde. Of these, belladonna probably leads most frequently to toxic symptoms. Occasionally patients, especially children, may develop delirium following the introduction of atropine into the eye. In addition to the usual physiological symptoms the patient manifests a delirium marked by fear, excitement and visual and auditory hallucinations. Prolonged use of chloral hydrate may lead to a delirium lasting two or more weeks.

BIBLIOGRAPHY

Angyal, A.: Predisposing factors in bromide intoxication. Arch. Neurol. & Psychiat., *49*:359–382, 1943.

Blackman, S. S., Jr.: Lesions of lead encephalitis in children. Bull. Johns Hopkins Hosp., *61*:1–61, 1937.

Byers, R. K., and Maloof, C.: Edathamil calcium disodium (versanate) in treatment of lead poisoning in children. Am. J. Dis. Child., *87*:559–569, 1954.

Clarke, L. D., Bauer, Walter, and Cobb, Stanley: Preliminary observations on mental disturbances occurring in patients under therapy with cortisone and ACTH. New England J. Med., *246*:205–216, 1952.

Curran, F. J.: Current views on neuropsychiatric effects of barbiturate and bromides. J. Nerv. & Ment. Dis., *100*:142–169, 1944.

Domzalski, C. A., Kolb, L. C., and Hines, E. A.: Delirious reactions secondary to thiocyanate therapy of hypertension. Proc. Staff Mtgs., Mayo Clinic, *28*:272–280, 1953.

Flinn, R. H., et al.: Chronic Manganese Poisoning in an Ore-Crushing Mill. U. S. Pub. Health Serv. Bull. 247. Government Printing Office, 1940.

Goolker, P., and Schein, J.: Psychic effects of ACTH and cortisone. Psychosom. Med., *15*:589–613, 1953.

Isbell, H.: Chronic Poisoning with Sympathomimetic Amine. In Cecil and Loeb, Textbook of Medicine, 9th ed., 1955, p. 578.

Jenkins, C. D., and Mellins, R. B.: Lead poisoning in children. Arch. Neurol. & Psychiat., 77:70–78, 1957.

Karpinski, F. E., Rieders, F., and Gersh, L. S.: Calcium disodium versenate in the therapy of lead encephalopathy. J. Pediat., *42*:687–699, 1953.

Lindemann, E., and Clarke, L. D.: Modifications in ego structure and personality reactions under the influence of the effects of drugs. Am. J. Psychiat., *108*:561–567, 1952.

Perkins, H. A.: Bromide intoxication. Arch. Int. Med., *85:*783–794, 1950.
Pleasure, H.: Psychiatric and neurologic side effects of isoniazid and iproniazid. Arch. Neurol. & Psychiat., *72:*313–320, 1954.
Ritchie, E. A.: Toxic psychosis under cortisone and corticotrophin. J. Ment. Sc., *102:*830–837, 1956.
Shillito, F. H., Drinker, C. K., and Shaughnessy, T. J.: The problems of nervous and mental sequelae in carbon monoxide poisoning. J.A.M.A., *106:*669–674, 1936.
Tillin, S. J.: Bromide intoxication. Am. J. Psychiat., *109:*196–202, 1952.

CHAPTER X

Alcoholism and Alcoholic Psychoses

"In the bottle, discontent seeks for comfort, cowardice for courage, and bashfulness for confidence."
SAMUEL JOHNSON (1709–1784)

ALCOHOLISM and the disturbances of metabolism often associated with it may lead to both acute and chronic brain syndromes. It seems desirable, however, to include a discussion of both of these syndromes in one chapter as well as that of various other aspects of indulgence in alcohol.

The subject of the use and effect of alcoholic liquors, whether considered from sociological, physiological or psychiatric points of view, still provokes much discussion and wide divergence of opinion. Unfortunately, moralistic implications have retarded the development of a scientific understanding and rational management of alcoholism. Perhaps there is no group of persons in greater need of understanding than alcoholics. It is estimated that there are about four and one-half million persons in United States on whose lives drinking has an adverse effect in one way or another, also that at least 12,000 alcoholics die each year from chronic alcoholism. Five out of six alcoholics are men between the ages of 30 and 55—the most productive years. Alcoholism, therefore, constitutes a major health problem.

Psychogenic Factors in Alcoholism

Psychological knowledge and experience show that a practice so universal as that of the use of alcohol must exist because it satisfies some deep-seated psychological need. This need, it often appears, is for relief from the tensions which have been induced by conflicts, resentments, frustrations and other sources of anxiety. Anxiety is such a constant and universal experience of mankind and alcohol is so effective in alleviating it that its use has become very wide. A well adjusted person has his anxieties but is able to manage them without resorting to measures that tend to disturb his personality. His personality is mature, relatively well organized, and his tolerance for anxiety, guilt and frustration is adequate. His need for relief from these factors is small and may be met by a few mildly neurotic traits. In contrast, if the individual is emotionally dependent and immature and his tensions are extreme or his tolerance for anxiety and frustration is low he may either develop a neurotic reaction or resort to excessive drinking, even to intoxication and its blotting out of reality, as an easy means of relief and of handling his difficulties. Any act that readily results in a reduction of anxiety tends to become a habit. All too frequently, therefore, the use of alcohol as a means of narcotizing anxiety becomes habitual. The strength of the habit depends upon the degree of anxiety which prompts it. At the same time, also, the alcoholic, below the level of conscious awareness, develops an obsessive nucleus of thoughts and feelings that drinking, and only drinking, will effectively quiet the maladjustments that make life uncomfortable or even unbearable. Alcohol serves, too, to create a vicious circle that aids in fixing the habit. Its use lowers the capacity for repression and tends to release inhibitions. Anxiety is therefore stimulated and even more alcohol is required for its relief. Thus, alcohol is liable to defeat the ends for which it is taken. As a result, too, of his excessive drinking, the alcoholic addict develops aggressive tendencies, also resentments and feelings of guilt and remorse. Such feelings and reactions constitute sources of more excessive indulgence.

Why, with the many neurotic, psychosomatic or psychotic methods of defense or escape equally available, the individual makes use of alcohol is not readily determined. A person with strongly developed defense mechanisms, although he may acquire a restricted personality through them, often becomes able to protect himself against anxiety through the development of character traits or other internal operation. A person who lacks such automatic protection against anxiety may develop either alcoholism or neurosis. Either or both may be established to deal with similar types of anxiety-producing problems. Somehow the alcoholic is unable to construct as defenses against anxiety the character traits which the relatively well adjusted person employs or the overt neurotic symptoms which the psychoneurotic constructs. Sometimes, moreover, a patient, after long use of alcohol as an anxiety-reducing measure, finds this expedient inadequate and he resorts also, as it were, to an overt anxiety neurosis, to psychosomatic symptoms or to a psychosis, as a more drastic measure for dealing with his anxieties, frustrations and conflicts. The psychopathologic conditions leading to alcoholism vary with the individual alcoholic. It would appear in many instances that the addictive drinker may have been psychologically traumatized very early in life and his personality remained fixated at an early, oral stage of development. Again alcoholism may occur in persons who through the absence of a desirable identification figure never developed a stabilizing superego. Lacking in responsibility and ego strength, they are closely allied to the character neurotic. Sometimes the periodic drinker seems by his alcoholic bout to be seeking for relief from an overly strict superego. In some instances there are presumably unconscious homosexual identifications and tendencies. If his drinking continues and the alcoholic pattern becomes established, the disregard of reality which it brings about begins to operate and serves as a further but undesirable defense.

From what has been said, it naturally follows that an understanding of the psychopathologic conditions associated with alcohol can only be obtained by taking into account the developmental organization of the individual personality and its sources of anxiety rather than by stressing any specifically poisonous properties of alcohol. The particular reaction manifested by the individual is usually, in effect, an unmasking or accentuation of his previous personality, of its conflicts and of its defenses. If excessive alcoholism is continued, a social deterioration and a disintegration of the patient's value system frequently results from his habit.

Social and cultural factors influence the amount of alcoholism. It is, for example, distinctly less frequent among Jews and Chinese. Doubtless in some instances heavy drinking is merely the result of a wish to conform to group mores and represents a needed prestige-giving activity. Broadly speaking, however, the causes of alcoholism are the same as are productive of neuroses in the nonalcoholic. If an individual with a low anxiety tolerance lives in a social set which imposes heavy social penalties on intoxication, he may take recourse to other and frankly neurotic escapes. In general, anxieties, frustrations, fixations in psychosexual development, prolonged strain of situational difficulties, are other mainsprings of unconscious motivations for alcoholism. While alcoholism is symptomatic of psychopathology it is a symptom which has become a disease.

Physiological Effects

While alcohol affects all cells of the body the most marked effect is on the cells of the brain and is therefore manifested in behavior. Since alcohol does not require prior digestion, it may be absorbed directly into the blood. The rate of absorption is much more rapid than its elimination, with the result that with heavy indulgence a considerable concentration may occur. While there is an individual tolerance it is generally accepted that a person showing a concentration of 150 mg. or more of alcohol in 100 ml. of blood, or its equivalent in urine, saliva or breath, should be considered as intoxicated. In the opinion of the National Safety Council Committee on Tests for Intoxication, this concentration so impairs judgment and performance in driving an automobile as to render the operation of a car unsafe.

The first stage in the oxidation of alcohol consists in the formation of acetaldehyde. While to some degree this occurs elsewhere, it largely takes place in the liver. With the use of disulfiram combustion of acetaldehyde is inhibited and may reach toxic levels. The second stage of oxidation of alcohol is from acetaldehyde to acetic acid. This occurs not only in the liver but in other organs as well. Finally acetic acid is oxidized to carbon dioxide and water.

As previously indicated, alcohol is used for its tension-reducing effect. Since it reduces his anxiety, the alcoholic seeks its use more and more frequently and to the exclusion of more acceptable methods. His addiction is manifested not only by this persistent use but also by the effects of its withdrawal. These results may be moderate such as increased anxiety, a craving for alcohol, weakness, tremor and perspiration but may be even serious and include anorexia, nausea, vomiting, fever, tachycardia, convulsions, hallucinations and delirium tremens.

Although alcohol has long been known to be a depressant to brain function, its method of action is still uncertain. It is thought that it may be by interference with synaptic transmission. The effect of alcohol on the brain is from above downward. Higher cortical functions such as judgment, memory, learning, self-criticism and environmental awareness suffer first. With depression of higher functions, lower parts of the brain are released from higher control. Thus the excitement frequently seen in an intoxicated person is doubtless a release phenomenon resulting from a depression of the highest brain functions. With the ingestion of excessively large amounts of alcohol, this gradually descending depressive effect may extend to the entire brain and inhibit not only the supramedullary areas but even the medulla with its respiratory, cardiac and vasomotor centers.

Alcoholism and Crime

It was formerly stated that alcoholism was directly responsible for a large, perhaps a major, part of crime. There is now an increasing tendency to consider that both alcohol and criminalism are caused by similar social and psychological factors. Emotional instability and other expressions of a poorly integrated personality characterize both the recidivous criminal offender and the alcohol addict. More frequently is the relation of alcohol to crime one of a common cause rather than of cause and effect. It should be added, however, that the drinking of alcohol tends to be accompanied by a release of sexual and aggressive impulses.

Alcoholism and Psychoses

The relation between alcohol and the so-called alcoholic psychoses is not as simple as formerly assumed. In many instances alcohol serves merely to release a reaction that is primarily psychogenic with factors intrinsic in the personality. In other cases there is such an interplay of psychogenic and metabolic factors that the picture becomes complex. In Korsakoff's syndrome and in chronic alcoholic deterioration, the psychosis is not, as formerly believed, caused by the toxic effects of the alcohol itself but by thiamine deficiency. Even in this, the structure of the personality influences the picture. It is important to remember, too, that alcoholism may be a symptom—sometimes the most obvious symptom—of another psychosis such as paresis or manic depressive psychosis.

Pathological Intoxication

Occasionally an individual of unstable personality may, on partaking of alcohol, suffer from a transitory mental state much more striking in the nature and severity of the symptoms than ordinary drunkenness, and known as pathological intoxication. The onset is dramatically sudden. Consciousness is impaired and the patient is confused, disoriented, suffers from illusions, hallucinations of sight and transitory delusions. Activity is exaggerated, impulsive and aggressive, even to the point of destructiveness. The emotional disturbances are profound and may consist of rage, anxiety or of depression, perhaps with suicidal attempt. The disorder lasts from a few minutes to a day or more and is usually followed by a prolonged sleep, after awakening from which there is an amnesia for the episode.

There is an increasing tendency to consider that such episodes with their disturbances of consciousness and perhaps crimes of violence are really instances of psychomotor epilepsy released by alcohol in persons predisposed to such seizures.

The behavior observed in "pathological intoxication" is in many ways illustrated by the following case:

N. W., aged twenty-eight, was seen in jail while awaiting trial on a charge of drunkenness and disorderly conduct. The patient's father had committed suicide as he was about to be sent to a hospital for mental diseases. The patient himself was described as being a friendly but quick-tempered and restless individual whose marriage had terminated in early divorce. He was said never to have been particularly alcoholic but on one July 4 he celebrated the holiday by drinking two bottles of beer and a glass of wine. Soon afterward he attempted to fling himself down an 80-foot embankment and was so greatly excited that he was taken to the police station for the night. The next morning he had no recollection of the affair. Ten months later the patient called late one afternoon to see friends who invited him to sample what they considered choice varieties of whiskey and gin. He accepted their invitation and drank somewhat more heavily than usual. Soon after leaving the home of his friends he was observed by a police officer to be acting strangely. As the officer spoke to him he attacked him. While the officer was calling for help, the patient disappeared. About fifteen minutes later two women were startled to see a strange man thrust his head through a closed window of their living room and shout, "Help! Murder!" It was the patient, who then ran on to another house where he rang the doorbell insistently. As the occupant answered the summons he again screamed, "Murder!" and ran to the street once more where he broke the windshields and headlights of several parked automobiles and tore out the seats and pulled parts from other cars. At this point he was seized and taken to the police station where, on awakening the following morning, he had no recollection of his experiences of the previous night.

Treatment of Acute Alcoholism

In many ways a satisfactory method of treating severe cases of acute alcoholism is by the use of insulin which accelerates the metabolism of alcohol in the body. Before administration, it is advisable to determine the blood sugar level to make sure that the insulin is not given during a hypoglycemic state. If there is no contraindication to its use, the patient is placed in bed and given 46 to 60 units of insulin hypodermically. If this amount is not sufficient to produce somnolence, thirst and diaphoresis in one and a half hours, 20 additional units may be given intravenously. Because of the possibility of convulsions, an experienced nurse should be in constant attendance. If the initial dose produces convulsions or deep coma, the patient should receive 5 to 10 gm. of glucose intravenously or

4 to 6 oz. of sweetened fruit juice by mouth. Treatment, with its relaxation and sleep, is continued for two and one-half hours and then terminated by the administration of 8 oz. of fruit juice to which an ounce of sugar is added. While under the influence of insulin, the patient is given large quantities of water to drink. Following the treatment, he receives a full meal. One treatment may be sufficient but two, three or four may be required. More than one treatment in the first twenty-four hours may be advisable.

In cases of prolonged drinking, the patient may be much dehydrated and be vomiting. In such a case liquids containing nutritional elements may be given intravenously. A saline solution containing 5 per cent of dextrose may be given in 1000- to 2000-ml. doses in the course of twelve to twenty-four hours. This may be repeated every day for three days if necessary. It is well to add an ampoule of vitamin B complex and ascorbic acid.

If the patient is extremely drowsy and somnolent or depressed as a result of excessive ingestion of alcohol, such effects can be counteracted by the use of caffeine and sodium benzoate, dexedrine, Benzedrine or Ritalin.

Other Drugs. The various barbiturates have been widely used. Today, however, the consensus is that these drugs are neither necessary nor desirable in the treatment of the alcoholic. Their habituating properties will often lead the addictive alcoholic to switch from his alcohol to barbiturates for relief. Another drug that has enjoyed great popularity is paraldehyde. It is little more than a hypnotic, however, and renders the patient sleepy and drowsy even after awakening. If it is desired to continue this drug with chlorpromazine, it should be remembered that the chlorpromazine has a potentiating effect on the sedative and but a fraction of the ordinary dose of paraldehyde should be given. For a long time the use of the aqueous solution of adrenal cortex extract was popular and is still used intravenously to some extent. The dosage varies from 10 to 30 ml. in 1000 ml. of saline solution injected over a period of several hours.

Chlorpromazine, or chlorpromazine and meprobamate combined, are now extensively used to relieve the symptoms of acute alcoholism. Used in relatively large doses they produce prompt control of motor excitement and of nausea and vomiting, permit restful, relaxed sleep and contribute to the relief of tension and anxiety.

Delirium Tremens

This is an acute psychosis that may develop in the chronic alcoholic following an unusually severe or prolonged debauch. The term *delirium tremens* was first used by Thomas Sutton in 1813 in what is regarded as the classic description of this disease. The nature of the factors that operate in its production is uncertain. It has long been considered as an acute psychosis developed during drinking. At the present time, however, some psychiatrists believe it is a withdrawal syndrome precipitated in the chronic alcoholic suddenly deprived of alcohol. In some instances, at least, this is probably the case as delirium has been produced in the experimental laboratory by the sudden withdrawal of alcohol in those consuming 12 oz. or more of the agent for 48 or more days. The withdrawal may be associated not only with delirium and sometimes with convulsions but also abnormalities in the encephalogram. On the other hand, the disorder may arise from metabolic disturbances including faulty carbohydrate metabolism, impairment of the detoxicating function of the liver, disturbed protein metabolism, acidosis, suboxidation of the brain, disturbed water balance and various nutritional deficiencies, particularly of vitamin B which the alcoholic usually takes in insufficient amounts and may not be able to absorb. Absorption of toxins from the gastrointestinal tract may also be a factor in producing the toxic state. The patient is usually dehydrated and the blood chlorides are low.

Delirium tremens is rare in a person under thirty years of age, or after less than three or four years of chronic alcoholism. The delirium is usually preceded by an aversion for food, restlessness, irritability and disturbed sleep in which terrifying dreams occur. Occasional illusions and hallucinations are soon followed by more frequent ones, usually of a fleeting, terrifying nature. Figures on the wallpaper become menacing animate objects; inkspots become insects which the patient attempts to seize and destroy. The visual hallucinations are often of objects that appear to be moving, and are particularly apt to represent loathsome animals of fantastic shapes which terrify the patient and from which he may struggle to escape. These imaginary animals may be of diminutive size. At times hallucinations can be suggested; the patient, for example, may be handed an imaginary thread which in response to instructions he will carefully wind about his finger. Tactile hallucinations, probably associated with a peripheral neuritis, are not infrequent. The patient feels as well as sees the insects on his skin. Olfactory hallucinations may occur. The patient may exclaim with terror that gas is being pumped into his room. While visual hallucinations are most numerous, yet auditory ones are not infrequently added.

As indicated, the mood is usually one of irritability, fear, apprehension and even of terror. Occasionally, however, it is one of euphoria, amusement, good-natured silliness or grim humor accompanied by the narration of preposterous confabulations.

Consciousness is clouded and the patient may be greatly confused with disorientation for time and place. Speech is often incoherent. Persons about the patient may be misidentified. Attention is fleeting and impressions are retained but a moment. Not rarely the delirium is of an occupational type. The motor restlessness is marked. The patient repeatedly gets out of bed to attend to some detail of his supposed occupation or to seize some imaginary object. Sleep is usually impossible.

On physical examination, the conjunctivae and face are ordinarily found to be congested. The pupils are dilated and often react slowly. A coarse tremor is an almost constant accompaniment. It is increased by muscular tension, such as extension of the fingers. The tongue is tremulous, as are also the muscles of the lips and face in well developed cases. The pulse is rapid and often irregular and weak. The temperature is elevated and in some cases may be high. The skin is moist, the face often showing marked perspiration. The tendon reflexes are usually increased although occasionally absent because of neuropathy. At times the nerve trunks and muscles may be painful to pressure. Albuminuria exists in about half the cases. Epileptiform seizures may occur. The cause of the seizures is somewhat uncertain. At times the patient is an epileptic in whom convulsions were precipitated by alcohol. Again they may be caused by toxic products in the alcohol or by cerebral damage that has resulted from its use. As mentioned before, convulsions may follow sudden withdrawal of alcohol in the chronic drinker.

Pathology

Changes both of a degenerative and of an inflammatory nature may occur. The brain is usually edematous. There is more or less liquefaction degeneration of nerve cells and an increase of glia with some round-cell infiltration. There is degeneration of myelin sheaths, especially in the cerebellum. Punctate hemorrhages occur and a mild degree of leptomeningitis.

Prognosis and Course

Delirium tremens usually runs an acute course terminating in from three to ten days. Convalescence is frequently preceded by a prolonged sleep following which consciousness becomes clear and the hallucinations disappear although brief periods of delirium may occasionally recur at night for a short time. The prognosis depends largely upon the presence or absence of coexisting disease. The existence of a myocardial degeneration, which is not uncommon in such chronic alcoholic patients, makes the prognosis much less favorable. The mortality in the type of case that reaches a hospital averages from 5 to 15 per cent, the two most frequent causes of death being heart failure and pneumonia. Occasionally, instead of terminating in death or recovery within the usual period the psychosis may merge into a Korsakoff's psychosis.

Treatment

It has been customary to withdraw alcohol at once but this practice is questionable. Gastric lavage is advisable both to remove any remaining alcohol and the mucus and other products of a chronic gastritis. It is of great importance that care must be taken to conserve the strength of a patient suffering from delirium tremens. The patient suffering from this disease should be placed in bed immediately and as he is usually fearful he should be constantly supervised and be reassured concerning his fears and hallucinations. Many a patient has died from exhaustion while struggling under mechanical restraint or from the depressing effect of sedative drugs. Restraint should therefore never be employed. Chlorpromazine, given in divided doses either orally or by the intramuscular route and up to 1.0 gm. in a twenty-four hour period, has proven effective in preventing overactivity, providing sleep and improving appetite. While it does not modify the delusional or hallucinatory state nor shorten the course greatly.

the anxiety is much relieved. The agent is contraindicated when serious infection or cardiac disturbance coexists or following the recent use of other drugs. Cardiac stimulation by means of caffeine is usually to be recommended. It is frequently desirable to give some of the less depressing hypnotics such as paraldehyde in 3- to 4-drachm doses one to three times a day. Other sedation should be avoided. Morphine should never be given. Corticotropin in 25-mg. doses at four-hour intervals may help to bring about a more rapid recovery. This can be given intramuscularly or intravenously in dextrose and saline solution.

It is generally agreed that the patient should receive large amounts of dextrose, the normal nutritive material of the brain. This may be given in the form of frequent, large quantities of orange juice or as intravenous administration of 100 ml. of 50 per cent glucose repeated, if necessary, every three hours. Thiamine chloride (50 to 100 mg.) and nicotinic acid (10 mg.) should be given immediately and repeated three times daily. These vitamins may be added to the infusions for intravenous use. Alcohol disappears from the blood more rapidly if the patient receives 15 units of insulin three or four times a day. The administration of sodium chloride is advisable both to combat dehydration and to increase the alkali reserve. Capsules containing 2 gm. of sodium chloride should be given every four hours. In those patients where delirium and marked tremor exist the possibility of a magnesium deficiency must be considered. With evidence of depression of the serum magnesium (normal 2.0 milliequivalent per liter), magnesium sulfate in a 5 per cent sterile solution may be given in doses up to 2.0 gm. four times daily for three days and then 1.0 gm. per day for an additional two or three days.

Unless the patient is also suffering from cardiac failure or other general medical contraindication he should receive 3000 to 4000 ml. of fluids a day. Orange juice is by far the most desirable form of liquid, since it combats acidity, supplies certain minerals and vitamin C, and perhaps helps to prevent or overcome infection. Milk should also be given freely. Many physicians recommend the use of high enemas twice a day both for the chronic constipation usually existing and for the additional fluids thus made available. The former practice of dehydrating the patient on the theory that he may have cerebral edema ("wet brain") is no longer followed. Likewise, very few physicians now recommend lumbar puncture for the purpose of withdrawing cerebrospinal fluid. The patient has usually eaten little or nothing for several days. Since his gastrointestinal tract suffers from catarrhal inflammation because of his long indulgence in alcohol, he has little appetite and may even be nauseated. It is, however, exceedingly important that he receive an abundant, soft diet, particularly of carbohydrates. If possible, it should contain from 3000 to 4000 calories a day and should be rich in vitamins. The administration of the entire vitamin B complex would seem especially advisable as a preventive of Wernicke's syndrome or nicotinic acid deficiency encephalopathy. One should not hesitate to employ tube feeding if necessary.

Korsakoff's Psychosis

Sometimes it will be noted in what, except for the absence of the usual critical sleep, appeared to be an ordinary case of delirium tremens that the hallucinations and acute delirium disappear but the clinical picture merges into one characterized by amnesia, disorientation for time and place and a falsification of memory, associated with the symptoms and signs of a peripheral neuropathy. At other times the syndrome develops in the chronic alcoholic who has not suffered from a preceding delirium tremens but has indulged excessively in alcohol for several years. This syndrome was described in 1887 by the Russian psychiatrist Sergei Korsakoff. Because of its frequent association with chronic alcoholism Korsakoff's psychosis has long been classified among the alcoholic psychoses. Strictly speaking, this syndrome should not be classified among them. It is but one of several syndromes that result from vitamin B deficiency, a form of deficiency to which the chronic alcoholic with his impaired gastrointestinal absorption, his diet largely limited to vitamin-free alcohol and his increased vitamin requirement resulting from the high caloric effect of alcohol, is especially prone. Vitamin B deficiency may, of course, exist under various circumstances. While a deficiency of other vitamin B constituents doubtless contributes to these syndromes, thiamine and niacin deficiencies are particularly responsible for them. The variations in these syndromes depend largely upon the parts of the nervous system in which the neuronal degeneration is localized. If this degeneration is largely in the cerebrum and the peripheral nerves, a Korsakoff's syndrome results. If the degenerative changes occur in the long peripheral nerves of the alcoholic, the result is known as "alcoholic neuritis." If the greatest deficiency is in niacin and the degeneration is marked in the cerebrum, less in the spinal cord and least in the peripheral nerves the vitamin deficiency encephalopathy assumes the form of pellagra. If the brain stem is the site of the degenerative process, the syndrome is that of Wernicke's disease. Frequently these syndromes are not sharply defined but merge one into another depending upon the vitamin in which the deficiency is greatest and upon sites and extent of the degeneration. For example, symptoms of Korsakoff's psychosis and of Wernicke's disease or of Wernicke's disease and of pellagra may be associated. In fact, in nutritional encephalopathy it is possible in the same individual to see delirium tremens, Korsakoff's psychosis, niacin deficiency encephalopathy and the Wernicke syndrome.

The nutritional encephalopathy is probably caused by the fact that in the absence of ample quantities of thiamine and nicotinic acid there is an impaired oxidation of pyruvic acid during the breakdown of glucose.

The histopathology of Korsakoff's psychosis consists of diffuse parenchymatous changes. Among these changes are axonal alterations, a deposition of excessive amounts of normal lipochrome pigment in the nerve cells, glia, microglia and around the blood vessels in the prefrontal and motor cortex, and acute chromatolytic changes in the larger nerve cells in these areas, especially in the Betz cells.

Symptoms

The most conspicuous symptoms have already been indicated. Superficially, consciousness may appear clear and the seriousness of the mental disorder not apparent. On questioning the patient, however, one is often surprised to discover the extent of mental impairment. While possessing a relatively good grasp of what is in sight he is disoriented as to that which is beyond immediate observation and dependent on memory. At first the memory loss is most marked for events occurring since the onset of the disease, but later the memory for remote events is lost also. The amnesia is anterograde and frequently the patient cannot recall what has just been said to him. He usually presents a superficial cheerfulness and often evades inquiries by jocularities. In his confabulation the patient relates fictitious memories which superficially conceal the actual amnesia. The pseudo reminiscences which usually vary from day to day can often be suggested and guided by leading questions with the result that the patient will narrate whatever fictitious reminiscence is proposed. Presumably the patient's confabulations serve as a defense against anxiety by concealing from himself his defective functioning. The patient characteristically presents a jovial mood and often misidentifies people about him. Disorientation, especially as to time, usually exists. The polyneuropathy, which is sometimes absent, is most marked in the legs, with pain, tenderness over the nerve trunks, absent knee jerks, and in severe cases foot drop and wrist drop. The disease is relatively more frequent in women.

Course and Prognosis

Many cases clear up after six or eight weeks with approximate restoration to mental health. If the process is not fully reversible, the disease continues for several months with a gradual improvement but without complete return of memory. In some cases there is a permanent impairment of efficiency and a certain degree of intellectual, emotional and esthetic deterioration. The neuropathy usually improves rather rapidly and often completely disappears. A Korsakoff-like amnesia with confabulations serving to fill in the losses of memory may occur in uremia, after brain trauma, in general paresis and in other organic and toxic diseases of the brain—conditions in which the pathogenesis does not seem related to dietary deficiency. If irreversible changes have not already occurred the active symptoms may rapidly disappear. Insight is not usually regained.

Treatment

The first step in treatment is the discontinuance of the use of alcohol. To correct the deficiency of vitamin B_1, 20 to 50 gm. of thiamine chloride may be given daily for a few days to be followed by 20 gm. of powdered brewers' yeast in iced milk three times a day. Milk, fruit, eggs, meat and other foods rich in vitamin B complex should be liberally provided. It is probably advisable to administer ascorbic acid also. If irreversible structural changes have already taken place, the symptoms are not affected by vitamins. As in other mental disorders associated with chronic alcoholism, daily doses of insulin are often advisable. When acute neuropathy exists, rest in bed is desirable. Care should be exercised to prevent a permanent foot drop. As soon as pain and tenderness in the legs have disappeared massage and electricity are of value. The patient should then be encouraged to move his feet.

Acute Hallucinosis

Since excessive indulgence in alcohol is the occasion of the symptom complex to be considered, it has usually been classified as an alcoholic psychosis. The present tendency is to look upon it as a psychogenic reaction liberated by alcoholic excess rather than as a purely toxic expression. It seems reasonably safe to state that the clinical characteristics are determined by personality factors. Many factors suggest a close relationship to schizophrenia, and in some cases lead one to believe that the disorder is a schizophrenic reaction released by alcohol. Cases diagnosed as chronic alcoholic hallucinosis ultimately become obvious paranoid schizophrenic reactions.

Symptoms

As in the case of delirium tremens, acute alcoholic hallucinosis develops only after the prolonged and excessive use of alcohol, although usually precipitated by increased indulgence. Descriptively the reaction may be summarized as one of auditory hallucinosis occurring in a clear sensorium accompanied affectively by marked fear. In content the hallucinations are usually accusatory, or threatening, or both. The voices are particularly apt to accuse the patient of homosexual practices and to call him indecent names. In women, as in men, the hallucinations are frequently accusatory and of sexual content. The voices, however, accuse the patient of heterosexual offenses rather than of homosexual ones as in men. The hallucinated voices often refer to the patient in the third person and threaten him with such expressions as, "Now shoot him." "Let's cut him up tonight." The patient may hear the firing of pistols or other sounds suggesting a threat of attack. Not infrequently in the case of the operator of some mechanical equipment the hallucinations appear at first to come from his machine and to be synchronous with the rhythmical sound of its operation. Olfactory hallucinations are not infrequently associated. Illusions of sight are not uncommon. Visual hallucinations may be intermingled to a slight extent but are rarely present in a typical case.

The patient's ideational content and his behavior are determined by the acceptance of his hallucinations as reality. Ideas of reference and misinterpretations are common. A delusional system is rapidly acquired while additions and elaborations are quickly introduced. The patient may appeal to the police for protection or arm himself in self-defense.

In contrast to its disturbance in delirium tremens, consciousness remains clear in alcoholic hallucinosis and the patient continues oriented, projecting his hallucinations into a real environment. In another respect, too, acute hallucinosis differs from delirium tremens: after recovery there is no amnesia for events occurring during its course.

The disturbance in mood is usually pronounced, being characteristically one of fear and apprehension. Terror-stricken by the threats of his imaginary pursuers, or reduced to despair by the accusing voices and his panic state, the patient may attempt to end his own life. The fear may at times be accompanied by anger or by depression. Not infrequently there is an element of irritability, while during the temporary cessation of the hallucinations the characteristic alcoholic humor may be manifested.

Course

Recovery from alcoholic hallucinosis usually occurs in five days to a month. Recurrences are common if the patient again indulges excessively in alcohol. Unlike delirium tremens, alcoholic hallucinosis is never followed by the Korsakoff syndrome. Occasionally the hallucinatory episode continues beyond the usual period and merges into a manifest schizophrenia.

Psychological Factors

Mention has already been made of the fact that acute hallucinosis is not an uncolored alcoholic psychosis. There seems reason to believe that if a certain type of personality takes large quantities of alcohol over a considerable period of time a psychogenic reaction of an acute schizophrenic nature may be liberated. The frequent history of unsuccessful heterosexual adjustment in the patient with alcoholic hallucinosis and the homosexual character of the hallucinations suggest that in some cases, at least, unrecognized homosexual tendencies may be the psychopathogenic factor which has both prompted the use of alcohol and determined the nature of the hallucinations. As to the psychogenic determination of the mood in alcoholic hallucinosis one may speculatively suggest that the unconscious sense of threat to the personality in the biologically destructive and socially prohibited homosexual impulse is greater than the feeling of guilt which this repressed impulse sometimes arouses, hence the mood is usually one of fear rather than of depression. From the standpoint of self-respect, too, fear is psychologically preferable to shame. If the sense of guilt is relatively strong then the patient exhibits the depression occasionally seen in the disease.

Treatment

The treatment consists in placing the patient under such supervision that he may neither commit an indiscreet act nor do harm to himself. All alcohol must of course be withdrawn. The continuous bath assists in calming the fear and anxiety. Chlorpromazine or related tranquilizing agents are useful for this purpose. The administration of food is not so difficult as in delirium tremens, but it should be given regularly and in abundance. It is well to give large amounts of orange juice, also vitamin B complex.

Alcoholic Paranoia

Clinically it is convenient to describe an alcoholic paranoia although its recognition as a true alcoholic psychosis is scarcely warrantable. Here, too, there may be a common factor—the repressed homosexual impulse—beneath both the alcoholism and the psychosis. Usually the patient has never established a wholesome, mature heterosexual relationship. In the prepsychotic life of the patient we often find the same incomplete developments, fixations, traits of personality and psychopathological processes as in other paranoid psychoses. In alcoholic paranoia the use of alcohol, prompted by these tendencies, weakens repression and causes the vicious psychopathological circle of homosexual conflict, alcoholic indulgence and paranoid delusion to continue without interruption. Psychologically the conditions were favorable for the development of a psychosis before the use of alcohol became excessive. In some cases one might almost say that a latent psychosis already existed and that the alcohol did no more than hasten its appearance. The previous personality pattern has been characterized by stubborness, suspiciousness, resentment, projection and other defensive mechanisms. The history of the future patient usually shows that he has accepted discipline poorly and that he has preferred the society of men.

Symptoms

This clinical manifestation is typically characterized by delusions of jealousy and infidelity. At first the patient is irritable, fault-finding and distrustful. To these unpleasant defensive characteristics are later added accusations of marital infidelity, as evidence of which are cited the most insignificant and absurd arguments. With his jealousy motivated by an unrecognized sense of guilt and fear based on the odious trends and impulses of his own personality, the suspicious husband devises numerous schemes to entrap his wife and her supposed paramour. A noncommissioned officer in the Army, whose enlistment had perhaps been prompted by an unrecognized homosexual interest, argued that he could not be the father of the child to which his wife had given birth inasmuch as it was born two hundred and seventy-nine instead of two hundred and eighty days following marital relations with her. As evidence that the family physician was the father of the child he cited the fact that on one occasion the doctor had not submitted his bill promptly. On several occasions he threatened the life of the physician and finally actually attempted to shoot him.

Because of their incompletely developed and poorly integrated personalities these patients are peculiarly inadequate for the sustained demands for social adaptation which marriage brings. By imputing to the wife, too, the interest which they fundamentally feel for other men they secure an alleviation of anxiety. The ideas which follow are psychologically protective but adjustively disruptive. At times, with the increased use of intoxicants, an impotence, produced by the toxic action of the alcohol on the central nervous system, increases the patient's sense of insecurity and incompetence, the prevention of any recognition of which requires a further development of ideas of infidelity.

Prognosis

The prognosis in the alcoholic paranoid state is not good. With the decrease in demands for adjustment that follows removal to a hospital, the patient may improve and no longer entertain his delusional ideas. At other times, having observed that the expression of his ideas has resulted in a deprivation of his liberty, he may dissimulate and maintain that he now recognizes he was in error and that he no longer doubts the fidelity of his wife. At any rate, after the return to the old situation, the former delusions and threatening behavior usually soon reappear.

WERNICKE'S SYNDROME

This encephalopathy, resulting from a deficiency in vitamin B, may be associated with alcoholic addiction or with other conditions in which this deficiency exists. It will be discussed in Chapter XIX, Chronic Brain Syndrome Associated with Other Disturbances of Metabolism, Growth or Nutrition.

Alcoholic Deterioration

A considerable number of persons who consume large amounts of alcohol over a prolonged period ultimately suffer a certain disintegration of personality, the change ranging from an impairment of emotional stability and control to a noticeable dementia. The principal organic damage that alcohol inflicts upon the human nervous system is caused by avitaminosis rather than by primary toxic injury itself. From the standpoint of anatomical pathology there is, in the more severe cases, a progressive, chronic parenchymatous nervous degeneration, sometimes affecting a considerable part of the neuraxis. As previously indicated, so-called alcoholic dementia is caused by a progressive atrophy of the cortex of the frontal lobes. The reaction seems to result from the toxic effects of ethanol rather than from malnutrition (avitaminosis).

Symptoms

One of the earliest mental symptoms of the abuse of alcohol is an increased tendency to act impulsively in accordance with primitive instinctive forces and the momentary affectivity. Because of various factors, particularly through a sense of rejection and frustration, the alcoholic patient develops resentment, hostility and feelings of guilt. Although, at least for a considerable period, a capacity for ethical sentiments remains, yet these are not sustained or applied with the result that ethical purposes and strivings suffer, will is weakened, perseverance of endeavor is lost, and the patient becomes untruthful and unreliable. His tendency to deception and to gloss over whatever is discreditable in behavior or character is but a part of a fundamental inability to face the facts of reality and of his own situation. He blames others for his failure and represents himself as abused and as the victim of circumstances for which he is in no way responsible, while at the same time he exaggerates his own achievements. Affection is lost and ambition disappears. The confirmed alcoholic becomes careless as to his personal appearance and neglectful of his family. With an increasing egocentricity, his former sense of social or other responsibility disappears, or rather is avoided by the process of evasively treating it facetiously and superficially. Usually the patient's mood is one of unwarranted euphoria and care-free good humor, but a word of implied reproval may evoke a violent and profane outburst of irritability. A word of commiseration calls forth a ready tear although, with a hearty slap on the back, it promptly gives way to a cheerful laugh. With his friends, the alcoholic may be a congenial and welcome companion who enters enthusiastically into their pleasures but at home be brutal, surly and without shame. In nearly every instance the patient's sex life is poorly adjusted, in some instances this failure serving as a cause of the alcoholism and in others representing a result. Not infrequently, this maladjustment operates to continue the vicious circle. A defensive attitude is assumed toward those who are not alcoholic in their habits, while the patient is touchy, irritable and critical in the presence of those who he believes do not approve his excesses. There is an increasing poverty of ideas, a growing incapacity for sustained attention and for more delicate discriminations. After a time memory becomes impaired and the insidious dementia finally becomes extreme. One patient, a physician, whose practice had been ruined by his habits, who had abused his children and accused his wife of neglect and infidelity, was unable to remember how long he had been in the hospital or give the name of his ward physician who had seen him daily for months. Psychometric examinations on alcoholic patients indicate that there is an impairment of the mental functioning of various abilities before there is any clinical evidence of brain lesion.

Course and Outcome

If the use of alcohol is discontinued as soon as any early character changes are noted, there may be a nearly complete restoration to former mental health which, however, must always remain precarious since the alcoholic was never well adjusted to life. Moreover, the alcoholic, in spite of his protests to the contrary, rarely wants to get well since alcohol provides the easiest way of escape from the difficulties which his inadequately integrated personality has precipitated. Deterioration of personality is permanent and any actual dementia is, of course, quite irremediable.

Treatment

Unfortunately alcoholism has long been regarded as simply a moral problem, with the result that the complex contributing factors have not received the scientific attention they have merited nor has attention to therapy been commensurate with the extent of the social problem. "Even mental disease, one of the most persistently misunderstood and mismanaged of our social problems, is accorded better treatment than inebriety. The schizophrenic, the paretic, the manic depressive, provided, of course, that they make themselves sufficiently obnoxious to be legally adjudged 'insane.' are hospitalized and given treatment in a state-supported institution. But the inebriate, who, in addition, may well be a schizophrenic, or manic depressive, and who certainly makes himself even more obnoxious, is sternly admonished to mend his ways and is sentenced to the workhouse, there to seek insight into his behavior."[1]

Alcoholism should be looked upon as a psychic illness rooted in a personality disorder or immaturity. The tension-producing factors which have led to the alcoholism may be of a wide variety. Sometimes there has been a close mother attachment with resulting personality fixations and immaturities, again there may be latent or frank sexual maladjustments. Pathogenic intrafamily relationships are not rare. As in the psychoneuroses, with which alcoholism has much in common, the patient is usually unaware of the particular personality problems from which he has sought relief through the escape and anxiety-relieving mechanisms which alcohol facilitates. Theoretically, therefore, the object of treatment should be directed toward preventing the patient from desiring alcohol rather than toward restraining him from it. He must recognize, however, that he should never drink again. No addictive alcoholic can ever become a moderate, social drinker. All too rarely, even in the early days of his habit, will the patient co-operate in any adequate dynamic study of his personality or adjustment, or aid in the adoption of emotional compensations or socialized psychological substitutes that will relieve his anxiety and other tensions. The patient should be approached with the attitude that his disorder is one of personality rather than of morality. The emphasis should not be on the alcoholism but on the individual in whom it occurs. Psychiatric treatment should have a basic routine program of active physical exercise, constructive occupational work, agreeable social relaxation and psychotherapy. The patient's mental life and experiences should be reviewed for the purpose of discovering the main factors which have caused him to become dependent on alcohol. One must therefore obtain a thorough understanding of the patient as a person and of his particular life situation. A psychoanalytically oriented approach based on a careful understanding of psychodynamics is the one that offers the greatest promise of success. Orthodox psychoanalytical techniques are usually not practicable with the addictive drinker, partly because of his instability and low tolerance to stress. Because of these characteristics he usually resumes drinking whenever painful, unconscious material begins to come to the surface. A constructive analysis of his personality difficulties must be accompanied by a prolonged re-educational effort.

The alcoholic is usually a dependent personality and therefore needs continuous support over a long period of time, frequently for years. Frequently, too, he is a hostile, anxious, guilt-ridden person. Primitive or restraining measures that increase the patient's sense of being wronged

[1] Hewitt, C. C.: A Personality Study of Alcohol Addiction. Quart. J. Stud. on Alcohol, *4*:368–386, 1943.

and stir aggressive and resentful feelings should be avoided. The therapist will not condone his patient's alcoholic habits yet he will not be critical or judging. His attitude should be objective and impersonal. It should be remembered that the patient's rationalized reasons for his alcoholism are not the real reasons. It is usually necessary that the treatment be carried out in an institution, although in one where the patient can lead as normal a life as possible. In those instances where there is a demonstrated dependent relationship upon a protecting person, often the mother, wife or lover, who provides the alcohol and gives in to the insatiable demands of the alcoholic, this individual must also come under treatment in order to break the pathological bond that perpetuates the habit. Better results are secured in special institutions for alcoholics where there is a planned psychotherapy. Psychotherapy is of course possible only in the habitué whose intellectual equipment is still sound. If dementia has occurred, he must usually be committed to an institution where he can no longer secure intoxicants and where both the patient and society may be protected from the results of his intellectual and moral defects.

Group psychotherapy of alcoholics is being increasingly employed and promises to become an increasingly useful method of treatment. The experience of being with other similarly afflicted people seems to make the alcoholic accept more readily treatment in the group environment. The interpretations offered by other members make the attainment of insight easier and less frightening. Individual psychoanalysis seems to be useful only in carefully selected cases. Its objectivity and depth of searching are apparently more than most alcoholics can tolerate.

Alcoholics Anonymous. In recent years an organization, Alcoholics Anonymous, established in 1935 in Akron, Ohio, and conducted by former alcoholics, has produced many temporary and even prolonged cures of alcoholic addiction. The organization now has over 100,000 members. Although organized without psychiatric guidance and although its movement is largely limited to a social-religious program, it has been of great value in re-orienting many addicts in a socially efficient way of life. This program, although very heavily weighted with an unrealistic optimism, has constructively utilized many principles of group psychotherapy. As a rule, members of Alcoholics Anonymous are above the average in intelligence, education and social status and their attitude toward the addict is tolerant and constructive. The organization offers the confirmed addict an opportunity to escape from his former psychosocial isolation, from the feeling that no one really understands or cares about him and that he can trust no one. In his group, the addict has a sense of belonging, of being understood and accepted and of sharing common convictions. In his allegiance to the group, the member develops a religious fervor and in answering a call to aid another alcoholic at the cost of inconvenience and self-denial, his religious devotion is constructively internalized. An inspirational and mass-suggestion approach is an important feature. By arousing a deep desire to help others and by creating a sense of responsibility for doing so, the organization contributes to the addict's cure. The opportunity to talk about himself in the group meetings affords the addict an opportunity for narcissistic satisfaction, for self-expression and for therapeutic catharsis. The program of Alcoholics Anonymous ignores the cause of the alcoholic's addiction and focuses directly on the drinking itself. The permanency of the organization remains to be determined but thus far it has escaped the dangers of sentimentalism and of misguided enthusiasm. Its methods of thinking are naive but have doubtless contributed to its success.

DISULFIRAM OR ANTABUSE THERAPY. In 1948 two Danish investigators, Jens Hald and Erik Jacobsen, in search of a vermifuge tried disulfiram (tetraethylthiuram disulfide). They observed that persons who had ingested this substance showed symptoms after consumption of alcohol which differed quantitatively and qualitatively from the common picture of alcoholic intoxication. The discomfort after alcohol consumption in persons taking this drug was so great that they decided to use it as a remedy for alcoholism. It is believed that this discomfort is caused by interference with the excretion of acetaldehyde, an intermediary product, as already indicated, in the oxidation of alcohol.

When a patient who has taken 0.5 to 1 gm. of disulfiram within the preceding twelve hours partakes of alcohol, he experiences within five to fifteen minutes a feeling of heat in the face soon followed by an intense vasodilation in the face and neck, the skin of which may assume a purple-red color. At the same time the conjunctiva is injected and the patient suffers from tachycardia. These symptoms are soon followed by headache, dyspnea, dizziness, chest pain, nausea, palpitation and vomiting. There is an initial rise of blood pressure followed by a fall, perhaps to 80 mm. Hg. The discomfort following the imbibition of alcohol so long as disulfiram is in the blood is so great that the patient does not care to drink. The dose of disulfiram should be individualized but usually 0.125 to 0.50 gm. once a day, preferably in the morning, is sufficient. Rarely 1.0 gm. is required. Initial treatment with a drug possessing such serious toxic potentialities should be under constant medical supervision. Cardiovascular complications, including myocardial infarction, may occur. While it was originally believed that persons suffering from marked disease of the liver, coronary disease, arteriosclerosis with hypertension or diabetes should not receive disulfiram experience with a large series of patients suggests that the only important contraindication is cardiac decompensation. There have been several reports of psychoses occurring during the administration of the drug.

Formerly the administration of disulfiram was not begun until after an abstinence from alcohol for one week but in recent years disulfiram has been given even when the patient is intoxicated. In such instances, the initial dose is one-half or less of the usual (7.5 mg. per kilogram of body weight) and is given with an antihistaminic drug, such as 25 mg. of Promethazine, and 5 gm. of sodium chloride in one-half glass of water.

A new agent, citrated calcium carbimide, is now under study. This drug shows effects similar to those of disulfiram; however, there are effects immediately after ingestion though there is little duration of action after the final dose. Citrated calcium carbimide may offer a useful substitute for certain patients.

Disulfiram therapy must be considered as a variation of the conditioned reflex aversion method. In contrast to other forms of conditioned reflex methods, the unpleasant effects are present not only each time the patient takes a small but adequate dose of disulfiram and drinks alcohol but they actually increase with continued treatment with the drug. If continued, it probably helps to overcome the craving for alcohol. For the treatment to be successful, however, it is necessary that the patient have a real desire to be helped, to be willing to take the drug with consistency and to co-operate in psychotherapy. Daily uninterrupted administration of disulfiram makes it physiologically impossible to continue to use this defense. To remove this protection, however, without at the same time eliminating its need by psychotherapy can scarcely lead to a cure of the patient. As long as the basic difficulties which led to the alcoholism are not resolved, the desire for alcohol will persist and together with it an unwillingness to take the medication. During psychotherapy the psychiatrist will aim to discover both the internal, anxiety-producing factors and any social and family conditions that led to the alcoholism. With the aid of a social worker it will doubtless be necessary, too, for the patient to change various habits and improve social adjustments.

BIBLIOGRAPHY

Alexander, L.: Neuropathological findings in the brain and spinal cord of chronic alcoholic patients. Quart. J. Stud. on Alcohol, *2:*260, 1941.

Armstrong, R. W., and Gould, Jonathan: The nature and treatment of delirium tremens. J. Ment. Sc., *101:*70–84, 1955.

Banay, R. S.: Pathologic Reaction to Alcohol. Quart. J. Stud. on Alcohol, *4:*580–605, 1944.

Brunner-Orne, Martha: Treatment and rehabilitation of alcohol addicts in a general hospital setting. J. Am. M. Women's A., *10:*193–195, 1955.

Courville, C. B.: Effects of Alcohol on the Nervous System of Man. Los Angeles, San Lucas Press, 1955.

Feldman, D. J.: The treatment of chronic alcoholism. Ann. Int. Med., *44:*78–87, 1956.

Ferguson, J. K. W.: A new drug for the treatment of alcoholism: I. Preliminary clinical trial of citrated calcium carbimide. Canad.M.A.J., *74:*793–795, 1956.

Flink, E. B., Stutzman, F. L., Anderson, H. K., Konig, T., and Fraser, R.: Magnesium deficiency after prolonged parenteral fluid administration and after chronic alcoholism complicated by delirium tremens. J. Lab. & Clin. Med., *43:*169–183, 1954.

Haggard, H. W., Ed.: Alcohol, science and society. New Haven, Quart. J. Stud. on Alcohol, 1945.

Hald, J., Jacobsen, E., and Larsen, V.: The sensitizing effect of tetraethylthiuramdisulfide (Antabuse) to ethyl alcohol. Acta pharmacol. et toxicol. *4:*285–296, 1948.

Hanfmann, Eugenia: The life history of an ex-alcoholic. Quart. J. Stud. on Alcohol, *12:*405–443, 1951.

Hewitt, D. W.: Alcoholism: A Treatment Guide for General Practitioners. Philadelphia, Lea & Febiger, 1957.

Himwich, H. E.: The physiology of alcohol. J.A.M.A., *163:*545–549, 1957.

———, ed.: Alcoholism: Basic Aspects and Treatment. Washington, Am. Assoc. for Advancement of Science, 1957.

Isbell, H., Fraser, H. F., Wikler, A., Belleville, R. E., and Eisenman, A. W.: An experimental study of the etiology of "rum fits" and delirium tremens. Quart. J. Stud. on Alcohol, *16*:1–33, 1955.

Jacobsen, E., and Martensen-Larsen, O.: Treatment of alcoholism with tetraethylthiuramdisulfide (Antabuse). J.A.M.A., *139*:918–922, 1949.

Jellinek, E. M.: Effects of Alcohol on the Individual. New Haven, Yale University Press, 1942.

Martensen-Larsen, O.: Five years experience with disulfiram in the treatment of alcoholics. Quart. J. Stud. on Alcohol, *14*:406–418, 1953.

May, Philip R. A., and Ebaugh, F. G.: Pathological intoxication, alcohol hallucinosis, and other reactions to alcohol. Quart. J. Stud. on Alcohol, *14*:200–227, 1953.

Myerson, D. J.: An active therapeutic method of interrupting the dependency relationship of certain male alcoholics. Quart. J. Stud. on Alcohol, *14*:410–426, 1943.

Pfeffer, Arnold Z., *et al.*: A treatment program for the alcoholic in industry. J.A.M.A., *161*:827–836, 1956.

Ritchie, O. W.: A sociohistorical survey of Alcoholics Anonymous. Quart. J. Stud. on Alcohol, *9*:119–156, 1948.

Schultz, J. D.: *et al.*: Chlorpromazine in the management of acute alcoholic states. Quart. J. Stud. on Alcohol, *16*:245–250, 1955.

Smith, J. A.: Psychiatric treatment of the alcoholic. J.A.M.A., *163*:734–738, 1957.

Strecker, E. A.: Psychotherapy in pathological drinking. J.A.M.A., *147*:813–815, 1951.

Sutton, Thomas: Tracts on Delirium Tremens, on Peritonitis, and on Some Other Internal Inflammatory Affections and on the Gout. London, Thomas Underwood, 1813.

Thompson, G. N., Ed.: Alcoholism. Springfield, Charles C Thomas, 1956.

Usdin, G. L., and Robinson, K. E.: Psychosis occurring during Antabuse administration. Arch. Neurol. & Psychiat., *66*:38–43, 1951.

Victor, Maurice, and Adams, R. D.: The Effect of Alcohol on the Nervous System. Vol. XXVII, Chapter XXVIII, Proceedings of Association for Research in Nervous and Mental Disease. Baltimore, Williams & Wilkins Co., 1953.

Wells, R. E.: Use of reserpine in the management of chronic alcoholism. J.A.M.A., *163*:426–429, 1957.

Williams, W.[1]: The society of Alcoholics Anonymous. Am. J. Psychiat., *106*:370–375, 1949.

---

[1] Co-founder with Robert H. Smith, M.D. (deceased) of Alcoholics Anonymous.

CHAPTER XI

Mental Disorders Caused by or Associated with Head Trauma

WITH THE mounting occurrence of accidents incident to industry and traffic and with the enactment of industrial compensation laws, there has been a marked increase in traumatic mental disorders and their medicolegal importance. For these reasons, the relationship of head trauma to the development of mental disorders often presents an important and difficult problem. Not infrequently the difficulty of this problem is increased by the fact that the clinical picture may become complicated by the addition of psychogenic symptoms to an organic syndrome. In order to arrive at an accurate diagnosis, it is often necessary not only to make detailed mental and neurological examinations but also to obtain a precise history of the patient's mental status prior to his injury. The opinion popularly entertained that injuries to the head are a frequent cause of mental disorders is an error. Undoubtedly severe trauma to any part of the body may occasionally serve as a contributing or precipitating agent in schizophrenia and manic-depressive psychosis in persons predisposed to these respective reactions. At times, too, trauma of the head, without recognizable injury to the brain, may activate an asymptomatic paretic process and lead to clinically active syphilitic meningoencephalitis. Such psychoses, however, are not included among the traumatic mental disorders.

The mental disturbances associated with head trauma are divided into those caused by acute brain disorder and those caused by chronic brain disorder. There will be some explanatory discussion of this classification as these disorders are considered.

Acute Disorders Caused by or Associated with Head Trauma

The acute (at times subacute) disorders following trauma of the head tend to fall into the following syndromes:

(*a*) Concussion
(*b*) Traumatic coma
(*c*) Traumatic delirium
(*d*) Korsakoff, or amnesic-confabulatory syndrome

Concussion Syndrome

In concussion, there is a momentary physiological interruption of cerebral processes because of head injury but there are no histological changes or clinical signs. Recovery is rapid and complete. There is not only an amnesia for the moment of injury but also for a period, usually seconds or moments, before the injury. Concussion follows the impact of a severe, functionally paralyzing force upon the head, especially of a force that causes abrupt acceleration or deceleration. In recent years it has been suggested that concussion may be the result of the cavitation phenomenon in the cellular fluids. Experiments show that an impulse applied to the skull by a severe mechanical blow or by an underwater explosion produces first a momentary positive pressure wave followed by a negative one. Although this negative wave is sustained for only an infinitesimal period of time it apparently causes minute bubbles to form momentarily in the cellular fluids. This phenomenon of cavitation with its molecular-disrupting action produces a momentary generalized cortical electric discharge that renders the patient unconscious. This discharge is followed by a depression of function. Recently brains of animals subjected to concussion and examined by finer techniques several days after the trauma have disclosed histological changes in nerve cells. These suggest that some of the remote symptoms following concussion may develop on the basis of nerve cell changes taking place some time after the concussion. The period of unconsciousness may be momentary or may continue for hours. Many patients vomit as they regain consciousness. There is apparently no relationship between the severity of the concussion as measured by the duration of unconsciousness and the severity of the psychiatric sequelae. In regaining consciousness the patient may wake up suddenly or may pass through a state of clouded consciousness and confusion. He will subsequently have a loss of memory (posttraumatic amnesia) for this period even though he seems alert and able to carry on a conversation. Usually recovery is complete in a short time but occasionally a chronic personality disorder may follow.

Contusing and lacerating injuries do not in themselves produce concussion although they may be associated with it. On the other hand, a severe injury may be sustained without concussion. The diagnosis of uncomplicated concussion can be made only in retrospect. Only after the regaining of consciousness can one be sure that no organic sequelae will follow. While cerebral concussion is an acute syndrome there is frequently an aftermath of variable, even prolonged, duration. These postconcussion symptoms will be discussed on page 219.

Traumatic Coma

A severe concussion without injury, or more frequently concussion accompanied by contusion (a mechanical disruption of tissue usually accompanied by minute capillary hemorrhages), or by laceration (a gross tearing of tissue), may produce prolonged coma. Coma is, of course, characterized by absence of response on stimulation. It may last for hours or for several days, the duration depending upon the degree and extent of the injury. In the absence of localizing signs of laceration or of pressure (as by subdural hemorrhage), coma for more than twenty-four hours usually means a major contusion. Following coma there is a period of stupor, restlessness and clouding of consciousness from which the patient may emerge into clear consciousness or at times pass into traumatic delirium. Coma is often interrupted by intervals of semistupor. Prolonged coma is frequently followed by a period of delirium succeeded by a longer period of amnesia or by the amnesic-confabulatory syndrome known as Korsakoff's syndrome.

Traumatic Delirium

If delirium follows the suffering of head trauma, it usually begins during the gradual emergence of the patient from traumatic stupor or coma. The underlying cause may be concussion, contusion, laceration, hemorrhage or increased intracranial pressure. In a majority of cases delirium is mild and consists of haziness, irritability, dreamy fabrications, restlessness and mild disorders of the sensorium. The patient does not grasp the finer points of situations and events of his surroundings. While most of the time he may realize that he is in a hospital, he does not remember how he came to be there, may not recognize persons about him or understand why he is detained. Other patients may be definitely bewildered. Not a few are apprehensive and fearful. In some cases the delirium is occupational in nature. Many patients are resistive, noisy, irritable, unco-operative, and verbally abusive. Some patients are belligerent, demanding and aggressive. If hallucinations occur, they are usually visual. In the more severe cases there may be such a confusional excitement and tendency to wander about that restraint becomes necessary. Violent, impulsive outbursts making the patient dangerous to himself or others may occur. As their noisy delirium subsides some patients remain talkative and show a perseveration of words. At times after the stage of irritability the emotional state may be characterized by a childish elation and happiness. As in delirium resulting from other causes, the course may be characterized by fluctuations between relative clearness and confusion. In some instances the syndrome may be that of a twilight or dream state instead of delirium. With or without preceding delirium, various degrees of post-traumatic defect may follow major contusions with their diffuse degenerations of ganglion cells. Delirium continuing for more than a week suggests considerable damage. An estimate of the final residual defect should not be given for at least six months. Delirium or coma of more than a month's duration usually means serious tissue destruction. An estimate of the final deterioration and other results of tissue destruction should not be made until twelve to eighteen months after the injury. The final mental defect will usually not be as serious as early symptoms suggest.

Korsakoff or Amnesic-Confabulatory Syndrome

A relatively frequent syndrome following head trauma is that first described by Korsakoff as associated with chronic alcoholism. The most striking feature of this syndrome is confabulation, although this is accompanied by disorientation and impairment of perception and of recent memory. The fabrication of memory may be a mixture of truth and fiction or purely new fabrications. Suggestive questions may often elicit contradictory statements. The patient may superficially appear alert but on closer examination it will be found that perception is greatly deranged. Many patients with Korsakoff syndrome show a serenity and mild euphoria or even facetiousness but readily become irritable on questioning. The polyneuritis resulting from thiamine deficiency and seen in some Korsakoff syndromes does not occur in the post-traumatic syndrome. Since polyneuropathy is not present as in the syndrome originally described by Korsakoff the term "amnesic-confabulatory syndrome" is more appropriate. The syndrome following trauma is of shorter duration than the alcoholic Korsakoff syndrome.

In practice it will be found that the acute and subacute symptoms of traumatic mental disorder do not usually occur in such distinct classificatory types as have been described. In severe cases one often observes mixed and transitional reaction types. Delirioid and Korsakoff symptoms are particularly apt to be associated.

Treatment of Acute Traumatic Mental Disorders

Except for the surgical procedures required in the case of definite injuries to the head, operative interference is to be avoided. The patient will be closely watched for any signs of increased intracranial pressure, also for the occurrence of any complication.

The initial objective is to quiet the patient. Rest in bed and as limited a use of sedatives as possible is important. Narcotics are contraindicated. In the acute stages careful note should be made as to the state of awareness and the presence or absence of signs of injury to the cerebral substance. Vital signs should be recorded at two- to four-hour intervals. Fluids and a soft or liquid diet may be administered if the patient is conscious and able to swallow. With the presence of coma, either feeding by a nasal tube or the administration of parenteral fluids is indicated. Daily dosage of penicillin is indicated to prevent pulmonary infection. Fluids and salt should be restricted but not to the point of leading to dehydration and acidosis. The fear of cerebral edema should not lead to their over-restriction. Patients with simple concussion require at least twenty-four hours of observation and may then return to their usual activities. The period of bed rest and convalescence of patients with more severe injuries is determined by the reactivity of the patient to the treatment. It is important that the severity of the injury not be overemphasized or the period of hospitalization unduly prolonged. There should be a gradual increase of activity with continuance of convalescence at home through the medium of graduated exercises. Active work should be deferred for two to three months following discharge from the hospital. Patients should be advised that alcohol tolerance is diminished following head injury.

Of utmost importance in the treatment of the acute traumatic mental state is the continued awareness of the possibility of severe complications. Such changes in the vital signs as slowing of the pulse and respiration, fluctuating states of consciousness, or the development of signs of focal disturbances of the brain including paresis, suggest strongly the possibility of serious pathology. In particular, the possibility of subdural hemorrhage must be kept in mind.

Subdural Hematoma

Following injury to the head subdural hematoma is said to occur in from one to 10 per cent of individuals. In a series of 3,100 consecutive autopsies of psychotic patients, 8 per cent showed evidence of subdural hemorrhage. Subdural hematoma may be associated with any variety of psychotic reaction but occurs particularly in the senile, epileptic, alcoholic, and paretic individual. Such patients are especially prone to head injury.

Subdural hematoma consists of a collection of blood between the dura and arachnoid in the subdural space. The bleeding in this space is of venous origin and follows tearing of small veins reaching the subdural space. The fluid in the space may be admixed with cerebrospinal fluid if the arachnoid tears. Blood extravasated into this area fails to be absorbed and eventually is organized and encapsulated by the dura. Fibroblasts proliferate from the inner surface of the dura and invade the clot when in contact with the dura. Capillaries extend into the clot and gradually absorb the liquefied fluid. If the clot is small it may become completely organized but if large fibroblasts may form an encapsulating membrane both by growing along the inner surface of the clot and on the surface adjacent to the dura.

Subdural hematomas may either occur acutely following the head injury or at later periods. In either case the symptomatology may be brought to the attention of the psychiatric consultant. Headache is invariably present. Perhaps most important is the variable state of consciousness. Following recovery from the initial coma the patient becomes irritable or confused. His mental status frequently changes from day to day or even from hour to hour. Focal signs of cerebral damage are not present in more than one-half of the cases. The most frequent signs are hemiplegia or central facial weakness. In chronic cases the symptoms are similar but in addition slight to severe intellectual impairment is usually noted. The initial trauma may not be remembered.

Cerebrospinal fluid is usually bloody and under increased pressure. Roentgenologic examination of the skull may or may not show evidence of a linear fracture. The electroencephalograph is often helpful in defining an abnormality on one or the other side of the brain. The diagnosis is firmly established only by placing a burr hole on both sides of the skull with discovery of the characteristic hematoma. Other complications that may follow head injury in the acute phase are extradural hemorrhage, intracerebral hemorrhage, subdural hygroma, and cerebral thrombosis. When a subdural hemorrhage or other traumatic vascular lesion is suspected, neurological and neurosurgical consultations are immediately indicated.

Chronic Disorders Caused by or Associated with Head Trauma

A definite classification of mental disturbances caused by or associated with head trauma into a group of acute disorders and a group of chronic disorders is somewhat arbitrary but in general there are two groups of syndromes both in respect to their temporal relation to the trauma and in respect to clinical features. The chronic disorders may also be divided into two subgroups. One subgroup consists of those disorders presenting symptoms which are the direct result of the trauma and the other in which the syndrome is only a secondary result of the head trauma. The following classification of the chronic traumatic disorders is therefore suggested:

I. Caused primarily by head trauma:
 Post-traumatic personality disorders
  a. of adults
  b. of children
 Post-traumatic defect conditions
  Traumatic encephalopathy of pugilists (punch drunk)
  Traumatic convulsive disorder (traumatic epilepsy)

II. Caused secondarily by head trauma:
 Psychoneurosis with head trauma

I. CHRONIC MENTAL DISORDERS CAUSED PRIMARILY BY HEAD TRAUMA

Psychopathology which occurs following lesions of the brain is now regarded not only as an expression of changes which the patient's personality undergoes as the result of cerebral lesions but also as an expression of the efforts of the brain-damaged personality to adapt to these defects and to those demands that can no longer be met because of these defects. In his work on persons with brain injuries consequent to war wounds Goldstein emphasized that various types of symptoms must be evaluated and understood in this context if a rational therapy is to be applied in the treatment of individuals with chronic disorders resulting from head injury.

The effort of such patients to find a new adjustment necessary because of the head injury results in three types of symptoms: The first expresses the conflict which the individual faces; the second reflects the tendency to build up substitutive performances so as to adapt to the demands of the environment in the most effective manner under the circumstances of the defect consequent to the injury; and a third group of symptoms is the direct result of the impairment of the brain-functioning itself. In the third group, the defect may be ameliorated by training, and it is here in particular that the impairment of the "abstract attitude" described by Goldstein is to be found.

Among the symptoms exposing the patient's defect is that now commonly known as the "catastrophic reaction." Confronted with a problem he cannot solve, the brain-injured individual becomes suddenly anxious, agitated, and may appear dazed. A change in his color may appear, he fumbles at the task and may present other evidences of autonomic disturbances, such as irregular pulse and changes in respiratory rate. If he were initially in good spirits he now becomes evasive, sullen, irritable, and even aggressive. The "catastrophic reaction" develops simultaneously with the attempt to perform the task in which he fails and not following the performance. Thus it does not represent the patient's response to the awareness that he has failed. As a consequence of such catastrophic reactions, a definite behavior pattern evolves in many of the brain-injured. Some, when confronted with tasks they cannot solve, lose consciousness. Others avoid exposing themselves to such situations by isolating themselves from individuals, or by avoiding tasks through apparent inability to understand directions. Some brain-injured attempt to prevent upsurges of anxiety by continuous activity which exposes the inability of the individual to adopt a reflective attitude to take himself for granted, or to place himself in the position of a detached spectator. The overactivity may be of the type commonly spoken of as "occupational delirium" seen in cases with dementia. Certain patients appear unable to follow directions and carry out tasks. Essentially they avoid the task in the anxious expectation of precipitating the unpleasant catastrophic response. Others adapt through an excessive orderliness. This may not only express itself in a meticulousness in relation to one's own property but also to that of others in the home.

The brain-injured person tends to suppress knowledge of his disability. Such denial, according to Goldstein, is more easily achieved in the patient with complete destruction of some function than in the individual with incomplete disturbance.

In addition to the efforts of the brain-injured person to avoid the catastrophic reaction by restricting his environment, his brain defect expresses itself through evidence of increase in the threshold of excitability with the result that greater stimuli are required to bring forth responses. At the same time the patient may appear unusually susceptible to exposure to various external stimuli because of his easy distractibility. Owing to his difficulty in discriminating between the object to which he is exposed and the background or setting in which the object is presented the brain-injured patient suffers doubt and anxiety in his perceptions of common objects presented under ordinary circumstances. Thus his capacity for solving problems is impaired as a consequence of this perceptual weakness.

Goldstein has described what he terms the "abstract attitude." He defines this as the capacity to assume a mental set voluntarily; to shift from one aspect of a situation to another; to retain simultaneously several aspects of a situation; to break up and isolate the whole into its constituent parts; and to abstract common properties, plan ahead ideationally and think or behave symbolically. The "concrete attitude," on the other hand, is a form of thinking fixed and unable to proceed beyond the stimulus of an immediate experience or object. To him the brain-injured is impaired in his ability to assume the "abstract attitude" and has difficulty moving easily from the "abstract" to the "concrete."

Post-traumatic Personality Disorders

While these personality disturbances are primarily a result of injuries to the cranial contents, psychological factors usually participate to a varying degree. A decision as to the relative importance of the brain injury, of environmental factors and of the previous personality pattern of the patient is not always easy. Sometimes the impression is gained that the patient has always had an immature attitude or as a result of the accident has reverted to such an attitude accompanied by a reluctance to face former responsibilities. Again the mental symptoms appear nearly all or entirely psychogenic and merge into a neurosis secondary to the trauma (accident neurosis).

Among the names applied to the personality syndrome caused directly by the head injury are "postconcussion syndrome," "post-traumatic general cerebral syndrome" (Foerster), "minor contusion syndrome" (Symonds), "traumatic constitution" (Meyer), "traumatic psychopathic constitution" (Ziehen), "traumatic encephalopathy," and others. In adults this primary post-traumatic personality syndrome may assume two forms: (a) a milder and more frequent form known as postconcussion syndrome or postconcussional neurotic state, and (b) a more serious disturbance to which the name post-traumatic personality disorder is applied in a narrower and more specific sense.

POSTCONCUSSION SYNDROME. Whether the injury that preceded this syndrome was mild or severe the presenting symptom is anxiety. Other symptoms are headache, vertigo, fatigability, oversensitivity to strong sensory stimuli, insomnia, impairment of memory and of ability to concentrate, a narrowing of interests, a lessening of spontaneity, aggravation of symptoms by heat, excitement or exertion and a reduced tolerance of alcohol. Headache and vertigo are aggravated by quick movement, by stooping or by psychological tension. Many patients are emotionally labile, irritable and easily moved to tears. Many patients complain of decreased sexual potency. Some become "head-conscious." This is perhaps to be expected since the head is the most significant part of the body-image. Head injury, therefore, is more commonly experienced as a form of psychic trauma than injury to almost any other part of the body. If the injury occurred under conditions of discontent or dissatisfaction psychogenic symptoms are particularly apt to follow.

Diagnosis and Prognosis. The chief problem in the diagnosis of the postconcussion syndrome is to determine when a postconcussional headache and other symptoms having an organic basis cease to be a result of organic causes and are carried on by psychological influences. The relative importance of psychogenic and physiogenic factors is often difficult to determine. If the headache is paroxysmal, throbbing, aggravated by postural alterations or physical exertion it may be that it persists from an encephalopathic rather than from a neurotic state. The same is true if mental functions tend to be sluggish, if the emotional status is sanguine and not characterized by gloom, ready annoyance and apprehension. If the symptoms are definite, constant, are not modified by suggestion and the patient's interest is in rehabilitation and not in indemnification, they are probably not of psychogenic origin. The postconcussive or neurotic state will be discussed later in this chapter. Most, but not all cases, of postconcussion syndrome recover if not complicated by too numerous or too severe psychoneurotic symptoms. Recovery may be delayed for one or two years.

Treatment. In certain respects the most important aspects of treatment are careful and adequate surgical and medical treatment at the time of injury combined with subsequent discreet management in adjusting the patient to his symptoms and to the general situation with which he is confronted. Too early return to strenuous labor should be discouraged, yet too long a rest may lead to a secondary neurotic syndrome. Nearly every concussion patient should have supportive and suggestive psychotherapy.

Post-traumatic Personality Disorder of Adults. In some instances the most conspicuous sequel of head trauma is a change from the original personality make-up of the patient. The amiable, placid individual may become irascible, irritable and impulsive. He may become quarrelsome and be subject to outbursts of rage, aggression and motor excitement. Family and other obligations and responsibilities are disregarded. Ambition and initiative are lost. The patient becomes petulant, resentful, self-centered, willful and selfish. Some become morose and tend to develop paranoid reactions toward persons about them. Others lose all interest in activities and withdraw from social contacts. Not uncommonly, some degree of organic mental deterioration accompanies these changes in the psychological structure of the personality.

Post-traumatic Personality Disorders of Children. In general, children withstand head injury better than adults. Not rarely, however, brain-damaged children may become serious behavior problems. Children without serious destruction of brain tissue may show much disorganization of behavior. The behavior disorders are similar to those seen following the epidemic encephalitis of the 1920's but more severe and of poorer prognosis. The previously normal child becomes disobedient, distractible, impulsive, aggressive, destructive, cruel, quarrelsome and antisocial. Constant restlessness and overactivity are the rule. There may be some degree of intellectual deficit. The child is dominated by instinctive and emotional impulses and shows no regard for the welfare of others. While there is little impairment of original intellectual capacity, the child does not concentrate, shows little interest in school work and does poorly in the classroom where he is intolerably disruptive. The usual methods of training and discipline are ineffectual and eventually the most serious delinquents become institutionalized.

While the emotional disorders seen in the brain-injured child probably have organic roots, they certainly have psychogenic ones. Because of his handicap, the brain-injured child is in need of emotional support. Parental feelings and their attitude toward the child's handicaps may greatly influence his behavior. Some parents may manifest a smothering overprotectiveness and others be unsympathetic and rejecting. An impatient attitude and unjustified blame by the teacher will increase the child's anxiety and result both in more disturbed behavior and in less ability to learn. Environmental pathology becomes, therefore, the crucial determinant of the disturbances in behavior.

Post-traumatic Defect Conditions

Mental deterioration (dementia) following severe head trauma may or may not have been preceded by a traumatic delirium. It not rarely happens that as consciousness returns following a delirium an impairment of former mental capacity will become manifest. In milder forms this may consist only of loss of initiative, mental slowing, loss of sense of responsibility and impairment of ability to recognize abstract relationships. In somewhat more serious disturbances memory is impaired, attention is reduced, reaction time is slowed and defensive confabulations may be expressed. Judgment is impaired and finer affective feelings are blunted. Social values are not appreciated. Tasks which were formerly performed easily become difficult or impossible. The patient may consider himself normal although it is apparent to his intimates that he has never been the same since his injury. The degree of dementia varies greatly according to the site of the lesion, the nature and extent of the injury and its secondary results (atrophy, meningoencephalic adhesions, distortion of ventricles). A permanent mental deterioration to a degree requiring institutional care is uncommon after contusion. If laceration has been extensive, the dementia may be great and associated with epileptiform seizures, paralyses, aphasia, deafness and other neurological signs.

Difficulty sometimes arises in differentiating post-traumatic mental deterioration from psychoses of arteriosclerotic origin complicated by head injury. Careful inquiry should be made as to any symptoms of arteriosclerosis existing before the injury. The possibility that the confusion of an arteriosclerosis or of a cerebral attack may have led to the injury should be kept in mind.

Severe, chronic dementia is hopeless yet caution should guide the therapist in expressing a prognosis in acute or subacute cases, since with time many patients show a surprising improvement.

Traumatic Encephalopathy of Pugilists (Punch Drunk)

A chronic post-traumatic personality disorder first described by Martland is that to which he gave the name "punch drunk." This syndrome occurs among pugilists who have sustained repeated severe blows on the head over a period of at least a few years. The more skillful the fighter the more probable that he will either escape the causative injuries or remain relatively free from them for a considerable period of time. The disorder probably results from successive and accumulative petechial hemorrhages and foci of necrosis deep in the cerebrum. The patient shows an insidious impairment of skill, a slowing of muscular action, a little uncertainty in equilibrium, slight confusion, deterioration in attention, concentration and memory. Speech becomes thick and hesitating. The patient "continuously simulates a person who is just a little drunk." Most patients are voluble and euphoric. Confusion and defects of memory become more marked and intellectual impairment continues to a disabling degree. The tremor, propulsive gait and masklike facies of the parkinsonian syndrome may appear. The symptoms progress for approximately a year then become stationary. The degree of deterioration depends upon the extent and degree of brain injury.

Traumatic Epilepsy

One of the sequelae of brain injury may be epilepsy. There is so wide a variation in statistics as to the incidence of epileptic seizures following head injury—4.5 per cent (Sargant) to 34 per cent (Denny-Brown)—that they are probably of little value. Study of 279 American personnel who sustained wounds of the brain in World War II showed that 36 per cent developed seizures within two years after injury and 41.6 per cent within three years after receipt of penetrating brain wounds. The incidence is greatest in patients who suffer a penetration of the dura. Penfield showed that the most frequent epileptogenic lesion in post-traumatic convulsive state is a cerebrodural or cerebral cicatrix and focal atrophy. Epilepsy is therefore more common after penetrating than after closed injuries and is not the result of generalized damage to the brain. Seizures do not develop after a simple concussion.

A lesion causing the convulsive state does so as a result of irritation of adjacent areas of the brain. The pattern of the attack and the march of motor phenomena during the seizure may betray the epileptogenic point of origin. Electroencephalography may be of much value in localization. In the typical focal or jacksonian seizure, consciousness is not lost. Clonic twitches develop in one part of the body and spread consecutively to other parts of the same side. In a large percentage of cases, however, consciousness is disturbed in the manner of either the petit mal or grand mal seizure. There may also be the same paroxysmal periods of depression or of exaltation or fugues. Mental deterioration may be slight or extreme.

II. CHRONIC MENTAL DISORDER SECONDARY TO HEAD TRAUMA: PSYCHONEUROSIS

Although Chapter XXX will be devoted to a description of the psychoneuroses, those associated with head trauma have features sufficiently significant to justify special mention in a discussion of mental disorders following head injury. It is not generally considered that traumatic neuroses are the direct result of anatomical or physiological changes produced by the trauma yet a subjectively disturbing postconcussion syndrome or other post-traumatic symptoms may facilitate or become the nucleus for neurotic attitudes. This is especially true if the trauma occurred at a time or in a setting in which anxiety-producing factors existed. There may, for example, have been economic insecurity, occupational dissatisfactions, family tensions, or inability to secure work. The circumstances under which the trauma was sustained—compensable accidents, in contrast to accidental falls in the home or injuries in sports—may have a significant etiological relation. There is also a contributing element in the fact that the head, particularly the brain, is an organ on which the patient sets particular value. If, therefore, the injury is followed by dizziness and headache, or if other physical symptoms are associated with it, a sense of insecurity and an associated anxiety may readily develop. Not rarely, complicating situational stresses arising out of or relating to the injury not only tend to create but also to perpetuate the neurotic symptoms. Feelings of discontent or of grievance predispose to their development. Fear, suggestion and wishful thinking may all be important psychological factors in the production of symptoms.

The onset of a psychoneurosis associated with head trauma is not at the time of injury but at a variable period after it. Not rarely there is a history that the patient recovered from the organic symptoms produced by the trauma and was about to return to his usual employment, or even did resume work for a brief period, when a return of headache, dizziness and other symptoms rendered employment impossible. This period between time of injury and the appearance of neurotic disability is often described as one of "incubation and contemplation." The patient who has had a resentful, dissatisfied attitude toward his work and was protected from resuming former responsibilities by reason of the acute physical symptoms that followed the head trauma is prone to the development of a neurosis. With the loss of the protecting physical disability other means of avoiding a return to a distasteful situation must be sought. This means is readily provided by a return of headache, vertigo, impairment of memory, fatigability, irritability and other symptoms. Likewise, both the man who is fundamentally covetous and indolent, or who was harassed by debts or other financial obligations before his injury, and the apprehensive, suggestible man fearful of losing compensation by return to work may develop similar psychoneurotic symptoms to assure a continuation of compensation. The sympathy and solicitude of friends, lack of occupation and interest, suggestive examinations, misdirected treatment, continued compensation and other subconscious motivations tend to fix the symptoms. Various factors, such as fears related to the injury, head-consciousness and accentuation and elaboration of pre-existing conflicts concerning occupational and financial problems, contribute to the development of anxiety which is often a conspicuous symptom. Other symptoms are physical and mental fatigability, depression, apprehension, neurasthenic and hypochondriacal reactions and a volubility and elaboration in expression of complaints. Symptoms tend to be vague, numerous and inconstant.

Undoubtedly the organic concussion syndrome with its disturbance of consciousness and subsequent dizziness and the feeling of insecurity connected with it facilitates the production and suggests the nature of neurotic symptoms. As organic symptoms continue, they often tend, therefore, to acquire an overlay of psychoneurotic ones. Frequently, indeed, the post-traumatic concussion syndrome becomes the basis for psychological elaborations of a hysterical type. As a result psychogenic symptoms may coincide or be interwoven with organic sequelae of head injuries. With this tendency of neurotic attitudes to crystallize around the nucleus of head injuries, the differentiation between organic and psychogenic symptoms is not always easy; every combination of organic and psychiatric symptoms may, in fact, exist. The relative significance of these two groups may be a matter of personal opinion.

Treatment

Since the pretraumatic personality and the setting and circumstances of the accident are often more significant than the severity of the injury in producing post-traumatic mental disability, apprehension should not be manifested either by the physician or the patient's relatives. Prolonged rest in bed after head injury suggests that the injury is serious, engenders anxiety and predisposes to the development of the post-traumatic syndrome. The stay in a hospital should not be prolonged and the patient should return to his work as soon as practicable. Planned activity even before return to regular employment is desirable. Reference has already been made to the fact that occupational and home worries and concern for compensation favor the persistence of symptoms. Gain from the injury in any way deters recovery. A speedy settlement of any compensation question is advisable. Since the association between head injury and psychiatric factors is close the "preneurotic interval" between the injury and the development of the neurosis is one in which preventive psychotherapy is advisable.

Rehabilitation of the brain-injured should commence immediately after the patient has become conscious. Such patients are often highly fearful and suggestible. Explanation as to the nature of the injury and reassurance as to outcome should be given. Efforts should be made to avoid inquiry concerning symptoms which are not spontaneously presented. As soon as the patient is able, he should move about and a carefully planned program of progressive activity should be established. Such a program should not overtax his capacities intellectually, emotionally or physically. Those with chronic defects require more than a regimen of occupational therapy, games and exercises even though such activities assist in restoring self confidence and an awareness of capacity for performance. Treatment is most effectively managed in hospitals with well established departments for rehabilitation including occupational, recreational and vocational therapies. Many advances have been made in the methods used in the re-education of those with chronic brain damage, particularly of those who manifest, in addition to disturbances of the abstract attitude, specific defects in the field of language, motor disabilities and perception, as Goldstein has indicated. Such patients require a careful psychological evaluation and then retraining by skilled persons. There is a continuing need for the insight of the psychiatrist and his assistants in dealing with the emotional problems of patients. However, in addition to this type of therapy, the utilization of the psychologist trained in the pedagogy of the brain-injured, also of the social worker where there are particular family needs, must be considered. The outcome varies according to the severity of the lesion and the pretraumatic personality of the individual. In some cases intellectual tests may fail to reveal serious disturbances, yet when the patient has returned to work his impairment in judgment and capacity for work may be demonstrated. Here the well established rehabilitation center with the opportunity for testing performance in a workshop is most useful in determining the eventual capacity of the individual for an occupation and the proper type of vocation for the future. In those rare cases of dementia with severe personality change, the prognosis is grave. No final assessment of the degree of damage should be made in less than twelve to eighteen months after the injury.

BIBLIOGRAPHY

Adler, Alexandra: Mental symptoms following head injury. Arch. Neurol. & Psychiat., *53:*34–43, 1945.

Allen, A. M., Moore, M., and Daly, B. B.: Subdural hemorrhage in patients with mental disease. New England J. Med., *223:*324–329. 1950.

Association for Research in Nervous and Mental Diseases, Vol. XXIV: Trauma of the Central Nervous System. Baltimore, Williams & Wilkins Co., 1945.

Blau, Abram: Mental changes following head trauma in children. Arch. Neurol. & Psychiat., *35:*723–769, 1936.

Bowman, K. M., and Blau, Abram: A revised classification of mental sequelae of trauma of the head. Arch. Neurol. & Psychiat., *41:*1270–1274, 1939.

Courville, C. B.: Commotio Cerebri: Cerebral Concussion and the Postconcussion Syndrome in their Medical and Legal Aspects. Los Angeles, San Lucus Press, 1953.

Critchley, Macdonald: Medical aspects of boxing. Brit. M.J., *5015:*357–364, 1957.

Denny-Brown, D.: The sequelae of war head injuries. New England J. Med., *227:* 771–780 and 813–821, 1942.

———: Disability arising from closed head injuries. J.A.M.A., *127:*429–436, 1945.

Ebaugh, F. G., and Brosin, H. W.: Traumatic psychoses. Ann. Int. Med., *18:*666–696, 1943.

Eisenberg, Leon: Psychiatric implications of brain damage in children. Psychiatric Quart., *31:*72–92, 1957.

Foerster, O.: Commotionsneurose. Beitr. z. Klin. Chir., *137:*647, 1926.

Friedman, A. P., and Brenner, Charles: Amnestic-confabulatory syndrome (Korsakoff psychosis) following head injury. Am. J. Psychiat., *102:*61–66, 1945.

Goldstein, K.: After-effects of Brain Injuries in War. New York, Grune & Stratton, 1942.

Guttmann, E.: Psychiatric aspects of head injury. J. Ment. Sc., *90:*328–350, 1944.

———: Late effects of closed head injuries. J. Ment. Sc., *92:*1, 1946.

Ingram, T. T. S.: A characteristic form of overactivity behavior in brain-damaged children. J. Ment. Sc., *102:*550–558, 1956.

Kasanin, J.: Personality changes in children following cerebral trauma. J. Nerv. & Ment. Dis., *69:*385, 1929.

Kozol, H. L.: Pretraumatic personality and psychiatric sequelae of head injury. I.

Arch. Neurol. & Psychiat., *53*:358–364, 1945. II. Arch. Neurol. & Psychiat., *56*:245–275, 1946.
McConnell, A. A.: The cephalic post-traumatic syndrome. J. Ment. Sc., *102*:330–335, 1956.
Martland, H. S.: Punch drunk. J.A.M.A., *91*:1103–04, 1928.
Meerloo, A. M.: Cerebral concussion. J. Nerv. & Ment. Dis., *110*:347–353, 1949.
Meyer, Adolf: The anatomical facts and clinical varieties of traumatic insanity. Am. J. Insan., *60*:373–441, 1904.
Penfield, W.: The mechanism of cicatricial contraction in the brain. Brain, *50*:499, 1927.
———: Epilepsy and surgical therapy. Arch. Neurol. & Psychiat., *36*:499, 1936.
Rowbotham, G. F.: The long-term results of injuries of the head. J. Ment. Sc., *95*:336–354, 1949.
Ruesch, J.: Intellectual impairment in head injuries. Am. J. Psychiat., *100*:480–496, 1944.
———, and Bowman, K. M.: Prolonged post-traumatic syndromes following head injury. Am. J. Psychiat., *102*:145–163, 1945.
Siegal, L. J.: Craniocerebral postconcussive personality states. Psychiatric Quart. Supplement, *24*:65–72, 1950.
Strauss, A. A., and Lehtinen, L. E.: Psychopathology and Education of the Brain-injured Child. New York, Grune & Stratton, 1947.
Tobias, J. S., Lowenthal, M., and Maringer, S.: Evaluation and management of the brain-damaged patient. J.A.M.A., *165*:2035–2041, 1957.

CHAPTER XII

Brain Syndromes Associated with Circulatory Disturbances

Circulatory disturbances such as cerebral embolism, arterial hypertension, cardiorenal disease and cardiac decompensation sometimes give rise to disorders of the sensorium with confusion and other organic brain syndromes. Emboli arising from the pulmonary circulation, from vegetations on the heart valves or from thrombi of the neck or head may occlude cerebral vessels with resulting disturbance of circulation and consequent softening. When such disturbances occur, the neurological and mental symptoms will depend upon the size and location of the vessels occluded. The onset is in the form of an apoplectic stroke, often accompanied by loss of consciousness followed by a confused or delirious period. In the wake of these acute symptoms are organic reaction symptoms of varying degrees and permanence. Among the usual ones are irritability, change of character, disorder of judgment, disturbance of memory, difficulty of grasp and of orientation and perhaps confusion.

Mental symptoms, some mild, will be observed in 5 to 10 per cent of patients suffering from serious cardiorenal or heart disease, particularly that with congestive heart failure. Common symptoms are insomnia and nocturnal restlessness with sudden starting in a state of fright and alarm if the patient falls asleep. Irritability, moodiness and emotional instability are common. Frequently the patient is confused and misidentifies those about him. In some instances there may be auditory and visual hallucinations, incoherent speech and even unintelligible muttering. In the delirioid states of heart disease, the trend, as is frequently the case with other organic reaction types, is determined by the prepsychotic problems and conflicts of the patient. Delirium associated with cardiac decompensation and resulting cerebral anoxia should be promptly recognized.

Anxiety is the most frequent pathological mental symptom in cardiac patients. It is not entirely equivalent to fear and a justified apprehension but is often a complicated emotion in which hostility is mobilized as a defense against fear. Sometimes excessive dependency needs or needs to control the environment may prolong an invalidism for secondary gain. As in the case of other disabling illnesses the patient may use his invalidism to escape from some emotionally troublesome situation and be reluctant to relinquish this defense as he improves physically. Again the threat of his illness may be so intolerable to the patient as to lead to an irrational and rebellious denial of its existence.

The treatment of mental disorders associated with disturbances of the circulation will be directed largely to the cause of the disturbance. In those associated with heart disease this will, of course, include rest and proper cardiac stimulation, particularly with digitalis preparations. Sedatives may be necessary but hypnotics should be avoided lest a drug delirium develop.

As may be inferred from what has already been said, the internist has been prone, in heart disease as in many other organic diseases, to forget the importance of associated emotional factors. With cardiac function already greatly disturbed by a serious somatic lesion, a load of anxiety added from the psychic side may be sufficient to throw the balance in the direction of decompensation. If a patient is found to have frequent breaks in compensation when there is but relatively slight damage of heart muscle, a search should be made for complicating psychic factors the elimination of which may determine the course of the illness. From the standpoint of the psychiatrist, the most important problem is the handling of the patient's anxiety. Frequently he is deeply threatened by his symptoms and by the implications, often irrational, conveyed by the diagnosis. The physician should utilize his knowledge of psychopathology in dealing with the lowering of personality defenses that may occur in the face of fear of possible impending death. A strong, dependable and constructive doctor-patient relationship should help the patient in handling both intrinsic and extrinsic tensions and the emotionally disturbing life situations that frequently exist. Emotional decompensation may occur after surgical procedures, such as mitral commissurotomy, with sudden increase in physical capacity associated with expectations of increased activity. Those patients who have become dependent through long invalidism or have utilized the illness to avoid anxiety-provoking situations are most prone to respond to the surgical procedure in this manner.

In heart disease, particularly in coronary thrombosis, the physician should seek to dissipate the patient's fear of the disorder as an incapacitating or fatal ailment. Unwarranted fear is too often fostered by the gloomy predictions of the physician.

BIBLIOGRAPHY

Drewry, Jr., P. H., and Wall, J. H.: Mental reactions and their management in patients with cardiac disease. Am. J. Psychiat., *94:*561–576, 1937.

Duncan, C. H., *et al.:* Life situations, emotions and paroxysmal auricular arrhythmias. Psychosom. Med., *12:*23, 1950.

Kaplan, S. M.: Psychological aspects of cardiac disease: A study of patients experiencing mitral commissurotomy. Psychosom. Med., *18*:221–233, 1956.
Lewis, N. D. C.: Psychic phenomena with cardiac failure. Arch. Neurol. & Psychiat., *37*:782–795, 1937.
Reiser, M. F.: Emotional aspects of cardiac disease. Am. J. Psychiat., *107*:781–785, 1951.
Sprague, H. B.: Mental adjustments to heart disease. J.A.M.A., *112*:2384, 1939.
Wolfe, T. P.: Dynamic aspects of cardiovascular symptomatology. Am. J. Psychiat., *91*:563–574, 1934.
———: Emotions and organic heart disease. Am. J. Psychiat., *93*:681–691, 1936.

CHAPTER XIII

Acute Brain Syndromes Associated with Metabolic Disturbances

While chronic brain syndromes are more frequently associated with diseases of metabolism, endocrine disturbances and vitamin deficiencies than are acute ones, reversible syndromes may also occur at times with these disorders.

Although they are complex and imperfectly understood, and although the psychological and physical interrelations of *endocrine derangements* are poorly correlated, it is apparent that mutually influencing reactions occur among the central nervous system, mental functioning and the endocrines. It is reasonable to assume that interactions between emotional and metabolic processes may produce endocrine disturbances and these, in turn, may affect cerebral functions and mental reactions. The psychological consequences of a given hormonal action is not uniform. A certain hormonal change may or may not have a psychological effect. If it does produce an effect, it is not necessarily the same in all cases but will depend upon the previous personality organization of the individual and upon all the other influences acting upon the personality. It is not clear, however, whether endocrine abnormalities will in themselves produce a psychosis. Some endocrine disturbances produce changes in brain function by influencing brain metabolism. Yet this is no indication that such changes are related to disturbances in behavior. This is well illustrated when thyroid function is considered. While psychotic and other types of reaction occur in association with hyperthyroidism, it has been shown by recent work that the cerebral metabolic rate is not elevated from normal in this condition. On the other hand, in myxedema there is a reduction of oxygen consumption by the brain and a slowing up of expression at the psychological level.

Hyperthyroidism

In the mental disorders associated with hyperthyroidism—an association in which there is a striking interaction between emotional and metabolic processes—it has long been noted that a special type of personality seems usually to have existed before the clinical signs of Graves' disease were apparent. This disease arises largely in sensitive, impressionable persons who react keenly to life, who have a marked feeling of insecurity and an unusual sense of responsibility. The general hypermotivity, emotional excitability, alertness to every sound and impression, the tendency to walk, talk and eat rapidly, and the mild anxiety, apprehensiveness and irritability commonly observed in Graves' disease and characterized by the laity as "nervousness," represent in many ways but an exaggeration of a previously existing pattern of response to ordinary life problems. In other words these persons have been anxious individuals with psychiatric problems giving rise to tension. In them it is frequently impossible to tell where anxiety stops and hyperthyroidism begins. Psychiatric studies have shown that usually long before the onset of the clinical symptoms of hyperthyroidism patients who succumb to this illness have suffered emotional and psychological maladjustment. The majority of those who have examined groups of patients indicate that the basic need of such patients is for the satisfaction of an exaggerated dependency relationship. With chronic frustration their response is aggressive and leads to the welling up of death wishes toward the hoped-for gratifying party. As a means of adapting to such wishes the patients may respond by an over-depressed relationship to the significant person or turn away from this person and attempt a striving at self-sufficiency which is often premature. Women with the illness have many conflicts and fears in relation to childbirth, yet at the same time manifest a strong desire for children. The dependency needs are satisfied while the child is small but when the time comes for the child to seek its own independence, the mother responds often with anxiety and anger or with the reaction formation of anxious overconcern. These psychological defenses are not specific for the hyperthyroid patient and may be seen with many other conditions. Nevertheless, the strivings of individuals with this type of personality structure relate well to those observations which show that the psychiatric problem frequently precipitating the hyperthyroid activity is that of the loss of a key person in the patient's life.

While the usual mental symptoms associated with hyperthyroidism are those of tension, overactivity and emotional instability already mentioned, yet in about 20 per cent of acutely thyrotoxic patients a psychotic reaction appears. In extreme cases a fairly typical manic excitement may develop as if in accordance with the increased tempo of all organic processes. In other instances there may be an acute hallucinatory delirium accompanied by great restlessness and insomnia. Other patients present depressed, anxious, agitated reactions. Paranoid states with systematized delusions may occur. In general the symptoms manifested are exaggerations and caricatures of the previous personality. It will usually be found that persons with recurrent hyperthyroidism after thyroidectomy are still struggling with serious and unresolved personality difficulties.

The treatment of hyperthyroidism is often a joint task for the psychiatrist and the internist. While the internist will direct his efforts to the restoration of the metabolic rate to normal limits, the function of the psychiatrist is of value in those patients who are disturbed emotionally in accepting the need for therapy through bringing insight to their denial of symptoms. Continued psychotherapy is indicated for those hyperthyroid patients who present clear evidence of psychological maladjustment prior to the onset. Here psychotherapy is an important adjunct in bringing about a permanent euthyroid state with reduction in emotional and psychological symptomatology described above.

Pituitary Disorders

In his original description of what has come to be known as Cushing's syndrome, a disease occurring in association with a basophile adenoma of the pituitary gland, Harvey Cushing called attention to the frequent coexistence of mental symptoms. The most frequent mental accompaniments associated with this disease or with adrenocortical hyperfunction are depression and irritability. At times schizophrenic reactions have been observed. The patient may also be retarded or show agitation, anxiety and nonco-operative behavior. The mental symptoms may be related to adrenocortical dysfunction and metabolic abnormalities. On the other hand, they may to a considerable extent represent a psychological reaction to the disfiguring alteration in the patient's appearance. As the disease progresses the patient's appearance may be changed from that of an attractive girl to that of an obese and bearded old lady whose activities are restricted by weakness and fatigue.

Hypoglycemia

It is now recognized that spontaneous—in distinction from therapeutically induced—hypoglycemic states may occasionally exist. At times the clinical picture of such hypoglycemic attacks may be dominated by mental symptoms, usually transitory in nature. There is no single psychic syndrome characteristic of the condition. Among the many mental phenomena that may be prominent are the following: apathy, irritability, restlessness, anxiety, negativism, somnambulism, confusion, disorientation, fugue states, delirium, syncope, stupor or coma. Thinking may be confused and retarded and speech disturbed. Grasp may be impaired and emotions unstable. Hallucinations and delusions may be present. The patient may complain of weakness, fatigability and hunger. He perspires and may suffer from tremor, unsteadiness of gait, diplopia and convulsions. There is no recollection of the attack. There is a tendency for the symptoms to appear after exertion or when the patient is hungry. Complete relief from the symptoms follows the administration of sugar. Hypoglycemia should always be suspected as the cause of any mental symptoms appearing in a diabetic who is receiving insulin. The diagnosis of spontaneous hypoglycemia is made on evidence of depression of the blood sugar level. Since the periods of hypoglycemia are transient it is often difficult to establish the diagnosis by simple study of the fasting blood sugar. A definitive diagnosis is evident if the blood sugar determination occurring during an attack falls below 50 or 60 mg. per 100 ml. If the attack is convulsive in nature the blood sugar may be elevated following the seizure. Glucose tolerance tests have limited value but may suggest the diagnosis if the blood sugar level falls to 50 mg. per 100 ml. three to five hours after the stimulating dose of glucose. When hypoglycemia is not demonstrated by these means a 24 or 48 hour fast should be instituted and blood sugar determinations made at 12-, 18- and 24-hour periods. With the onset of symptoms and their prompt alleviation by the use of intravenous glucose, the diagnosis is established. Electroencephalographic changes occur in association with such attacks and show local or widespread dysrhythmias which again are relieved on ingestion or intravenous application of glucose.

Once the diagnosis of hypoglycemia is established, its etiology must be determined. While the majority of such patients will be found to suffer from hyperinsulinism caused by islet cell tumors of the pancreas, the functional cases with an associated neurosis are of particular interest to the psychiatrist. It has not been determined whether this type of condition may occur as a somatic manifestation of a psychoneurosis or whether the majority of such cases fall into the group of induced hypoglycemic states symbolic of a sado-masochistic neurotic conflict. A number of such induced hypoglycemic cases have been observed, usually in women and most frequently nurses who have had experience with the utilization of insulin. The diagnosis was established on one occasion by tagging the insulin used by the patient with radioactive phosphorus and then detecting the excretion of the radioactive material in the urine the following day. In some instances the patient suffered from diabetes and had numerous unexplained attacks of hypoglycemia though denying the use of insulin.

The following case history illustrates such a problem and its management:

> The patient, a 44-year-old married nurse, with a history of episodic attacks of hunger, weakness, sleepiness, sweating, vertigo and occasionally unconsciousness was referred for study. The attacks were always aborted by eating. They were so severe that six months previously the patient had to give up a fast. Another physician had diagnosed an islet cell pancreatic tumor and advised surgery. The patient refused operation stating that she had gained weight and was not suffering any pain. She consulted other physicians in an attempt to obtain a different diagnosis. She expressed her fear to these physicians that if operated upon she would become diabetic and require insulin.
>
> A careful medical examination failed to reveal any evidence of tumor. The patient sustained a fast without the development of hypoglycemia. In view of previous experiences with patients who had induced hypoglycemia, the patient's room was searched while she was having a diagnostic test and several bottles of insulin and a syringe were found. At this point a psychiatric examination was requested.

In consultation the patient reported that her mother who died two years previously had been a diabetic and had been nursed in her terminal illness by the patient. The patient had lived a restricted life and had entered nursing to relieve herself of her loneliness. Some four years previously she had undergone a hysterectomy performed by the physician who had advised her that she had an islet cell tumor.

Following the initial psychiatric interview the patient stated that she proposed to sign out of the hospital. Since it was considered that her condition was dangerous in the sense that she was exposing herself to a potentially major surgical procedure the psychiatric consultant concluded that it was advisable to suggest the possibility of induced hypoglycemia to the patient. This was done by informing her of the conclusions reached by the medical service on the basis of finding the bottle of insulin and the previous experience of the hospital with others with similar conditions. The patient was gently told that if this were the case she must have some underlying emotional problems which had led her to the desperate expedient of the self-administration of insulin and that she might therefore wish to solve the major conflicts which had driven her to such action. The suggestion was met by immediate denial. When seen the following day the patient asked assurance that any information given by her would be considered inviolate. When this was given she broke down, cried and gave the following information:

She stated that her drive for the self-administration of insulin began about four months previously during the period of a fast when she felt weak and unable to continue her work. Believing that she might obtain a dispensation from a religious fast from the physician who had removed her uterus some years earlier, with whom she worked and toward whom she had a strong positive attachment, she asked if he would assist her in securing a dispensation for medical reasons. He replied that he would do so if he found her to be suffering from hypoglycemia. Shortly before blood was to be drawn for the determination of its sugar content the nurse, without the knowledge of the physician, took her first injection of insulin. Naturally a hypoglycemia was found. The physician therefore gave her the desired recommendation that dispensation be granted from the obligation of fasting before communion.

The nurse then revealed that she had developed a feeling of depression after her hysterectomy. She worried that she had not healed properly and wondered whether she would develop a cancer. Her father had died of cancer and had suffered from fears relating to mental disease. He was given insulin to relieve his depression. The patient herself had given insulin in mental hospitals and recalled her anxiety on being shown the brain of a patient who had died during insulin shock therapy. Throughout her life she had felt hungry, had been an extremely heavy eater and fasting had caused her to feel weak. The patient had always devoted herself to the care of her mother and an aunt and had spent months at home each year nursing them for their various ailments. The mother would write her that she should provide nursing services not only for herself and the aunt but also for her brothers if she really loved her family. She always seemed fearful of losing the love of her relatives. Perhaps it was not surprising that upon the death of her parents she expressed the sentiment that her brothers "beat her out" of her patrimony.

The nurse declared that she had devoted the same amount of attention to the care of her physician's patients as she had to her own family. She admitted that her response to his rejection of a request for a medical dispensation had been one of anger and resentment. On the other hand she felt so anxious concerning the possibility of losing his respect and good will and so guilty in relation to the church that she was forced to continue the self-administration of insulin when faced with another medical examination. Following these revelations which were responded to with sympathetic interpretation of her emotional responses and their origin, the patient returned home to her profession and made a satisfactory adaptation with no recurrence of the hypoglycemic attacks.

Acute Vitamin Deficiency Syndrome

Chronic mental syndromes are not exceedingly rare in cases of chronic avitaminosis, particularly in thiamine deficiency, but acute mental syndromes are quite uncommon. Jolliffe, however, called attention to what he called "acute nicotinic acid deficiency encephalopathy." This syndrome is characterized by delirium, sucking and grasping reflexes, cogwheel rigidities and irregular jerking movements of the extremities. This readily disappears when treated with niacin.

Exhaustion Delirium

At times acute, confusional, delirioid reactions accompany marked states of exhaustion. Since such reactions are not associated with infection, they may best be considered in a discussion of acute syndromes resulting from disturbances of metabolism. Exhaustion delirium is not common but is occasionally associated with hemorrhage, unusual and extremely prostrating physical exertion, starvation, prolonged insomnia under conditions of stress or emotional tension and debilitating effects of a chronic wasting disease such as carcinoma. This acute hallucinatory confusion ("confusion mentale") was described by Chaslin under the term primary mental confusion and by Meynert under the designation *amentia*, a term still applied to this syndrome by English and German but not by American psychiatrists who occasionally employ the word as synonymous with feeblemindedness. The onset is usually with insomnia, some clouding of consciousness, mild confusion, difficulty in collecting one's thoughts, perplexity, perhaps of a distressed type, vague fears, restlessness, illusions, fleeting hallucinations and changing delusions. The patient's mood varies with his thought content. The environment appears obscure and distorted. As the condition increases in severity, the patient becomes more bewildered; his perceptions more impaired, he misidentifies persons and objects and becomes disoriented. Sometimes speech production is of a question and answer form. Frequently the patient may seem to be groping in a mental fog as if attempting to differentiate his confused, dreamlike world from that of reality and gain a point of contact with his previous normal life. Sometimes he may be comparatively clear for a period only to return to his previous confusion. This confusional, toxic-exhaustive state may continue for several weeks but recovery finally takes place. After his recovery the patient may be able to give considerable retrospective interpretation of his delusions and hallucinatory experiences.

Postoperative Neuroses and Psychoses

Since metabolic changes (acidosis, acetonuria, glycosuria, hypoglycemia and hepatic insufficiency) may in some instances act as contributory agents to many postoperative mental disturbances these should be included among acute brain syndromes resulting from metabolic and endocrine disorders. It is probable, however, that other factors, both somatic and psychogenic, are of equal or more importance. Postoperative anxiety and other neurotic states are, too, more frequent than postoperative psychoses. Their source is to be sought in emotional factors.

Physical agents, other than metabolic changes, may include the anesthetic, sedative drugs, toxic and infectious complications, also nutritional disturbances with associated dehydration, ketosis or avitaminosis. Among psychological factors are fear and apprehension preceding the operation. The fear of mutilation, of loss of part of one's body and of possible death is important. The strangeness of the setting, the sights and sounds in the operating room and all the other preoperative procedures including anesthesia with the fear of losing consciousness contribute to the tension and apprehension. The importance to the patient of the particular organ operated upon will affect the possibility of a postoperative psychosis and will influence the character and content of any psychotic ideas. Psychotic reactions are most frequent following operations upon the eyes and the genitals. There is usually a postoperative interval of three to ten days before the onset of the psychosis. The most frequent type of postoperative syndrome is delirium with its confusion, disorientation, hallucinations, paranoid delusions, fear, apprehension and restlessness. Similar disturbances may follow amputations of limbs and other external appendages. In these instances, the clinical picture is complicated by the patient's reaction to the "phantom phenomenon" (described in Chapter XXIX). A not uncommon postoperative mental syndrome is that which occasionally follows the removal of a cataract. The patient becomes suspicious and confused and manifests fear and panic-like excitement, particularly at night. The loss of familiar landmarks adds to the sense of insecurity.

Manic states, depressions and schizophrenic reactions determined by long-standing personality factors may be released by emotional, toxic or other agents incident to the operation.

Surgery may be accompanied not only by trauma to the body but also to the personality. Psychological factors such as those mentioned may also act in the production of anxiety and occasionally of hysterical syndromes. In addition to these factors ill-considered remarks by the surgeon or his assistants, technical bedside discussions or the demonstration of charts or roentgenograms that create apprehension on the part of the patient may produce alarm in the insecure personality. Pelvic evisceration in the woman highly desirous of bearing children may prove so frustrating that a permanent neurosis results. While scarcely pertinent to the present topic, it should be borne in mind that many a failure of surgery to relieve a disabling symptom is because an attempt has been made to remove surgically the somatic expression of an emotional illness. All too often such attempts merely lead to their repetition.

BIBLIOGRAPHY

Abeles, M. M.: Postoperative psychoses. Am. J. Psychiat., *94*:1187–1200, 1938.

Association for Research in Nervous and Mental Disease, Vol. XXII: The Role of Nutritional Deficiency in Nervous and Mental Diseases. Baltimore, Williams & Wilkins Co., 1943.

Bleuler, M.: Endokrinologische Psychiatrie. Stuttgart, Georg Thieme Verlag, 1954.

Brown, W. T., and Gildea, E. F.: Hyperthyroidism and personality. Am. J. Psychiat., *94*:59–72, 1937.

Harn, G. C., et al.: Dynamic Aspects of the Personality Features and Reactions Characteristic of Patients with Graves' Disease. In Proceedings of Association for Research in Nervous and Mental Diseases, Vol. XXIX. Baltimore, Williams & Wilkins Co., 1950.

Himwich, H. E.: Brain Metabolism and Cerebral Disorders. Baltimore, Williams & Wilkins Co., 1951.

Kepler, E. J., and Moersch, F. P.: The psychiatric manifestations of hypoglycemia. Am. J. Psychiat., *94:*89–108, 1937.

Kleinschmidt, H. J., Waxenberg, S. E., and Cuker, R.: Psychophysiology and psychiatric management of thyrotoxicosis. J. Mt. Sinai Hosp., *23:*131–153, 1956.

Lidz, Theodore: Emotional factors in the etiology and therapy of hyperthyroidism. J. Mt. Sinai Hosp., *20:*27, 1953.

Mandelbrote, B. M., and Wittkower, E. D.: Emotional factors in Graves' disease. Psychosom. Med., *17:*109–123, 1955.

Rome, H. P., and Braceland, F. J.: Psychological response to corticotropin, cortisone, and related substances. J.A.M.A., *148:*27–30, 1952.

Rynearson, E. H.: Hyperinsulinism among malingerers. M. Clin. North America, *477:*480, 1950.

Sokoloff, L., Wechsler, R. L., Mangold, R., Balls, K., and Kety, S. S.: Cerebral blood flow and oxygen consumption in hyperthyroidism before and after treatment. J. Clin. Investigation, *32:*202, 1953.

Thethowan, W. H., and Cobb, Stanley: Neuropsychiatric aspects of Cushing's syndrome. Arch. Neurol. & Psychiat., *67:*283–309, 1952.

CHAPTER XIV

Chronic Brain Disorders

THE MENTAL syndromes discussed in Chapters VIII to XIII inclusive are, for the most part, the result of temporary, reversible, diffuse impairment of brain tissue function. In the present and in several succeeding chapters we deal with chronic organic syndromes resulting from relatively permanent, more or less irreversible, impairment of cerebral tissue function. Usually some impairment of "intellectual" functions, such as memory, comprehension and judgment, as well as affect, persists permanently.

Syphilitic Meningoencephalitis

The chronic brain syndrome associated with syphilitic meningoencephalitis, and formerly known as general paresis, general paralysis of the insane, or dementia paralytica, is a disorder produced by a progressive syphilitic meningoencephalitis leading to a degeneration of brain parenchyma with an infiltration of interstitial elements. Clinically, general paresis is characterized by a comprehensive but variable syndrome of neurological and mental disturbances associated with fairly constant serological changes.

History

Although Haslam of Bethlehem Hospital, in a monograph entitled "Observations on Insanity," described in 1798 the associated mental and physical symptoms that occur in general paresis, yet the credit for its recognition as a clinical and pathological entity belongs to the French psychiatrist, A. L. J. Bayle, who published his thesis in 1822 at the age of twenty-three. An opinion that paresis was caused by syphilis was first expressed in 1857 by Esmarch and Jessen. At first this theory received but little credence. Finally it became accepted that syphilis was a cause in some cases, although many psychiatrists continued to believe that other causes might be operative, an opinion maintained by only a few after Alzheimer and Nissl in 1904 demonstrated the histopathology of the disease. Later the development of the Wassermann reaction indicated the existence of syphilis in practically all cases of paresis. Any remaining doubt that syphilis is the sole determining cause was dispelled in 1913 when Joseph W. Moore of the Central Islip (New York) State Hospital, confirmed by Hideyo Noguchi of the Rockefeller Institute, demonstrated the Treponema pallidum in the brains of paretics. It is now possible to demonstrate treponemata in fresh paretic brains taken at necropsy and studied by darkfield illumination. They may also be discovered in brain tissue obtained by puncture in living paretics.

The disappointment arising from the failure of the brain lesions to respond to arsphenamine as did the signs and symptoms of syphilis elsewhere in the body stimulated research into other forms of treatment. In 1917 Wagner-Jauregg of Vienna found that artificial fever induced by inoculation with malaria resulted in an arrest of the paretic process and an improvement of the patient. Within the next few years other methods of producing artificial fever, some of them equally effective, were developed. In 1919 the discovery of tryparsamide, a pentavalent arsenical, by Jacobs and Heidelberger at the Rockefeller Institute added a valuable chemotherapeutic agent. In 1943 penicillin was found to be an active spirocheticidal agent and has since then proven to be an effective means of treating both general syphilis and neurosyphilis. Thanks to these discoveries and to the more widespread use of lumbar puncture as an early diagnostic measure, paresis, instead of being an invariably fatal disease, can now be prevented in a vast majority of cases if treatment of syphilis is early and active. If paresis arises because of the absence or inadequacy of treatment, it can nevertheless be arrested in 70 to 80 per cent of cases and if treated early 50 per cent of cases can be restored to their former station in society.

Frequency

Prior to 1920, 8 to 10 per cent of patients committed to public hospitals in the United States were suffering from general paresis whereas at the present time about 2 per cent of first admissions are suffering from this disease. This decline in admissions is probably a result of both a decrease in syphilis and of earlier and more adequate treatment.

The Treponema pallidum is one of the few microorganisms which can penetrate the blood-brain barrier with ease. It is now believed that during the period of generalized spirochetemia this invasion of the neuroaxis occurs in most if not all patients infected with syphilis. In the majority of cases, this original invasion never produces symptoms, physical signs, or changes in the cerebrospinal fluid; the organisms which have penetrated the nervous system are spontaneously eliminated by obscure immune processes not yet understood. The reason for the development of paresis in some luetics while others remain free from the disease is not known but perhaps the incidence is determined by the virulence of the infection and by immune factors in the host. There probably is not a special neurotropic strain of treponemata. Abnormalities of the spinal fluid found to persist for more than two years after infection suggest that the central nervous system may be seriously involved. Even though the patient then shows no clinical signs or symptoms of neurosyphilis he is extremely likely to do so later and is particularly prone to develop paresis. It is therefore exceedingly important that examinations of the spinal fluid be continued during the first three years following infection and, if found positive, that treatment continue until it is negative. A normal spinal fluid three years after the primary lesion, whether therapy has been given or not, is nearly always assurance against future parenchymatous neurosyphilis. With adequate treatment of syphilis in its early stage followed by prolonged observation, general paresis can be prevented in almost 100 per cent of cases.

Paresis occurs four times more frequently in men than in women. The cause for this strikingly higher incidence in men is uncertain since the probable ratio of primary syphilis infection among men as compared with women is not greater than 2 to 1 (Moore and Merritt). Parenchymatous neurosyphilis is also much less frequent among Negroes than among whites in spite of the greater incidence of syphilis among the former. Not a few persons develop syphilitic meningoencephalitis without previous knowledge of their luetic infection.

Pathology

The basic pathology of paresis is a chronic syphilitic meningoencephalitis in which two pathological components—inflammation and degeneration—are at work. The process with its progressive degeneration of nerve cells begins largely in the frontal region but as the disease progresses any part of the cortex, cerebellum or bulb may become involved. The pia is typically thickened, edematous and infiltrated, often presenting a cloudy, frosted appearance. Frequently it is firmly attached to the surface of the brain so that on attempting to remove it portions of the brain substance are torn away with the result that the cortex may present a flaking appearance. The thickening of the meninges is largely a result of infitration with lymphocytes and plasma cells and proliferation of the endothelial cells. Because of a diffuse atrophy of the cerebral cortex the sulci are widened and the convolutions less distinct than in the normal brain. The atrophy is greatest in the frontal lobes and progressively decreases toward the posterior poles of the hemispheres. There is an increase in both the subarachnoid and the ventricular cerebrospinal fluid. The ventricular ependyma is thickened, and often, particularly on the floor of the fourth ventricle, presents a frosted or granular appearance known as granular ependymitis.

Microscopically the perivascular lymph spaces of the vessels are crowded with proliferated endothelial cells, occasional mast cells, and most important of all, lymphocytes and plasma cells. The pia is similarly infiltrated with lymphocytes and plasma cells. A sprouting of the capillaries produces increased vascularity, while the "cuffing" of these capillaries by the perivascular infiltration mentioned gives rise to one of the important histopathological features of paresis, although it is not confined to general paralysis but occurs also in epidemic encephalitis and in trypanosomiasis. The ganglion cells are cloudy, suffer degeneration, and many disappear, particularly in the middle layer of the frontal cortex. It has not yet been determined whether the degenerative changes are caused by the action of the spirochetes themselves or by their toxic products. The usual cortical architecture with its lamination and column formation of the neuron cells is disorganized. The glia is proliferated. Scattered about through the cortex are numerous cylindrical-appearing cells known as rod cells or stäbchenzellen, first described by Franz Nissl—"An extraordinary long cell, whose cell body does not appear plainly or adheres to both poles in the form of a single thread."

Another constant finding in the brain of the paretic is the presence of iron pigment in the walls of the blood vessels and in the cortical microglia. Many pathologists consider that the presence in the rod cells of a substance giving a Prussian blue reaction is to be considered as characteristic and pathognomonic of general paresis. Spirochetes are found in about 80 per cent of untreated cases. The greatest number are usually to be found in the second and third layers of the anterior frontal cortex but may exist in nearly all gray matter of the brain. They have never been found lying free in the white matter. According to Jahnel, spirochetes have never been satisfactorily demonstrated within ganglion cells. Blood cultures of a patient with general paresis have never shown a growth of treponemata.

The degree of the brain changes is believed to be dependent upon the multiplication of the parasites and, perhaps, upon the production of a toxin. Probably of significance is the increased permeability in the barrier between the blood vessels and the cerebrospinal fluid observed in general paresis by Malamud. The fact that in paresis the resistance of this barrier in the walls of the cerebral capillaries is lowered, or, stated differently, that the permeability from the blood into the cerebrospinal fluid is increased (as determined by the passage of bromides) suggests that the toxins of syphilis may more easily and freely secure entrance into the brain tissue. Perhaps this index of permeability may be an indicator of the condition of the capillaries and small vessels and therefore a link between the clinical and histological pictures. Bielschowsky expresses the opinion that the altered permeability is due to inflammatory changes in the walls of the vessels.

Incubation Period

General paresis develops from five to thirty or more years after the primary infection with syphilis. In one half of the cases, the incubation period is from ten to twenty years; in one fourth the period is under ten years, and in one fourth it is over twenty years. The peak in the curve of incidence occurs between the ages of thirty-five and forty-five. This long period of incubation does not mean that the nervous system of a person who develops general paresis is not invaded long before the appearance of clinical symptoms. The invasion, in fact, probably occurs in the first few months of the infection although the serological changes in the cerebrospinal fluid characteristic of the disease do not develop until later. Invasion of the nervous system by Treponema pallidum is first manifested by a rising cell count. Three to six months later the protein becomes elevated and this is then followed by the development of a positive Wassermann and colloidal reaction. If the nervous system has not been invaded by the end of the second year of the disease it is unlikely that it will ever be involved. How long the serological changes of the paretic formula antedate the appearance of clinical symptoms is uncertain. It is established, however, that there is such a preclinical period during which the only evidence of the disease consists of spinal fluid findings characteristic of the disease. Clinical symptoms have not yet developed. During this period the patient may be said to be suffering from *asymptomatic paresis*. It should be regarded as the forerunner of clinical paresis. In fact the difference between the asymptomatic phase and the symptomatic one is only a matter of degree. It would be highly desirable if the disease could be discovered and treated during this asymptomatic stage. For this reason every patient having a positive Wassermann reaction of the blood serum should also have an examination of the cerebrospinal fluid even if there are no signs or symptoms of central nervous system involvement. Also a spinal fluid examination should be made on every patient with early syphilis within 12 to 24 months after completion of treatment.

Trauma and Paresis

The question as to whether trauma may play a precipitating role in the production of general paralysis in a person already suffering from syphilis is one which occasionally confronts industrial accident and other boards exercising similar judicial functions. There are medical evidence and judicial precedent to connect head trauma with development or acceleration of the paretic process. The limits usually set for this causal relationship are six weeks to three months as a minimum and two or three years as a maximum. There is, however, divergence of opinion as to the severity of injury necessary for a relationship between the injury and the development of the disease. To justify the opinion that trauma precipitated or aggravated the general paralysis, it must be shown that the trauma involved the head and was of sufficient intensity to injure the brain by concussion, or more likely by contusion. It is not probable, in such a case, that the injury initiated the paretic process but that the trauma activated an asymptomatic paresis and caused clinical symptoms to appear. It cannot be stated whether or not, in the absence of trauma, a person in such a preclinical stage would have developed general paresis. At times the trauma does not activate a pathological process but perhaps aggravates one that already existed although its symptoms had thus far not been recognized. Probably most psychiatrists feel that the role of trauma in the precipitation or aggravation of the symptoms of general paresis has not been adequately established on a scientific basis. Since there is basis for controversy in individual cases, the therapist should be conservative in expressing any conclusions as to relationship. By far the most frequent relation between trauma and general paresis is that the injury was sustained in an accident that resulted from the impairment of judgment, apperception or co-ordination produced by the unrecognized existence of the disease. Such accidents serve to call attention to the menace in industry of the early paretic, the existence or nature of whose symptoms has escaped recognition.

Symptoms and Signs

The description of syphilitic meningoencephalitis may conveniently be considered under the following headings: (*a*) mental symptoms, (*b*) neurological signs, and (*c*) serological changes.

Mental Symptoms. Mental symptoms are usually first in calling attention to the disease although inflammatory and degenerative changes have previously taken place. Serological changes have already existed for a considerable period. The clinical findings often fail to reflect the extent of the pathological process. Frequently the mental symptoms develop so insidiously that the patient's family has not recognized that a deteriorating change in personality has been taking place. The physician often has difficulty in determining the exact time when symptoms first existed. The early symptoms may consist largely of an extension and exaggeration of previous personality traits. Other early symptoms may be irritability, fatigue, difficulty in concentration, depression, periods of confusion, disturbed sleep and headache. Not rarely the early paretic is opinionated and perhaps quarrelsome. Frequently he becomes neglectful of his dress, unkempt in appearance, inconsiderate of others, forgetful of social amenities and proprieties and manifests an insidious breakdown of higher ethical and cultural sentiments and standards. The moderate user of alcohol may become dissipated; sexual activities may become excessive. The man whose previous life has been quite exemplary may not only suddenly show some surprising defect of character but feel no concern for his dereliction. Early in the disease there is often an impairment in professional skill or in craftsmanship. Unaccustomed slips and failures in the discharge of ordinary duties occur. The consequences of errors are not foreseen. The patient may conceive ambitious schemes of an extremely impracticable and extravagant nature. The business man may not only no longer show his former capacity for successful management but because of failing judgment may dissipate the resources upon which the livelihood of his family depends. There is often a contented indifference–an apathy and unconcern that at first may be mistaken for laziness. Not infrequently there is a tendency to drowsiness. The patient becomes incapable of submitting his impressions and conclusions to a critical examination nor does he recognize the insidious deterioration that is going on in the intellectual, feeling and social aspects of his personality. The man previously regarded as possessing an acute and well-trained mind and sound judgment surprises his acquaintances by his failure to grasp the finer shades of meaning or by some puerile, inept remark. Associations are characterized by their slowness, superficiality and poverty. A change of mood is common in the early stages, frequently taking the form of apathy or depression. Sometimes the early stages are characterized by anxiety. In some cases euphoria and expansiveness exist from the beginning but more often these mood trends appear somewhat later. Momentary periods of confusion or an inability to grasp a situation and to act promptly and correctly not rarely lead to automobile accidents in early paretics whose mental disorder has not yet been detected. One paretic whose disorder had not yet been recognized left his home dressed only in night clothes, coat and hat to attend the funeral of a friend. Occasionally, particularly in the early stages of the disease, there may be a tendency to a Korsakoff type of confabulation, the content of which is characterized by the narration of fantastic experiences.

Delusions occur at some period of the disease in a majority of paretics. It has usually been emphasized that the delusions are grandiose, yet not more than 50 per cent of paretics express delusions of this nature. Expansive delusions may reach the height of absurdity. The patient may declare, for example, that he owns a railroad freight train each car of which is loaded with million-dollar treasury notes. Ideas of boundless benevolence may be expressed, including fantastic schemes for the welfare of all mankind. Not rarely, however, delusions are depressive, self-accusatory, nihilistic or persecutory. Hallucinations occasionally occur but are not of diagnostic significance. In the very early stage of the paretic process, individuals who before the development of the psychosis showed a definite tendency to schizoid or cyclothymic manifestations frequently at the onset of the mental disturbance exhibit features suggestive of schizophrenia or manic-depressive psychosis.

The dementia of general paresis, even at a comparatively early stage, tends to be of a diffuse type involving memory, judgment, emotional life and conative expressions. Intelligence tests show a mental deterioration with defective reasoning and an impairment of social ability, memory and learning. Unlike the dementia of senility, it is not at first limited largely to memory. As the disease advances, the dementia becomes progressive. Affectivity and emotional response suffer impoverishment, inadequacies of perception prevent contact with the environment, memory fails, associations become slow and limited, apperception is destroyed, spontaneous activities cease and finally the mental processes, devoid of conscious participation, are reduced to those at the reflex and vegetative level.

Physical and Neurological Signs. As numerous and varied as are the mental symptoms that may exist in paresis, the physical and neurological symptoms are equally so. During the stage of onset the patient may become easily fatigued and perhaps lose weight. Numerous somatic complaints referred to the various bodily systems are frequent in the early course of the disease. Many paretics have been diagnosed as suffering from neurasthenia. Many patients complain of headache, caused probably by the thickening of the meninges and by an increase in pressure of the cerebrospinal fluid. Because of the loss of tone in the facial muscles, the lines of expression become smoothed out. This relaxation of the facial muscles together with the blunting of emotional response gives the facies a vacant, fatuous appearance. There seems reason to believe that this loss of expression, the tremors and the spasticity to be mentioned later may well be a result of changes in the basal ganglia and substantia nigra.

Disturbances, varying greatly in degree, occur almost certainly at some period in the eye, or in its innervation or reflexes. Papilledema, syphilitic retinitis or primary optic atrophy may occur. Bruetsch reports that complete optic atrophy occurs in 2 per cent of cases and that incipient and intermediate stages of atrophy occur in 62.5 per cent of paretics. Probably optic atrophy is the end result of direct infection and inflammation of the optic nerve and chiasm causing destruction of nerve fibers, disappearance of nerve fibers, disappearance of myelin sheaths and connective tissue and glial overgrowth. More frequent than optic atrophy are the disturbances of the pupils, which may be unequal in size, irregular in outline, much contracted or widely dilated. Reaction to light is often sluggish or lost as may also be the convergence reaction. The pupil first described by Argyll Robertson in 1869 will be found in over one half of paretics. This is a miotic pupil which contracts when the eyes converge and accommodates for near vision but which does not contract when strong light is suddenly thrown on the eye. Occasionally there may be some degree of ptosis of one lid or a weakness of one of the external muscles of the eye, especially the external rectus. It is to be distinguished from Adie's myotonic pupillary response which also is seen associated with absent deep reflexes. The myotonic pupil is never miotic but dilated, sometimes oval, and after a period in the dark it slowly contracts with exposure to light.

A progressive weakness and inco-ordination of all voluntary muscles occurs. There is a tremor of the facial muscles, first observed in the lips when the patient attempts to speak or show his teeth. As enunciation becomes more difficult, there is an overactivity of all the facial muscles when speech is attempted. The tremor of the tongue is coarse and is best demonstrated when it is protruded. This muscle weakness and inco-ordination lead to the disturbance of speech which, when associated with the blandly inane facial expression already noted, constitute a syndrome so characteristic that the experienced psychiatrist can often make a diagnosis as the patient speaks. At first this speech defect is often manifested in the form of a hesitation, drawl or slurring. Later there is omission, reduplication or transposition of syllables. The speech disturbances are often best demonstrated by asking the patient to repeat polysyllabic words or phrases containing labial or dental types of consonants (as "electrical artillery brigade"). Omission of syllables, slurring, a terminal clipping of words and even a forgetting of some of them will often be demonstrated if the patient is requested to repeat the words three or four times. As the disease progresses the speech may become quite unintelligible. Transient, incomplete aphasic attacks may occur, at times rather early in the disease.

Deterioration in handwriting is often an early clinical symptom. Because of loss in delicate muscular co-ordination it is often tremulous. There may also be reduplication or elision of letters in syllables. Characters show irregularity in spacing or size, a diminutiveness of which is particularly common. As the disease progresses the patient usually becomes unable to write at all from dictation, and if he attempts to form characters he produces only an unintelligible scrawl.

Muscular inco-ordination gives rise also to many other symptoms. Among early ones is a tremulous inco-ordination of finer movements of the hand. Later the patient is unable to button his clothing or even to dress himself. As the disease progresses, station and gait become uncertain, all movements are clumsy, and finally because of his weakness and ataxia, the patient is confined to his bed. The muscles of deglutition do not escape involvement with the result that difficulty in swallowing may occur.

Disturbances of the deep tendon reflexes are the rule. More frequently these are exaggerated, when ankle clonus and spasticity are usually present, but if, as not infrequently happens, a tabetic process coexists the knee jerks are absent. Disturbances of the rectal and vesical sphincters are common in the terminal stages. Not infrequently the bladder may become greatly distended, resulting in a dribbling of urine caused by an overflow of retention. Rupture of such a bladder may occur upon receipt of slight trauma. Trophic changes may occur in the bones with the result that they may be easily fractured.

It is not uncommon for the paretic suddenly to develop a marked rise in temperature without evidence of infection or of additional somatic disease. These apparently causeless fevers are probably a result of disturbances of the heat-regulating centers.

About three fourths of all paretics suffer from convulsions at some time during the course of the disease. Occasionally a convulsion, particularly of an abortive type, may be the first symptom to attract attention to the disease, although more frequently convulsions do not occur until the disease is well developed. The occurrence of a convulsion in a person of early middle age who has never previously suffered from a seizure should always suggest the possibility of general paresis. The seizures may show numerous variations in type but are most frequently of an epileptiform nature. Convulsions in syphilitic meningoencephalitis must be considered of serious significance as not a few patients die during or soon after a seizure. The cause of these convulsions is not known but they are perhaps a result of sudden deprivation of oxygen at some area by reason of vascular disturbances.

Another form of episodic attack is apoplectiform in type. These attacks are sudden in onset, are accompanied by disturbances of consciousness and followed by hemiplegia or more localized paralyses. These paralyses are usually temporary in nature, often clearing up without residuals in a few days. Less frequently a hemorrhage occurs, leaving a permanent paralysis.

Serology. Serological changes provide important diagnostic evidence as to the existence of general paresis. The spinal fluid syndrome provides the best guide to the activity of a syphilitic infection of the central nervous system and to the effect of treatment. In nearly all cases of untreated paresis, the Wassermann reaction on the blood serum is positive. Of much greater importance, as indicating not only the presence of neurosyphilis but also its parenchymatous nature, are certain changes in the cerebrospinal fluid. In general paresis, the patient usually suffers less headache and discomfort following the withdrawal of 10 ml. of the fluid than does the person with intact nervous system. The normal limits of pressure of the cerebrospinal fluid when the patient is prone are generally considered to be from 70 to 160 mm. of water. In general paresis this pressure may be increased, and in approximately 8 per cent of cases it will exceed 200 mm. of water. The important tests in the examination of the cerebrospinal fluid for the existence of general paresis are the Wassermann reaction, protein tests, the cell count, and a colloidal test, preferably the gold test. In untreated syphilitic meningoencephalitis, the Wassermann reaction in the cerebrospinal fluid is positive with 0.2 ml. of the fluid in 90 per cent of the cases and is always positive with 1 ml. A positive Wassermann reaction does not, of course, signify that the neurosyphilis is of the paretic type nor does it necessarily indicate that the process is active. Under ordinary conditions, the protein content of the spinal fluid is chiefly albumin and globulin in the ratio of 4 to 1. An increase of protein to 50 to 150 mg. per 100 ml. (normal, 25 mg.) with a disproportionate increase of globulin is the rule in paresis although these increases are merely indicative of a disorder—not necessarily syphilitic—within the nervous system. The total protein and the amount of globulin are greater in general paresis than in any other type of neurosyphilis except acute meningitis. The more active the paretic process, the larger the amount of these substances. The normal cell count of the spinal fluid varies from one to five small lymphocytes per cubic millimeter. In paresis, the number of cells in the spinal fluid may remain normal or may reach one hundred, the average being twenty-five to fifty. An excess of this number indicates that a syphilitic meningitis also exists. The cell count affords the most valuable information as to the activity of the infection. It is also the first abnormality to return to normal as a result of treatment.

Given a positive Wassermann of the spinal fluid and other evidence of neurosyphilis, one of the most valuable tests in determining its type is the colloidal gold test described by Lange in 1912. This test depends on the precipitation and varying degrees of decolorization of a solution of gold chloride by a series of dilutions of the cerebrospinal fluid. The precipitation is considered to be caused by globulin, the curve of precipitation depending on the relative amounts of globulin and albumin present in the arachnoid fluid. Since, of the various forms of neurosyphilis, paresis shows the largest amount of globulin in the cerebrospinal fluid, it would be expected that the greatest precipitation of gold chloride would be in this form. This is found to be true, the precipitation in the various dilutions of cerebrospinal fluid in parenchymatous neurosyphilis following what is known as the paretic, or first zone curve. The precipitation is complete in the first three to six tubes which contain the most cerebrospinal fluid, becoming progressively less complete with the greater dilutions. Degrees of precipitation show as changes from the normal salmon red color of the solution, ranging through a slight change to deeper red, to lavender, violet, red-blue and the colorless solution representing complete precipitation of the gold. For convenience, these shades of color are graded by numbers, the colorless fluid of total precipitation being represented by 5, red-blue 4, violet 3, lavender 2, deeper red 1, and the transparency of a brilliant salmon color with no precipitation by 0. Changes which are graded as 1 or 2 are not usually of pathological significance but a grade of 3 or higher always indicates an abnormal fluid. An intense paretic reaction might be as follows: 5555554432; while one less marked might be: 5543211000. In multiple sclerosis, Schilder's disease and in other types of neurosyphilis, the decolorization curve with colloidal gold may follow that of general paresis. The colloidal gold reaction is no longer thought to be diagnostic of any particular disease of the central nervous system but is simply an indication of an abnormality of the protein content of the fluid. It does not reflect the activity of the disease. This, as previously stated, is best indicated by the cell count.

Clinical Types

Because of the conspicuousness of certain presenting symptoms, different clinical types of syphilitic meningoencephalitis are usually described. Such a division into forms is artificial and possesses the merit of descriptive convenience only. Some cases, too, do not fit into such a classification and in others the symptoms may shift during the course of the disease.

SIMPLE DEMENTING TYPE. In this form the chief symptom is an insidious, progressive dementia with few, if any, delusions and no psychomotor disturbance except the declining activity indicative of the failing interest and capacity. Following closely upon the gradual loss of ambition and of mental alertness there appears the flabby, vacuous facies, presenting a syndrome that can scarcely be mistaken. This type of paretic often puts on weight during the early stages of his disease, maintaining the additional flesh until his disorder is far advanced. Remissions are rather uncommon in the simple dementing form. Someone has said that the paretic patient lives apathetically in the present whereas the patient suffering from senile dementia lives in the past.

The following brief abstract indicates the general clinical picture often occurring in the simple dementing form:

> A woman of twenty-six was brought to the hospital because she had become lost when she attempted to return home from a neighboring grocery store. About seven months before the patient's admission her husband noticed that she was becoming careless of her personal appearance and neglectful of her household duties. She often forgot to prepare the family meals, or, in an apparent preoccupation, would burn the food. She seemed to have little appreciation of time and would not realize when to get up or go to bed. The patient would sit idly about the house staring uncomprehendingly into space.
>
> At the hospital the patient entered the admission office with an unsteady gait. There, by way of greeting, the physician inquired, "How are you today?" to which she replied in a monotonous, tremulous tone, "N-yes-s, I was-s op-er-a-ted on for 'pen-pendici-ci-tis." She never made any spontaneous remarks and when, a few days after her admission, she was asked if she were sad or happy she stared vacantly at the physician and, with a fatuous smile, answered, "Yeah." The patient would sit about the ward for hours, taking no interest in its activities.

Sometimes she would hold a book in her lap, aimlessly turning the pages, never reading but often pointing out pictures like a small child and showing satisfaction when she found a new one to demonstrate. Neurological examination showed dilated pupils that reacted but slightly to light and on convergence. There was a tremor of lips and facial muscles on attempt to speak. The protruded tongue showed a coarse tremor. All deep tendon reflexes were hyperactive. The Wassermann reaction was strongly positive in both blood serum and cerebrospinal fluid. There were 24 cells per cu. mm. of spinal fluid, the Pandy reaction of which was two plus, as was also the Ross-Jones reaction. The colloidal gold curve was 5555543210.

EXPANSIVE TYPE. The expansive form, while no longer emphasized as distinctly characteristic, is nevertheless regarded as one of the most important of the clinical types. In the early stages the patient is self-satisfied and has a superficial good humor, but becomes easily irritated. If handled with good-natured and tactful suggestion he is quite amenable, but if interfered with his resentment may lead to violence. Although his grandiose ideas may be most absurd, the paretic sees nothing incredible in them.

The following will illustrate the defective judgment and grandiose ideas of the expansive type:

M., aged forty-one, a roofing salesman, was transferred to a state hospital from the jail to which he had been sentenced for violation of the motor vehicle laws. The prodromal symptoms of the patient's oncoming disease were apparently slight as the informant, his sister, who however had seen him but infrequently, stated that she had not noticed any change in the patient except that for a year he had seemed somewhat "worried." While driving his car he disregarded the collector at a toll bridge and drove across the structure at high speed. When overtaken by a police officer, the patient was found to have no license to drive an automobile, the permit having been revoked several years previously. Three days later, while awaiting trial for this offense, he was again arrested for driving an automobile without a license. He was given a short sentence in jail where a physician soon recognized the patient's disorder and had him committed to the hospital. On arrival at the admission office of the hospital he told the office attendant that he was going to give her a million dollars because she was "a nice lady." As he was being questioned for the usual admission data he began to boast of his wealth, claiming that he had three automobiles, thousands of dollars in the bank, a "diamond watch" and much other valuable jewelry. His son, he said, was Lieutenant Governor of the State, was soon to be Governor and later would be President of the United States. After having expressed various absurdly grandiose plans, he added, "I have another plan, too. I'm going to the wardens of the prisons in this state and all the other states and I'm going to buy the prisoners. I'll have an agreement with the warden to take their prisoners and put them to work on farms and I'll charge each prisoner $300 for doing it and for getting him out of jail. I made $105,000 with prisoners just last week and when I get going I'm going to make plenty of money." The neurological signs were all consistent with those of syphilitic meningoencephalitis and the serology was in all respects typical of the disease.

As a subgroup of the expansive type may be mentioned an excited or galloping form which includes those who show great motor excitement, often with confusion. Some of these cases run a rapid course, quickly exhaust themselves and die within a few weeks after the appearance of the excitement.

DEPRESSED TYPE. Not particularly uncommon are the depressed forms, characterized by melancholia and frequently by hypochondriasis or by nihilistic delusions. Some such paretics have ideas of persecution and many have ideas of unworthiness and attempt suicide. In spite of the depression, there is often a certain element of apathy, and observation usually detects some dementia.

B. J., a woman of thirty-seven, was admitted to the hospital in September, 1949. The date of her infection is uncertain but in 1939 at the out-patient department of a municipal hospital she was discovered to have a positive Wassermann but failed to secure treatment. Six months before her commitment the patient became depressed, declared she had tuberculosis, refused food because, she said, her stomach was too small to contain any food. On one occasion she drank iodine and again attempted suicide but failed through lack of resolution.

On arrival at a public hospital her facies was noted to be ironed out, her hair unkempt, her clothing loosely arranged and soiled, her posture was stooped and her movements slow. The Wassermann reaction was positive in both blood and cerebrospinal fluid. The latter contained 97 cells per cubic millimeter, an excess of albumin, the presence of globulin and the colloidal gold curve was read 554432100. It was often impossible to secure any replies to questions and those obtained were given with considerable delay and incompleteness. She left her tray of food untouched because her stomach was not "working any more." She looked fixedly toward the floor, declared that her condition was hopeless and that her blood was "all gone." She said, "Look at what a mess I have made around here. The only way I can be happy is down there," pointing downward. When a specimen of blood was taken for the Wassermann test she appeared to enjoy it, adding that she "ought to suffer." Later she became assaultive, often attacking the nurses, all of whom, she said, God had told her to kill.

CIRCULAR TYPE. Interesting, but not particularly common, are the circular forms of paresis presenting alternations of mood that in their course and clinical manifestations resemble manic-depressive psychosis. It has been suggested that the organic disease is superimposed on a cyclothymic personality.

J. T., was admitted when fifty-three years of age. The informant, who either did not know or was unwilling to divulge much concerning the patient's earlier life, stated that for three months he had been irritable, childish, forgetful and would go to sleep when callers were present. He went to a city in a neighboring state to look for work, but was arrested for carrying a concealed weapon when he visited the city police department and exhibited a revolver. After a short term in jail he was committed to an institution for mental diseases from which he was transferred to a state hospital. In the admission office he was friendly, talkative and exalted. With a marked pressure of speech he insisted on telling about his various activities as a detective for numerous police departments, for the United States Government, and as a crusader against the anarchists. He owned, he said, the largest arsenal in the world, used exclusively for the purpose of entertaining his distinguished friends. On the ward he was superior and patronizing in his manner. When not otherwise engaged he was busy writing letters to the officials of various organizations and to women of his acquaintance, particularly to the nurses connected with the hospital from which he had been transferred. He declared his love to them and proposed marriage to two of them. The neurological and serological findings were typical of paresis.

In less than two months from the date of his admission, the patient had so improved that he was given freedom of the hospital grounds and placed in charge of the laboratory animals. For a month the patient appeared practically well; then he gradually grew depressed, slept poorly and lost much weight. He was preoccupied with ideas about his body and expressed depressive, nihilistic and persecutory delusions. "Something has gone wrong with me. My gizzard has been cut. I can only breathe that gas you are putting in me. I am the worst person in the world. I wish you would take me out and kill me." One day he was found with a table cover tied about his neck. Gradually he gained weight and strength but eighteen months after the depression began he was still melancholy.

LISSAUER'S TYPE. This is a form with atypical clinical and pathological features named after the pathologist by whom, in collaboration with Storch, it was first described. Pathologically this form, in addition to the usual lesions of syphilitic meningoencephalitis, is characterized by unilateral localized atrophies, macroscopically apparent, and located particularly in the precentral, postcentral, occipital and rolandic areas, thus giving rise to the focal symptoms to be mentioned later. A specific feature of these lesions is their laminar distribution. Microscopically these atrophic areas are characterized by extreme pathological changes in the cortex causing these foci to present a moth-eaten appearance known as status spongiosus. In these areas, all parenchymatous components of cortex at the focus involved may be destroyed, the only tissue remaining being fibrous glia. Demyelination of infracortical white matter may be extensive. The cause of status spongiosus is unknown but it may be of local vascular origin. Clinically, in addition to the symptoms associated with the usual forms of paresis, there are localizing signs and symptoms determined by the foci of maximum atrophy. We therefore find aphasic speech disorders, epileptiform attacks confined to one side of the body, unilateral facial paralysis, hemiplegia, hemianopia, hemianesthesia, apraxia, unilateral astereognosis, cortical deafness, etc.

TABO-PARESIS. Not rarely patients with neurosyphilis show evidence not only of the parenchymatous involvement of the brain seen in general paresis but also symptoms and signs of involvement of the posterior columns met with in tabes dorsalis. The coexistence of both of these diseases is known as tabo-paresis. The symptoms of tabes usually precede those of paresis.

The tabo-paretic patient manifests not only the mental symptoms of general paresis but also the ataxia and other physical evidence of tabes. Frequently there is a history of difficulty in walking in the dark, of "shooting" pains in the legs. The knee jerks are absent. A Romberg's sign is present and there is a loss of sense of position in the lower extremities. Primary optic atrophy may occur. The colloidal gold curve may be of the second zone type.

JUVENILE PARESIS. This form which occurs in the child or adolescent suffering from congenital syphilis was first described by Clouston in 1877. Infection is transmitted from the mother to the offspring by the transplacental route after the fifth month of pregnancy. It is estimated that rather less than 1 per cent of cases of congenital syphilis develop general paresis. The age of the juvenile paretic at the time of the onset of symptoms corresponds approximately to the length of the incubation period in adult paresis. The child will generally, therefore, be from five to twenty years of age at the time of onset of symptoms. In about one third of the cases, there is a retardation of physical development. Many, perhaps 40 per cent, will be found to have always been feeble-minded. In those who have been markedly feeble-minded the onset is usually so vague that it is impossible to set a time of onset. In the moderately feeble-minded, and in those who have a period of normal development before the onset, there is an insidious but definite failure of previously learned accomplishments followed by a progressive dementia. Not rarely, therefore, the child's history reveals that he had attended school and had acquired knowledge with fair success until eight to fourteen years of age when insidious dementia began to develop. Many patients show confusion and restless, purposeless behavior. Because of the impairment of intelligence and the appearance of convulsions, not a few are diagnosed as epilepsy or idiocy with epilepsy. Delusions and euphoria are much less frequent in the juvenile than in the adult form of paresis. Trophic and other neurological disturbances are often conspicuous. Optic atrophy is not uncommon. Remissions of the type seen in paresis resulting from acquired syphilis are uncommon. The average duration of the disease is four to five years. In the final stages, the child is mute, untidy, emaciated and lives at merely a vegetative level. Treatment is less effective than in adult forms.

The following is a fairly illustrative case of juvenile paresis:

J. C. was admitted to a hospital in 1929 when seventeen years of age. The first pregnancy following his parents' marriage terminated at seven months, the child dying almost immediately. The patient was the next child in order of birth. His early development was said to have been normal. He attended school from six to thirteen years of age and is said to have been promoted each year. The first symptoms appeared in October, 1925, when, as his father explained, the boy "became draggy and droopy" and "didn't want to serve his paper route as before." In December, 1925, the teacher reported that he was failing in school. In the spring of 1926 the patient "began to talk funny and was thick-tongued." At practically the same time the parents noticed a weakness of the left leg and arm. His difficulty in walking increased, his speech became almost unintelligible and he occasionally soiled himself.

On admission to the hospital the patient was found to be of rather small stature but fairly well nourished. He walked somewhat in the manner of a mechanical doll, with his elbows pressed close to his ribs, his forearms extended straight before him and his fingers separated. His steps were short and shuffling, with his feet widely separated as if to maintain his balance. His pupils were widely dilated (the right more than the left), were irregular and did not react to light, but showed a little contraction on convergence. Both nerve heads were found to be somewhat atrophic. His tendon reflexes were exaggerated, there was a bilateral Babinski reaction and he showed a tremor of the fingers. Coordination in fine movements was defective. Attempts to secure the finger-to-nose tests were unsuccessful as the patient could not be made to comprehend the instructions. The Wassermann reaction was positive on both blood and spinal fluid. The latter contained 19 cells, an excess of globulin and showed a colloidal gold curve of 5555422210.

Mentally the patient's manner suggested that of a high-grade idiot. His facial expression was smoothed-out and he frequently exhibited a silly grin. He cooperated in the eager, ineffective manner of a mentally defective and responded to all questions with "Huh?" He could not utter a single intelligible word but obeyed simple requests, such as "Shut your eyes," "Close your mouth." The Wassermann reaction on the father's blood was found to be positive.

Because of the active effort now made to ascertain if pregnant women are infected with syphilis and the efficacy of treatment with penicillin, cases of congenital syphilis are relatively rare. Juvenile paresis is therefore now an uncommon disease.

Psychological Considerations

General paresis is an organic disease entity but in its early stages psychological factors may color the clinical picture. The organic damage to the central nervous system produced by the paretic process may permit less restrained expression of previous personality maladjustments and often releases tendencies which had formerly been successfully repressed. In the early stages, therefore, important symptoms may not be the direct result of damage to the brain but to a considerable extent may be determined by the individual's previous personality features, its organization, motives, problems and experiences. It seems obvious that neither the spirochete nor the destruction of brain tissue can explain the grandiosity of one case, the stupor in another, or the paranoid delusional system in a third. Some symptoms may be the expression of attempts on part of the personality to cope with threats to its integrity. The patient's delusions, for example, may well be looked upon as psychologically reparative and defensive processes on the part of a personality the integrity of which is threatened with disorganization because of the destructive assault upon its organic aspect. Finally, the defect and other symptoms caused by the progressive organic disease of the brain come to overlie and more or less conceal the underlying deviation in personality. Since because of his age a desire for wealth or social distinction has not come to be a matter of such concern to him as to the adult, the juvenile paretic patient's ideas are rarely expansive.

The paretic is not aware of the insidious dissolution going on in his personality. Kinnier Wilson tells of a psychiatrist who suffered from paresis yet never realized that he was succumbing to the disease on the histology of which he was an acknowledged expert.

Course and Prognosis

If not treated, syphilitic meningoencephalitis leads inevitably to dementia and death and if not arrested within a reasonable period it produces a permanent but varying degree of dementia and economic dependence. In the absence of treatment, death usually occurs from two to five years after the first appearance of symptoms. The course may be interrupted, however, by spontaneous remissions in slightly over 10 per cent of untreated cases. The clinical improvement that may occur in these remissions may seem almost miraculous and often leads the patient's relatives to the erroneous conclusion that improvement will be permanent. Remissions are more frequent in those cases in which the onset has been comparatively sudden and stormy. The duration of the remissions is quite variable, extending from one or two months to five or six years. The average life expectancy in the untreated patient is four years. The prognosis in the treated patient depends upon the promptness and thoroughness of treatment. Active treatment with adequate doses of penicillin during the asymptomatic stage should prevent the development of clinical symptoms in at least 85 per cent of cases. If treatment is begun in early clinical stages 60 or more per cent of patients will improve sufficiently to permit return to work. It is generally believed that a spinal fluid negative after three years from the date of infection will not become positive. In hospitals where patients are admitted in all stages of the disease the number recovering rarely exceeds 30 per cent, the death rate is 20 to 30 per cent and further progress is arrested in 30 to 50 per cent of patients.

Symptoms which may be described as organic are caused by the changes produced in the central nervous system by the spirochete; some changes are of an inflammatory nature, while others are degenerative. If the spirochetes can be destroyed by treatment, it is probable that the inflammation caused by them will subside and the symptoms attributable to inflammatory lesions will disappear but those caused by degenerative changes will persist. The prognosis depends therefore upon the relative extent to which degenerative changes have occurred before the activity of the paretic process is arrested by treatment. Frequently the relative extent to which these two processes exist cannot be ascertained until treatment has been undertaken. The results of structural injury already suffered cannot be remedied.

Diagnosis

The data presented by mental, neurological and serological examinations constitute a syndrome that can scarcely be mistaken. If the neurological signs alone are considered, cerebral arteriosclerosis may at times be confused with demential paralytica. The mental symptoms in the early stages of paresis may suggest neurasthenia or one of the phases of manic-depressive psychosis. Dementia, slurring speech, tremors, epileptiform seizures and even pupillary disturbances may occur in chronic alcoholism but the serological changes of dementia paralytica are of course absent. Finally, the diagnosis of syphilitic meningoencephalitis should not be made until the results of mental, neurological and serological examinations are available. Unless all these examinations are made, paresis may be confused with Alzheimer's disease, Pick's disease, multiple sclerosis, senile dementia, cerebral tumor or other diseases producing cerebral damage, particularly to the frontal lobes.

The spinal fluid findings constitute the most important differential criterion. In order of diagnostic value and activity of process, these are: (a) increased cell count, (b) increased concentration of protein, (c) positive serological reaction for syphilis, and (d) abnormal reaction in the colloidal gold test. The results of these four tests, interpreted as a whole, give reasonably accurate information as to the presence or absence of neurosyphilis and as to its type and activity. A normal number of cells and normal amount of protein indicate that the process is inactive even though Wassermann and colloidal reactions are normal.

Treatment

Ever since its introduction, penicillin has been increasingly employed in the treatment of syphilitic meningoencephalitis. For a considerable period it was believed that it should be supplemented by fever therapy.

It is now generally agreed, however, that fever therapy should be avoided until penicillin has been proved deficient in a particular case. Usually a course of penicillin, repeated if necessary, is effective in a large proportion of both symptomatic and asymptomatic forms of the disease. With experience, the dosage of penicillin has been gradually increased until now a patient receives a total of 12,000,000 to 15,000,000 units. Different types of penicillin are used by different clinics. Many physicians use 600,000 units daily of procaine penicillin G given intramuscularly for twenty days.

The results of the spinal fluid tests serve as a guide for both the activity of the paretic process and the effect of treatment. The spinal fluid should be examined four to six months after the completion of treatment. The first change in the cerebrospinal fluid following penicillin therapy is a reduction in number of cells which usually reach normal limits within six months. This is followed by a drop in total protein level. If the increased cell count has reverted to normal or near normal, the amount of protein has decreased, and the patient seems improved, no further treatment is needed. The complement-fixation reaction and results of the colloidal test may not revert to normal for several months or years and cannot be used to gauge adequate treatment. If the cell count and protein value remain high a second course of treatment is mandatory. The second course should be the same as, or more intensive than, the first one. When the response is favorable, the spinal fluid should be examined at intervals of four to six months for the first year after treatment, then yearly until the spinal fluid is no longer abnormal. Less reliance is placed upon clinical features than upon spinal fluid changes as a guide to further treatment.

In greatly overactive patients, also in those with prominent affective components, it is often well that the administration of penicillin be preceded by a course of electroshock treatments.

Fever Therapy

If two courses of penicillin fail to effect good results, a few physicians use fever therapy, but it is rarely employed. However, malaria, or another antibiotic such as chlortetracycline, is sometimes administered to the patient.

Employment of Recovered Paretic

Frequently the question arises as to when the paretic who has become free of clinical symptoms through treatment may resume activities involving the safety of others. It should be advised that he not operate an automobile until his cerebrospinal fluid is negative in every respect. Should his occupation involve still greater responsibility, such as that of locomotive engineer, he should probably never resume it.

Treatment of Juvenile Paresis

The treatment of juvenile syphilitic meningoencephalitis is less satisfactory than the usual adult form of the disease. It is generally considered, however, that the most complete and most persistent remissions are secured by penicillin. Spinal puncture should be done in all cases of congenital syphilis, followed by treatment in the manner described if the cerebrospinal fluid suggests involvement of the central nervous system.

Treatment of Asymptomatic Paresis

Attention has been called to the fact that every case of symptomatic general paresis is preceded by an asymptomatic stage when examination of the spinal fluid reveals the paretic formula but clinical manifestations are still absent. It is therefore of course axiomatic that no patient suffering from systemic syphilis should, regardless of serological tests on his blood, be discharged from treatment until the cerebrospinal fluid has been examined and found to be normal. Even without treatment the treponemata may be eliminated from the central nervous system within the first five years of infection. Examinations of the cerebrospinal fluid should, however, be made annually for five years. Should the spinal fluid at any time show the paretic formula, the patient should, even though there be no clinical signs or symptoms of paresis, at once receive penicillin therapy. With adequate treatment the prognosis of asymptomatic paresis is excellent.

BIBLIOGRAPHY

Alzheimer, A.: Histologische Studien zur Differentialdiagnose der progressiven Paralyse. Histologische und histopathologische Arbeiten über die Grosshirnrinde, Bd. 1. Jena, G. Fischer, 1904.

Bayle, A. L. J.: Recherches sur l'arachnitis chronique, la gastritie et la gastroentérite chronique, et la goutte, considérées comme causes de l'aliénation mentale. Didat Le Jeune, Paris, 1822.

Bruetsch, W. L.: Penicillin in Neurosyphilis. New York, Grune & Stratton, 1949.

Clouston, T. S.: A case of general paralysis at the age of sixteen. J. Ment. Sc., *23:*419–420, 1877.

Curtis, A. C., Horne, S. F., and Norton, D. H.: Neurosyphilis. Am. J. Syph., Gonor., & Ven. Dis., *33:*527–536, 1949.

Dattner, Bernard, Thomas, E. W., and de Mello, L.: Treatment of neurosyphilis. J.A.M.A., *141:*1260, 1949.

Haslam, J.: Observations on Insanity with Particular Remarks on the Disease and an Account of the Morbid Appearance on Dissections. London, 1798.

Jahnel, F.: Die progressive Paralyse, ihre Pathogenese, ihre Diagnose und Therapie. In Berliner Klinik, Leipzig, Fischer, 1930.

Lissauer, H., and Storch, E.: Ueber einige Fälle atypischer progressiver Paralyse. Monatschr. f. Psychiat. u. Neurol., *9:*401, 1901.

Menninger, W. C.: Juvenile Paresis. Baltimore, Williams and Wilkins Co., 1936.

Merritt, H. H., and Solomon, H. C.: Relation of trauma to syphilis of the nervous system. Ann. Surg., *117:*623, 1943.

Moore, Merrill, and Solomon, H. C.: Contributions of Haslam, Bayle, and Esmarch and Jessen to the history of neurosyphilis. Arch. Neurol. & Psychiat., *32:*804, 1934.

Nissl, F.: Zur Histopathologie der paralytischen Rindenerkrankung. Histologische und histopathologische Arbeiten über die Grosshirnrinde, Bd. 1, Jena, G. Fischer, 1940.

Noguchi, H., and Moore, J. W.: A demonstration of Spirochaeta pallida in the brain in cases of general paralysis. J. Exper. Med., *17:*232, 1913.

Robertson, G. M.: Discovery of general paralysis. J. Ment. Sc., *69:*1, 1923.

Rose, A. S., and Solomon, H. C.: Penicillin in the treatment of neurosyphilis; a study of one hundred cases followed twelve months or more. J.A.M.A., *133:5*, 1947.

Smith, R. H. F.: Permeability of the blood-brain barrier to penicillin in cases of parenchymatous neurosyphilis. J. Ment. Sc., *97:*340–361, April, 1951.

CHAPTER XV

Mental Disturbances with Other Forms of Syphilis of the Central Nervous System

IN SYPHILITIC meningoencephalitis we deal with a form of neurosyphilis in which the important pathological lesions are confined largely to the cerebral cortex, the inflammatory and degenerative processes being mainly limited to the parenchyma. Frequently, however, the lesions of neurosyphilis are predominantly interstitial, the parenchyma escaping the syphilitic process. Except for the comparatively rare cases of discrete gummata, this interstitial involvement is meningovascular in distribution. By common consent the meningovascular forms of brain syphilis in distinction from the meningoencephalitic forms of brain syphilis are spoken of as cerebral syphilis and any psychotic reactions that are associated with them are referred to as psychoses with cerebral syphilis. This distinction from parenchymatous brain syphilis is important not merely from the standpoint of pathology but because the symptoms, course and prognosis of meningovascular brain syphilis are typically quite different from those of the meningoencephalitic form. In many cases both meninges and blood vessels are diffusely involved while again the pathological changes may be largely confined to one or the other of these mesoblastic structures. The mesoblastic forms of syphilis of the central nervous system tend to produce distinguishable groups of symptoms, yet no clear distinction can always be drawn. Partly because of this tendency and partly for ease of description, the symptoms of the more characteristic pathological processes will be presented as if the lines of distinction were more clearly drawn than often obtains. It should be remembered, however, that while syphilis of the central nervous system is classified pathologically into meningeal, vascular and parenchymatous according to the element most seriously involved, yet these classifications are not mutually exclusive and many cases show a mixture of two or all three types.

Syphilitic Meningitis

It is customary to divide syphilitic meningitis into three types depending on the site of selective involvement.

Acute Syphilitic Hydrocephalus. This is a relatively rare form of neurosyphilis and is not characterized by selective involvement. Signs and symptoms include headache, nausea, vomiting, choked disc, stiffness of the neck and Kernig sign. The symptomatology is caused by an excessive formation of cerebrospinal fluid and an impairment of the absorption of the fluid resulting from the inflammatory reaction.

Basilar Meningitis. In this form the inflammatory process is concentrated around the base of the brain. Basilar meningitis, which is one of the commonest forms of neurosyphilis, usually develops from one to three years after the primary infection. Thickening and infiltration of the pia occur in the cerebellopontine angle and in the interpeduncular space. With the infiltration of the former region the sixth, seventh and eighth nerves are affected and as exudative processes occur in the latter space the second and third nerves are involved. Headache and perhaps dizziness appear; the patient shows mental hebetude, impairment of memory for recent events, sleepiness, difficulty of comprehension, perhaps clouding of consciousness, confusion and delirium and occasionally stupor. The degree of disturbance of consciousness and of impairment of the more strictly intellectual functions varies roughly with the extent to which intracranial pressure is increased as well as the degree to which the cortex is involved. The mental symptoms, however, if present, are usually so clearly of an organic type, are associated with obvious neurological signs and yield so quickly to treatment that comparatively few patients reach the mental hospital. Signs resulting from involvement of the optic nerve and of the nerves controlling the extrinsic muscles of the eye appear early and are perhaps fluctuating and inconstant at first. We therefore find ptosis, diplopia, strabismus, pupillary disturbance, papilledema and choked disc. Loss of corneal reflex, facial anesthesia, peripheral facial palsy, deafness, or signs of involvement of other cranial nerves may occur. Even in the absence of treatment the mental symptoms may disappear, only shortly to reappear.

Vertical Meningitis. This type of cerebral syphilis usually occurs later than the more focal forms of syphilitic meningitis and involves the meninges of the convexity rather than of the base of the brain. Severe paroxysmal headache, often worse at night, is common. Dizziness is frequent. Sometimes the mental symptoms are so indefinite and combined with such an ineffectiveness of personality that the patient is thought to be neurasthenic. More frequently there is an irritability, loss of ability for sustained effort, progressive hebetude, slow thinking, inertia, amnesia and other signs of intellectual impairment. There is often much irregularity in the impairment of intellectual functions, some being retained much better than others. The nucleus of the personality is less impaired than in syphilitic meningoencephalitis. Retarded speech, brief attacks of aphasia and other speech difficulties occur. Generalized or jacksonian convulsions may appear and hemiplegia is not uncommon. Confusion, delirium and stupor may be present in relatively acute cases. Paranoid reactions may exist but here, as in the other forms of nonparenchymatous forms of brain syphilis, there is less disturbance of behavior, judgment and social reactions, and fewer delusional trends than in paresis.

Syphilitic meningitis is accompanied by a positive Wassermann reaction in both blood serum and cerebrospinal fluid, cells are markedly increased, there is an excess of albumin and globulin is present. Typically the precipitation of colloidal gold is greatest in the second zone, giving what is called the "luetic curve" (0123443210).

Vascular Neurosyphilis

This type of cerebral syphilis may begin to give rise to symptoms within a few months after infection or as late as ten or twelve years after the primary lesion, the majority of cases appearing in the first three to five years of the disease. Vascular involvement in the early stages of syphilis is usually an accompaniment of syphilitic meningitis and consists of a thrombosis secondary to the inflammatory reaction around the vessel. Vascular symptoms during later stages are caused by a thickening of the intima and adventitia with such damage to the walls that thrombosis, obliteration, miliary aneurysm or hemorrhage may occur, leading to atrophy, softening and degeneration of brain substance.

SYMPTOMS. Among the early symptoms is intermittent headache, often worse at night, and aggravated by mental or physical effort. Dizziness is another troublesome symptom, as is insomnia. Periods of intense sleepiness or of stupor may occur. The patient becomes irritable, emotionally unstable, shows loss of interest in and lack of capacity for work, an increasing apathy and impairment of memory. With or without the prodromal symptoms mentioned, the majority of cases of vascular cerebral syphilis develop symptoms or neurological signs of a focal nature. Since these vascular accidents are usually thrombotic, the signs are ordinarily of slow onset and are quite variable in their intensity and permanency. Consciousness is often not lost and there is a surprising tendency for serious neurological disturbances to recover. Hemiplegias are common, the particular syndrome depending on the site of the lesion—cortical, capsular, pontine, etc. Aphasias, usually transient, are frequent. After these apoplectic attacks, the patient is frequently left with a certain impairment of effectiveness and of intellectual capacity. Subarachnoid hemorrhages may also occur as a result of syphilis of the meningeal vessels. The Wassermann reaction of the blood serum is, of course, usually positive. This reaction is frequently positive in large amounts of cerebrospinal fluid but may be entirely negative, a fact that should be borne in mind. Protein is usually increased and cells may or may not be increased. The colloidal gold reaction in vascular neurosyphilis is quite uncertain, since while it often gives a curve of the luetic type it may not be distinctive or may even be negative. It will thus be seen that the serology in the vascular form of cerebral syphilis may be conclusive but that the absence of positive findings may not exclude its existence.

The following abstract will illustrate a case of mental disorder resulting from interstitial brain syphilis the lesion of which was probably vascular in nature.

J. L. was admitted to a public mental hospital in October, 1928, at forty-eight years of age. In 1920 he had contracted syphilis. In May, 1924, he had suffered a "clot back of his eyes." For a short period he was nearly blind but soon recovered. About this time a change in personality occurred. He lost interest in his home, drank heavily, began to gamble and was discharged from the position he had satisfactorily held for twenty-two years. In October, 1924, the patient suffered an apoplectic stroke with hemiplegia of the right side. He was described as semiconscious for three or four weeks following which he had difficulty in talking. Following another stroke in February, 1925, the patient became sullen, irritable, suspicious, threatening and at times abused his wife. Early in October, 1928, he threatened his daughter with a knife and drove his family from the house. The following day he refused to eat, declaring that his food was poisoned.

On arrival at the hospital the patient was found to be fully oriented and well in touch with his environment. His memory was fair but his fund of information was impaired and his capacity for apperception was faulty. Neurologically he showed a slight ptosis of both upper lids, slight external strabismus of the left eye and the pupils were unequal but reacted to light and convergence. His speech was characterized by dysarthria, the right arm and leg were moderately spastic and presented exaggerated tendon reflexes and the right foot showed ankle clonus. The Wassermann reaction on the blood serum was positive, but was negative on cerebrospinal fluid which contained 2 cells per cu. mm., gave a "suspicious" Pandy reaction and the following gold curve: 1122110000. Under treatment the serology became entirely negative. Four years later he was still in the institution, where he was well behaved, had freedom of the grounds and worked in the hospital industrial shop. His higher intellectual functions were obviously much impaired, however, and he was quite incapable of supporting himself or adjusting independently in the community.

TREATMENT. It should be borne in mind that no clinical symptoms of neurosyphilis, whether meningeal, vascular or parenchymatous develop without previous laboratory evidence of involvement of the central nervous system. It is therefore highly important to detect the existence of neurosyphilis during this asymptomatic period, *i.e.*, before the infection has spread to the blood vessels, to the brain parenchyma or has involved the meninges to an extent sufficient to produce clinical symptoms. For this reason the cerebrospinal fluid should be examined in all patients with syphilis. A patient undergoing treatment for early syphilis should receive an examination of the cerebrospinal fluid after treatment for a year to a year and a half. A negative finding previous to a year of treatment does not necessarily mean that there will not be later involvement; also positive findings previous to that time would not materially influence the treatment. The presence of a positive fluid after a year and a half of treatment or in an untreated patient requires that treatment be continued until the cerebrospinal fluid becomes entirely normal, even if there have been no clinical symptoms of neurosyphilis and even if serological tests on the blood have become negative. The treatment of asymptomatic and of meningeal and vascular forms of neurosyphilis will be the same as that of the meningoencephalitic form, *i.e.*, with penicillin. Treatment by this antibiotic is usually followed by excellent results unless vascular or meningeal inflammation has already caused permanent damage to the nervous tissue. Routine laboratory examinations of both blood and cerebrospinal fluid should be made every six months.

BIBLIOGRAPHY

Dattner, Bernhard: Penicillin in Neurosyphilis. New York, Grune & Stratton, 1949.

Merritt, H. H.: The early clinical and laboratory manifestations of syphilis of the central nervous system. New England J. Med., *223*:446–450, 1940.

———, Adams, R. D., and Solomon, H. C.: Neurosyphilis. New York, Oxford University Press, 1946.

CHAPTER XVI

Brain Syndromes Associated with Cerebral Arteriosclerosis

"It is not a divinity but the mystery of arteriosclerosis that shapes the earthly endings of most lives."[1]

THE DESIGNATION "Psychoses with Cerebral Arteriosclerosis" is, strictly speaking, a misnomer. The term *arteriosclerosis* may still be used in a generic sense applied to a group of vascular diseases characterized morphologically by hardening of the vessel wall. It does, however, place undue emphasis upon the hardening aspect of the changes that occur with age in the walls of blood vessels. It is now known that the hardening *per se* is a relatively benign process which produces little if any interference with the flow of blood. On the other hand, the process known to the pathologist as atherosclerosis is vastly more serious since it is characterized not so much by hardening of the vessel wall as by the *narrowing* or *obliteration of the lumen.* It is an occlusive disease that affects the nutrient vessels of the brain, heart or kidney, and by progressively choking off the flow of blood leads to functional alteration and even to disability or death. When, therefore, the term arteriosclerosis is used in this chapter it should be borne in mind that the real nature of the pathological vascular process is an atherosclerosis with its distinctive morphological feature of stainable lipid within the atheromatous lesions. The part played by age in the genesis of atherosclerosis has been discussed at great length by pathologists. While it is now generally agreed that arteriosclerosis (atherosclerosis) is not a necessary result of age it is indirectly related to the aging process in the sense that it is a cumulative

[1] The "little strokes," New England J. Med., *246:*155, Jan. 24, 1952.

and slowly progressive disease that becomes increasingly manifest with the passage of time. It is therefore quite natural that with the progressive lengthening of the life span during the present century there should have been a great increase in the number of persons suffering from arteriosclerosis. There is perhaps no better evidence of this fact than the striking increase in the number of admissions to public mental hospitals of persons suffering from mental disorders incident to this disease. Persons suffering from brain syndromes associated with cerebral arteriosclerosis constitute approximately 22 per cent of first admissions to New York State psychiatric hospitals.

With the progressive diminution in caliber of the relatively narrow vessels of the brain, the flow of blood is slowly throttled and the nutrition of the parenchyma affected. Ganglion cells gradually deteriorate and areas of atrophy develop around the constricted arterioles. Hemorrhage or thrombosis and embolism with infarction may occur. Thrombosis is much more frequent and probably accounts for 85 per cent of vascular accidents.

Symptoms

The age of onset of the arteriosclerotic psychoses varies widely but in general it is between fifty and sixty-five. Prodromal symptoms in the form of fatigue, headache, dizziness, diminution of capacity for prolonged concentration, drowsiness in the afternoon or evening, and an insidious impairment of physical and mental abilities are common. Not rarely latent character features are revealed or previous trends become pathologically exaggerated. Any apparent change in character in a person over fifty should suggest the possibility of cerebral arteriosclerosis if syphilitic meningoencephalitis is excluded. The old question as to whether or not "spasm" occurs in arteries of the brain remains unsettled. There is, however, much evidence that states of prolonged vasoconstriction do occur in the brain and that they are of great functional significance. In somewhat more than half of the cases, a sudden attack of confusion is the first obvious mental symptom. Episodes of confusion or of excitement or, particularly, of their combined association, constitute a frequent symptom of the arteriosclerotic syndrome. There is clouding of consciousness, incoherence and restlessness, sometimes extreme. In other cases the onset is insidious and represents what has been descriptively characterized as "a slow dying at the top." Among such symptoms are easy mental fatigability, a lessening of initiative, an impairment of attention, emotional instability with outbursts of weeping or laughter and perhaps a tendency to depression. Some patients are irritable, aggressive, meddlesome, quarrelsome, obstinate, jealous and paranoid. Finer sentiments, such as affection, may be destroyed. Some patients become garrulous. Memory is impaired to varying degrees. At first it may consist merely of difficulty in recollecting names, but later may become general. The facies may become increasingly immobile and inanimate. Nocturnal attacks of bewilderment, of delirious, anxious states or of violence may occur. Not infrequently the arteriosclerotic patient becomes neglectful of his personal appearance, his clothing may not be clean and he may fail to bathe. Delusions may be expressed and are particularly apt to be of a persecutory nature although ideas of ruin and hypochondriacal delusions are not uncommon. The patient may be distressed by ideas of jealousy concerning his wife or other members of his family. His ideational content, like other expressions of his psychosis, is influenced largely by former types of mental mechanisms and other patterns of personality expression. Occasionally a patient is noted who expresses ideas of grandeur representing a compensation for failing sexual capacity. As in senile dementia, defective judgment and decreased inhibition may result in sexual indiscretions or offenses.

Characterological changes representing alterations in adaptive mechanisms and personality defenses may occur. Defenses against feelings of dependency may, for example, be replaced by acceptance of these needs. Hostile impulses that were previously suppressed may be released. Premorbid defensive drives, such as for perfectionism, may be relaxed.

Among persons with more advanced cerebrovascular disease are those subject to "the little strokes" (Alvarez). Such individuals may become intermittently psychotic or subject to periods of delirium. In the case of sclerosis of the large cerebral vessels, the first gross symptom may be an apoplectic stroke, aphasic attack or other focal disturbance, although other evidence of vascular disease usually appears first. Vertical headaches that are worse in the morning, giddiness, short periods of confusion, and fleeting loss of power in arm or leg, or momentary aphasias or apraxias usually give warning of subsequent more serious focal lesions. Station becomes insecure, its base wide, the gait uncertain and the steps short and spastic. Pupillary inequalities are not uncommon, although recent studies have shown that there is no close relationship between retinal atherosclerosis and sclerosis of the small arteries supplying the brain. Coarse tremors may appear, and the patient may finally experience much difficulty in feeding himself. Cardiovascular disease in the form of cardiac hypertrophy, coronary sclerosis or chronic valvular disease is common. Numerous paralytic lesions appear—evidence of focal destruction of nervous tissue by occlusion or by rupture of a vessel of considerable size. Upper motor neuron paralyses and various aphasias and apraxias are most frequent. Paraphasia, or confusion of words, may occur. Deterioration and dementia are hastened by these focal lesions, especially by those that result in serious speech disturbances. Certain intellectual functions may be much impaired while others remain comparatively intact. Epileptiform attacks, either jacksonian or general, may occur, caused, some believe, by temporary anemia or edema.

Sands has called attention to the fact that patients with cerebral arteriosclerosis are peculiarly apt, on the occasion of a mild infection, to suffer from episodes characterized by confusion, disorientation, misidentification of persons, anxiety, fear reaction, suspiciousness and delusional trends.

Contrary to the dementing senile patient, the arteriosclerotic patient, at least in the early stages of his deterioration, recognizes that there is a decline in the quickness and accuracy of his mental functions. He often feels keenly his difficulty in finding a word, his weakness of memory and the diminution of physical and mental capacity.

The following abstract of a patient's clinical record illustrates some of the more frequent symptoms resulting from the physiological disturbances of brain function through arteriosclerotic changes:

W. B., aged 66, a bookkeeper by occupation, was brought to a mental hospital in 1941 from the Ab. Hospital to which he had been admitted one month previously. The family physician reported that the patient had had elevated blood pressure for ten years. Three weeks before admission to the general hospital he suddenly suffered from an attack of vertigo and severe headache lasting for about twenty minutes. He then resumed his daily task although he felt weak and tired. On the following day "for no reason that he can explain, as he claims he was not dizzy," his brother reported, "he just lost his balance and fell downstairs." He was then referred to the hospital for study and diagnosis.

The patient's brother added that eighteen months previous to this episode the patient first showed a change in behavior. He talked much less and "would often sit and look at absolutely nothing for long periods. For the past year he had been saying rather peculiar things. He became silly, flighty and confused." While in the general hospital to which he had been admitted he was constantly worrying over loss of his money although there was no basis for such a belief. The brother described the patient's behavior in the general hospital as follows: "He was very confused. He would not remain in bed, and instead of getting out of the side of the bed he would crawl over its foot to get out."

Upon arrival at the mental hospital his systolic blood pressure was found to be 240 and the diastolic fluctuated from 100 to 140. He said he had come from the B. General Hospital and had never heard of the Ab. Hospital. When asked the dates when he became ill he maintained that he had not been ill. He gave his age, his birth year and the current year correctly but when asked the present date he replied, "The New York Giants won the first game, Brooklyn won the second game and the third game was going home when I went." A month after admission he conversed freely and usually rationally with other patients and showed concern about the condition of the feeble ones. He continued, however, to manifest difficulty in concentration, in apperception and in memory for recent events. He was then fully oriented as to time and place and recognized that his memory was impaired. He remarked to his physician, "I don't know. If I have to keep on this way maybe the good Lord ought to take me." Four months after admission he was described as having periods of memory loss. Although the United States was then intently preoccupied with World War II he took no interest in the world situation and important events. At times he showed difficulty in choosing the proper word and occasionally became quite irritated at himself for having this difficulty. Although he had completed three years of college he was unable to answer simple mathematical questions and failed in an attempt to subtract from 100 by using 7 as the subtrahend and the successive differences as the minuend. Under the simple routine of hospital life and freedom from responsibility, the patient improved still further. Five and a half years after admission he was described as discussing his business affairs intelligently and as showing an interest in hospital activities and as being well informed on current events. In 1949 there developed periods of twenty-four hours duration during which he became excited, screamed at anyone who approached him and often became quite threatening although he never did violence to them. At such times he was somewhat confused. In 1953 he was continuing to have periods of irritability and confusion sufficiently disturbing to make his return to his family inadvisable.

Prognosis

The prognosis is naturally unfavorable but the course is not always uninterruptedly progressive. It frequently happens that a patient, particularly if he has cardiac and general vascular disease also, will enter an institution in a greatly confused, perhaps excited, state, so that he appears quite demented. After rest and several days or a few weeks of the simple regime of hospital life, the patient may become clearly conscious and apparently recover from the acute symptoms. There is constant danger, however, that an apoplectic stroke or another confused episode may occur at any time. Many patients, nevertheless, retain considerable, although impaired, capacity for several years before dementia or physical helplessness removes them from the scene of activity. In many cases death is hastened by a general arteriosclerosis associated with cardiorenal disease.

Diagnosis

The mental disorder from which the differentiation of an arteriosclerotic psychosis is most frequently required is senile dementia. Since the two forms of deterioration are often associated and the manifestations of both about equally prominent, a differentiation may be difficult or impossible. In such cases, preference for statistical purposes should be given to arteriosclerotic disorder. Arteriosclerotic psychosis occurs somewhat more frequently in men than in women while senile dementia occurs more frequently in women. Arteriosclerosis usually arises earlier in life than senile atrophy. Usually there is less intellectual impairment in arteriosclerosis. Headache, dizziness or apoplectic phenomena occur in about one half of cases of arteriosclerotic psychosis. Fainting attacks, convulsive seizures or attack of cardiac dysfunction likewise suggest an arteriosclerotic origin. Sudden attacks of confusion often occur in arteriosclerotic psychoses. In younger persons the clinical picture may be strongly suggestive of syphilitic meningoencephalitis but laboratory tests quickly provide differentiating data. When depression and anxiety are present the differentiation from a depressed phase of manic-depressive psychosis or from involutional melancholia may not be easy. While in all three disorders the presenting picture may be an affective one, yet in arteriosclerotic disease there will usually be evidence of an underlying organic impairment of mental capacity or of signs of beginning vascular disease. Fluctuations in the sensorium and other episodic manifestations are often significant of involvement of the cerebral vessels. It should be remembered that acute confusional states resulting from toxic and biochemical factors are not uncommon among the aged, associated, at times, with dehydration.

Treatment

Since our knowledge concerning the causes of cerebral arteriosclerosis is so limited, little can be done to prevent its development. The milder psychoses with cerebral arteriosclerosis may be cared for at home; the severe ones require institutional treatment. In either case a carefully regulated mode of life is a fundamental requirement in treatment. While neither heavy manual labor nor mental tasks involving burdensome responsibilities or emotional stress should be permitted, an agreeable occupation of simple type should be continued as long as possible, due attention being paid to recreation and physical rest. It should be borne in mind that suicide is not rare in arteriosclerotic depressions. The arteriosclerotic patient will be wise to refrain from alcohol. Any inadequacies of nutrition should be improved and attention be directed to any associated cardiorenal or other pathologic condition. The value of low cholesterol, low fat diets, estrogens, heparin, choline or inositol as a means of influencing the presumed disturbed lipid metabolism remains controversial. Hydrotherapy in mild forms, carefully supervised, may be employed, but measures that are too long or too vigorous may be harmful. Chlorpromazine has been helpful with some patients in reducing nocturnal insomnia and restlessness, confusion, excitement and aggressive, destructive behavior, but care must be taken in the case of the arteriosclerotic patient because of the possibility of a hypotensive reaction following administration of the drug. For this reason oral administration is preferred, commencing with small doses (10 mg. three times daily) and gradually increasing. The use of other sedatives often may be discontinued. The dosage needed and tolerated is highly variable. Psychotherapy should not be forgotten in the anxious patient. Barbiturates will sometimes aggravate the confusion associated with cerebral arteriosclerosis and hypertensive encephalopathy. Reese and Kant report that the dizziness, headache, insomnia, confusion and delirious confusion occurring in these disorders is often relieved by the administration of aminophylline in doses of 4 grains each four times a day. Nicotinic acid or its amide is often used to improve the cerebral circulation.

BIBLIOGRAPHY

Allen, E. B.: Psychiatric aspects of cerebral arteriosclerosis. New England J. Med., *245*:677, 1951.

———: The management of cerebral arteriosclerosis: psychiatric aspects. Bull. New York Acad. Med., *31*:366–475, 1955.

Apter, N. S., Halstead, W. C., and Heimburger, R. F.: Impaired cerebral function in essential hypertension. Am. J. Psychiat., *107*:808–813, 1951.

Binger, C. A. L.: Personality in Arterial Hypertension. New York, R. Brunner, 1945.

Malzberg, B.: The expectation of psychoses with cerebral arteriosclerosis in New York State. Psychiatric Quart., *19*:122–138, 1945.

Pollack, B.: The addition of chlorpromazine to the treatment program for emotional and behavior disorders in the aging. Geriatrics, *11*:253–259, 1956.

Raskin, Naomi, and Ehrenberg, Ruth: Senescence, senility and Alzheimer's disease. Am. J. Psychiat., *113*:133–137, 1956.

Rothschild, David: Neuropathologic changes in arteriosclerotic psychoses and their psychiatric significance. Arch. Neurol. & Psychiat., *48*:417–436, 1942.

———: Premorbid personality in arteriosclerotic psychoses. Am. J. Psychiat., *100*:501–505, 1944.

———: The clinical differentiation of senile and arteriosclerotic psychoses. Am. J. Psychiat., *98*:324–333, 1941.

Simon, Alexander, et al.: Lipoproteins in general and cerebral arteriosclerosis. Am. J. Psychiat., *108*:663–668, 1952.

Wright, I. S., and Luckey, E. H., Eds.: Cerebral Vascular Diseases. New York, Grune & Stratton, 1955.

CHAPTER XVII

Brain Syndromes Associated with Convulsive Disorders (Epilepsy)

"*As for this disease called divine, surely it too has its nature and causes whence it originates, just like other diseases, and is curable by means comparable to their cure.*" HIPPOCRATES

THE TERM *epilepsy*, derived from the Greek word meaning to seize or fall upon, has long been applied to a group of explosive reactions formerly believed to constitute a disease *sui generis*. The name has persisted although it is now generally agreed that epilepsy is not a disease entity but is a symptom-complex characterized by periodic, transient episodes of alteration in the state of consciousness which may be associated with convulsive movements and/or disturbances in feeling or behavior. The following may be regarded as a reasonable clinical definition of epilepsy: "Episodic, recurrent, limited periods of altered consciousness with or without involuntary movements, not the result of bodily disorders such as failure of circulation, low blood sugar, emotional disturbance, or use of soporific drugs or intoxicants."[1]

Physiologically, epilepsy may be regarded as a disturbance in the electro-physico-chemical activity of the discharging cells of the brain, a disturbance that may be produced by a variety of irritative stimuli im-

[1] J.A.M.A., *164*:1706, 1957.

pinging upon them from within or from without. This physiological disturbance may be expressed in the form of: (*a*) a change in electric potential as recorded in the electroencephalograms, (*b*) varied disorders of consciousness, (*c*) disordered functioning of the autonomic nervous system and (*d*) convulsive movements or psychic disturbances. The nature of the disturbance of the internal milieu which in so-called idiopathic epilepsy alters the activity of the cortical neurons or of basal gray matter and precipitates an abnormal discharge of electrical energy in the brain is unknown, but there is much to suggest that biochemical changes which increase the excitability of neurons may be the pathophysiological abnormality. Epilepsy, therefore, is probably neurogenic rather than psychogenic although psychogenic factors may precipitate a seizure in a person who has a tendency to them. Presumably psychological factors may act physically on the organism. In female epileptic patients, the occurrence of a seizure in association with the menstrual period is common, but it is not known in what way the premenstrual hormonal interplay acts to precipitate attacks. The final metabolic derangement which results in a seizure is probably not the same in all patients or even the same at all times in any one patient. If the equilibrium of the internal milieu is in delicate balance, an attack may be precipitated by a minor physiological disturbance, such as that produced by hyperventilation.

Electroencephalography

Although the occurrence of an abnormal discharge of energy in the cerebral cortex coincident with epileptic attacks has only relatively recently been proved by electrical methods, Hughlings Jackson (1834–1911), the father of clinical neurology, conceived the idea nearly seventy-five years ago that such a discharge must be the basis of epilepsy. In 1929 Hans Berger of Jena discovered that by perfecting technical methods of amplification he could record through the intact skull the changes in electric potential already known to accompany cortical activity. The electroencephalogram (EEG) indicates alterations in electrical, and thus physiological, activity within the brain. Further study showed that normally about ten electrical impulses originate in the brain every second and that when these currents are recorded in the electroencephalogram they show a pattern of voltage and frequency (height and rate of the waves) more or less characteristic of the individual. It was then found that in epilepsy there are paroxysmal bursts of abnormal cortical activity with resulting changes in the rhythmic pattern of the EEG indicating abnormalities in both rate and voltage of these currents. For this reason Lennox introduced the term "paroxysmal cerebral dysrhythmia" as applicable to epilepsy. While abnormalities are to be observed in the electroencephalogram in many conditions other than epilepsy yet in this disorder these abnormalities tend to assume certain patterns. Further, these patterns are distinctive for certain types of seizures. The electroencephalogram reveals the presence of these dysrhythmic discharges but fails to reveal their pathogenesis. Gibbs states that when the focal discharging lesion is in the parietal, occipital or frontal lobes, the symptomatology is largely neurological; if the disorder is in one or both temporal lobes, the symptomatology is largely psychiatric or that of psychomotor epilepsy.

It is generally estimated that 5 to 10 per cent of normal persons exhibit abnormalities of their electroencephalograms similar to those seen in epileptics. It is believed that such persons are predisposed to epilepsy although the disturbance in cortical electrodynamics as represented by the EEG is not so serious as to result in seizures unless the cerebrum suffers some pathological alteration. It has also been found that about 85 per cent of persons with a history of epilepsy show abnormalities of electroencephalographic rhythm during a fifteen-minute recording in the interval between convulsions as compared with 10 per cent in the average population. When such abnormalities of the EEG exist in the interparoxysmal period they tend to be of the same general type as those observed in the form of seizure from which the patient usually suffers. These types will be described later. There are, however, undoubted epileptics in whom abnormal tracings have never been obtained even by repeated examinations.

It will thus be seen that the electroencephalogram has its limitations. Although the finding of seizure discharges creates a presumption that clinical seizures have occurred or will occur, a negative report (no seizure discharges) does not rule out epilepsy. This is because (*a*) seizure discharges can be present in the depths of the brain and not appear in standard recordings from the surface of the head and (*b*) discharges may occur so infrequently that there is almost no likelihood of one occurring during the relatively short period of recording required in a routine examination. In the waking state, but more especially during sleep, seizure discharges occur, as evidenced by the electroencephalogram, which are not immediately associated with clinical symptoms. Eighty per cent of patients with a history of convulsive epileptic seizures have nonconvulsive seizure discharges while asleep. When not asleep only 35 per cent have subclinical seizure discharges.

To be of value it is essential that the making of an encephalogram be carried out with meticulous care by a thoroughly trained technician. The requirements in this respect are far more exacting than for other diagnostic procedures in common use. Artifacts resulting from technical errors or mechanical defects may easily arise. Even greater technical knowledge and experience is required in the interpretation of the encephalogram. The individual who interprets the record must have all the information available regarding the patient if the test is to be really useful and dependable. With the possible exception of a minority of cases of idiopathic epilepsy, it is rarely if ever possible to make a conclusive diagnosis on the basis of an EEG alone. Gibbs, Gibbs and Lennox conclude that in about 48 per cent of persons with a history of seizures, a routine EEG is of great value in diagnosis and in about 42 per cent it is of little or no value.

Idiopathic and Symptomatic Epilepsy

In many instances clinical seizures develop in persons with pre-existing cerebral dysrhythmia but in whom no visible or otherwise demonstrable alteration of cerebral tissue can be discovered. For this reason seizures of unknown origin have long been known as *idiopathic epilepsy*. It is now generally acknowledged, however, that epilepsy is not a disease in itself but rather a symptom of some underlying cerebral disorder. Perhaps in the so-called idiopathic, or better cryptogenic, epilepsy there is some metabolic disorder of the brain cells as a result of which they are apt to discharge in an explosive way. This may happen at any time and without apparent cause. About 77 per cent of all epileptics fall among those in whom no cause of the condition can be found. Cases in this group tend to manifest themselves early in life. In other instances tumors, trauma, inflammation or other discoverable lesions precipitate seizures in a person who may or may not have had a pre-existing cerebral dysrhythmia. Those seizures in which a cerebral lesion either brought out a subclinical dysrhythmia or produced seizures in the absence of pre-existing dysrhythmia are known as *symptomatic or acquired epilepsy*. A growing recognition of the multiplicity of etiological and contributing factors continues to displace the traditional idiopathic *versus* symptomatic point of view.

Frequency of Epilepsy

It is generally estimated that the incidence of epilepsy in United States is 1 in 200 of the population. This means that there are over 700,000 epileptics in this country. Because of the development of new drugs in recent years for the treatment of the disorder, fewer patients than formerly require institutional care. For the most part these epileptics are chronic, mentally deteriorated patients. The incidence in males is slightly greater than in females, probably because of the greater frequency of head trauma in the male both at birth and in adult life.

Age of Onset

"Idiopathic" epilepsy may develop at any age but a majority of cases appear between the ages of ten and twenty. Not a few occur before ten years of age but the first appearance of a seizure after twenty requires study by all known methods before the conclusion is reached that it is idiopathic. Infantile convulsions appearing without obvious cause should be regarded with apprehension. Thom reported that infantile convulsions associated with fever or other physical disturbance increase the chances of epilepsy five times.

Inheritance

The exact degree to which heredity influences the development of seizures is a controversial subject. The work of Lennox and his associates strongly suggests that it is of considerable influence while Alstrom, a Swedish epileptologist, although believing epilepsy to be a symptom and not a disease *sui generis*, concludes that it is rarely gene-determined. After a careful study of 897 families in which one or more members suffer from the disorder, he concluded that the incidence of epilepsy among close relatives of epileptics does not significantly exceed that of the general population. Lennox, Gibbs and Gibbs, on the other hand, found from an electroencephalographic examination of parents of epileptics that these parents had abnormal brain waves much more frequently than did control persons. In the opinion of these authors, the "presence of abnormal brain waves in the parents of epileptics is presumably evidence that the cerebral dysrhythmias associated with epilepsy are inheritable and that parents who show such cortical dysrhythmias are 'carriers' of the disorder." These authors found that 60 per cent of near relatives of noninstitutional epileptics had dysrhythmia and 2.4 per cent of them had a history of seizures. Of their controls 10 per cent showed dysrhythmia. Of course none had seizures. It has been found that amongst identical twins idiopathic epilepsy occurs eight times more frequently in both individuals than it does in both of fraternal twins. It is estimated that epilepsy occurs about five times more frequently among near relatives of idiopathic epileptics than it does in the general population. The existence of a predisposition to the disease in the child of an epileptic is often demonstrable in the form of cerebral dysrhythmia. There is also a striking likeness of brain wave abnormalities in epileptics with the same heredity. A person afflicted with epilepsy who marries a nonepileptic may, however, expect only one child in fifty resulting from the union to suffer from convulsions.

Not infrequently the psychiatrist is asked concerning the advisability of marriage for the epileptic or the probability that his children may inherit the disease. Lennox[2] points out the following factors as tending to minimize the chances of the disease in the child of an epileptic: a family history devoid of epilepsy or migraine for the spouse as well as the patient; a minimal abnormality of their electroencephalograms; some acquired condition that is at least partially responsible for seizures; late onset of the illness, and a normal mental endowment. In his opinion the genetic factor in epilepsy is probably no greater than it is in many other common diseases.

Types and Their Symptoms

Three major types of clinical seizures are usually described: grand mal, petit mal and psychomotor seizure or psychic equivalent. Heredity is of importance in determining the pattern of seizure. The seizures of all types are irregular and unpredictable. There are many variants of epilepsy which, because they depart so far from the "usual" forms of seizures, are apt to escape recognition. Loss of consciousness with or without convulsive spasm is the criterion of epilepsy. It is probably not sufficiently appreciated that in many attacks consciousness is not lost but is merely disturbed. The patient may be aware of all that is going on around him, may hear and understand what is being said but is for the time being unable to collect his thoughts or reply to a question. Not rarely the occurrence of a major epileptic fit suddenly renders clear the meaning of obscure minor events that may have existed for years. These may have been myoclonic, local muscle spasms, defects of attention, "absences," dreamy states, or brief periods of mental inhibition when mental processes seem to be arrested and the mind a blank. The form that epilepsy

[2] Lennox, W. G.: The Heredity of Epilepsy as Told by Relatives and Twins. J.A.M.A., *146*:529–534, 1951.

takes depends not so much on the pathological features of the lesion as upon its site and upon the violence of the neuronal discharges in the neighborhood of the lesion and the extent of their spread to the rest of the brain.

GRAND MAL. The grand mal seizure with its intense spontaneous neuronal activity is the most dramatic of the epileptic manifestations. Seizures of this type tend to be accompanied by an increase in speed and voltage of brain waves which are recorded in the electroencephalogram as sharp spikes, often at the rate of twenty-five per second. From a moment to several seconds before the loss of consciousness about one half of patients with grand mal type of attack have an *aura*, or warning, that a seizure is immediately imminent. The aura is not really a premonition but the first manifestation of the neuronal discharge. The form of the aura depends primarily upon the site of the epileptogenic focus. Lesions of the precentral region generally give rise initially to motor phenomena and of the postcentral region to sensory phenomena. The aura may consist of numbness, tingling, uncomfortable sensations, of a feeling of distress in the epigastrium, perhaps passing up toward the head, or of a hallucination of the special senses, such as flashes of light, certain noises or olfactory hallucinations. The aura is usually affectively unpleasant. Sometimes the aura is motor in nature and consists of a twitching or stiffness in a certain group of muscles preceding the loss of consciousness. The loss of consciousness is sudden and complete. The patient falls at once and as there is rarely any opportunity to protect himself he may sustain serious injuries. As he falls the entire voluntary musculature goes into a continuous contraction, remaining in this *tonic* phase from ten to twenty seconds. The muscles of the chest often contract at the same time as do those of the larynx; air is thereby forcibly expelled and results in the peculiar sound known as the epileptic cry. At first the face is pale but as the muscles rigidly contract the superficial veins become engorged. At the same time the chest becomes fixed and the aeration of the blood ceases, thus adding to the cyanosis of the face. During this tonic phase and for a variable period afterward the pupils are dilated, do not react to light and the corneal reflex is absent. The Babinski reflex is present and the tendon reflexes absent or decreased. During the general muscular contraction, the bladder is often emptied and occasionally the rectum. The tonic stage is followed by intermittent or *clonic* muscular contractions, at first rapid but gradually growing less frequent. If at this time the tongue happens to fall between the teeth during a relaxation it may be bitten when a clonic contraction follows. As respiration returns the saliva, which could not be swallowed, may become intermixed with air and thus appear in a foam, perhaps tinged with blood. In the *postconvulsive coma* the pupils are rigid, tendon reflexes are absent, respiration is stertorous, the face is congested and covered with perspiration and the lips are cyanosed. If an arm or leg be lifted and then released, it drops heavily as in a state of flaccid paralysis. If left undisturbed, the patient may sleep for an hour or two, complaining of headache, fatigue and perhaps of a painful tongue on awaking. As the patient emerges from the coma, he is often bewildered and may perform semiautomatic acts, move aimlessly about, exhibit chewing movements, fumble at his clothing or attempt to remove it. Sometimes clouded states persisting for a few days may develop after several successive convulsions. They are more frequent in men than in women.

Some patients have convulsions during sleep as well as in their waking hours, while in some patients the convulsions are always nocturnal. Many have their seizure just as they are falling asleep. It should be remembered that occasionally an epileptic who is subject to nocturnal seizures is suffocated by burying his face in a pillow during a convulsion.

Status Epilepticus. Sometimes a patient may pass from one seizure into another without intervening recovery of consciousness. This condition, known as status epilepticus, always involves danger to life. It is sometimes precipitated by abrupt withdrawal of medication, particularly if the patient has been receiving phenobarbital. It may follow alcoholism or excessive fatigue but frequently no precipitating factor is evident. It is not rare after cerebral operations on epileptics. If preventive measures are not taken the temperature may rise to dangerous heights. The patient may become profoundly exhausted, lapse into coma and die from cardiac dilation or pulmonary edema.

Petit Mal. Abortive seizures of various degrees and types occur in all of which there is usually some disturbance of consciousness. The most frequent of the minor forms is that of petit mal which is characterized by a transient interruption of the stream of consciousness. The electroencephalogram of petit mal consists of a slow, round wave followed by a quick, sharp spike. Groups of these alternately slow and fast waves occur three times a second. It is the most distinctive of any of the epileptic brain wave records. The details of these minor attacks differ widely among individual patients but the most frequent form consists of a loss of consciousness lasting from five to thirty seconds. They begin and end abruptly and are without warning or sequel. The patient does not fall. He may become pale, his posture become fixed, his eyes be staring and expressionless, his attention cannot be secured, he may suspend his occupation and through loss of muscle tone drop whatever article may be in his hand. Usually there is a little rhythmic twitching of eyelids, eyebrow or head. After a few seconds, consciousness abruptly returns and the patient resumes his activities. Most patients recognize that an attack has occurred but some remain unaware of this "absence." The onset of petit mal is usually between four and eight years of age. After 18 years of age it tends to disappear or to be replaced by other types of seizure. Petit mal attacks usually occur much more frequently than grand mal seizures. From one or two to a few hundred attacks may occur in a day. The two forms frequently coexist. Two of every three children with petit mal subsequently develop grand mal. Many children with petit mal are often socially and emotionally maladjusted. This maladjustment often appears to be explained on the basis of an impaired parent-child relationship which affects the child's personality formation. The impaired relationship apparently grows out of a conscious or unconscious parental rejection. The lack of basic security occasioned by the impaired parent-child relationship tends to extend and pervade all relationships. Sometimes the child, believing that all adults are like his parents and that all experiences will be frustrating, develops a pattern of antagonism and rebellion.

Usually included in the petit mal form are myoclonic twitches in which single contractions of flexor muscles of the arms occur without loss of consciousness, also akinetic attacks in which there is a sudden falling with muscular hypotonia. Like the classical petit mal, the latter two forms show a wave-and-spike rhythm of electrical discharge. Formerly the term pyknolepsy was given to what was believed to be a special type of seizure allied to petit mal. It is now considered to be a true petit mal. The name should therefore be dropped.

PSYCHOMOTOR EPILEPSY. Psychomotor epilepsy is characterized clinically by trance-like attacks and confusional episodes and is much more common in adults than in children. The patient is not unconscious but has no memory of the episode. Some patients describe brief affective states of fear, vague alarm, terror, rage and occasionally of well being or pleasure. The patient's behavior is appropriate to his mood. Other episodic but sustained moods may be in the form of extreme irritability, depression, ill humor or bad temper. Sometimes the psychomotor seizure takes the form of a clouded state characterized by confusion, bewilderment, excitement with hallucinations, outbursts of violence, or occasionally ecstatic moods with religious exaltation. Clinically the clouded state suggests a delirium with liberation of aggressive, and occasionally, self-destructive impulses. Acts of violence may be committed in these automatisms and may be of a strikingly brutal nature, the patient pursuing his crime to a most revolting extreme. These furors are characterized by their suddenness, absence of premeditation and of precaution and by amnesia for them. The extraordinary degree of discrimination and judgment displayed in the psychomotor attack often gives the patient's acts a misleading appearance of deliberation. It may be difficult to accept the fact that the author of the crime was not responsible for his acts. Usually these psychomotor seizures continue for only a few minutes but they may go on for hours or even days. Sometimes the seizure may assume the form of a fugue. Occasionally the patient may report feelings of loneliness or strangeness or typical "déjà vu" phenomena as if he had undergone the same experience in the dim past. Psychomotor seizures may occur in pure form but in many cases grand mal seizures may also be present. Their frequency increases with age.

Probably to be included among the psychomotor epilepsies is the syndrome known as *epilepsia cursiva* ("running fit"). This is an episodic alteration of awareness associated with running. Consciousness may be clouded to a variable degree. Sometimes the running fit occurs immediately after a grand mal seizure. There may or may not be an aura. The duration of the running is brief. Frequently one finds a history of conflicts with members of the family that seem to have acted as precipitating factors.

The distinguishing feature of the electroencephalogram in the psychomotor seizure is the presence of spike seizure discharges at the rate of from four to eight a second. It is believed that the focus of electroencephalographic activity is the anterior part of the temporal lobe. There is an increasing tendency to use the term *temporal lobe epilepsy* as a synonym for the psychomotor type, or to refer to the seizures characterized by hallucinations, memory disturbances and automatisms as "temporal lobe" in preference to "psychomotor." Penfield and his coworkers, by stimulation of the cortex of the temporal lobe in patients with temporal lobe epilepsy, produced complex hallucinations, vivid memories and dreams which were often identical with the content of the seizures.

The following case is fairly illustrative of the type of epileptic that enters institutions for mental disorders:

T. C. was admitted to a state hospital at the age of thirty-one. He was described by his family as having a rather bad temper, being somewhat stubborn and inclined to boast. At seventeen he began to suffer from mild seizures with loss of consciousness but without generalized convulsive movements. Not until twenty-seven did seizures occur more than two or three times a year. At that age they began to occur once or twice a month. At twenty-nine the seizures became more severe with marked convulsive movements and longer periods of unconsciousness. Because of a seizure at his place of employment he lost his position in an ice factory. Unable to find other employment, the patient became somewhat depressed, worried, irritable and "hard to get along with." His seizures became more frequent and severe. One day following a period of moody preoccupation during which he seemed unaware of his wife's presence, he said to her, "Catherine, I've done good today. I've made my fortune." He then added, "Call the doctor and the priest, I'm afraid I am going to die." That night he walked about all night, talking constantly about becoming rich, quoted passages from the salesmanship instructions issued by a concern for which he had recently attempted to canvass, and paid little heed to his environment. The following night he became so uncontrollable that at his family's request he was taken to the police station and on the following day committed to the state hospital. He was brought to the institution in straps and in the admission office shouted in a loud tone, "I drank a lot. I don't need that fellow. I thought an awful lot of that fellow. I think an awful lot of my mother. I told them plenty, I said 'No! No!'" At intervals he struggled violently to escape from the two officers who were holding him. When asked any questions he would shout, "None of your business."

On examination at the hospital he was noted to be a tall, ungainly individual, his large ears standing out prominently at nearly a right angle to his skull. The conformation of his facies suggested that he was a biological variant. He remained clouded for about six weeks, at times apparently hallucinated, sometimes preoccupied, mute and having to be tube-fed, again talking in a loud angry tone. When not in the continuous bath he was usually to be found in his room, frequently with his prayer beads hanging from his mouth, often nude, and when approached would spontaneously make such remarks as: "I'm–I'm trying to solve the problem. I'm trying to find the solution. Irish! Irish! Captain I, an eye for an eye, and a tooth for a tooth. I've tried to save my soul."

After this prolonged clouded state the patient remained clear for two months, occasionally suffering from a convulsion. Four months after admission he again became cloudy. At times he was stuporous, at times excited, and on several occasions attempted suicide. Nine months after admission he was paroled to his family and for seven months remained well except for occasional light convulsions. At the end of that period while attending church he suddenly arose during the services and began to pray loudly. He held a crucifix high above his head, and when led from the building seemed much confused. The patient was then returned to the hospital where the clinical course was much like that of the first residence.

Narcolepsy

The term *narcolepsy* was introduced in 1880 by Gélineau to describe a "rare neurosis characterized by an invincible need for sleep, ordinarily of short duration, occurring at longer or shorter intervals of time, often several times a day, forcing the subject to fall to the ground or to lie down in order to avoid falling." It has often been described as a variant of epilepsy. Probably, however, this is not the case and it should be considered as a special clinical type in a group of sleep disorders. In many cases a history of previous epidemic encephalitis has been obtained. In some instances narcolepsy may be a sequel or a continuing form of that disease. Narcolepsy is characterized by a sudden, irresistible desire to sleep. Regardless of the situation in which he may be placed or of the activity in which he may be engaged the patient falls fast asleep. The sleep is apparently natural; the patient may be awakened but the period of sleep usually lasts from seconds to thirty minutes. After he has awakened the patient usually states that he feels refreshed. Nocturnal sleep is not modified. Narcolepsy is most frequent in young male patients. Sexual impotence, obesity and lymphocytosis are often associated symptoms. It is generally believed that some anatomical pathologic condition, the result of localized encephalitis, trauma or neoplasm, exists in the gray matter surrounding the third ventricle at the level of the ocular nuclei or in the hypothalamus. Lesions of the hypophysis may be secondary. Cases supposed to be psychogenic have been reported. Psychometric studies in certain groups of patients with the narcoleptic syndrome have shown a common background of emotional conflict. The individuals felt caught in a life pattern which they resented but felt obligated to conformity. Frustrated in their efforts to achieve an autonomy in another pattern of their own choosing because of their dependent emotional attachments, the narcoleptic complex emerged relieving the anxiety of open conflict. Many consider narcolepsy as a syndrome that may occur in several pathological states. It is probably not a disease *sui generis*. Electroencephalographic records do not show the cerebral dysrhythmia of epilepsy. On the contrary, they are practically the same as those observed in ordinary nocturnal sleep. Narcolepsy does not respond to bromides, phenobarbital or other sedatives but is controlled by dextro amphetamine sulfate (10 to 50 mg. twice daily) or racemic amphetamine sulfate (10 to 50 mg. twice daily). If taken after midday such drugs may produce insomnia. Since this disorder may have psychogenic determinants or be confused with hypersomnia as a symptom of an emotional disturbance, careful psychiatric evaluation is indicated in all suspected cases. Psychotherapy is reported helpful in certain instances.

Cataplexy

Apparently related to narcolepsy are the paroxysmal attacks known as cataplexy in which, under the influence of emotional excitement, there is a paralysis of voluntary movements, a postural collapse of the whole body. The patient suddenly loses power and tone of all skeletal muscles, his knees give way and he sinks helplessly to the ground. Many patients are unable to speak during the episode although consciousness is fully preserved during its existence. Laughing, in particular, appears to provoke an attack although anger, anxiety or annoyance may act similarly. Narcolepsy and cataplexy are probably allied reactions, since cases of a transitional nature including narcoleptic attacks provoked by emotion are observed. Some writers consider cataplexy as a symptom of narcolepsy. The attacks of narcolepsy and cataplexy constitute what is often spoken of as the narcoleptic-cataplectic syndrome.

Epileptic Personality

Reference is often made to a so-called epileptic personality. The idea, however, of an "epileptic personality" as a precursor and essential background of epilepsy has been discarded. Undoubtedly some epileptic children are overly aggressive, irritable, restless, overactive, moody, stubborn, oversensitive, shy and may manifest such conduct disorders as lying, stealing, fighting, sex misbehavior, cruelty and destructiveness. By no means all epileptic children show these characteristics. If they exist they are probably a result of bad home environment and of the frustrations, social rejection, state of insecurity, constant anxieties and other emotional difficulties arising from the child's handicap. Psychiatrists whose contacts with adult epileptics are limited to institutionalized patients usually assert that the epileptic patient has a rigid, unpleasant, irritable, self-centered personality given to rage on frustration. On the other hand, physicians who see no epileptics except those met in office and clinics report that their patients do not exhibit more undersirable traits than do persons free from the disease. Undoubtedly, however, the patient who feels that he is handicapped through his disorder, who is constantly struggling for a place in his community, who fears exposure and is convinced that he is destined to be an abnormal member of the family has periods of irritability and depression. The sense of resentment which he often feels may produce unhappiness, add to his problem of adjustment and perhaps create antisocial tendencies. Discouragement and hopelessness may lead to contraction of interests and mental slowness. The religiosity shown by some epileptics may have its origin in a search for security, solace and self-esteem.

Epileptic Deterioration

In a certain number of epileptics the range of interests narrows as the convulsive reaction continues. A psychic slowness develops, attention, intellectual processes and emotional responses become increasingly dull, and comprehension and memory become impaired. The patient suffers from a poverty of ideas, shows a tendency to stress the trivial as much as the important, to become circumstantial in his ideational expression, to disregard the interests of others, to become selfish, affectively self-satisfied, boastful, lazy, careless in appearance and his facies to be characterized by expressionless vacuity. His speech comes to be slow and monotonous, with but little variation as to accent or tone, and his vocabulary becomes limited. The degree to which dementia progresses, if it occurs, varies greatly. In extreme cases this dementia is great, the patient existing at a purely vegetative level, having no interest in and no intelligible communications with his social environment. Dementia is a much more frequent outcome in those who develop epilepsy in early childhood than in those in whom it appears in later years. Deterioration occurs less frequently if the patient was mentally normal at birth and if his seizures are of the petit mal or of infrequent grand mal types. It is more frequent in institutional patients than in the noninstitutional ones. Of the latter, about one third show some degree of mental impairment, although in only about 10 per cent is it so gross as to be immediately evident.

It is possible that deterioration may, in fact, be the result of the repeated anoxia and increased intracranial pressure that accompany repeated convulsions. In part it may be the result of prolonged toxic effect of drugs; and in considerable part as response to the problems and situations which the very nature of the disease creates. The social and intellectual ostracism from which the epileptic often suffers, the deprivation of normal educational advantages, his feelings of inferiority and his discouragement and hopelessness lead to a contraction of interests and to an impoverishment of personality.

Diagnosis

If witnessed by the physician or by a trained observer, the diagnosis of the typical grand mal with its unconsciousness and sequence of tonic cramp, cyanosis, clonic convulsive movements separated by intervals of gradually increasing length, stertorous breathing, perhaps automatic activity, stupor, and hebetude, is comparatively easy. In the case of petit mal or of an atypical and incompletely developed seizure, the diagnosis may be difficult. One should inquire for a history of migraine, of fainting attacks, and ascertain if any disturbances of consciousness have been accompanied by biting of the tongue, relaxation of the sphincters or injury to self. If observed by the physician the discovery of fixed, dilated pupils, of loss of corneal reflex and the presence of a Babinski reflex may confirm suspicion as to the epileptic nature of the paroxysm. The diagnosis of epilepsy is, however, not always easy. Attacks of loss of consciousness, of muscle-twitching, of feelings of faintness or of unreality will usually suggest epilepsy, but often a diagnosis must be based on retrospective facts found by careful questioning of patient and observers.

The electroencephalogram is of assistance in establishing a diagnosis but the evidence supplied by it must be supplemented by clinical observation. It must be remembered that about 5 per cent of persons who never suffer from seizures of any kind show minor dysrhythmia in the EEG, and occasionally the EEG in such normal persons may be characteristic of the records made in epileptics between attacks. This is particularly true in the relatives of epileptics. In rare instances an epileptic with definite clinical seizures may in intervals between convulsions show an entirely normal EEG. It is estimated that the chances are nine in ten that any disturbances of consciousness occurring in a person with a positive EEG are epileptic. Activation of the abnormal electrical potentials may be induced on occasions by hyperventilation, or by small doses of metrazol intravenously. It is of interest that mescaline and diethyl lysergic acid diethylamide (d LSD 25) are incapable of activating the attacks or the typical electroencephalographic abnormality in those with temporal lobe seizures.

Hysterical patients with attacks resembling epilepsy usually have normal electroencephalograms. The seizures of the hysteric occur in the presence of others and there is often some fairly obvious gain or domination to be secured by the paroxysm. The hysteric rarely injures himself in a seizure. It is important to remember the make-up of the hysteric with his tendency to histrionic poses and simulation of symptoms. While there may be a history of emotional disturbance just prior to an epileptic convulsion, yet any dramatic staging of a seizure points strongly toward hysteria. The hysterical seizure is usually grotesque in its manifestations, lacks the characteristic "march" of phases seen in epilepsy and is not accompanied by ocular signs indicated in the previous paragraph, by sphincter incontinence, Babinski sign or by so deep a loss of consciousness. In hysteria there is never any biting of the tongue as in epilepsy. There may be difficulty in the differential diagnosis of temporal lobe epilepsy and hysterical amnesic periods with automatism. The presence of psychogenic factors and the absence of the psychomotor type of electroencephalogram will point to the latter. It is often said that no epileptic attack is "motivated" and that no motivated act is epileptic.

The diagnosis of syncope from epilepsy is not always easy. The loss of consciousness in epilepsy is primarily caused by paroxymal discharges within the brain, while in syncope it results primarily from a fall in blood pressure. In syncope a cause—postural, emotional or physical—seems apparent. In syncope there is a fairly long warning. The patient often comments "I feel faint," and adopts some protective action, such as sitting. Pallor and hot or cold sweating are apparent. Consciousness usually returns without any confusion or sequel except sweating. The epileptic's loss of consciousness is usually followed by drowsiness and frequently associated with headache. In a Stokes-Adams attack, syncope and a convulsion may be closely linked. Here a rapid fall of blood pressure caused by cardiac arrest produces convulsions through cerebral anemia.

Course and Prognosis

Today the average epileptic enjoys an incomparably brighter prognosis than he did 20 years ago. Credit belongs mainly to the widespread availability of the electroencephalograph for diagnosis, to an ever-expanding group of nonsedative drugs that in many cases suppress epileptic phenomena, and to an increasing education of the public concerning the disorder with a resulting lessening of the rejection and social stigma from which the epileptic suffers.

The institutional physician may acquire altogether too pessimistic a view as to the prognosis of epilepsy. Most epileptics are intelligent and normal persons apart from their attacks and are quite able to earn a living. A large percentage of the patients seen by the private physician either do not deteriorate at all or but slightly. This does not mean that essential epilepsy is not a serious symptom complex, one in which the prognosis must always be guarded and in many instances is absolutely bad. The prognosis is usually most unfavorable if the onset is in childhood. The prognosis as to recovery is worse in petit mal than in grand mal but, contrary to general opinion, the mental life does not suffer so much in petit mal.

To a considerable extent the prognosis is dependent upon the promptness of diagnosis and treatment. Both rate and extent of deterioration vary greatly but tend to be influenced by the age of onset, the frequency of seizures and the effort made to maintain wholesome, constructive, satisfying, unselfish interests and constant employment. The emotional handicap produced through faulty attitudes such as shame or overprotectiveness on part of the patient's family may operate against recovery. In its more malignant forms the deterioration may proceed until the patient lives at an essentially vegetative level. A few epileptics become psychotic and require care in a hospital for mental diseases. However, with the use of anticonvulsant drugs now available, complete control or total abolition of grand mal seizures can be secured in 80 per cent of patients.

Treatment

General Management

The medical profession is beginning to modify its fatalistic attitude toward the epileptic syndrome. In a minority of cases, epilepsy leads to a devastating impoverishment of personality but much more frequently it is not incompatible with the functioning of the patient as a normal citizen. The social handicap remains, however, out of all proportion to the seriousness of the disease.

One of the fundamentals of treatment is the maintenance of optimum physical health. Physical and mental activities should be encouraged, especially those that afford a combination of muscular exercise, intellectual interest and pleasure. It should be remembered that conscious or unconscious parental rejection may seriously warp the developing personality of the child. He should not be the object of oversolicitous fear and overprotection. Petit mal attacks, even if frequent, should not prevent attendance at school, nor should infrequent major attacks. The epileptic patient should be employed, but at a job wherein his own safety or that of others would not be jeopardized should he suffer a seizure. If possible, safety should not be purchased at the cost of active participation in life. Although it is usually necessary to raise the seizure threshold through medication, psychiatric treatment should not be omitted. Emphasis should be placed upon the relief of emotional or other psychic stress and upon the promotion of a normal life within the limits of the patient's psychobiological equipment. He should be given opportunity to preserve his self-respect, develop his abilities and maintain social usefulness. Many epileptics tend to daydream and to indulge in idle dissipations that increase the frequency of their seizures and hasten deterioration. The epileptic should be encouraged to plan his own work, studies and activities. Sustained work is often a difficult habit for him to establish but one of great importance.

There has often been an unnecessary restriction of the epileptic's diet. Ordinarily he should eat the same food as other members of the family, but attacks may be precipitated by hypoglycemia. The patient should therefore not go too long without food. The ingestion of an abnormal amount of fluid at one time may precipitate an attack. Food should be moderate in amount, and alcohol should be avoided.

Drug Therapy

The aim in treatment is to give medicine which will counteract the explosive tendency of the brain cells. For over sixty years *bromides*, first suggested in 1857 by Sir Charles Locock, constituted the principal form of medication. They have now been largely displaced by newer drugs.

Phenobarbital, or phenylethylbarbituric acids, first recommended by Hauptmann in 1912, is one of the drugs most widely used for raising the convulsive threshold of the epileptic. In persons twelve or more years of age, one may begin with a 0.1 gm. dose once a day. In adults this may, if necessary, be increased to 0.3 to 0.4 gm. administered in divided doses. In children under five 0.05 gm. may be used. If the seizures are nocturnal, it may be given at bedtime. If they are diurnal, it may be taken in the morning. Should seizures be frequent and severe, the patient may receive the drug three times a day. Even ordinary doses may produce drowsiness at the beginning of its use but this effect usually disappears in a few weeks. Toxic doses may produce apathy, slow mental reactions, ataxia, slow speech and muscular weakness. A sudden discontinuation of its use usually leads to an increase in number of seizures and even to status epilepticus. Phenobarbital, nevertheless, is usually the most effective drug in alleviating grand mal seizures and least frequently produces toxic symptoms. It is of little value in petit mal which should usually be treated by Tridione. Methylethylphenylbarbituric acid (mephobarbital or Mebaral) acts similarly to phenobarbital but is more effective with certain individuals. For adults the dosage is 0.3 to 0.6 gms. daily.

In 1937 Merritt and Putnam introduced sodium diphenylhydantoin sodium, generally known as Dilantin, an anticonvulsant that has proven of great value. Not being a hypnotic it does not cause drowsiness as is so often the case with phenobarbital. The usual dose is 0.1 gm. capsule three times a day. The maximum amount that adults tolerate is approximately 0.6 gm. daily. If necessary for the control of seizures, this may be increased somewhat. In psychomotor seizures, it is the most efficacious of the antiepileptic drugs and in grand mal may be effective in some cases where phenobarbital has failed. There is apparently a synergism between phenobarbital and Dilantin sodium which makes the combination more effective than when either drug is used alone. In toxic amounts Dilantin causes gastric distress, a symptom which usually ceases after one or two weeks of treatment. Less frequently it causes dizziness, ataxia, tremors, nystagmus, diplopia, drowsiness, and hyperplasia of the gums. Its sudden, complete discontinuance may induce status epilepticus.

Another anticonvulsant which is now rather extensively used is Mesantoin. The usual doses are 0.1 gm. three times a day for children and 0.2 gm. for adults. Since it may be toxic, blood counts should be made once a month. Combined with Dilantin or phenobarbital it may be effective in cases resistant to other drugs. Its combination with Tridione is to be avoided.

Trimethadione, introduced in 1945 under the trade name Tridione, has been found to produce gratifying results in the treatment of petit mal but may aggravate other types. The starting dose of trimethadione is 0.3 gm. three times a day for adolescents and adults. Gradual increases in dosage are carried out until therapeutic effect is obtained, usually between 1.5 and 2.7 gm. daily. In children under two years of age 0.15 gm. two or three times is the initial dosage with increments of 0.15 gm. Toxic symptoms in the form of skin eruptions, "glare phenomenon," a photophobia in which objects appear to shimmer, blurring of vision, drowsiness, dizziness and headache may occur. Toxic action on the blood-forming elements of the bone marrow followed by death has been reported. For this reason the blood should be examined once a month for agranulocytosis. For some persons paramethadione dimethylethyloxazolidine dione (Paradione) is more effective than Tridione. *N*-methyl- *alpha*-phenylsuccinimide (Milontin) may also be used for petit mal though it is less effective than the diones. For adults the dose is 0.9 to 3.0 gm. daily and for children 0:6 to 1.8 gm. daily.

Another drug which has been increasingly employed in therapeutically resistant convulsive disorders since 1949 is Phenurone (phenacetylcarbamide). This may be used in both grand mal and psychomotor seizures, but seems to be more effective in the latter type. It may be given in 500 mg. doses three times a day. After the first week of treatment an additional 500 mg. may be taken on rising. One-half the adult dose is recommended for children from 5 to 10 years of age. It seems to be especially useful in combating drowsiness and lethargy in patients who are affected in this manner by phenobarbital and other drugs. Patients receiving Phenurone should be watched carefully for the possible development of serious damage to the hematopoietic system and to the liver. Primidone (Mysoline) is safer than Phenurone and is reported to be of much value in the treatment both of psychomotor epilepsy and grand mal. Dosage range is from two to eight 250-mg. tablets a day.

All types of seizure patients show some improvement under anticonvulsant therapy and those with focal and grand mal seizures respond best.

Phenobarbital and Dilantin usually give the best results in seizures of those types.

Because of the danger of status epilepticus, anticonvulsive drugs should not be withheld abruptly. The occurrence of status epilepticus constitutes a medical emergency and is best handled in a hospital. Prolonged status epilepticus may lead to irreversible cerebral changes and even death. The patient must be heavily sedated and kept in deep sedation for 24 hours. This is best accomplished with a solution of amobarbital sodium 1.0 gm. in 20 ml. for injection given slowly intravenously at the rate of 1 or 2 ml, per minute until the seizure stops and deep sleep results. Sleep is maintained with a continuous intravenous drip of 0.5 gm. amobarbital sodium (Amytal) in 500 ml. of isotonic saline solution. The patient should be turned every half hour to prevent hypostatic and aspiration pneumonia. Mild Trendelenburg position is maintained, and mechanical aspiration of secretions is often necessary. Oxygen is given through a nasal catheter when indicated. Additional sedation may be obtained without depressing respiration with the use of paraldehyde suppositories each containing 4.5 ml. of paraldehyde, repeated every four hours. A parenteral preparation of diphenylhydantoin sodium (Dilantin) is now commercially available and may be injected either intramuscularly or intravenously. This has been found valuable in status epilepticus in dosage not to exceed 500 mg.

In the case of seizures secondary to meningocerebral cicatrix formation resulting from trauma or infection, relief has at times been secured by surgical removal (Penfield) of the cicatrix. Surgery is being increasingly employed in the treatment of seizures of focal nature.

Benzedrine sulfate seems to be the drug of greatest value in the narcoleptic and cataplectic syndromes.

Because of the physical hazards involved the epileptic should be safeguarded from obvious environmental and occupational risks.

It is agreed that an epileptic whose disorder is not well controlled should not be permitted to operate a motor vehicle. In many states a known epileptic is forbidden by law to operate one. In recent years there has been a tendency to be more permissive in the case of persons with well controlled epilepsy. In 1949 the Wisconsin legislature, with the support of the state medical society, enacted legislation to allow the person with controlled epilepsy to drive a motor vehicle subject to the following provisions:[1] When the epileptic can present medical certification that he has been completely free of attacks for two years he can obtain a driver's license, renewable every six months, upon application to the motor vehicle division. Medical forms are sent to him to be filled out by his physician attesting to the fact that his condition has been completely controlled for over two years. This license is automatically renewable every six months upon application and medical certification that the patient's condition has remained under complete control during the previous six months.

It is reported that, during the period 1949–1957, 553 licenses to operate

[1] J.A.M.A., *164:*1705–6, 1957.

a motor vehicle were granted, that 96 licenses were denied after review by the medical review board and that but one accident occurred during the period because of an epileptic seizure by a driver.

BIBLIOGRAPHY

Adrian, E. D., and Yamigiwa, K.: The origin of the Berger rhythm. Brain, *58:*323–351, 1935.

Barrow, R. L., and Fabring, H. D.: Epilepsy and the Law. New York, Paul B. Hoeber, Inc., 1956.

Barsa, J. A., and Kline, Nathan S.: Reserpine in the treatment of psychotics with convulsive disorders. Arch. Neurol. & Psychiat., *74:*31–35, 1955.

Berger, H.: Ueber das Elektronkephalogram des Menschen. Arch. f. Psychiat., *87:* 527–570, 1929.

Bickford, R. G., Whelan, J. L., Klass, D. W., and Corbin, K. B.: Reading epilepsy; clinical and electroencephalic studies of a new syndrome. Tr. Am. Neurol. A., *100:*102, 1956.

Bradley, Charles: Behavior disturbances in epileptic children. J.A.M.A., *146:*436–441, 1951.

Brazier, M. A. B.: Electrical Activity of the Nervous System. New York, The Macmillan Co., 1951.

Bridge, E. M.: Epilepsy and Convulsive Disorders in Children. New York, McGraw-Hill Book Company, 1949.

Davidson, Jr., D. T., and Lombroso, C.: Epilepsy. New England J. Med., *251:*853–858, 897–903, 1954.

DeJong, R. N.: "Psychomotor" or "temporal lobe epilepsy." Neurology, *7:*1–14, 1957.

Denny-Brown, D.: The clinical aspects of traumatic epilepsy. Am. J. Psychiat., *100:* 585–592, 1944.

Drake, F. R.: Narcolepsy: Brief review and report of cases. Am. J. Med. Sc., *218:*101–114, 1949.

Falconer, M. A., et al.: Treatment of temporal lobe epilepsy by temporal lobectomy. Lancet, *268:*827–835, 1955.

Fox, J. T.: Social aspects of epilepsy. Lancet, *1:*775, 1947.

Gélineau, J. B. E.: De la narcolepsie. Gaz. d. hop., *53:*626–628, 1880.

Gibbs, F. A.: Ictal and non-ictal psychiatric disorders in temporal lobe epilepsy. J. Nerv. & Ment. Dis., *113:*522–528, 1951.

———, and Gibbs, E. L.: Atlas of Encephalography. Addison-Wesley Press, Inc., Cambridge, Mass., 1950.

Gill, A. W.: Idiopathic and traumatic narcolepsy. Lancet, *1:*585–592, 1944.

Glaser, G. H., and Dixon, M. S.: Psychomotor seizures in childhood. Neurology, *6:*646–655, 1956.

Hill, Denis, et al.: Personality changes following temporal lobectomy for epilepsy. J. Ment. Sc., *103:*18–26, 1957.

Hoch, P. H., and Knight, R. P., Eds.: Epilepsy; Psychiatric Aspects of Convulsive Disorders. New York, Grune & Stratton, 1947.

Jasper, H. H., and Penfield, W.: Electroencephalograms in post-traumatic epilepsy. Am. J. Psychiat., *100:*365–377, 1943.

Kaye, Irving: What are the evidences of social and psychological maladjustment revealed in a study of seventeen children who have idiopathic petit mal epilepsy? J. Child Psychiat., *2:* Section 2, 115, 1951.

Langworthy, O. R., and Betz, B. J.: Narcolepsy as a type of response to emotional conflicts. Psychosom. Med., *6:*211–226, 1944.

Lennox, W. S.: The genetics of epilepsy. Am. J. Psychiat., *103:*457, 1947.

———: Tridione in the treatment of epilepsy. J.A.M.A., *134:*138, 1947.

———: Psychiatry, psychology and seizures. Am. J. Orthopsychiat., *19:*432–446, 1949.

———: The heredity of epilepsy as told by relatives and twins. J.A.M.A., *146:*529–536, **1951.**

Livingston, S.: The Diagnosis and Treatment of Convulsive Disorders in Children. Springfield, Illinois, Charles C Thomas, 1954.
Penfield, Wilder, and Erickson, T. A.: Epilepsy and Cerebral Localization. Springfield, Illinois, Charles C Thomas, 1941.
———, and Jasper, H. H.: Epilepsy and the Functional Anatomy of the Human Brain. Boston, Little, Brown & Co., 1954.
Pond, D. A.: Narcolepsy: A brief review and study of eight cases. J. Ment. Sc., *98:*595–604, 1952.
Ruskin, I. W.: Medico-Legal Aspects of Epilepsy. Dis. Nerv. System, *13:*166–174, 1952.
Russell, W. R., and Whitty, C. W. M.: Studies in traumatic epilepsy. J. Neurol., Neurosurg. & Psychiat., *15:*93–98, 1952.
Schwab, R. S.: Electroencephalography in Clinical Practice. Philadelphia, W. B. Saunders Co., 1951.
Schwarz, B. E., Bickford, R. G., Mulder, D. W., and Rome, H. P.: Mescaline and LSD-25 in activation of temporal lobe epilepsy. Neurology, *6:*275–280, 1956.
Symonds, Sir Charles: Epilepsy. Brit. M. J., *1:*533–537, 1948.
Taylor, James: Selected Writings of John Hughlings Jackson. London, Hodder and Stoughton, 1931.
Walker, A. E.: Prognosis in post-traumatic epilepsy. J.A.M.A., *164:*1636–1641, 1957.
Yahr, M. D., and Merritt, H. H.: Current status of the drug therapy of epileptic seizures. J.A.M.A., *161:*333–338, 1956.

CHAPTER XVIII

Senile Psychoses

"He who is of a calm and happy nature will hardly feel the pressure of age." PLATO

IN 1900, 1 in 25 living persons was over the age of 65; in 1950 this ratio had changed to 1 in 13. The total population of the United States doubled between those years but the number of persons of sixty-five years or over almost quadrupled and is said to be increasing at the rate of 1000 per day. This has naturally been reflected in the number of aged people who develop mental disorders. In the past 30 years the number of first admissions to New York state hospitals of persons aged 60 or more has increased from 19.1 per cent to 40 per cent of all admissions.

A gradual wearing down of energy, a decline in responsiveness, a waning of initiative and of creative imagination, a narrowing of interests, an increase in egocentricity and a certain warping of personality must be looked upon as a normal involutional process operating with the passage of time. With advancing age there is a progressive loss of physical and mental resources, a loss which tends to arouse feelings of helplessness. These feelings serve to create anxiety which the individual tries to overcome by mechanisms which he has long employed in making his adjustments. As one grows older, therefore, he "grows more like himself." The stress of increasing physical and mental limitations, loneliness resulting from the loss of friends and relatives and perhaps rejection by children produce an anxiety which may evoke various protective mechanisms. Among them may be a turning to and perhaps embellishment of the past, a paranoid projection or a self-assertiveness to the point of being domineering. Other elderly persons, through feelings of insecurity or inadequacy, become ill-natured and contentious or regress to a dependent state. Both biological and sociopsychological factors contribute therefore to the personality changes of old age.

From these mild, senescent mental changes, there is a sliding scale to the extreme impoverishment of mental resources that characterizes senile dementia. The dividing line may be a matter of individual opinion.

Often the senile dementia patient is one who has not felt secure and whose pattern of living has long been constricted. The person of cheerful disposition who maintains contact with the outside world, has been well adjusted in previous years, and has built up emotional and intellectual resources may well escape the dementia of senility. The person who develops senile dementia has often been characterized by rigid and static habits. Persons who have always had difficulty in adjusting to the demands of life are prone to react to the inevitable retirement from business and professional posts of honor, to deaths of friends and relatives and the loosening of family and social ties that accompany old age by the development of mental symptoms. The more immature and maladjusted, too, have been the adaptations of earlier life the smaller is the stress required in old age to produce disorganized or disturbed behavior. That social activities and a wholesome variety of mental occupation may retard mental senility has long been recognized. In one of his famous dialogues Cicero said, "Old men retain their intellects well enough if they keep their minds active and fully employed." It will therefore be seen that although of great importance organic disease of the brain is often not the only factor in the development of senile psychoses. It is increasingly recognized that frequently they result from the interaction of organic and psychological factors.

Pathology

It is generally accepted that the anatomical changes associated with senile dementia are a result of deficiencies in cerebral blood flow with a concomitant decrease in brain metabolism and available oxygen. In many cases arteriosclerotic changes apparently equal in extent to those observed in senile dementia are found in elderly persons who manifest little or no dementia. It would appear, therefore, that not all the factors producing senile dementia are known. Perhaps there are predisposing constitutional ones. As already indicated, psychological factors may also contribute to personality breakdown of the aged.

The gross pathology of the brain in senile dementia is typically characterized by cerebral atrophy but frequently this is not easily demonstrated. If atrophy is apparent, it will be greatest in the frontal lobes where wide sulci and narrowed gyri may give the brain a wrinkled appearance. In extreme cases, the ventricles are widened and the ependyma presents granular excrescences. On section, the gray matter may be less atrophied than the white. One of the most significant histopathological changes, if demonstrable, is the reduction in number of cells. Occasionally, however, more severe neuropathological disturbances are found in brains of senile dementia patients who are not psychotic than are found in the brains of those suffering from unquestioned senile dementia. On the other hand, psychotic seniles may show only mild histological changes in the brain. In other words, there is not always a correlation between the degree of histological changes and the degree of intellectual impairment.

Symptoms

The transition from usual old age to senile dementia is ordinarily gradual and any decision as to when the imaginary line is passed must often be an arbitrary one. A dislike of change, a reduction in ambition and activity, a tendency to become constricted and self-centered in interests, an increased difficulty in comprehension, an increase in time and effort necessary for the performance of familiar duties, an increasing difficulty in adapting to new circumstances, a lessened sympathy for new ideas and views and a tendency to reminiscence and repetition are scarcely signs of senile dementia, yet they pass imperceptibly into mental destitution and personality regression. Many elderly people have little capacity to express warm and spontaneous feelings toward others. During relatively early stages and before mental impairment is advanced, periods of reactive depression following some specific event are not uncommon. Physical illness or severe emotional disturbance may quicken mental deterioration. Rarely are the symptoms of waning mental capacity sufficiently marked to warrant the diagnosis of senile dementia until after sixty years of age. The decreased impressionability, impaired registration and declining interest in environment and in present affairs predispose to the loss of memory for recent events that often serves as the earliest clinical criterion for the diagnosis. Limitation of ideas and impairment of capacity for abstract thought usually appear early as may also an indifference to the ceremonies and courtesies of social life. The patient resents what he considers as interference by younger persons and may complain that he is neglected. Some show a hostile but anxious and fearful dependence. Natural affections become blunted and may turn to hatred. A certain tendency to isolation occurs. This tendency to self-isolation and to hostility toward some living person is most frequent if some close member of the family has been lost. Altruistic sentiments are usually lost early, while egoistic, selfish ones are intensified and, like the instinctive ones, may be crudely manifested. Irritability, either as an expression of egocentric trends or a defensive reaction to the impairment of memory, is common. Exaggerated sexual activities or sexual indecencies may be exhibited, in which case they usually represent not merely a weakening of inhibitions but a defensive effort at psychological compensation for the waning of a fundamental function. Some senile dementia patients become careless in habits of toilet and dress; pride of appearance is forgotten. At times there is a tendency to be distrustful, prying and suspicious. Hoarding and delusions of theft, of poisoning, of poverty or of not being wanted are common. Exaggerations and caricatures of the previous personality betray its earlier tendencies. Anxiety, irritability, timidity and other personality changes frequently seen in senility are not attributable solely to changes in the brain. Many of them are caused by the fact that the individual has been shoved into a position that frustrates his wishes and deprives him of his usefulness and of his status as an autonomous person. A failure to find the satisfactions necessary to replace those the elderly person had when he felt needed, important and productive tends to lead to regressive changes.

While not rarely occurring to some degree these regressions of personality are less constant and less progressive than the impairment of the more strictly psychic functions. Accompanying, or even preceding the amnesia, is a tendency to reminiscence, the theme being characteristically personal. As memory for recent life sinks further away from recollection, the limits of recall are forced back further and further until the patient with the loss of his ability to assimilate new ideas and experiences, comes to live in the distant past, often in the period of his childhood. The patient may speak of parents or grandparents as still living and persons are often misidentified. Any recollection for the simplest events of recent life may be lost. This retention of memory for remote events and loss for recent ones seems reasonable in view of the theory that the hypothetical neuronal circuit patterns responsible for memories become more strongly established with time. The longer, then, the pattern has been established the more strongly does memory resist degenerative states such as those of senility. Orientation becomes defective and in his confusion the patient may wander away and become lost. Judgment becomes impaired; the personal hazards of traffic or other situations are not recognized. Frequently the patient forgets where he has placed articles and accuses other persons of having stolen them. He may leave the gas jet burning and is careless with matches and fire. He may become the victim of unscrupulous persons, particularly if their technique involves an appeal to the patient's vanity either in matters of competence or of sex. Many are restless at night and either wander about the house or engage in some aimless, perhaps destructive, activity in a confused manner. Through the day, on the other hand, the patient may sleep much of the time. Hoarding of articles of no value is common, quantities of worthless objects being carried in the patient's pockets or jealously guarded in some cherished hiding place. Hallucinations may occur; in some cases absurd delusions are conspicuous.

Physical Symptoms

Physically, the patient usually exhibits conspicuous signs of senility. The skin is often thin, atrophic and wrinkled. In advanced forms the special senses lose in acuity, weight is lost, the muscles are wasted, the gait becomes unsteady and shuffling, the voice harsh and speech slow. The handwriting becomes tremulous, while tremors of head and hands are common. Coexisting sclerosis of the cerebral arteries frequently gives rise to headache, dizziness, and the episodic and focal disturbances incident to vascular accidents.

Clinical Types

Different clinical types, such as simple deterioration, delirious and confused, depressed and agitated, paranoid and presenile types are described but there is frequently so much overlapping that the assignment to any particular group is an arbitrary matter.

Simple deterioration is the most frequent form of senile psychosis, and is characterized largely by progressive memory defect, at first for recent events but later for remote ones, a narrowing of interests, loss of initiative, sluggishness of thought, apathy, irritability and nocturnal restlessness. Contact with the environment becomes less and less, and a vegetative, mildly stuporous state may finally develop.

The nature of the *delirious and confused type* is indicated by its name. The onset of this delirioid and confused reaction is comparatively acute and may accompany a variety of physical illnesses. Among them are alkalosis, anoxia, hypoglycemia and urinary infection. An incautious use of bromides, morphine, barbiturates or other drugs may precipitate an attack. The reaction may be associated with dehydration occurring in fever or following a surgical operation (such as prostatectomy) requiring general anesthesia. Less frequently it may be caused by vitamin deficiency. In milder cases the patient is perplexed, disoriented and perhaps inaccessible. Insomnia is marked and hallucinations are frequent. In more severe cases the patient is restless, resistive, noisy and may exhaust himself. Strictly speaking, such a reversible process is not a part of senile dementia but represents a reaction to which the elderly person is particularly prone. Some seniles, however, present a chronic confusional state. Such a person may present a bewildered expression, move about in a vague and aimless fashion and be only dimly aware of his whereabouts.

The *depressed and agitated type* presents not merely the memory loss and intellectual impoverishment of senile dementia but also a marked egocentricity, persistent agitation and melancholic, hypochondriacal and nihilistic delusions.

The *paranoid type* is distinguished by the conspicuousness of delusions, most frequently of a persecutory nature. Sometimes helplessness is used as an effective means of power and of wielding it. Many paranoid seniles are irritable, quarrelsome, hostile and demanding. Complaints of bad treatment are nearly always expressed. This type of behavior usually occurs in persons whose life personality pattern has been characterized by dissatisfaction, projection and other defensive mechanisms. As its physical substratum suffers the degenerative changes of senility, the personality is no longer able to cope with its problems, its former defensive and compensatory mechanisms are exaggerated and delusional beliefs falsify reality to protect the personality and maintain its self-esteem. Memory loss may be absent or comparatively insignificant for a long time. As memory defect appears, delusional extension and further defensive emotional reaction may take place in an attempt to repair the additional psychobiological defect. Similarly, as judgment fails the delusions become more absurd, partly because beliefs are no longer subject to any critical scrutiny, and partly because the damaged personality requires more fantastic beliefs for its support. Hallucinations and illusions occur more frequently than in any other type of senile psychosis. Consciousness is not disturbed and orientation usually remains unimpaired. Of the various types of senile psychosis already mentioned, the paranoid form stands out most clearly as a special type. Transitions and admixtures of the various types described are common.

Presbyophrenia. The presbyophrenic type is characterized largely by a defect of retention with confabulation. It is doubtful if it should be accorded a special classification but rather should be regarded as a somewhat precocious form of senile dementia exhibiting certain clinical symptoms. It occurs rather more frequently in women than in men. Usually it will be found that the premorbid personality was characterized by cheerfulness, energetic activity, a certain vivaciousness and a good adjustability. The previous personality is fairly well retained and the patient continues to manifest a warm emotional response but with a tendency to be suggestible and to vacillate between friendliness and irritability. Most presbyophrenic patients are talkative individuals with an apparent alertness, who, however, when addressed are found to be quite out of touch with their environment. Impressibility and retention are defective, and memory is greatly impaired. Without the slightest realization of his memory fault, the patient supplies the deficiencies with confabulations, often accepting with good humor and amplifying as facts the fabrications that are suggested to him. His absurd contradictions and repetitions pass unnoticed by the patient. Many presbyophrenic patients are constantly busy with a restless, unproductive, even destructive, activity. With a certain amiable eagerness, as if occupied with his usual vocation, the patient intently disarranges or destroys his bed. The fabrication and memory disturbances are suggestive of the Korsakoff syndrome but the age of the patient, the gradual onset, complacent loquacity, progressive deterioration and absence of neuritic symptoms serve to differentiate presbyophrenia from Korsakoff's psychosis.

The following case history abstract is illustrative of simple senile dementia with an admixture of paranoid features—a not uncommon association:

H. S. was admitted to a public hospital for mental disorders when seventy-two years of age. When six years old she sustained a fracture of the hip. Four years later an operation was performed in an effort to correct the deformity and disability. "She had to be strapped to the bed for six months following the operation." The functional results of this operation were disappointing and the patient was always self-conscious concerning the considerable degree of disability that persisted. She always felt that people did not wish to mingle with her because of this infirmity and did not seem comfortable in the presence of others. It is quite possible that the few paranoid features accompanying the patient's senile dementia may have had their origin in this defensive characteristic.

Five years before her admission her adopted son with whom she resided noted that the patient was becoming forgetful, especially concerning her usual household duties and recent incidents. She hoarded articles and sometimes said that someone had stolen them. She remembered events of her childhood quite well and at times was somewhat boresome in her accounts of early experiences. Her adopted son noted that she became increasingly neglectful of her personal appearance. For many months prior to her admission she would not bathe unless reminded to do so. Recently she often went to bed without removing either clothing or shoes. At times she put on her clothing "inside out." For four years prior to admission she seemed to find it difficult to prepare meals at accustomed times. On many occasions she completed the preparation of the mid-day meal at 8 a.m. and insisted that the family should eat at that time. In preparing coffee she often put sugar instead of coffee in the coffee pot but failed to recognize her error. In a few instances she wished to pay bills that she had already paid. She was restless at night but often slept during the day. The patient became increasingly confused in surroundings with which she had formerly been quite familiar. Often when crossing the street she paid no attention to approaching automobiles. At times she wandered away from home. There were periods during which she constantly packed and unpacked her clothing. During recent months she had often failed to recognize friends. The patient became increasingly suspicious, said that neighbors were talking about her, spoke of them in extremely derogatory terms, maintained that her son lied to her, had tried to poison her and that her neighbors had threatened to kill her. She claimed that her son and an elderly woman who had been employed to exercise protective care for her had been secretly married. The patient complained that everyone was trying to control her activities and threatened to commit suicide if not permitted to do as she wished.

When the patient was brought to the mental hospital she rose to meet the admitting physician, shook his hand, asked him where he was and if there was anything she could do for him. She knew her name but could not give her address or other identifying data. She claimed that her son, who had really been extremely devoted to her, had ejected her in order to secure possession of her house which was located "down the hill." At the time of this writing she has been in the hospital for eighteen months. Affectless and placid she sits in a rocking chair all day paying little or no heed to her environment. Her existence is now but little above a vegetative level.

Prognosis and Course

The prognosis of advanced senile dementia is manifestly hopeless. No well-defined remissions are to be expected although in the excited types subsidence may occur. The course is progressive; the patient gradually becomes more demented although life may continue for ten years or even longer before death supervenes. Not a few mental disorders in the aged are, however, precipitated by exhaustion and toxic and nutritional factors. Many of these are quite amenable to appropriate therapy.

Diagnosis

In well-developed, simple senile dementia, the age of the patient, the progressive egocentricity and the characteristic memory loss, particularly for recent events, makes the diagnosis easy. In the paranoid form, the memory loss and evidences of dementia may be comparatively slight. Since these senile paranoids have usually had a life pattern of a defensive, paranoid type, the matter of deciding when this exaggerated pattern crosses the psychotic line may be one of arbitrary decision to be determined largely by social criteria and by the interpretation and values accorded reality. In such paranoid personalities, their exaggeration to a psychotic degree may, in both arteriosclerotic and senile disease of the brain, follow from the threat to the integrity of the personality contained in the degenerative, structural changes taking place in the organ which constitutes the important physical substratum of the personality. When arteriosclerotic changes in the brain, rather than the histological ones of senility, are the basis for such paranoid psychoses, the patient usually suffers from easy mental fatigability, dizziness, or slight confusion suggestive of changes in the smaller vessels of the cerebrum. Some depressed and agitated types suggest involutional melancholia. The differentiation must be made largely by the age of the patient and particularly by the presence or absence of deterioration. Differentiation from arteriosclerotic psychoses was discussed in Chapter XVI. A restricted diet in the old may lead to an avitaminosis suggestive of senile psychosis. Toxic psychoses are frequently mistaken for senile dementia. It should be remembered that, in the aged, mental disturbance may be caused by uremia, anemia, decompensated heart disease or by pulmonary disease rather than by senile dementia. The differentiation of presbyophrenia from Korsakoff's disease has already been mentioned.

Treatment

The discussion in the early part of the chapter has already suggested the importance of prophylactic factors in the prevention of the senile psychoses. It is therefore highly desirable that the aged person maintain a feeling of emotional security and a sense of dignity. One will accordingly attempt to see that the old person's needs for affection, for a feeling of belonging, for achievement and for recognition and approval are met.

The milder form of senile dementia should be cared for in the home. It is there that the patient's roots are deeply imbedded. Unless circumstances are such that either the safety of the patient or that of the family is endangered it is well to attempt to care for him in the usual and familiar environment. The patient is ordinarily happier there than in the unaccustomed and rather rigid routine of an institution where the habits of a lifetime have to be reconstructed. It is true, however, that the patient's inability to recognize his failing physical and mental vigor may present a serious problem to his family. In not a few cases, too, hospital care becomes necessary because of nocturnal restlessness, disturbing reponse to paranoid delusions, marked irritability, assaultiveness, sexual play with children, exhibitionism or ill-considered plans for marriage. Impaired judgment in business affairs may make the appointment of a legal guardian necessary. Care must often be exercised to prevent the confused patient from setting fire to clothing or furniture, to prevent wandering from home or from falling with resulting fracture of the neck of the femur. Because of the danger of suicide patients suffering from depressed or agitated types should receive hospital care. Mild hypnotics may be required at night. Chlorpromazine is often useful in the treatment of agitation, restlessness, irritability, confusion and delirium. The dosages and problems of treatment are similar to those described in Chapter XVI, Brain Syndromes Associated with Cerebral Arteriosclerosis. If appetite has been poor or diet restricted, it is advisable to prescribe ascorbic acid, thiamine chloride, niacin and glutamic acid. Preparations are now available supplying the latter agent in its utilizable form, monosodium L-glutamate. Vitamins are frequently of value in confused and delirious senile states. In the depressive forms, electroshock therapy can often be used safely and with great success.

BIBLIOGRAPHY

Busse, E. W., Barnes, R. H., et al.: Studies of the processes of aging. Am. J. Psychiat., *111:*896–901, 1955.
Clow, H. E.: Psychiatric factors in the rehabilitation of the aging. Ment. Hyg., *34:* 592–599, 1950.
Diethelm, O., and Rockwell, F. V.: Psychopathology of aging. Am. J. Psychiat., *99:*553–556, 1943.
Doty, E. J.: The incidence and treatment of delirium reactions in later life. Geriatrics, *1:*21, 1946.
East, W. N.: Crime, senescence and senility. J. Ment. Sc., *90:*835–850, 1944.
Ebaugh, F. G.: Age introduces stress into the family. Geriatrics, *11:*146–150, 1956.
First National Conference on Aging: Man and his Years. Raleigh, N. C., Health Publications Institute, Inc., 1951.
Kay, D. W. K., and Roth, Martin: Physical accompaniments of mental disorder in old age. Lancet, *2:*740–745, 1955.
Kolb, Lawrence: Mental hospitalization of the aged: is it being overdone? Am. J. Psychiat., *112:*627–636, 1956.
Lansing, A. I., Ed.: Cowdry's Problems of Aging, 3rd ed. Baltimore, Williams & Wilkins Co., 1952.
Lemkau, P. V.: The mental hygiene of aging. Public Health Reports, *67:*237–241, 1952.
Litin, E. M.: Mental reaction to trauma and hospitalization in the aged. J.A.M.A., *162:*1522–1524, 1956.
McFarland, R. A.: The psychological aspects of aging. Bull. New York Acad. Med., *52:*14–32, 1956.
Newton, R. D.: The identity of Alzheimer's disease and senile dementia and their relationship to senility. J. Ment. Sc., *94:*225–249, 1948.
Pollack, B.: The addition of chlorpromazine to the treatment program for emotional and behavior disorders in the aging. Geriatrics, *11:*253–259, 1956.
Proceedings of Association for Research in Nervous and Mental Disease: The Neurologic and Psychiatric Aspects of the Disorder of Aging, Vol. XXXV. Baltimore, Williams & Wilkins Co., 1956.
Rothschild, D.: The clinical differentiation of senile and arteriosclerotic psychoses. Am. J. Psychiat., *98:*324–333, 1941.
Sands, I. J.: The neuropsychiatric disorders of the aged. New York State J. Med., *51:*2370–2375, 1951.
Stieglitz, E. J.: The Care of the Aging and the Aged, 2nd ed. Philadelphia, W. B. Saunders Co., 1949.
Titchener, J., Zwerling, I., Gottschalk, L., and Levine, M.: Psychological reactions of the aged in surgery. Archiv. Neurol. & Psychiat., *79:*63–73, 1958.
Wilson, D. C.: The pathology of senility. Am. J. Psychiat., *111:*902–906, 1955.

CHAPTER XIX

Chronic Brain Syndromes Associated with Disturbance of Metabolism, Growth or Nutrition

Alzheimer's Disease

In 1906 Alois Alzheimer (1864–1915) described the case of a woman who had died at fifty-one following a rather rapidly progressing dementia and in whose brain a conspicuous tissue reaction was the development of tangled threadlike structures occupying much or all of the body of many cortical ganglion cells. These agglomerated neurofibrils stain black and silver. This degenerative change may involve even a fourth of the ganglion cells although it is now known that they are not limited to this disease but may be observed in senile dementia and even in the brains of the normal senium. There is an accompanying diffuse gliosis and an abnormal amount of fatty pigment in the nerve cells. Another histopathological change that practically always exists is the presence of senile plaques with their amorphous and homogeneous core. Plaques are most frequent in the frontal cortex and in the cornu Ammonis. In Alzheimer's disease the cortical degeneration is diffuse and involves the outer layers of the cortex, especially those of the frontal and temporal lobes. The cerebral atrophy can be demonstrated by pneumoencephalography. Changes in the basal ganglia are regularly found. Air encephalograms show a dilation of the ventricular system and increased cortical markings.

The onset of Alzheimer's disease is usually between fifty and sixty years of age although earlier appearances have been reported. The disease begins insidiously with a reduction of spontaneity, a progressive intellectual deterioration and alterations in behavior. There is no characteristic pattern in either the intellectual impairment or the behavioral disturbances. Disorientation, memory impairment, defects in calculation, general information, emotional lability, and in concreteness in thinking are present in varying degrees and combinations. Pronunciation is difficult, spoken language is comprehended poorly and errors are made in reading and writing. The patient makes mistakes in the routine details of his everyday life, words are forgotten and speech disorders are common. A not infrequent disturbance is a perseveration of speech in the form of logoclonia. In advanced stages of the disease speech becomes an incoherent jargon without sentence formation. Prolonged periods of restless overactivity, anxiety and depression may occur. Agnosia, apraxia and temporary hemiplegic or paraplegic weakness may exist. Syncopal and epileptic attacks are common. A Parkinson-like difficulty in gait is often seen. Facial paresis and hypertonicity of muscles are frequent and in late stages there may be contractures of the extremities. At this stage the patient becomes extremely demented, is entirely out of touch with his environment and becomes reduced to a mere vegetative existence. The usual duration of the disease is five to ten years, but the course may be characterized by remissions.

Little is known concerning the factors contributing to this form of presenile dementia. The clinical diagnosis from Pick's disease is often difficult and at times impossible. Certain symptom differences will be mentioned in the discussion of the latter disease in Chapter XXI. The following is a rather typical clinical history of a patient suffering from this disorder:

W. M. was admitted to the Norristown State Hospital in March, 1943, at the age of 52. The patient's early life, including medical history, does not appear to have been significant. The onset of his mental disorder was so insidious that his wife was able to give only an approximate date. About five or six years before his admission he began to show less affection toward his family. His wife added that at about the same time "he grew lazy and his interests gradually dulled. He had a habit of just sitting around the house. For years he has not mentioned the payment of the interest on his mortgage or his taxes." About three years before admission his wife noticed that he could not tell time correctly and that he would make errors in writing a check. "He would set out for the store to buy feed for his cows and forget to do so. One time he wanted to walk to his father's place, thinking that it was just down the road whereas it was a matter of sixty miles. He grew confused and on one occasion he stopped the car in the middle of an intersection. He would put on his trousers backward and his overalls inside out. Sometimes when a dish of food was put on the table for the whole family he would eat the entire amount himself."

The pre-admission history is obviously that of an insidiously developing and progressive dementia. On admission the patient appeared to be older than he actually was. He was completely disoriented for time and place. He did not know whether his home was in Pennsylvania or New Jersey. On the day of admission he said he was thirty-four years of age and on the following day gave his age as twenty-five and a few weeks later gave it as eighty. He was careless and untidy in dress and wandered about the ward in a confused and bewildered manner often mistaking the nurse for his wife.

On admission a general hyperreflexia was noted but no other neurological abnormalities. Prior to his death his extremities showed spasticity. The patient became incontinent of urine, gradually grew weaker and even more demented. In August, 1945, nearly two and one-half years after admission he suffered a rather typical epileptic seizure. About September 1, 1945, he became comatose and died nine days later.

At autopsy the brain weighed 1250 gm. A coronal section through the frontal lobes showed pronounced cortical atrophy with enlargement of the sulci. The island of Reil was also atrophic. On microscopic examination, a marked cortical atrophy was found, also a decrease in amount of subcortical white matter. In some convolutions the white matter was reduced to a narrow band. The subcortex showed a moderate general demyelination. Sections through the plane of the substantia nigra showed this to be depigmented. A section further caudad showed the posterior horns of the ventricles to be considerably enlarged at the expense of the white matter. Stained sections showed a focal and general loss of ganglion cells, the presence of ghost cells, severe degenerative changes in the cells that remained, and a uniform gliosis. Special silver stains demonstrated numerous senile plaques, also neurofibrillary degeneration of many ganglion cells. These showed thickening and agglutination of the neurofibrils, their displacement to the periphery of the cells and their bizarre arrangement within the cells.

Vitamin Deficiency Syndromes

In recent years it has become recognized that there is a common factor operative in various mental and neurological phenomena which had been previously regarded as unrelated entities. This common factor is a vitamin deficiency, particularly a deficiency of vitamin B. The localization of the pathological process produced in different parts of the nervous system by the deficiency determines the neurological signs and releases the mental symptoms. The nature of the symptom or syndrome depends upon the particular member of the B complex in which the deficiency is relatively greatest and upon the part of the nervous system predominantly affected by the deficiency. If the deficiency of nicotinic acid is greatest, the clinical picture produced is that of pellagra. If, as is not rare, a peripheral "neuritis" is also associated or if a Korsakoff syndrome is observed, a deficiency of thiamin exists also. If, because of chronic alcoholism, the patient suffers from thiamin deficiency he may suffer from a painful thiamin neuropathy, or "alcoholic neuritis." If at the same time there is nerve cell degeneration in the cerebral cortex resulting from deficiency of other member or members of the B complex (probably niacin), the patient will present an alcoholic Korsakoff syndrome.

Wernicke Syndrome

In 1881 Wernicke described a syndrome consisting of ophthalmoplegia, memory loss, confabulation, apathy, progressive dementia, ataxia, clouding of consciousness and even coma. It is now known that it is invariably associated with thiamin deficiency and that usually there is a deficiency of niacin also. Because of the thiamin avitaminosis, there is an impaired oxidation of pyruvic acid which is formed during the breakdown of glucose. As a result pyruvic acid accumulates in the blood.

Wernicke's "encephalitis" mainly affects chronic alcoholics but has also been described in pernicious anemia, hyperemesis gravidarum, gastric cancer and in prisoners of war. Delirium usually precedes its development. Wilder reports that the Wernicke syndrome formerly observed occasionally in pernicious vomiting of pregnancy or after abdominal or pelvic operations when solutions of glucose were administered in considerable amounts is now seen much less frequently, apparently because thiamin is given with the glucose as a usual procedure. Jolliffe states that this syndrome which before 1942 was frequently seen among alcoholics admitted to Bellevue Hospital, New York City, has almost disappeared since that date. He ascribes this disappearance to the fact that enrichment of bread and flour began in that year.

The pathological changes are mainly in the brain stem and involve the mammillary bodies and the regions adjacent to the aqueduct and to the third and fourth ventricles. The lesions are characterized by various degrees of necrosis of both nerve cells and nerve fibers, together with reactive changes of microglia and astrocytes, alteration of small blood vessels and, in some instances, petechial haemorrhages.

The ocular disturbances take the form of horizontal and vertical nystagmus and various degrees of paralysis of conjugate gaze and of the external recti.

H. B., aged 62, a chronic alcoholic who had been arrested many times for drunkenness was taken to a general hospital October 1, 1951, because of confusion and difficulty in walking. There was a history that following a long alcoholic debauch he had been taken into custody by the Salvation Army. For several days the supervision of this organization made it impossible for him to secure alcohol. He then remained at its hotel for several days more, performing light duties until his physical disabilities made employment impossible. Soon after entering the general hospital he became confused, restless, demanding and was noisy at night. He was then transferred to a psychiatric hospital where the confusion soon subsided. On neurological examination he showed a marked bilateral ptosis, his pupils reacted very slightly to light and he was totally unable to follow a light in any direction. His speech was thick and slurred, there was a great defect in co-ordination of his extremities, all tendon reflexes, except the biceps, were absent. The calves of both legs were tender and he was unable to walk unaided. A diagnosis of Wernicke's syndrome plus a peripheral neuritis was made. He was at once placed on large doses of thiamin. He soon began to improve but the evidence of ophthalmoplegia did not completely disappear for seven months.

If the thiamin deficiency produces a peripheral neuropathy, cardiac hypertrophy, myocardial weakness and edema, the clinical manifestation is that of beriberi, a form of deficiency without mental accompaniment. Beriberi may, however, be associated with Wernicke's encephalopathy. An uncomplicated thiamin deficiency without any associated neurological phenomena may produce a neurasthenic syndrome characterized by feelings of weakness, easy fatigue, emotional instability, irritability, moodiness, quarrelsomeness, forgetfulness, apathy, mild depression and vague fears. These symptoms soon disappear after the intake of thiamin is increased.

In nutritional encephalopathy, there is almost never a single vitamin deficiency. In the same individual one may see delirium tremens (the cause of delirium tremens is uncertain but it is probably a result of a disturbance of cerebral metabolism incident to vitamin deficiency), Korsakoff's psychosis, nicotinic acid encephalopathy (pellagra) and the Wernicke syndrome. There may also be a neuropathy in the form of an "alcoholic neuritis."

Psychoses with Pellagra

Although pellagra was first described in 1735 by a Spanish physician, Gasper Casal, under the name *mal de la rosa,* he attributed the disease to a poor diet, but not until 1915 was its dietary origin conclusively demonstrated by Goldberger. Not until 1937 was it discovered that nicotinic acid (niacin) is the pellagra-preventive vitamin. The principal deficiency, therefore, is in nicotinic acid although it appears that the disease may also result from a deficiency in the amino acid, tryptophan. Usually there are also other associated deficiencies, particularly of thiamin and riboflavin. Often, too, there is a deficiency of ascorbic acid. Many of the neurological symptoms in pellagra are presumably a result of the associated thiamin deficiency.

Pellagra occurs most frequently in communities where the prevailing low economic status leads to extensive nutritional deficiencies. Isolated cases occur among chronic alcoholics whose food has consisted largely of alcohol and has therefore been deficient in vitamin B complex. It is not rare in aged, destitute people who, living alone and in deprivation, suffer from vitamin deficiency. Sporadic cases may also occur in persons suffering from intestinal lesions that interfere with the absorption of food.

It should not be forgotten that pellagra may develop in persons who are already psychotic. This was formerly not uncommon in institutions for mental diseases. With more abundant and better balanced diets such institutional cases are no longer common.

Morbid Anatomy

There is but little experimental evidence indicating that uncomplicated niacin deficiency results in injury to the nervous system. In well developed cases, neuronal and capillary changes are found distributed throughout the neuraxis, usually most marked in the cerebrum. In the frontal lobes and in the hippocampus the ganglion cells lose their Nissl substance and may eventually disappear. There may be proliferation of glia cells and of capillary endothelium. The similarity of these changes to those of Meyer's "central neuritis" and to those of Wernicke's syndrome has long been noted. There now seems reason to believe that the same factor is common to all these conditions, that the histopathological changes in all of them are caused by thiamin deficiency or by a polyavitaminosis of the vitamin B complex since it is known that single vitamin deficiencies rarely if ever occur. Until the pathological changes become somewhat advanced they may be reversible.

Symptoms

The early mental symptoms of pellagra are often regarded as psychoneurotic and consist of vague headache, irritability, difficulty in concentration, forgetfulness, restlessness, apprehension, and a feeling of inability for mental or physical effort. These early symptoms are followed by those of an organic syndrome and consist of memory defects, confusion, disorientation, intermittent delirium, Korsakoff's syndrome and dementia. Some patients show a manic excitement while others may be depressed, anxious, apprehensive or paranoid. While organically released the particular type of such reactions will be determined by the patient's previous personality pattern. Later in the disease there may be evidence of irreversible neurological impairment resulting from advanced deficiency encephalopathy. This may be in the form of stupor, convulsions, incontinence, muscular rigidity, irregular involuntary movements, hypertonia, defective sensation and muscle paralysis.

Mild mental symptoms are usually the first evidence of pellagra but after some months these are followed by stomatitis and by a glossitis in which the tongue is red and painful and the papillae atrophic. Digestive disturbances with achlorhydria and diarrhea are common. An early erythema of the skin is followed by coarse scaling and a deep red-brown pigmentation. The dermatitis occurs characteristically on the extensor surface of the extremities, vulva and inner surfaces of the thighs.

Prognosis

If treatment is begun early before irreversible neuronal changes have taken place the prognosis is good but in neglected cases permanent impairment of memory and a persistent dementia result.

Treatment

Mild, ambulatory cases of pellagra are relieved by 100-mg. doses of niacin or niacinamide given three to six times a day. Extremely severe cases should receive 1200 to 1500 mg. a day for several days. Sodium nicotinate may be given intravenously or intramuscularly in 100 mg. doses. Parenteral liver extract given intramuscularly in doses of 20 cc. three to five times daily is indicated in severe cases. Since a thiamin deficiency usually coexists, this vitamin should also be given. The patient should receive from 40 to 200 gm. of powdered brewers' yeast daily, best tolerated in iced milk. The diet should be liberal and include a quart of milk daily, wheat germ, lean meat, liver and such green vegetables as lettuce, spinach, asparagus, fresh peas, cabbage and tomatoes. Diets high in carbohydrate and fat are contraindicated. The patient should receive and retain a diet of approximately 4000 calories daily.

Mental Syndromes Associated with Pernicious Anemia

Although Addison in his original descriptions of pernicious anemia in 1849 and in 1855 spoke of the occasional "wandering of the mind," the mental disorders associated with the disease have received less attention than have the associated neurological disturbances incident to the accompanying degeneration in the spinal cord first recognized by Lichtheim in 1886. Mental symptoms, however, are not at all rare in the disease. They are probably secondary to disturbances in cerebral metabolism. It is estimated that 35 per cent of patients with pernicious anemia manifest minor mental symptoms. If the patient is observed for delirioid reactions, mental changes will be noted more frequently than has usually been reported. Symptoms of a degree sufficient to be called psychotic have been reported by various clinics as occurring in from 4 to 15 per cent of patients suffering from the disease. With the effective and early treatment now available, these symptoms are encountered less frequently. Mental symptoms may be present alone or in association with cord disturbances.

Morbid Anatomy

Degenerative foci in the white matter of the brain similar to the degenerative plaques in the cord were first demonstrated by Barrett although they are not always present. Areas of degeneration occur also in the gray matter, the pyramidal cells undergoing disintegration with the presence of rod cells and other changes, particularly an increase in glia, increase in lipoid products in cells, swelling and proliferation of intimal cells in cerebral blood vessels and miliary hemorrhages. Ferraro and his associates have pointed out that the pathological changes both in their location and in their nature are suggestive of those found in Wernicke's encephalopathy.

Symptoms

The time of onset of mental symptoms in relation to the course of pernicious anemia is variable. Although any associated psychosis was formerly thought to be a terminal condition, it is now recognized that mental symptoms may also occur early, even before the typical blood picture of pernicious anemia is established. Except sometimes in the case of confusion there is no relationship between the degree of anemia and the intensity of the mental symptoms. While there is no mental syndrome characteristic of pernicious anemia, the mental picture tends to fall into one of the following groups: (*a*) acute delirioid state; (*b*) paranoid condition; (*c*) affective reaction; (*d*) organic deterioration. Probably the organic changes release a psychosis the type of which is predetermined by previous psychogenic factors and psychological mechanisms.

Characteristics of the respective groups are as follows: (*a*) The acute confusional, delirioid state is the most frequent form of psychosis. It is characterized by fluctuations in degree of consciousness, by illusions and by transitory and terrifying hallucinations. The patient may show drowsiness with incomplete awakening, impaired ability to maintain attention and decreased ability to utilize abstract concepts. As in delirium resulting from other causes, the content of thought and of hallucinations and of frustrating dreams is more dependent upon the previous life experience and psychological development of the patient than upon the nature of the underlying physical cause. The delirious states may continue for several weeks or even longer. Because of the occasional failure to recognize the source of these states in pernicious anemia, it is well in the case of a toxic-infectious type of reaction of undetermined origin in a person over forty years of age to look for a glossitis, a disturbance in vibratory sense and other signs of cord sclerosis and to make a careful blood examination. (*b*) Patients with mild paranoid reactions present an irritable, complaining, discontented attitude with a tendency to be verbally abusive to persons charged with their care. Others become suspicious, state that their food has been poisoned or develop other ideas of persecution based on affective and other psychological factors. As a result of these delusions the patient may become restless, noisy and abusive. Not rarely the patient's delusions center around members of his family. In one of the authors' cases the patient developed delusions of persecution concerning his daughters, with the result that he excluded them from the list of beneficiaries named in his will. (*c*) Affective reactions are usually in the form of depression, agitation and apprehension. In rare cases the patient may end his life. (*d*) In patients with the organic deterioration syndrome there is a gradual disintegration of intellectual functions with impairment of memory and judgment and, at times, periods of confusion.

There is a tendency for mental symptoms to improve with liberal doses of liver extract, or with cyanocobalamine, vitamin B_{12}. Both should be administered parenterally. During the first week of treatment 30 micrograms of vitamin B_{12} or its equivalent as liver injection USP should be given intramuscularly each day. Thereafter the same dose is given twice weekly. After two months, if the response is satisfactory, a single injection every other week is sufficient.

Porphyria

This condition, first described in 1911 by Günther, is a constitutional metabolic disorder resulting in the production of abnormal types of porphyria which appear in the urine. Three types of porphyria are usually described: the congenital, acute intermittent, and the mixed. The congenital type is seen only in childhood and the mixed has mostly dermatological symptoms. The acute intermittent type is the one with which mental symptoms are most frequently associated.

The acute intermittent type is commonly familial and thought to be inherited through a Mendelian dominant trait. Congenital porphyria, on the other hand, appears to be transmitted as a Mendelian recessive. Biochemically, it has been suggested that inhibited synthesis of purines with consequent overproduction of porphyrins and their precursors takes place as a consequence of poisoning of the succinate glycine cycle. In this cycle α-amino levulinic acid is the common precursor of both porphyrins and purines. Inhibition of the oxidative de-amination of this acid may block purine synthesis and lead to overproduction of the porphyrins. This biochemical explanation remains to be confirmed.

Pathologically the changes in the nervous system have consisted of patchy areas of demyelinization with or without the destruction of axis cylinders, particularly in the spinal nerves. Retrograde degeneration of the motor cells occurs in the central nervous system and the sympathetic ganglia. These findings are inconstant and nonspecific. In rapidly fatal cases no changes may be evident in the central nervous system. The liver may show fatty degeneration, cirrhosis or cell injury. In the hematopoietic type the bone marrow is hyperplastic and normoblastic. Splenomegaly and hemolytic anemia exist. The teeth may be reddish brown, as are the bones, as a result of uroporphyrin deposit.

Symptoms and Signs

Porphyria occurs much more frequently in women than in men. The disease may be suspected in a patient who presents a combination of abdominal, neurological, psychiatric and at times dermatological symptoms. The acute attack often starts with colicky abdominal pain, sometimes associated with nausea, vomiting and constipation. The gastrointestinal symptoms often suggest appendicitis with the result that a laparotomy is performed. The patient continues to complain bitterly of abdominal pain, becomes anxious, irritable, argumentative and perhaps obviously psychotic. As the disease progresses, the patient loses much weight and may become quite cachectic.

Psychiatric manifestations are varied and may be the most prominent presenting symptoms. They are probably due to a direct, possibly reversible, metabolic effect of the disease. They usually precede the neurologic symptoms. Agitation, depression, disturbances of memory and of the sensorium with delirious and psychotic-like hallucinatory and delusional experiences are among the most common.

The neurological manifestations are greatly varied. Perhaps the most frequent are motor weaknesses which may be irregularly distributed but are most frequent in the exteremities and less so in the muscles of the trunk and abdomen and in the muscles innervated by the cranial nerves. Of the latter the facial and oculomotor muscles are most often involved. The motor weaknesses may be accompanied by severe pain and paresthesias but there is usually little or no objective sensory disturbance. The paralysis is flaccid and tendon reflexes are usually absent or depressed. Convulsions may occur. Cases of both receptive and expressive aphasia have been reported. Bulbar involvement with dysphonia, dysphagia, tachycardia and respiratory and vasomotor dysfunction may occur.

The following case report illustrates the acute intermittent form:

A woman registered for examination at a medical clinic at the age of 40 with a history of five attacks of pain in the right upper abdominal quadrant during the previous eight months. The attacks of pain were described as continuing from a half hour to two hours. Results of the general physical examination were essentially normal. A cholecystogram made at this time was reported as disclosing nothing abnormal. A brief note by the medical consultant suggested the existence of an emotional disturbance associated with an unsatisfactory marital relationship. The diagnosis of porphyria was not made at this time. A history of brief attacks of pain in the right upper abdominal quadrant recurring periodically over a period of eleven years was obtained. The present attack began ten days before the patient's visit to the clinic. This attack was more severe than usual, was accompanied by fever and persisted much longer. The severity of the pain was such that for the first time the patient allowed her physicians to administer narcotic agents by hypodermic injection. These consisted of one scopolamine and morphine tablet administered nine days before admission and 100 mg. of meperidine hydrochloride (Demerol) on the following days, when she was placed in a hospital elsewhere. No further sedatives were administered. Penicillin was given and plans were made to remove her gall bladder after the fever had subsided. The patient and her family, because of their religious beliefs, were opposed to this or any surgical procedure. Four days before her clinic visit her family noticed that she wrote unusual letters and displayed peculiar, incessant to-and-fro movements of her hands and arms to the extent that she had no rest. She withdrew from contact with others. The day before her admission to the clinic she refused to accept food or fluids.

At the time of her registration, the patient held herself in a rigid position, with her right arm stiffly raised in a cataleptic pose. Her hands were clenched tightly, her eyes were closed and she muttered incoherently. When she was spoken to she closed her eyes more tightly and repeated in a rhythmic way, "Are they laughing at her"? She resisted attempts to change her position by strong muscular contractions wherever she was touched. When she was left alone she opened her eyes; occasional jerky, sucking movements of her mouth were observed. Results of the neurological examination were essentially negative. With great difficulty she was examined by a surgeon who found no evidence of an acute abdominal lesion.

The patient's history was obtained from the husband. She was the eighth of eleven children. The father was alcoholic until fifteen years before his death at 85 (four years prior to the time of this report). The parents' attitude toward surgical treatment had always been, "What God put there was meant to stay." The patient had repeatedly refused cholecystectomy. She had been in good health except for the repeated attacks of pain in the right upper abdominal quadrant previously mentioned. Information about the patient's relatives indicated that in general they had lived to advanced age and had been free of abdominal complaints and mental symptoms.

During the first seven days in the hospital repeated physical examinations failed to disclose abnormalities except for the behavior disturbance. The patient's temperature remained persistently elevated between 99.6° and 102.8° F. Oliguria was present. The specific gravity of the urine was 1.030. Grade 4 albuminuria was noted. The value for urea nitrogen was 68 mg. per 100 ml. of blood. After the subcutaneous administration of fluids the output of urine increased, there was a decrease in the content of albumin in the urine and a rapid decrease in the level of the blood urea nitrogen. On the third hospital day qualitative study of the urinary porphyrins showed no uroporphyrins, but the presence of coproporphyrin. On the fourth and fifth hospital days the patient was mute. On the sixth day she was either crying out incoherently or whispering and muttering unintelligibly. On this day the diagnosis of porphyria was established by the detection of porphobilinogen in the urine. (Quantitative porphyrin test, twenty-four units; uroporphyrin, none; porphobilinogen, 2.6 Ehrlich units; coproporphyrin, 333 micrograms.) The patient's rectal temperature reached 105° F. on the seventh hospital day. She remained withdrawn, mute and uncommunicative until the twelfth hospital day when she began to talk irrelevantly. Visual and auditory hallucinations occurred on the fourteenth hospital day. She sang and talked inhoherently, and screamed for long periods. She soiled and smeared herself with feces. She spoke of being crucified, of sinning so terribly that she would never be forgiven and of committing sexual misdemeanors. On the nineteenth hospital day results of qualitative tests for urinary porphyrins were reported negative. The behavior disturbance remained unchanged. Electroshock treatment was initiated on the twentieth hospital day. Immediately after this treatment the patient inquired as to where she was and what she was doing. She declared she wished "to get better." Following the second electroshock treatment the patient spoke to the ward personnel and began to eat without assistance. She declared that she had burning sensations (paresthesias) and complained of pains in the distal portions of her extremities. Her verbal production still indicated suspicion and misinterpretation of her environment.

Six electroshock treatments were administered between the twentieth and thirtieth hospital days. After the fourth treatment the patient's temperature again became normal. She was oriented and was able to recall recent and past events except for the period of acute illness, although she did not recall her fright and some of the hallucinations which occurred in this period. At this time there was slight increase in the sensitivity of her feet to touch and pinprick. She was returned to her home thirty-three days after admission.

Diagnosis

The diagnosis depends upon the finding in the urine of uroporphyrin and/or porphobilinogen in excess. Porphobilinogen is found only in patients showing combined abdominal and nervous manifestations. With the excretion of large amounts of uroporphyrin, the urine attracts attention because of its characteristic red port wine color. Spectroscopic examination readily permits identification of the uroporphyrin. It is important to stress the fact that the presence of reddish urine is by no means a general rule. Frequently a fresh urine specimen is nearly normal in color while in other instances it is light yellow or dark amber. When porphyria is suspected it is unwise to discard a sample of urine merely because it fails to show the characteristic port wine color. Such specimens should be kept in the light; they will then darken and appropriate laboratory tests for uroporphyrin may be performed. Porphobilinogen may be detected in fresh urine by means of the Ehrlich aldehyde test. Excessive coproporphyrin may be found in such urines. Recently α-amino levulinic acid has been found also.

The triad of variable abdomen pain, gradually increasing paralysis of the arms and legs, and toxic-organic mental symptoms should suggest the possibility of this rather uncommon and not rarely misdiagnosed disease.

Prognosis

The outlook for life is relatively good in the erythropoietic and in the dermatological or photosensitive types; in the intermittent acute variety the mortality is relatively high, particularly in those with symptoms referable to the bulbar nervous system.

Treatment

Chlorpromazine is the most helpful remedy thus far available in the treatment of acute porphyria. It does not affect established paralyses, may not prevent fatalities from bulbar or respiratory paralyses and does not appear to influence porphyrin metabolism directly. At the outset it may be necessary to give as much as 100 mg. four to six times in 24 hours intramuscularly; however, it is usually possible to reduce this dose quite rapidly and often to discontinue it entirely. There are some cases in which a small maintenance dose is necessary. Electric shock therapy has been tried in several patients with psychotic symptomatology, and the response has been variable. Conflicting reports have been expressed concerning the effectiveness of cortisone and of corticotropin (ACTH). Alcohol, barbiturates and other toxic agents should be avoided. It is important also that emotional stresses be avoided insofar as possible. These are often decisive in precipitating attacks.

Myxedema

Although Ord, in 1877, first proposed the term "myxedema," Gull, four years earlier, had presented a paper entitled, "On a cretinoid state supervening in adult life in women." Accompanying mental changes were noted in the early descriptions of the disease. Among the most frequent mental symptoms are slowness and difficulty in apprehension, thought and action. These retardations together with indecision and listlessness may suggest depression. Memory may be impaired, the defect being more marked in respect to recent events. Speech is frequently slow and changes in articulation may occur. Recently these clinical findings have been interpreted as resulting from an impairment of the level of awareness leading to defects in attention, concentration, endurance and conceptual use without sensory activation. In cases showing such manifestations, there is associated an electroencephalographic abnormality with diminution in mean frequency and voltage resulting from impaired cerebral metabolism. The serial subtraction test is said to expose the defect in awareness most effectively. Associated with their hebetude many patients show an unusual fretfulness, irritability and a paranoid trend. The clinical picture is determined largely by individual emotional and personality factors. There may, therefore, be paranoid characteristics, delusions of persecution and hallucinations. Mild degrees of thyroid insufficiency are not infrequently seen in middle aged persons who complain of fatigue, pains, headache and are pessimistic.

Treatment with thyroid extract not only relieves the above symptoms but corrects the electroencephalographic disturbance in those without permanent cerebral damage. Treatment with the extract should be iniated with caution, is best carried out in a hospital under careful observation, and commenced with low dosages of 15 mg. daily. The sudden changes in metabolism are particularly dangerous for those with cardiovascular disorders.

Acromegaloid Personality

Manfred Bleuler (son of Eugen Bleuler) of the Zurich Psychiatric Clinic, Burghöltzli, has called attention to the fact that, while acromegaly does not in itself lead to a psychosis, it is quite regularly accompanied by an alteration of personality. This change consists mainly of a lack of initiative and spontaneity and a change in mood. Some patients show brief periods of moodiness without apparent cause, sometimes manifesting cheerfulness, self-satisfaction and elation with passivity and indifference. Again, the mood may at times be anxious, resentful, tense and unpleasant. In advanced acromegaly, even without increased intracranial pressure, there are slow reactions and a slowness in stream of thought. There is no intellectual impairment except that referable to apathy and slowness of thought and action. The patient's social attitude is usually characterized by egocentricity, lack of consideration and interest in other people, impatience, irritability and oversensitivity during social contacts. Bleuler does not mean that this type of personality is specific to acromegaly but speculatively raises the question whether the endocrine disturbance of acromegaly and the emotional and other psychological disturbances may not, as in other fields of psychosomatic medicine, be merely different aspects of a single life process. To support this hypothesis, Bleuler calls attention to the fact that it is now conceded that psychogenetic factors are of importance in many forms of hyperthyroid disorders, in Cushing's disease and other endocrine derangements.

BIBLIOGRAPHY

Addison, T.: Anemia: Disease of the suprarenal capsules. London Med. Gaz., *43:*517, 1855.

Alzheimer, A.: Ueber eine eigenartige Erkrankung der Hirnrinde. Centralbl. f. Nervenh. u. Psychiat., *18:*177, 1907.

———: Ueber eigenartige Krankheitsfälle des spateren Alters. Ztschr. f. d. ges. Neurol. u. Psychiat., *4:*356, 1911.

Association for Research in Nervous and Mental Disease. Vol. XXII. The Role of Nutritional Deficiency in Nervous and Mental Disease. Baltimore, Williams & Wilkins Co., 1943.

Bailey, F. W.: Histopathology of polioencephalitis haemorrhagica superior (Wernicke's disease). Arch. Neurol. & Psychiat., *56:*609, 1946.

Barrie, H. J.: Wernicke's encephalopathy in surgical practice. Lancet, *2:*278, 1947.

Bleuler, Manfred: The psychopathology of acromegaly. J. Nerv. & Ment. Dis., *113:* 497, 1951.

Browning, T. B., Atkins, R. W., and Weiner, H.: Cerebral metabolic disturbances in hypothyroidism. Arch. Int. Med., *93:*938–950, 1954.

Brunsting, L. A., Mason, H. L., and Aldrich, R. A.: Adult form of chronic porphyria with cutaneous manifestations. J.A.M.A., *146:*1207–1212, 1951.

Cleghorn, R. A.: Endocrine Influence on Personality and Behavior. In the Biology of Mental Health and Disease. New York, Paul B. Hoeber, Inc., 1952.

Ferraro, A., Arieti, S., and English, W. H.: Cerebral changes in the course of pernicious anemia and their relationship to psychic symptoms. J. Neuropath. & Exper. Neurol., *4:*217–239, 1945.

Freeman, J. G., and Kolb, L. C.: Acute intermittent porphyria: Associated psychiatric symptoms treated by electroshock. Proc. Staff Meet. Mayo Clin., *26:*401–406, 1951.

Granick, S., and Van den Schrieck, H. G.: Porphobilinogen and α-amino levulinic acid in acute porphyria. Proc. Soc. Exper. Biol. & Med., *88:*270, 1955.

Grünthal, E.: Zur hirnpathologischen Analyse der Alzheimerschen Krankheit. Psychiat.-Neurol. Wchnschr., *30:*401, 1928.

———, and Wenger, O.: Nachweis von Erblichkeit bei der Alzheimerschen Krankheit nebst Bemerkungen über den Altersvorgang in Gehirn. Monatschr. f. Psychiat. u. Neurol., *101:*8, 1939.

Harris, Seale: Clinical Pellagra. St. Louis, C. V. Mosby Co., 1941.

Hierous, Raymond: Changes in the nervous system in acute porphyria. Brain, *8:*176–192, 1957.

Himwich, H. E.: Brain Metabolism and Cerebral Disorders. Baltimore, Williams & Wilkins Co., 1951.

Holmes, J. M.: Cerebral manifestations of vitamin B deficiency. Brit. M. J., *2:*1394–1398, 1956.

Korsakoff, S. S.: Ueber eine besondere Form psychischer Störung, combiniert mit multipler Neuritis. Allg. Ztschr. f. Psychiat., *46:*475, 1890.

Martin, W. J., and Heck, F. J.: The porphyrins and porphyria. Am. J. Med., *20:*239–250, 1956.
Melby, J. C., Street, J. P., and Watson, C. J.: Chlorpromazine in the treatment of porphyria. J.A.M.A., *162:*174–178, 1956.
Money, John: Psychologic studies in hypothyroidism. Arch. Neurol. & Psychiat., *76:*296–309, 1956.
Newton, R. D.: The identity of Alzheimer's disease and senile dementia and their relationship to senility. J. Ment. Sc., *94:*225–249, 1948.
Samson, D. C., et al: Cerebral metabolic disturbance and delirium in pernicious anemia. Arch. Int. Med., *90:*4–14, 1952.
Spillane, J. D.: Nutritional Disorders of the Nervous System. Baltimore, Williams & Wilkins Co., 1947.
Stengel, E.: A study on the symptomatology and differential diagnosis of Alzheimer's disease and Pick's disease. J. Ment. Sc., *89:*1–20, 1943.
Visher, J. S., and Aldrich, C. K.: Acute intermittent porphyria. Psychosom. Med., *16:*163–168, 1954.
Wernicke, C.: Lehrbuch der Gehirnkrankheiten, Vol. 2, p. 289. Berlin, T. Fischer, 1881.

CHAPTER XX

Chronic Brain Syndrome Associated with Intracranial Neoplasm

BRAIN tumors with accompanying mental disorder seem to be more frequent than formerly believed. In a review of the records of 2000 consecutive necropsies performed at St. Elizabeths Hospital in the period from 1923 to 1935, Hoffman[1] found that there had been 69 brain tumors discovered in the series—an incidence of 3.45 per cent. This is a somewhat higher figure than has usually been reported. The number of brain tumors discovered at necropsy is much larger than the number diagnosed correctly antemortem. The evidence seems to indicate that the prevalence of brain tumor patients in mental hospitals is approximately the same as among patients in general hospitals. Probably in only a minority of early cases of brain tumor are the mental symptoms so pronounced as to form a conspicuous part of the clinical picture of the neoplasm although there are few cases that remain entirely free of manifestations of mental disorder. There is need to recognize that the initial symptoms of tumor may be masked by pre-existing or concomitant mental and emotional disturbances. There is a great statistical disparity both as to the frequency and nature of mental symptoms in case of brain tumor. Clouding of consciousness and disturbance of memory are the two most frequent symptoms. There is, however, no symptomatic picture which may be considered characteristic of a brain tumor.

The genesis, pathological structure, neurological signs and electroencephalographic records of brain tumor will not be discussed. Generally speaking the symptoms and signs of brain tumor fall into three groups: (*a*) Headache, vomiting and papilledema; these manifestations are not

[1] Hoffman, J. L.: Intracranial neoplasms; their incidence and mental manifestations. Psychiatric Quart., *11*:561–575, 1937.

really indicative of tumor but of increased intracranial pressure. (*b*) Focal neurological symptoms and signs determined by the location of the tumor. (*c*) Psychiatric symptoms which tend to fall into two types. Symptoms of the first type, which often appear early, perhaps before those caused by increased intracranial pressure or the site of the tumor, are psychogenically determined by the characteristics of the patient's premorbid personality structure and his particular stresses, conflicts and defenses. In some cases the first and, perhaps for a time, the only symptoms may be psychiatric and consist of accentuations of personality tendencies. In some cases there is a loss of inhibitions with blunting of social or moral sense, egotistic tendencies, shamelessness and even gross sex or other misbehavior. Psychiatric symptoms of the second group stem from cerebral damage incident to the tumor and to increased intracranial pressure. These are of an organic reaction type and consist of impaired functioning.

Among early organic symptoms may be absent-mindedness, later becoming an obvious memory defect especially for recent events, easy fatigability, a raising of the threshold of consciousness, disturbances of sensorium, difficulty of grasp, impairment of calculation and of reasoning abilities, defective attention, hebetude, drowsiness, confusion and disorientation. Psychomotor retardation is not uncommon. Fluctuations of consciousness may occur. Sometimes the patient may confabulate as in Korsakoff's psychosis. Loss of libido is common.

A flattening of affect coupled with a growing apathy concerning personal and business affairs is frequent. Other emotional disturbances are instability, irritability, depression and anxiety. Euphoria and facetiousness (Witzelsucht of Oppenheim) are probably a little more frequent in tumors of the frontal lobe but are not specific for any one location in the brain. It well may be that this lightness of spirit and tendency to be witty is merely a defense reaction against the threat to the integrity of the organism by the destructive growth.

Fleeting auditory hallucinations occur in a minority of cases and are more apt to be in the form of ringing, whistling or grinding noises than of spoken voices. If visual hallucinations occur, they are more frequently associated with tumors above the tentorium and are apt to consist of flashes of light or of colored lights. Moving objects may be hallucinated. Complex visual and auditory hallucinations are more frequent in tumors of the temporal lobe. Olfactory hallucinations in the form of disagreeable odors may occur in the case of tumors on the undersurface of the hemispheres. It is generally agreed that tumors of the corpus callosum are accompanied by intellectual impairment, difficulty in concentration and in thinking and failure to respond to stimuli, particularly to auditory stimuli.

Although psychiatric symptoms are commonly considered to be associated more frequently with tumors of the frontal lobe than with intracranial neoplasms elsewhere, yet such symptoms are probably associated just as often with tumors of the temporal lobe. Tumors of the frontal lobe anterior to the motor areas seem particularly prone to produce insidious, subtle changes in personality.

The conspicuousness of the symptoms and, to some extent, their nature are determined by the rate of growth of the tumor. In the case of slowly growing meningiomas, there may be simply a slowly developing mental deterioration. In rapidly developing gliomas (spongioblastoma), there may be an active delirium suggesting a toxic state with confusion, disorientation and perhaps stupor. In those that develop unusually rapidly both the mental and neurological signs may suggest an inflammatory lesion.

If increased intracranial pressure appears suddenly and develops rapidly, mental symptoms are usually produced and may be severe. If pressure increases slowly, there may be no mental symptoms. Many tumors, because of their site and the particular structures they injure, produce neurological signs of great localizing value. Mental symptoms by themselves have, however, little or no value in localizing a tumor of the brain. It is stated that mental symptoms are nearly twice as frequent in case of supratentorial tumors as in infratentorial growths. In case the brain tumor causes convulsions, difficulty may arise in evaluating the mental symptoms with the result that they may be attributed to idiopathic epilepsy. Convulsions occur in about 8 per cent of cases and may be either grand mal or petit mal type. Seizures are rare in cerebellar tumors and most frequent in those of the parietal and temporal lobes. Difficulty in diagnosis may also arise if the patient suffered from cerebral arteriosclerosis prior to the appearance of the mental symptoms. If the patient suffers from sensory or motor aphasia or from apraxia by reason of the location of the tumors, the resulting inability of the patient to communicate his ideas adequately may make it difficult to determine the presence or extent of mental symptoms. In the terminal phase the patient may be stuporous and lose control of both rectal and vesical sphincters. The electroencephalogram is an invaluable aid in detecting those tumors present in "silent areas" or not productive of increased intracranial pressure early in their course. The use of the electroencephalogram has been recommended as a routine procedure for patients admitted to mental hospitals. However, its serial application is necessary in many instances to insure detection of tumors.

BIBLIOGRAPHY

Association for Research in Nervous and Mental Disease. Vol. XVI: Tumors of the Nervous System. Baltimore, Williams & Wilkins Co., 1937.

Bailey, P.: Intracranial Tumors, 2nd ed. Springfield, Illinois, Charles C Thomas, 1949

———, Buchanan, D. N., and Bucy, P. C.: Intracranial Tumors of Infancy and Childhood. Chicago, University of Chicago Press, 1939.

Davidoff, L. M.: Mental symptoms among brain tumor patients, and brain tumors among insane. New York State J. Med., *30:*1205, 1930.

Henry, G. W.: Mental phenomena observed in cases of brain tumor. Am. J. Psychiat., *12:*415, 1932.

Kanzer, Mark: Personality disorders with brain tumors. Am. J. Psychiat., *97:*812–830, 1941.

Keschner, Moses, Bender, M. B., and Strauss, Israel: Mental symptoms in cases of tumor of the temporal lobe. Arch. Neurol. & Psychiat., *35*:572, 1936.

———, ———, ———: Mental symptoms in cases of subtentorial tumor. Arch. Neurol. & Psychiat., *37*:1–18, 1936.

———, ———, ———: Mental symptoms associated with brain tumor. J.A.M.A., *110*:714–718, 1938.

Soniat, T. L. L.: Psychiatric symptoms associated with intracranial neoplasms. Am. J. Psychiat., *108*:19–22, 1951.

Strauss, Israel, and Keschner, Moses: Mental symptoms in cases of tumor of the frontal lobe. Arch. Neurol. & Psychiat., *33*:986, 1935.

Waggoner, R. W., and Baychi, B. K.: Initial masking of organic brain changes by psychic symptoms. Am. J. Psychiat., *110*:904–910, 1954.

CHAPTER XXI

Chronic Brain Syndromes Associated with Diseases of Unknown or Uncertain Cause

Demyelinating Diseases

WHILE demyelinization within the nervous system occurs as the consequence of vascular lesions, infectious illnesses and nutritional and toxic disturbances, this type of pathological lesion is not the primary phenomenon in these disorders. Multiple sclerosis and the various forms of diffuse sclerosis (encephalitis periaxialis diffusa of Schilder, encephalitis periaxialis concentrica of Balo, and the several forms of progressive cerebral sclerosis) form the group of primary demyelinizing disorders. The etiology of these structural disturbances of the nervous system is unknown. Their importance to the clinical psychiatrist springs from the concomitant personality disturbance noticed in the course of the illness, or the behavioral abnormalities often confused with other disturbances of personality. Their differentiation is important for therapeutic and prognostic reasons.

Multiple Sclerosis

Although multiple sclerosis is definitely a structural disease of the nervous system, a considerable percentage of patients show personality problems at the onset or during the course of the disease. Both in multiple sclerosis and in Parkinson's syndrome enough concomitant psychiatric symptoms may be present to mask the organic picture with the result that a psychiatric instead of a neurological diagnosis is made. Psychotic symptoms that require commitment are, however, rare. There is no characteristic syndrome determined by the organic pathology of the disease. The general nature of the symptoms tends to be dependent upon the personality make-up of the individual patient. Not rarely therefore we see paranoid, depressive, hypomanic or expansive reactions. Previous personality patterns of these types may, through the damage sustained by the personality at the organic level, become exaggerated. As a compensating psychological reaction to the disorganizing, destructive effect of the disease, one often observes a pathological complacency, cheerfulness and even euphoria. These symptoms occur so frequently that they have often been erroneously regarded as a particular feature of the disease process itself. Sometimes the patient's reaction to his disability is marked by an irritability or emotional instability that seriously disturbs interpersonal relationships. Impaired control over the expression of laughter and of crying resulting from bilateral upper motor neuron defects is often a significant feature. The former is associated with the clinical impression of intellectual impairment. If the explosive and forced laughing or crying occur, the patient does not feel any affect such as the emotional signs suggest. A few patients manifest serious behavior disorders. These are occasionally observed in patients who are impotent but nevertheless have an increase in sex urge. Emotional lability and intellectual impairment are often found in patients with marked neurological disability.

Examination of cerebrospinal fluid will reveal some abnormality in cell count, total protein or colloidal reaction in a majority of cases. The electroencephalogram is abnormal in one-half of patients although there is no pattern specifically diagnostic.

Diffuse Sclerosis

The most common type is that known as Schilder's disease which occurs as a rapidly progressive disorder productive of various mental symptoms, convulsions, loss of vision and motor or sensory defects. Fatal cases show extensive demyelinization of the cerebral hemispheres. The signs and symptoms are inconstant from patient to patient and depend upon those areas of the cortical hemispheres involved. Headache, vomiting and vertigo are common. Memory defects, apathy or irritability, personality changes or confusion with disorientation and dementia may occur. The neurological signs are extensive. Cortical blindness is common. Hemianopia, optic atrophy and choked discs have been observed. All varieties of motor and sensory disturbances with the associated defects in neurological examinations may occur. Occasionally these conditions are confused with brain tumors caused by the increase in intracranial pressure. Early in the course of these illnesses they have been confused with hysterical or schizophrenic reactions. The spinal fluid shows no consistent changes. In the majority of instances, these illnesses are clinically progressive and terminate fatally following the development of dementia and quadriplegia with decerebrate rigidity. Remissions occasionally occur. Treatment consists presently in providing symptomatic care and nursing.

Paralysis Agitans

In his "Essays on Shaking Palsy," published in 1817, James Parkinson, himself a victim, described the disease of late middle life now known as paralysis agitans. With its degenerative lesions of the extrapyramidal system, particularly of the corpus striatum and substantia nigra, the neurological symptoms are the conspicuous features of the clinical picture. The chronic progressive muscular rigidity, the immobile facies, the posture of flexion of neck, trunk and extremities, the poverty of movement and the slow, rhythmic tremor affecting the extremities to varying degrees constitute a striking syndrome. In many cases there are no mental symptoms. Most patients present a good natured complaisance but some, in reaction to their disability, are irritable, peevish and dissatisfied. The fact that the patient finds himself in a continuously contracting environment in which he becomes more and more dependent on other members of the family creates many emotional problems.

Drugs of the solanaceous group have been used for over eighty years in the treatment of this disease. Recently several synthetic antispasmodic drugs have been introduced of which trihexyphenidyl (Artane) is now most widely employed. The initial dose is 1 mg. on the first day, increased to 1 to 2 mg. daily up to a total of 4 to 8 mg. divided into three or four doses. Elderly patients usually can take only 1 to 2 mg. daily. Toxic effects of these drugs are dryness of the mouth, excessive mydrioses, gastrointestinal upsets and rarely a delirious reaction.

In cases of severe muscle rigidity, contracture and spasm the powerful muscle-relaxant action of benztropine methanesulfonate (Cogentin) may prove helpful. It is longer acting than other antispasmodics and can be taken in doses of 0.5 to 1 or 2 mg. in older patients and 1 to 4 mg. in younger patients, usually once a day on retiring.

Procyclidine hydrochloride (Kemadrin) is one of the newest of the synthetic antispasmodic drugs. It combines antirigidity action with a strong cerebral-stimulating action that is helpful in patients with somnolence and depression. The initial dose is usually 2.5 mg. three times daily, gradually increasing to 5 mg. three times daily.

Another anti-Parkinson drug which has been increasingly employed is orphenadrine hydrochloride (Disipal). The average dose is 50 mg. three times a day. It is a harmless preparation with minimal side reactions. Its chief drawback is the tendency for the good effects to wear off in the course of months.

Since changes may be produced in the basal ganglia by infections (virus, spirochetal), by toxins (carbon monoxide, manganese) and by trauma, a symptomatic Parkinsonism may be produced by various pathological agents.

Huntington's Chorea

Huntington's chorea is a degenerative disease of the central nervous system resulting from a dominant mutation. The first distinctive description of the disease was given in 1872 by Dr. George Huntington whose father and grandfather had practiced medicine at East Hampton, Long Island, for a period conjointly covering seventy-eight years and had observed families among the adult members of which an incurable chorea had existed for generations. No person, not descended from a progenitor so tainted, has ever been known to develop the disease. It is inherited as a pure mendelian characteristic. It behaves as a dominant with the result that from one-fourth to one-half of the offspring of a sufferer will develop the disease. Kennedy quotes over 1000 cases in the United States as having been traced to three individuals who emigrated from an English village in 1630. Its organic basis was demonstrated by Alzheimer. The essential pathology consists of a slow degeneration of the cells of the caudate nucleus, of the putamen and of the cerebral cortex.

Symptoms

The onset of Huntington's chorea is insidious and, generally speaking, occurs between thirty and forty-five years of age. Frequently a change of character antedates or accompanies the appearance of the choreiform symptoms. The patient may be irritable, obstinate, moody and lack initiative. In other cases the picture may be one of fatuous euphoria. Esthetic and ethical senses are blunted. Many patients become fault-finding, spiteful, irascible and even destructive and assaultive. There is an increasing lack of spontaneity in activity, of concern as to the disease, and of solicitude as to obligations of conscience, affection or ideals. Suspiciousness, jealousy and paranoid trends, even to the extent of well developed delusions of persecution appear. Some patients experience hallucinations. With the increasing emotional deterioration there is a coincident impairment of attention, memory and judgment. Interest in life becomes progressively narrower. There is also a poverty of ideas and a disorderliness of thought. The dementia may become extreme.

The choreiform movements usually appear first in the upper extremity, neck and face. These involuntary movements are clumsy, irregular, jerky, stretching ones. In the early stages it appears as if the patient were merely inattentive or careless in his movements which gradually increase in intensity and inco-ordination. The contractions of the facial muscles result in grimaces while those of the tongue, lips and respiratory muscles lead to a hesitating, explosive, poorly articulated type of speech which in advanced cases is difficult to understand. The choreiform movements result in a shuffling, dancing type of gait associated with irregular movements of the trunk. The movements usually cease during sleep. As the disease progresses there is interference with swallowing, walking becomes impossible and the patient may become bedridden. The tendon reflexes are increased. Suicide is not uncommon.

R. A. was admitted to a mental hospital at the age of 56. The familial incidence of Huntington's chorea is striking. A maternal grandmother, a maternal uncle and his daughter, the patient's mother and four of the patient's siblings exhibited definite symptoms of Huntington's chorea. Two members of the family committed suicide after they had developed the disease. Prior to her illness the patient seems to have been an attractive, well adjusted person. She was a Girl Scout leader and took part in community affairs. Shortly before she was thirty-five years of age the patient began to show an insidious change of personality. She discontinued her church, Girl Scout, card club and other activities, but she lost interest in her family and would wander away from home, returning at night but giving no information as to where she had been. At about the same time she began to drop articles and to show a twitching of her hands. The patient became neglectful of her personal appearance, refused to comb her hair, to bathe or change her clothes. She refused to launder soiled garments and would hide them in closets or corners. The choreiform movements increased in extent and she occasionally fell. At times she showed a temporary alertness and interest in anticipation of a visit from her daughter but after one or two days would drift back into her former seclusiveness and deteriorated habits. On many occasions she threatened and even attacked her husband, sometimes with a knife, and on one occasion inflicted a four-inch scalp wound. She became profane and her favorite term in addressing her husband was "You G - d - fool." The patient was subject to tantrums in which she would threaten to jump from a window. She came to be known to the children in the neighborhood as "the old witch on the third floor." Finally the choreiform movements became so extreme that it was difficult for her to go up and down stairs and she often fell.

On arrival at the hospital her facial expression was vacant and she showed such unco-ordinated and choreiform movements of her legs that she had difficulty in walking without assistance. There were gross choreiform movements of head and all extremities. The constant grimacing, blinking of her eyes and twitching of her fingers were quite striking. The co-ordination of her hands was so poor and the movements of her head so extreme that she had difficulty in eating. Her speech was explosive and difficult to understand. Although somewhat irritable, demanding and distrustful she adjusted to the hospital environment without serious difficulty.

Treatment

There is no effective treatment. The average duration of life is fifteen years.

Pick's Disease

This uncommon chronic brain syndrome first described by Pick of Prague in 1892 is characterized pathologically by atrophy and gliosis in the associative areas. The motor, sensory and projection areas are relatively unchanged. Several reports of multiple cases in one family suggest that the disease may be a heredodegenerative disorder but it does not show any simple mendelian pattern. The involvement is of cortical areas which are relatively younger genetically, areas which are concerned with higher associative functions. The mechanisms of speech and of thinking are therefore especially impaired. It has been suggested that the disease is a premature and localized neuronic aging, a senile process limited to a genetically younger area. The frontal lobe may look as if a constricting band had been applied to it. The clinical symptomatology is the result of a combination of the diffuse and focal processes. The majority of cases have been in persons between forty-five and sixty years of age, the youngest being thirty-one. Local areas of the brain, particularly the frontal and temporal lobes, may be severely atrophied and the total weight of the brain be reduced to less than 1000 gm. (the average normal male Caucasian brain weighs 1340 gm.). The whole depth of the cortex may be involved. Microscopically the lesions are found to be degenerative and not inflammatory. Usually there is distortion in the arrangement of the cytoarchitectural layers of the atrophic convolutions. Chromatolysis of the nerve cells is marked, there is a progressive disappearance of the chromatic substance, the nucleus becomes pale, is displaced to the periphery and the granulations are lost. Ballooned cells, not found in Alzheimer's disease, are regularly seen in Pick's disease. The loss of ganglion cells become marked and many of those remaining are swollen and show argentophilic granules. There is hypertrophy of the neuroglia and the microglia presents a swollen appearance with relatively numerous fatty granules. Senile plaques and Alzheimer fibrillary changes frequently found in senile dementia and Alzheimer's disease are rarely found. The white matter atrophies early. Changes in the basal ganglia are regularly found in Alzheimer's disease but are rare in Pick's disease.

Pick's disease occurs twice as frequently in women as in men. Among the earliest symptoms are lack of spontaneity, loss of memory, difficulty in thinking and concentration and a blunting of emotions. The patient becomes taciturn, indifferent, bewildered and is unable to deal with new situations. The memory for the execution of normal, concrete tasks is relatively well preserved but the capacity for abstract behavior is more seriously impaired. Dementia is usually well established within a year. Some patients show a euphoric contentment, while others are irritable, depressed and suspicious. Apraxia, alexia, agraphia or aphasia are common focal symptoms until such time as their characteristics are obscured by general dementia. The patient may have difficulty in naming objects although he may remember their use and properties. A rather important characteristic of these aphasias is that they are of gradual rather than of sudden onset and that the patients do not present the spontaneous logorrhea often found in aphasia due to vascular disease. Echolalia and stereotyped reactions are not infrequent. The pupils, other reflexes and spinal fluid are not disturbed.

As the disease progresses the patient becomes asthenic, confined to bed and scarcely moves. Dementia becomes extreme, sphincter incontinence develops, the capacity for speech practically disappears, cachexia becomes marked and the patient usually dies in from four to six years of some intercurrent infection.

Diagnosis

Clinical differentiation of the disease from Alzheimer's disease is extremely difficult. Many clinicians believe that this differentiation can be made only on postmortem examination of the brain. The age period, slowly progressive course and intellectual impairment are similar in both diseases. Convulsions, facial paresis, and muscular rigidity common in

Alzheimer's disease are rare in Pick's disease. Aphasic disturbances with perseveration and logoclonia are frequent in Alzheimer's disease but rare in Pick's. Motor impulsiveness and aggression are more common in Alzheimer's. Indifference is common in Pick's disease and anxiety in Alzheimer's disease. Defects of memory seem to occur earlier in Alzheimer's disease and in late stages of the latter disease memory may be practically obliterated whereas some retention of it continues in Pick's disease. Delusions, hallucinations and confabulations, rather frequent in the former disease, are not common in Pick's disease. Hyperactivity is common in Alzheimer's disease whereas in Pick's disease the patient tends to be underactive. Many believe that emotional, and especially habit, deterioration, progress more rapidly in Pick's than in Alzheimer's disease. In the former neurological signs are more frequently focal than in the latter. Finally, Pick's disease occurs much less frequently than does Alzheimer's.

Cerebral arteriosclerosis can usually be differentiated by the antecedent history of headache, dizziness, apoplectic phenomena and other evidences of vascular disease.

Lupus Erythematosus

To a psychiatrist practicing in the general hospital lupus erythematosus disseminata is now frequently encountered as a condition presenting with various reaction formations, or with delirious and psychotic manifestations. This condition, once considered rare, is now frequently diagnosed on the medical services because of the increasing awareness of the symptomatology and a better knowledge of the tissue and cellular pathology, including the existence of the now well known "LE cell." Lupus erythematosus disseminata is one of the group of conditions now known as diseases of the collagen tissues. In lupus the primary damage is to the subendothelic connective tissue of capillaries, small arteries and veins and the endocardium and synovial membranes. Approximately 85 per cent of all clinically recognized cases occur in women. The onset of the illness usually takes place in childhood but is most commonly recognized during adolescence and early adult life. The pathological changes are found in the ground substance and collagen which serves as a matrix and binding substance for the capillaries and small blood vessels in various parts of the body. Gross thickening is found in the endocardial and pericardial tissues while the small arteries and arterioles of various organs, including the brain, show a fibroid degeneration and necrosis in the connective tissue matrix of the vessel wall. In certain of the affected areas of connective tissue, the intercellular ground substance shows deep metachromatic staining or the presence of eosinophilic masses thought to be a result of the swelling and fibroid degeneration of collagen fibers. Certain deep purplish staining material found in some of the affected areas has been identified histochemically as desoxyribonucleic acid. This is apparently the abnormal chromatin material found in the so-called "LE" cells of the blood and bone marrow on dry smears.

In a recent series of patients followed at the Presbyterian Hospital in New York over a fourteen-year period, 50 per cent presented delirious or psychosis-like phenomena at some time during the course of their illness. Another small group developed neurosis-like symptoms while a considerable number had neurological signs at one time or another. The early symptoms of the condition are easy fatigability, malaise and fever. The so-called butterfly rash that occurs across the bridge of the nose and on the cheeks, often considered a traditional lesion of the disease, is not present nor necessary for the diagnosis of systemic lupus erythematosus. Commonly the initial signs are those of migratory joint and fibrous tissue reactions simulating rheumatic fever or rheumatoid arthritis. Examination sometimes discloses anemia, lymphadenopathy and edema or signs indicating pathology involving the pleura, lungs, heart, pericardium or gastrointestinal tract. The differentiation of the illness from rheumatic fever or rheumatoid arthritis is suggested on finding hematuria. The "LE cell" is found in stained blood of bone marrow smears particularly those made from clotted blood or the buffy layer of heparinized blood. They consist of phagocytes containing masses of chromatin material which stain deep purple with Wright's or Giemsa stain. Usually there are leukopenia, elevation of sedimentation rate of the erythrocytes and occasionally intermittently or falsely positive serological reactions for syphilis.

At the onset of the illness anxiety is often evident and the patients may manifest personality changes which are frequently considered to be reflective of the personality structure. Phobic, depressive and schizophrenic pictures have been seen as well as delirioid reaction. The psychiatric disorders have been thought by many to be related to the use of steroid therapy in the course of this illness. In the Presbyterian Hospital series, the psychotic reactions were usually apparent some twelve days after the institution of steroid therapy, with a maximum of thirty days and a minimum of two. It must be concluded, however, that the steroid therapy *per se* is not related to the occurrence of the disturbance of mental functioning. In this group of patients a large number recovered from the initial delirioid psychotic reaction only to have an active recurrence of lupus at a later time. The majority, when placed on an equivalent dose of ACTH or cortisone, did not again present the mental aberration. Exacerbation of the lupus erythematosus itself, rather than the usage of the steroids, appeared to increase the possibility of the occurrence of psychiatric disturbances.

While remissions may occur, and cortisone and ACTH have proven effective in inducing prompt improvement, most sufferers ultimately die from renal insufficiency and intercurrent pneumococcal or streptococcal infection. The majority who present psychotic disturbances have characteristic lesions in the cerebral hemisphere at autopsy.

The behavior disturbances associated with this illness often require protective hospitalization and careful nursing. Cortisone and ACTH should be administered. The former is usually given in dosages of 0.025 gm. every six hours intramuscularly. Cortisone may be administered orally in dosages of 0.15 to 0.30 gm. in four divided doses during the day. Following seven to ten days on this dosage, the agents may be gradually reduced each succeeding two or three days until a maintenance level is reached below which evidences of clinical activity are observed to recur. The majority of patients require a small maintenance dosage for indefinite periods. The careful collaboration of a psychiatrist and the internist is often indicated in the treatment of disseminated lupus erythematosus.

J. M.: Five months before her admission to a general hospital this 18-year old girl noticed fatigability, sore throat and fever associated with pain on movements of the ankles, fingers and joints. These symptoms improved. About four weeks before admission she suffered nausea, a loss of appetite and intermittent vomiting. Eleven days before admission she developed double vision on lateral gaze, at first intermittent, but later constant. A few days later her vision was blurred. On admission her temperature was 98.8° F., pulse 82, respiration 14. She had lost 22 pounds in weight.

At this time her behavior and mental status were not unusual. She appeared thin, showed some unsteadiness in standing and had double vision on lateral gaze, but otherwise there seemed to be no conspicuous physical disturbances. Her urine contained albumin, there was evidence of liver dysfunction with a positive cephalin flocculation test. Electroencephalogram was abnormal with disorganization and slowing in the temporal areas and periods of low voltage, 4 to 7 per second activity. At this time sedimentation rate equalled 82 mm. per hour. Bilateral papilloedema developed. A medical consultant suggested that the patient either had rheumatoid arthritis or possibly disseminated lupus erythematosus. An interior carotid arteriogram was normal. Treatment was commenced with cortisone. The spinal fluid contained 460 mg. per cent of protein. The patient's symptoms increased, particularly those referred to the joint pains. When she finally received 100 mg. of cortisone daily two months after admission her symptoms subsided quickly. She was then discharged home on cortisone 75 mg. daily.

She remained well at home until three months later when she became very elated and overactive. She spoke of her body and brain shrinking, said that she was becoming a baby again and would shortly die. Her return to the hospital was precipitated by a series of convulsions. She then seemed quiet, rather suspicious, but occasionally called out for help in a loud voice. She failed to recognize certain physicians who had treated her before. The cortisone dosage was reduced from 125 to 75 mg. and her symptoms remitted. Later the patient recounted that the psychotic disturbance occurred when she had the impression that she "was getting much better on the cortisone. I was getting stronger. About 8 p.m. when I was watching television I suddenly got the feeling that I was going to change into a baby. Previously I talked to my relatives about this but they didn't pay any attention to it. I felt that I was going to be bald, that all my hair was inside of my head and that they couldn't operate to let the hair out. I felt that I was cramped up and couldn't move." (At this point she assumed the fetal position.) "I felt that I was going to die like a girl that I knew while in the hospital. I was in a dream." She declared that she felt when blood was being drawn from her arm the purpose was to drain every drop of blood from her. "I felt that all the people in the ward were German spies. One of them had an Irish accent but I felt it was a German accent. They were trying to electrocute me. When my mother came to visit me I tried to push her off the bed so that she would not be electrocuted but she didn't understand this. I felt that all of the nurses were traitors–German spies." She seemed to interpret the slightest remark or facial expression as something of significance to her, was frightened when the doctors approached her. Her sensorium was clear. Some five day later the psychotic picture disappeared. A blood smear showed "LE cells." The encephalogram performed at the time of the behavior disturbance revealed an increase in the abnormality. Patient was discharged on 75 mg. of cortisone daily.

Because of increased weakness, joint pains and general debility she was readmitted to the hospital several months later. At this time no psychotic disturbance was evident although she was carefully followed by a psychiatrist. She was from time to time preoccupied by a fear of death and freely called for psychiatric help when most anxious. No recurrence of psychiatric symptoms took place on elevation of the daily dose of cortisone to 87 mg. per cent. Following another period at home she returned to the hospital two months later with a hemiparesthesia and expired shortly thereafter. Necropsy disclosed the typical pathology of lupus erythematosus.

BIBLIOGRAPHY

Bowman, L.: Diffuse Sclerosis: Encephalitis Periaxialis Diffusa. Bristol, John Wright & Sons, Ltd., 1934.

Braceland, F. J., and Griffin, M. E.: Mental changes associated with multiple sclerosis. Assn. Res. Nerv. & Ment. Dis., *28:*450, 1950. Baltimore, Williams & Wilkins Co., 1951.

Clark, E. C., and Bailey, A. A.: Neurological and psychiatric signs associated with systemic lupus erythematosus. J.A.M.A., *160:*455–457, 1956.

Davies, D. L.: Psychiatric changes associated with Friedreich's ataxia. J. Neurol., Neurosurg. & Psychiat., *12:*246–250, 1949.

Dunlap, C. B.: Pathologic changes in Huntington's chorea. Arch. Neurol. & Psychiat., *18:*867–943, 1927.

Greenfield, J. B., et al.: The pathology of parkinsonism. J. Nerv. & Ment. Dis., *122:* 200–201, 1955.

Hargraves, M. M., Richmond, H., and Morton, R.: Presentation of two bone marrow elements. The 'tart' cell and the 'LE' cell. Proc. Staff Meet., Mayo Clin., *23:25*, 1948.

Huntington, George: On chorea. Med. and Surg. Reporter, *26:*317, April 13, 1872.

Malamud, N., and Saver, G.: Neuropathologic findings in disseminated lupus erythematosus. Arch. Neurol. & Psychiat., *71:*723–731, 1954.

———, and Waggoner, R. W.: Genealogic and clinicopathologic study of Pick's disease. Arch. Neurol. & Psychiat., *50:*288–303, 1943.

McClary, A. R., Meyer, E., and Weitzman, E. L.: Observations on the role of the mechanism of depression in some patients with lupus erythematosus. Psychosom. Med., *17:*311–323, 1955.

Neumann, M. R.: Pick's disease. J. Neuropath. & Exper. Neurol., *8:*255–282, 1949.

O'Connor, J. F.: Psychiatric manifestations in patient's with lupus erythematosus. Arch. Neurol. & Psychiat., *77:*166–167, 1957.

Parkinson, J.: An essay on the shaking palsy. London, Sherwood, Neely, and Jones, 1817.

Pick, A.: Ueber die Beziehungen der senilen Hirnatrophie zur Aphasia. Prag. Med. Wchnschr., *17:165*, 1892.

———: Ueber einen Symptomenkomplex der Dementia senilis bedingt durch umschriebene Hirnatrophie. Monatschr. f. Psychiat. u. Neurol., *19:*97, 1907.

Polatin, P., Hoch, P. H., and Horwitz, W. A.: Presenile psychosis. Am. J. Psychiat., *105:*96–101, 1948.

Pratt, R. T. C.: An investigation of the psychiatric aspects of disseminated sclerosis. J. Neurol., Neurosurg. & Psychiat., *14:*326–335, 1951.

Raskin, Naomi, and Ehrenberg, Ruth: Senescence, senility, and Alzheimer's disease. Am. J. Psychiat., *113:*133–137, 1956.

Ross, A. T., and Reitan, R. N.: Intellectual and affective functions in multiple sclerosis. Arch. Neurol. & Psychiat., *73:*633–677, 1955.

Sofer, L. J., and Bader, R.: Corticotropen and cortisone in acute disseminated lupus erythematosus. J.A.M.A., *149:*1002, 1952.

Sjogren, Torsten, et al.: Morbus Alzheimer and morbus Pick: A genetic, clinical and patho-anatomical study. Acta Psychiatrica et Neurologica, Supplement 83. Copenhagen, Ejnar Munksgaard, 1952.

Stengel, E.: A study on the symptomatology and differential diagnosis of Alzheimer's disease and Pick's disease. J. Ment. Sc., *89:*1–20, 1943.

CHAPTER XXII

Mental Deficiency

Definition

By mental deficiency is meant such a defect in mental competency, resulting either from an innate fault in developmental potentiality or from an arrest in developmental progress, that it is impossible for the patient to make an adequate and independent social adjustment. According to this definition the mental capacity possessed by the average person has not been attained by the feeble-minded person, either because an innate relative poverty in his capacity for mental development has retarded his mental growth *ab initio*, or, as is now believed to be more frequently the case, disease or injury of the brain has caused a retardation in mental development. It will thus be seen that mental deficiency is not in itself a clinical entity but rather a symptom present in a large number of diseases of varying etiology. The group of mentally retarded is therefore by no means a homogeneous one but is marked by great dissimilarities etiologically, clinically and pathologically, although with the common criterion of intellectual inadequacy. Intellectual impairment that has developed because of brain injury or disease after adolescence is not regarded as mental defect but as dementia.

The mentally deficient show a defect in ability to reason, to plan or to construct. They exhibit a poverty of general information, are suggestible and show defects in foresight and judgment. They have but limited ability to modify behavior through experience and previous efforts to solve a problem. Probably the term *intellectually inadequate* would be more accurate than such terms as *mentally defective* or *mentally retarded* since "mind" or "mental" connotes much more than cognitive "faculties." These are only a part of "mind" which includes not only the intellectual processes but also conative and emotional ones. (See definition of "mind" in Chapter I: "A collective designation for certain functional activities of the organism, particularly those of the organism as an individual personality.") Some persons who are intellectually defective are emotionally mature and well adjusted, whereas many who are intellectually average or superior are emotionally undeveloped. As misleading as the term *mental deficiency* is, it is still the one customarily applied to the condition here under consideration.

It is estimated that from 1 to 2 per cent of the total population is feeble-minded and that about 3 per cent of the school population is mentally deficient. Any given city or state will probably find that another 5 per cent of its elementary school population will need special instruction in classes for the borderline subnormal (I.Q. from 60 to 85).

It is estimated that among the children in the United States up to 18 years of age there are about 1,500,000 who are mentally retarded. Many are fairly well adjusted in their communities but many more require training. About 150,000 are in special institutions for the mentally handicapped. There is considerable variation in the prevalence of mental deficiency from place to place and from one type of population to another. In areas where there is a high degree of illiteracy and of culture isolation it is difficult to evaluate mental deficiency since most tests presuppose certain common levels of education and culture. It is estimated that one bed per 1000 population should be provided in public institutions for the mentally defective. Eugenicists frequently point out that civilization tends to preserve the unfit and that therefore a general decline of physique and intelligence is to be feared. Penrose, an outstanding English investigator of mental deficiency, is of the opinion that the number of defective and subnormal individuals is not steadily increasing. He concludes that propagation of the unfit is not a danger to the community because such persons tend to be those who cannot propagate. He states that decisions about segregation or other disposition of high-grade defectives should be based solely on medical, psychological and social grounds; that the equilibrium with respect to biological fitness and intelligence level will be retained. Probably the only areas where the average intelligence is falling are certain small rural communities where there has been inbreeding of poor mental stock with a rapid emigration of better stock. The incidence of mental defect, particularly at the moron level, it distinctly higher in rural than in urban areas.

Causes

The causes of mental deficiency may be considered from many aspects. Perhaps, however, it is most convenient to divide them into those operating prior to birth, into those resulting from injuries at birth, and into those resulting from injuries or disease occurring after birth but before mental development has been fully attained.

Causes Acting before Birth. Probably from 50 to 65 per cent of cases of feeble-mindedness arise from poorly understood causes existing prior to birth. It is now agreed that hereditary transmission of mental defect plays a much less important role than was formerly believed.

It is often difficult to determine whether a mental defect was caused by factors inherent in the genes or whether toxic, infectious, endocrine, traumatic, nutritional and other prenatal pathogenic factors operating on the germ cell or within the pregnant mother tended to weaken or distort developmental capacity of the brain. Among prenatal factors may be pertussis, mumps and other virus infections, particularly the virus of rubella, which late in the first trimester of pregnancy may pass through the placenta and damage the brain. Anomalies of various organs often coexist with the defect. Other causes may be toxoplasmosis, the Rh factor (usually if the fetus is Rh-positive and the mother Rh-negative), the influences responsible for mongolism, also damage to the fetus by therapeutic doses of roentgen rays. Fetal oxygen deficiency as a cause of brain damage and subsequent mental defect usually occurs during labor but may happen earlier also. The mental deficiency of cretinism may either be caused by thyroid deficiency at a very early prenatal age or be coordinated to the hormonal defect rather than caused by it. Toxic, anoxic deficiency and infectious states which in the adult nervous system may be reversible or completely recoverable can produce permanent neural changes in the fetal neural structures leading to impairment of developmental potentiality. There are doubtless many possible causes for a failure of, or for accident to, neural evolution in intra-uterine life but they are inadequately understood. The extent to which feeble-mindedness is caused by congenital syphilis is uncertain but probably does not exceed 1 per cent. It is now a much less frequent cause than formerly.

In a certain number of cases in which the individual has developed from a hereditarily defective or a devitalized germ cell, the body may contain other evidence of germinal imperfection known as stigmata of degeneracy.

Causes Acting at Birth. Birth trauma resulting in either mechanical injury to the brain or in asphyxia with resulting anoxia may be a cause of mental defect. In recent years the surgical removal of subdural hematomas has prevented some degree of mental defect which would otherwise have followed birth injury. The most frequent immediate causes of cerebral hemorrhage at birth are prematurity and difficult labor. It is now recognized that asphyxia at birth is a common cause of mental defect. If the resulting anoxemia exists sufficiently long, it will produce permanent degeneration of the ganglion cells of the cerebral cortex with resulting impairment of mental capacity. It is estimated that about 8 per cent of mental defect results from causes acting at birth. Probably, however, 50 per cent of children showing clinical evidence of brain injury are not mentally defective.

Causes Acting after Birth. The various forms of virus and bacterial encephalitis and of meningitis are the most frequent factors acting after birth in the production of feeble-mindedness. While head trauma with brain damage in infancy or early childhood occasionally results in feeble-mindedness, yet this is much overemphasized by the laity. In institutionalized mental defectives, it will be found that in about 1.5 per cent of the inmates the defect is the result of postnatal cerebral trauma. Toxemia and vitamin deficiency in infancy and early childhood may, if long continued, produce irreversible changes in the cortex with varying degrees of mental retardation. Convulsive disorders often accompany mental defect resulting from organic disease of the brain.

In the congenitally blind and deaf, the reduced number of stimuli received from exteroceptors results in a certain degree of mental defect unless compensatory training is provided. It is generally agreed, too, that retardation in intellectual development may be caused by emotional factors without organic defect. Probably from 25 to 30 per cent of feeble-mindedness is a result of causes acting after birth.

Clinical Types

MICROCEPHALY. Among the relatively small number of feeble-minded persons who exhibit distinctive characteristics of skull or general bodily conformation or of brain structure that entitle them to recognition as clinical varieties are the microcephalics. Arbitrarily those defectives, mostly imbeciles or idiots, whose skulls on completion of development do not exceed 17 inches in circumference, are designated as microcephalic. Those of this clinical variety show not only a peculiarity in size of the head but also in its shape, which is characterized by a receding forehead and a flattening of the occiput. The hair which is wiry in texture extends low on the forehead. The scalp is greater in amount than is necessary to cover the cranium with the result that the excess becomes arranged in corrugations. The chin is usually receding and the stature short. As might be expected from the limited cranial capacity, the brain of the microcephalic is markedly underdeveloped. Histological defects are the rule while gross anomalies besides those of size are common.

MONGOLISM. A fairly frequent but as yet inadequately understood clinical variety of mental deficiency is that presented by mongolism, a name applied by Langdon-Down[1] to a certain group of defectives whose physiognomic features are suggestive of those normally exhibited by the Mongolian race. It is estimated that in each thousand of newborn infants from three to four will be mongoloid.

The cause of mongolism is still a matter of controversy but there is an increasing belief that mongolism is connected with anomalies in the transition from the first nutritional period under the influence of corpus luteum hormones into the second period under the domination of the placenta—the period of passage from embryonic to fetal life. The critical neofetal period during which undetermined, but perhaps toxic, conditions inherent to the mother interfere with developmental progress of the fetus is between the sixth and twelfth week of pregnancy. Statistical reports seem to show clearly that it occurs in relatively older mothers. The defect is almost certainly not inherited but acquired *in utero*. Usually both of monozygotic twins are affected but the coincidence is not invariable. It occurs in dissimilar twins in a higher percentage of cases than would be expected from statistical calculations. Repetition of the defect in the same family is so rare that the risk is ordinarily no contraindication to subsequent pregnancies. From 5 to 10 per cent of all defective individuals are mongoloids. The original name of the disorder was "mongolian idiocy" but this is misleading, as the mental retardation is frequently at the imbecility rather than at the idiocy level.

Clinically the mongol is characterized by short stature and a small round skull with a flattening both of the occiput and the face. The hair

[1] Langdon-Down, J. L. H.: Observations on an Ethnic Classification of Idiots. Clin. Lectures and Reports, London Hospital, *3*:259, 1866.

is scanty and coarse. The palpebral fissure is narrow and oblique with the inner end lower than the outer; a fold of skin continued from the upper eyelid over the inner angle adds to the Asiatic countenance. The tongue is large and fissured, its papillae hypertrophied, and it is often constantly protruded and withdrawn through the open mouth. The nose is short and broad with a depressed bridge; the hands are large and stubby, the fifth finger being particularly short and often incurved. The joint ligaments are lax and the muscles hypotonic, giving the joints an unusual mobility. The palate is often deformed, the abdomen large and the genitalia underdeveloped. The mongol's good disposition and tendency to imitativeness often conceal at first the seriousness of his mental defect. Most mongoloids have an I. Q. between 15 and 40 with an upper limit in the 50's.

TUBEROUS SCLEROSIS. This clinical form of feeble-mindedness, sometimes known as epiloia, is characterized by epilepsy, mental defect and by cutaneous nodules resembling sebaceous adenomas but really consisting of hyperblastic connective and vascular tissue. The disease results from a congenital blastomatous malformation involving the neuroectodermal system particularly. The brain shows diffuse disturbances in cytoarchitecture and localized neoplastic glial formations.

PHENYLKETONURIA. In 1934 Fölling,[1] a Norwegian biochemist, described a hitherto unrecognized type of familial mental deficiency associated with the excretion of phenylalanine and its derivatives, phenylpyruvate and phenyllactate, in the urine. Its frequency is estimated at about one per cent in institutions for retarded children.

Phenylpyruvic acid can be easily detected in the urine by adding a few drops of ferric chloride to an acidified specimen. An intense green color develops in the presence of phenylpyruvic acid. Phenylalanine is also found in increased amounts in the blood, spinal fluid and perspiration. The defect seems to be inherited as a simple recessive trait and is the result of an inborn metabolic defect. At present the defect seems to be caused by a blockage in the conversion of phenylalanine into tyrosine, the unmetabolized amino acid accumulating in the body fluid and as such or as its deaminated products—phenylpyruvic, phenyllactic and phenylacetic acids. There is a marked loss of myelinization of the nervous system. Accompanying the marked mental deficiency and the metabolic error are neurological manifestations generally regarded as an extrapyramidal syndrome. The posture of the patient is usually that of general flexion with bent head and body, both flexor and extensor muscles are rigid, the deep reflexes are active and many patients show hyperkinetic or dyskinetic manifestations such as tremor and athetosis. Encephalograms suggest that the extrapyramidal signs may be referred to cortical atrophy of the frontal lobe. Dermatitis, fair hair, a musty odor and convulsive seizures are often associated with the disorder.

Recently a few patients treated with phenylaline-restricted diets have

[1] Fölling, A.: Ueber Ausscheidung von Phenylbrenztraubensaure in den Harn als Stoffwechselanomalie in Verbindung mit Imbezillität. Ztsch. f. physiol. Chem., *227*:169, 1934.

shown objective improvement in behavior and mental functioning, a diminution in the abnormality of the electroencephalogram and a reduction in the amount of phenylalanine in the serum.

Congenital Galactosemia, or galactose diabetes, a specific metabolic defect productive of profound disturbance in growth and development, leads to mental retardation or deficiency unless recognized early and properly treated. The eventual effects of galactosemia relate to the amount and duration of galactose consumption and are reversible by removal of this substance from the diet. The infant born with galactosemia seems to be normal for several days but shortly commences to show difficulty with feedings, vomits and may develop diarrhea. If milk feeding is continued, there is noticed jaundice, enlargement of the abdomen because of ascites and hepatomegaly, nuclear cataracts and the indications of mental defect in delay in standing, walking and talking. Sugar is present in the urine. This is nonfermentable with yeast. Galactose tolerance tests are abnormal and the cephalin flocculation is elevated. If milk is eliminated from the diet and soy bean or casein hydrolyzate substitutes utilized in its place, the symptoms subside. Diagnosis early, with proper treatment, may prevent permanent cerebral damage.

Other Forms. Other clinical varieties are those associated with amaurotic family idiocy, hepatolenticular degeneration (Wilson's disease), encephalitis periaxialis diffusa or Schilder's disease, hypothyroidism, pituitary dystrophy, Friedreich's ataxia and Fröhlich's adiposodystrophy.

Mention should also be made of Heller's disease, dementia infantilis, first described in 1908. In this disorder the child develops normally for about two years then loses the ability to speak, has no interest in his toys and deteriorates rapidly to the point of idiocy. Biopsies show wide areas of ganglion cell degeneration and shrinkage of the cell processes. Therefore, it probably should be grouped among the organic degenerative disorders related to the Tay-Sachs disease group. Infantile autism will be discussed in Chapter XXVII, entitled Schizophrenic Reactions. Attention was called to the fact that while children with this disorder are of normal or better than average intelligence they behave almost as idiots because of withdrawal and emotional block.

Degree of Intelligence Defect

Perhaps before mentioning degrees of its defect a definition of intelligence should be discussed. Intelligence has been defined in different ways and no single definition has attained anything like universal acceptance. Most psychologists, however, are agreed that intelligence, no matter how defined, involves the following elements: the ability to learn, the ability to think or reason, the ability to deal effectively with one's environment and, finally, to profit from experience.

The official diagnostic and statistical manual of the American Psychiatric Association classifies the degrees of intelligence defect as *mild*, *moderate* or *severe*. An impairment of *mild* degree is such as would be expected in a person having an I.Q. of approximately 70 to 85. *Moderate* is used for a degree of functional impairment that will require such special training and guidance as would be expected in a person having an I. Q. of 50 to 70. *Severe* refers to a degree of defect such that the individual requires custodial or complete protective care. Usually this will apply to I. Q's. below 50. The degree of defect should not be determined solely by psychological test scores but should take into consideration cultural, physical and emotional determinants as well as school, vocational and social effectiveness. Usually a person having an I. Q. between 70 and 90 may be said to be of *borderline* intelligence.

There is a desirable tendency to discontinue the use of the descriptive terms *idiot, imbecile* and *moron*. Since, however, they are still occasionally used, their definition, as adopted in 1934 by the American Association on Mental Deficiency, may be quoted: "An *idiot* is a mentally defective person usually having a mental age of less than three years, or if a child, an intelligence quotient less than 25. An *imbecile* is a mentally defective person usually having a mental age of three years to seven years, inclusive. A *moron* is a mentally defective person usually having a mental age of eight years or upwards, or if a child, an I. Q. of 50 or more." As for the I. Q., the Association stated: "As a rule the upper limit for a diagnosis of mental deficiency should be an I. Q. of 69, but this limit should not be adhered to in cases where medical, social and other factors clearly indicate that the patient is mentally defective."

Several writers, notably Kanner, have called attention to a group of children who have often been neglected. This is composed of those who may be described as *apparently feeble-minded* or *pseudo-feeble-minded.* In many cases persons have been declared feeble-minded solely upon the basis of their intelligence quotient. While usually the I. Q. correctly measures a person's intellectual capacity, at times conditions may mask a child's intellectual potentialities. Among such conditions are blindness, deafness, spasticity, specific reading or numerical disability or emotional blocking with consequent inhibition of intelligent behavior or of responses in psychometric tests. The child with sensory defects often leads an isolated existence, full of frustrations and confusion and deprived of certain necessary types of stimulation and information with the result that he may not demonstrate his real intellectual potential. Sometimes a learning difficulty actually caused by emotional retardation may be mistaken for an organic deficiency. Occasionally the awkwardness of the examiner stimulates a negativism that prevents an accurate assessment of intelligence. The author is familiar with the case of a child whose admission to the public school system was refused because of his alleged imbecility as demonstrated by psychometric tests. The boy's parents, knowing that he was not feeble-minded, sent him to a private school where he soon demonstrated that he was of superior intelligence. At the usual age he entered a university from which he graduated with honors.

Determination of Intellectual Defect

In order to determine if a child who is suspected of being mentally retarded really is, and in order to outline constructive treatment, one should study the many factors which led not only to his intellectual defect but to his unique personality pattern. If one or both of the child's parents are known to be defective, it may be found that heredity has been an important factor. It should be kept in mind, however, that intellectually defective parents not only contribute defective genes but usually a home atmosphere deficient in intellectual, social and personality-forming influences which promote the potentiality of mental growth.

In many defectives there is some evidence either of a general biological inferiority or of the sequelae of former traumatic or inflammatory processes in the central nervous system. Other evidences of a biological inferiority are anomalies of the skull, such as microcephaly, oxycephaly or tower-shaped skull, hydrocephalus, the spherical skull of the mongol and asymmetry of the skull. Low fronto-temporal hair line, asymmetries of the face, malformations of the external ear, anomalies of the eye and its appendages, uncomeliness of the nose, thickness of the lips, receding or protruding mandible, imperfectly formed or irregularly erupted teeth and malformations of the palate are much more frequent than among persons of average intelligence.

In most mentally retarded children there will be a history of delay in the development of physiological, psychological or social functions. There usually exists, for example, an important relation between intelligence and the capacity for development of correct and distinct speech. The degree of intelligence is closely indicated by the age of acquisition of speech; by the character of articulation, *i.e.*, as to whether the articulation is clear, slovenly, slurring or jerking; by lalling, or the substitution of one consonant for another; and finally by the extent of vocabulary, since this measures rather well the stock of ideas. Usually the normal child should be speaking a few words at one year and should articulate clearly between three and four. A more valuable indication of the presence or absence of defect than is either the history of school progress or an examination in school work is the practical knowledge and general information possessed by the individual. Here we find that the ability for breadth and accuracy of observation, and the capacity for comparison, planning and discrimination essential for the successful solution of the practical problems connected with occupation and the business life, are inadequate in the mentally defective. His range of knowledge, too, concerning common objects and events in his environment is limited. The defectives often vary in their ability to apply their intelligence to concrete life situations.

In considering the field of social history and behavior, it should be kept in mind that social incompetency does not necessarily mean social delinquency. Such chronic social problems as pauperism, slumdom and recidivism are associated not so much with mental defect as with a population of borderline intelligence. The extent to which criminality is a result of mental defect is usually overestimated. Studies by English psychiatrists show that the percentage of criminals who are definitely feeble-minded is about 3.5. Probably the percentage in United States is about the same. The percentage of criminals of borderline intelligence is doubtless higher. While acquisitive crimes are the most frequent both among the feeble-minded and those of normal intelligence, it is estimated that serious sexual offenses are nearly ten times as common among defectives as among ordinary criminals.

Individual psychological as well as social factors contribute to delinquency among the feeble-minded. In the borderline defective, especially, it will be found that the precipitating factors of his delinquencies are emotional ones. Some behavior disorders may represent a rebellion against, or a flight from, a difficult environment. If the feeble-minded child is rejected by his home, feelings of hatred and resentment may be stimulated and transferred to all parental surrogates. Again aggressive and destructive behavior may represent a compensation for an underlying sense of inadequacy. Some defective individuals, through their wish to gain self-recognition, are easily led into delinquency by stronger, dominant personalities. Because the defective person obtains thrills and satisfactions so quickly, he is apt to follow those who show evidence of bold and vicious behavior.

While many who are not feeble-minded may rate low in economic efficiency, yet because the feeble-minded cannot successfully compete with those of higher intelligence the degree of economic efficiency possesses a certain practical value in determining intellectual endowment.

Psychometric Tests

From what has been said it will be realized that in ascertaining an individual's intellectual capacity one should make a comprehensive study of his personality in many fields. While psychometric tests reveal little information concerning his personality characteristics or emotional maturity, they do yield important information concerning the patient's native intellectual endowment. Not until 1905 was there any standard psychological criterion for the determination of intellectual capacity. At that time Binet, a French psychologist, and Simon, a psychiatrist, his associate on a commission appointed to study the matter of instruction of defective children, developed standard procedures for measuring intelligence and devised a plan for ascertaining mental age irrespective of chronological age. They drew up a set of graded problems constituting a progressive scale arranged in steps of increasing difficulty. These problems constituted tests of imagination, attention, comprehension, suggestibility, logical memory, language functions, common information, of ability to discriminate concepts, to detect absurdities and to solve problems. These tests, first introduced into the United States in 1910 by Henry Herbert Goddard of the Training School for feeble-minded children at Vineland, New Jersey, were devised after studying the abilities of children of all ages up to sixteen years, after which age it was found that there was little increase in native intelligence as distinguished from knowledge. The Binet scale was restandardized in United States in 1916 by Lewis M. Terman of Stanford University who developed the idea of the intelligence quotient. This Stanford test was last revised in 1937 when some of the previous shortcomings were eliminated, new problems were introduced and the scale extended both for the higher and the lower mental ages. Most intelligence tests, particularly the revised Stanford-Binet, are now based on the assumption that full maturation of intelligence is reached at fifteen years of age. In the application of a test the patient is given a standardized series of graded groups of tests (such as the Stanford-Binet), each successively more difficult than the preceding. The tests are grouped according to the age at which they are usually passed. Each succeeding group should be solved by a child one year older than he who solved the preceding one. One group of the series, for example, should be successfully solved by a child of six and the next most difficult group in the series by a child of seven. The mental age of the person examined is the average of the series of tests which he can successfully pass, the lowest age group used in determining the average being that one all the problems of which he successfully solved and the highest one being that in which he solved at least one problem. When this mental age is compared with the person's actual chronological age if he is fifteen or younger, or with fifteen if he is older, a measure of his retardation is secured. (The age of fifteen is used for comparison since, as already stated, there is probably no further development of native intelligence after that age.) This measure of intellectual development is usually expressed in terms of what is known as the intelligence quotient. The intelligence quotient, or I. Q., is obtained by dividing the mental age of the patient by his chronological age (or by fifteen if he is more than fifteen years of age) and multiplying the quotient by 100 for the sake of eliminating decimals. It should be remembered that since intelligence tests are expressed in terms of numerical findings their apparent definiteness is apt to be misleading. It should be remembered, too, that an adult who is, say, ten years old mentally but forty years old chronologically is a very different person from a child of ten. He may not be able to do any more with his intellect than a ten-year old child but he has had thirty more years of experience in living and his emotional experiences, conditionings and maturity may be very different. Routine intelligence tests are inadequate, too, to represent capacity for making a variety of social adjustments or, with proper training, for full or part adjustment to selected occupational or communal responsibilities.

Intelligence tests fall roughly into two classes, one largely verbal, the other performance. The degree of deviation from the average as revealed by a verbal intelligence tests is not necessarily the same as that revealed by a nonverbal test. Neither tells one the nature of intelligence any more than an ammeter tells one the nature of electricity. Performance tests consist of various kinds of puzzles which do not have to be solved in language terms and are therefore particularly applicable in illiterates and those not adequately familiar with the language in which the test is given. In the past the criteria employed in determining cognitive endowment have too often been confined to measurements of verbal intelligence. The performance tests indicate how well concrete material is handled and do better justice to the child whose powers of verbal expression may be poor. Among the best known performance tests are the Arthur scale, the Pintner-Patterson scale and the Cornell-Coxe performance ability scale.

A verbal and performance test which is frequently used is the Wechsler-

Bellevue Intelligence Scale developed by David Wechsler as a means of measuring the intellectual capacity of adults. This test obviates the necessity for resorting to tests devised primarily for the classification of children. In addition to the advantages of item selection and standardization on an adult population with allowance for changes with age, it permits direct comparison in equated terms of verbal ability and performance ability. The verbal division includes tests of information, comprehension, digit span, arithmetic and similarities; the performance division includes picture arrangement, picture completion, object assembly, block designs and a digit symbol test. A vocabulary test is also included in the scale. It is more reliable than the Stanford-Binet test in estimating average intelligence in adults.

The question naturally arises as to whether in applying intelligence tests one is measuring native endowment solely or whether to some extent the subject's kind of experience and the results of it are being measured also. While such tests as the Stanford-Binet, dealing with composite aspects of intelligence, are largely tests of innate endowment, they undoubtedly measure in part the use the subject has made of his experiences. The results of these tests will therefore be modified somewhat by the home environment and social status of the subject. Although these tests largely measure native endowment it is important to remember that it is in the main a measurement of ability to manage ideas rather than of the ability to handle or manipulate concrete objects or to get along with other people. They are useful as guides to educational policy, and to some extent to the complexity of the social and occupational situations to which adjustments may be expected. If the subject's score gives him a mental age of less than ten years it is not to be expected that he will be both self-supporting and capable of an unsupervised adjustment in an urban community. While we can scarcely identify the various attributes and qualities that enter into what we call intelligence, yet there appears to be a number of more or less distinct components in mental ability each of which can be measured by appropriate tests. Aptitude tests have been devised designed to discover evidence as to one's fitness for certain types of professions or occupations but any conclusions based on them must be accepted with great discretion.

Not infrequently in medicolegal matters the question arises as to the responsibility of an alleged feeble-minded person. In general it may be said that no limitation of responsibility should be recognized if the offender has a mental age exceeding ten years.

The various intelligence tests fall, also, in two groups insofar as technic of application is concerned. Some, like the Stanford test, must be given to one person at a time. Others, like the Army Alpha or the Kuhlman-Anderson, can be administered to groups.

Of the individual tests the Stanford-Binet, Standard Revision, has been most extensively used but has the disadvantage that it was based on results obtained by the examination of a group of individuals who were of more than average intelligence. As a result its standard intelligence quotient of 100, although supposed to represent the general average intelligence, is too high. An intelligence quotient of 87 on this scale more nearly represents the general average at fifteen, the age when the Stanford test assumes that full intellectual development has been obtained. A child found on the Stanford-Binet scale to have an I. Q. of 30 and a mental age of five cannot be expected successfully to complete school work more difficult than that of kindergarten grade. An I. Q. of 45 and a mental age of seven will permit one to complete the second grade of school. An I. Q. of 50 and a mental age of eight are required for the completion of the third grade; an I. Q. of 65 and a mental age of ten are necessary for the completion of fourth grade. An I. Q. of 80 and a mental age of twelve should enable one to complete the fifth or sixth grade. Persons with an I. Q. between 80 and 90 can sometimes complete grade school. Those with an I. Q. between 90 and 110 can often complete high school; those between 110 and 120 can complete college, and those above 120 can successfully pursue specialized graduate or professional training.

Psychoses with Mental Deficiency

It is generally agreed that most of the mental disorders that afflict persons of normal intelligence may also afflict the mentally defective. Sometimes, also, defectives suffer from psychoses of an acute transitory nature presenting episodes of excitement with depression, paranoid trends or hallucinatory experiences. They are often situational in origin.

Treatment of the Intellectually Retarded

While the limits of development of those aspects of the organism that we call intellectual are for the most part fixed, yet to a narrow extent intelligence grows by use and atrophies by disuse. It has been found that if identical twins are separated soon after birth and one is provided with educational opportunities definitely superior to the other he will develop an I. Q. higher than the one placed in a less favorable environment. Even though the intellectual capacity cannot be materially increased, the social capacity can be improved where it is most needed, *viz.*, in the higher grade defective. It should be remembered that the development of a normal personality requires not only a certain native intellectual endowment but also such emotional essentials as affection, security, social recognition, achievement and new experiences. So, too, the retarded or defective child should be led to feel that he is loved, approved and wanted as a member of the family and of groups outside the family. Surrounded with affection, handled with devoted patience and psychologically stimulated through fondling and play, such a child should acquire the feeling of significance and security essential to the development of a stable personality.

The emotional problem created for the parents by the retarded or defective child may be a difficult one and the manner in which it is met have much influence upon its future development. The knowledge that one's child is not developing normally often comes slowly and the mother may refuse to face the situation and develop a sense of personal shame, failure and even guilt. Her tearfulness and the father's angered disappointment may leave the child confused, frustrated and isolated. Again if he is rejected, emotionally deprived, coerced and perhaps beaten, the child will be restless, insecure, aggressive, hostile and perhaps become delinquent. Feelings of frustration and futility are more common among parents of the mentally retarded child than among parents of the physically handicapped. The latter can often experience a feeling of compensation in the child's intellectual and emotional growth. Such satisfactions are lacking in the case of the mentally arrested or retarded with the result that the underlying problems of the parents are intensified and often expressed in their attitude toward him with the result that he develops hostility and behavior problems. Many, perhaps most, defective individuals, like normal individuals, have their conflicts regarding their hopes, fears, anxieties and frustrations. The manner in which these are met by parents and teachers will have much influence on their behavior and social adjustment. Many mentally defective persons are more incapacitated by their emotional difficulties than by their intellectual deficit. As with children of normal intellectual endowment frustrations, humiliations, ridicule, anxieties, emotional deprivations and insecurities may be expressed in delinquent behavior.

In the field of education, teachers should concentrate from the start on those abilities and aptitudes with which the child is most fully endowed. Perhaps nothing is so devastating to the mental health of a defective child as to be offered lessons which are beyond his powers of comprehension.

The social training of retarded children is of immense importance and of far more significance to them than mere educational attainments. The extent to which they are accepted as agreeable individuals by and in a community is directly proportionate to their social adjustment. This attitude of the community has a direct relation to the mental health of the growing child. If he is accepted, he will feel that he has fulfilled his main ambition of being somebody in the eyes of others. If he is not accepted, he has a feeling of failure and frustration, or grievance and ill will against society, all of which breed discontent and unhappiness, leading to emotional difficulties and maladjustment and perhaps even to delinquency and crime.

Lack of intelligence is not by any means a bar to gainful employment. In many unskilled occupations, what counts in obtaining and retaining a job is not so much skill, literacy or information as steadiness, reliability, honesty and the ability to get along well with workmates and the foreman. With happiness will come mental health; and a child who has good mental health, even if he is intellectually defective, is an asset to the community.

It should be considered an obligation of the state to discover, classify and provide suitable education for all retarded children as early in their careers as possible. In some states an attempt is now made to meet this obligation by requiring an examination of all public school children who are retarded three years or more in their classes and by directing that special classes shall be provided for such children. Probably in cases of most of these defectives it would be better if they were discovered and assigned to special classes earlier. By assignment to a special class the child is removed from too difficult a curriculum in which he has no interest, from critical classmates, perhaps from an antagonistic teacher and other humiliating conditions that create feelings of inferiority, destroy a sense of security and lay the foundations for the easiest method of defense, that of overt, unsocialized behavior and socially maladaptive compensations. Since the child in the special class can compete with his fellows, the undesirable reactions mentioned are not only not stimulated but there is created a feeling of security, self-reliance, satisfaction and success that has great constructive value in personality formation. Approbation, attention and praise afford great satisfaction and within reasonable limits may produce a desirable, stimulating effect on the individual's effort to fit into a world that is always going to be beyond him. Feebleminded children should be encouraged to take part with normal children in all those games in which the defective child can compete on equal terms with the normal one.

In many ways the first persons who should be selected for admission to the institutions for feeble-minded are children of the moron level for whom special classes are not available or who are deficient in social adaptation. Among the beneficial results of institutional training are an improvement in attitude, stabilization of emotions and development of habits of industry. It is especially desirable that young, mentally defective children who are beginning to form antisocial habits should be placed in an institutional school before these habits become fixed, particularly if the home environmental influences cannot be modified. Provision should also be made in the institutional schools for the training of those children of the lowest mental levels. The number of persons who have been trained in the state institutions and placed in the community as useful, often self-supporting, members of society has increased in recent years. It is now estimated that 50 per cent of those admitted to the state schools can be returned to the community socially improved. Such institutions should therefore be looked upon as important parts of the public educational system. There are many who cannot be prepared for living successfully in the community, and yet in the routine, protected life of the institution become useful citizens.

The problem of treatment of the idiot and of the low-grade imbecile is simple and consists largely of physical care and custody. In the low-grade imbeciles efforts should be directed at training the child to dress and undress himself, at improving his habits of feeding himself, at bathing, curbing destructive tendencies, in teaching the child to avoid ordinary dangers, to associate common objects with their names, to pronounce a few easy words and to express simple wants. At best the object can be merely so to train the child that his care will be less burdensome. Whether this simple training will be undertaken at home or in an institution will depend on many factors, such as the capacity of the mother for training, the size of the family, its economic status, etc. In the case of these low-grade defective children, the efforts of the mother may usually be more profitably devoted to the rearing of her other children, to the duties of the home or to such other activities as may contribute to the welfare of her community and the development of her own personality. With institutional care of the low-grade defective child its family is usually able to make a better economic and social adjustment. From a community point of view these low-grade defective individuals do not constitute an important problem. Their number is small compared with that of the higher grade and many die at an early age. They do not constitute a eugenic problem since the defect is rarely of familial origin and very few ever procreate.

Some institutionalized low-grade defectives are noisy, overactive, aggressive and destructive. In such cases reserpine often exerts a desirable sedative effect. Opinions as to the value and wisdom of sterilization of the intellectually defective are not unanimous but it is no longer regarded as a panacea. Suggested as a means of preventing feeble-mindedness, its eugenic value is much more limited than was at first appreciated. We probably know too little about the inheritance of mental defect to apply sterilization in any but the lower grades of that condition where, in fact, the likelihood of procreation is the least. The legal provision for sterilization applies in most states to those committed to public institutions, but experience shows that a large proportion of morons, who of all defectives are most frequently of the familial type, are not committed to institutions. In the morons, too, the social adjustment is determined fully as much by social and family influence and environment as by the intelligence. Experience has thus far shown that even when the law provides for their sterilization only a few of those defectives who are supported by their families are subjected to this operation. The upper levels of the subnormal group are the most highly reproductive. Contrary to the opinion of many, most morons are not prolific and statistics show that but a very small percentage of male defectives who are committed and subsequently discharged ever marry or have children. Experience indicates that a majority of the detrimental behavior on the part of mental defectives is not their sex irregularity and reproduction but vagrancy, dependency and delinquency. Recent studies show that the mortality rate among feeble-minded is so high that the danger from their unrestrained propagation is thereby reduced much more than has been realized. It is now recognized, too, that society does not need protection from the feeble-minded girl as much as the defective girl needs protection from society. Many advocates of sterilization forget that it does not increase the patient's sense of social responsibility, that social adjustment is the end sought, and that even if discharged sterilized but without training in socialized habits the main object has been lost. It is becoming increasingly accepted that as a eugenic measure sterilization has on the whole been disappointing. This is not to say that in selected cases sterilization may not be wise, particularly as a social measure, since not a few feeble-minded couples will live a successful, happy life if not burdened with the financial, physiological and other strains incident to raising a family, yet many suffer social and economic collapse if obliged to assume these burdens. Much neglect and ill-treatment of children would be forestalled if persons intellectually or emotionally unfit to rear children could be sterilized but such a measure can scarcely be determined solely on the basis of the I. Q. Its usefulness is more individual than social. Finally, sterilization as a general policy is a superficial method of approaching the problem of feeble-mindedness since it ignores the need for special investigation and research as to its cause and prevention.

BIBLIOGRAPHY

Alford, A. F.: Mental health and mental retardation. Lancet, *268:*1233–1235, 1955.

American Association on Mental Deficiency: Statistical Manual of the American Association of Mental Deficiency; Part 1, Etiological Classification. Fourth ed. Willimantic, Conn., Am. Assoc. on Mental Deficiency.

Arthur, G.: Pseudo-feeblemindedness. Am. J. Ment. Deficiency, *52:*137, 1947.

Benda, C. E.: Mongolism and Cretinism, 2nd ed. New York, Grune & Stratton, 1949.

———: Developmental Disorders of Mentation and Cerebral Palsies. New York, Grune & Stratton, 1952.

———: Prenatal maternal factors in mongolism. J.A.M.A., *139:*979–985, 1949.

Bourne, Harold: Protophrenia. Lancet, *269:*1156–1163, 1955.

Bradley, Charles: Pediatrics, mental retardation and delinquency. J.A.M.A., *157:*101–108, 1955.

Clay, P. R., and Potter, C. T.: A case of galactosaemia with special reference to mental development. Arch. Dis. Childhood, *30:*147–149, 1955.

Cowie, Valerie: Phenylpyruvic oligophrenia. J. Ment. Sc., *97:*505–531, 1951.

Cross, T. N.: Porphyria–a deceptive syndrome. Am. J. Psychiat., *112:*1010–1014, 1956.

Davies, D. L.: Intelligence of patients with Friedreich's ataxia. J. Neurol., Neurosurg. & Psychiat., *12:* No. 2, 34–49, 1949.

Eustis, R. S.: Specific reading disability. New England J. Med., *237:*243, 1947.

Gesell, A., and Amatruda, C. S.: Developmental Diagnosis. New York, Paul B. Hoeber, 1941.

Grebler, A. M.: Parental attitudes toward mentally retarded children. Am. J. Ment. Def., *56:*475–483, 1952.

Hafemeister, N. R.: Development of a curriculum for the trainable child. Am. J. Ment. Deficiency, *55:*495–501, 1951.

Heller, T.: Über Dementia infantilis. Archiv für Kinderforsch., *37:*661–667, 1930.

Horner, F. A., and Streamer, C. W.: Effect of a phenylalanine restricted diet on patients with phenylketonuria. J.A.M.A., *161:*1628–1630, 1956.

Illingworth, R. S.: Mental retardation in the infant and preschool child. Brit. M.J., *4930:*1–6, 1955.

Itard, Jean-Marc-Gaspard: The Wild Boy of Aveyron. Translated by George and Muriel Humphrey. New York, Century Co., 1932.

Kalckar, H. M., Anderson, F. P., and Isselbacker, K. J.: Galactosemia, a congenital defect in a nucleotide transferase. Proc. Nat. Acad. Sc., *42:*49–51, 1951.

Kanner, Leo: A Miniature Textbook of Feeblemindedness. New York, Child Care Publications, 1949.

———: Problems of nosology and psychodynamics in early infantile autism. Am. J. Orthopsychiat., *19:*416, 1949.

———: Child Psychiatry, 2nd ed. Springfield, Ill., Charles C Thomas, 1948.

———: Emotional interference with intellectual functioning. Am. J. Ment. Deficiency, *56:*701–707, 1952.

Kelman, H. R.: The function of a mental clinic for mentally retarded children. Social Casework, *37:*237–241, 1956.

Knobloch, Hilda, et al.: Neuropsychiatric sequelae of prematurity. J.A.M.A., *161:* 581–585, 1956.

MacGillivray, R. C.: Gargoylism (lipochondrystrophy). J. Ment. Sc., *98:*687–696. 1952.

Milner, K. O.: Delinquent types of mentally defective persons. J. Ment. Sc., *95*:842–859, 1949.
Parotte, Irene: Modern trends in education for the educable mentally handicapped. Am. J. Ment. Deficiency, *53*:558–561, 1949.
Penrose, L. S.: The Biology of Mental Defect. London, Sidgwick and Jackson, 1950.
———: The supposed threat of declining intelligence. Am. J. Ment. Deficiency, *53*:114–118, 1948.
———: Observations on the etiology of mongolism. Lancet, *267*:505–509, 1954.
Rettig, J. H.: Chlorpromazine for the control of psychomotor excitement in the mentally deficient. J. Nerv. & Ment. Dis., *122*:190–194, 1955.
Richards, B. W.: Childhood schizophrenia and mental deficiency. J. Ment. Sc., *97*:290–311, 1950.
Stacey, C. L., and DeMartino, M. F., Eds.: Counseling and Psychotherapy with the Mentally Retarded. Glencoe, Illinois, The Free Press, 1957.
Terman, L. M., and Merrill, M. A.: Measuring Intelligence. Boston, Houghton Mifflin & Co., 1937.
Thompson, L. J.: Special disabilities in children with organic brain pathology. North Carolina M. J., *8*:224–228, 1947.
Townsend, E. H., Mason, H. M., and Strong, P. S.: Galactosemia and its relation to Laennec's cirrhosis. Pediatrics, *7*:760–773, 1951.
Wechsler, D.: The Measurement of Adult Intelligence. Baltimore, Williams & Wilkins Co., 1939.
Wright, S. W.: Phenylketonuria. J.A.M.A., *165*:2079–2083, 1957.

CHAPTER XXIII

Disorders of Psychogenic Origin

IN THE preceding fifteen chapters there has been discussion of mental disorders associated with diffuse impairment of cerebral tissue function. It was pointed out that if the brain lesion is reversible, the associated mental reactions are temporary and recoverable with no residual damage to the personality. On the other hand, if the damage to cerebral tissue is not fully reversible, a variable but permanent impairment of its function with resulting disturbance of memory, judgment, orientation, comprehension and affect will result.

Several of the chapters to follow will be devoted to a discussion of disorders which are not associated with any physiological or structural change in the brain as far as is known at the present time. The present belief is that they represent the result of symbolic, emotional and interpersonal factors acting on the organism. In other words, the group to be discussed includes those in which psychogenic factors are responsible for the malfunctioning of the personality. These psychogenically produced disorders may be divided into four groups:

a. Psychotic disorders
b. Psychophysiological autonomic and visceral disorders ("psychosomatic" disorders)
c. Psychoneurotic disorders
d. Personality disorders

a. Psychotic Disorders

These disorders are characterized by a varying degree of personality disorganization. To different degrees, too, the patient may break with reality or fail to test and evaluate it correctly. As a result his capacity for effective work and for adapted relations with other people is temporarily and in some instances permanently impaired or destroyed.

b. Psychophysiological Autonomic and Visceral Disorders

In this group we deal with disorders in which organ and visceral symptomatology is produced by emotional factors acting through the autonomic nervous system. Such a visceral expression of affect may serve to prevent it from becoming conscious. Long continued deranged physiological states of viscera produced in this way by emotional factors may eventually lead to structural changes—to peptic ulcer, for example.

c. *Psychoneurotic Disorders*

These disorders represent either a symptomatic expression of "anxiety" or the psychological mechanisms unconsciously and automatically adopted to control it. There is no material disorganization of the personality and no gross distortion or falsification of external reality as seen in the psychoses in the form of delusions and hallucinations. General types of psychoneuroses are recognized, the form being determined by the way in which the patient attempts to deal with the threatening danger felt in the conscious area of his personality but arising from the unconscious portion.

d. *Personality Disorders*

Disorders in this group are not characterized by mental or emotional symptoms but by developmental defects or pathological trends in the personality. In its classification of psychiatric disorders the Revised Psychiatric Nomenclature divides personality disorders into three groups:

a. Personality pattern disturbance
b. Personality trait disturbance
c. Sociopathic personality disturbance

In disorders included in this classification, the personality, in its efforts at adjustment to internal and external stresses, utilizes patterns of action or behavior and not measures or symptoms expressed in the mental, somatic or emotional spheres.

The first disorders of this psychogenic group to be discussed are those which are classified by the Revised Psychiatric Nomenclature as psychotic reactions. It defines such disorders as those in which "the personality in its struggle for adjustment to internal and external stresses utilizes severe affective disturbance, profound autism and withdrawal from reality, and/or formation of delusions or hallucinations."

CHAPTER XXIV

Psychotic Disorders

Involutional Psychotic Reactions

THE involutional psychoses tend to fall into two types. One is characterized largely by depression, the other by paranoid ideas. A depression occurring in the involutional period should usually not be included in the involutional psychotic reactions if there is a history of a previous manic-depressive reaction. In spite of the feature of depression common to both manic-depressive and involutional reactions there are such special physiological and psychological factors in the latter that it is no longer considered as a modified manic-depressive reaction occurring at a particular physiological epoch.

Involutional Depressive Reaction

The incidence of the depressive type of involutional psychosis is two to three times greater in women than in men. Among first admissions to hospitals for mental diseases it is exceeded in frequency only by schizophrenia, senile dementia and syndromes associated with cerebral arteriosclerosis.

Age Factors

While subject to considerable individual variation in the age of incidence, the involutional psychoses occur most frequently in women during the late forties and in men during the late fifties. It will be noted that this is the period when the endocrine and reproductive glands begin to suffer a decrease in functional activity—the age generally known as the involutional period. As the activity of these glands declines, there are extensive changes in the metabolic and vegetative activities of the body. With the cessation of ovarian activity there may be a change in functioning of other parts of the endocrine system involving an increased irritability of the sympathetic nervous sytem. Just what part these changes in essential physiological functions play in the genesis of the psychosis is uncertain, but there is much to suggest that they are not so important *per se* as are their psychological implications. The threat to the personality through the loss of prized biological functions and the imminence of the aging process with all it connotes may be more disturbing to the personality than endocrinological changes. The period is one of psychophysiological stress and one when increasing threats to an insecure personality are prone to elicit anxiety, depression and/or paranoid reactions, a period which threatens the security that has been established at a time when the individual can least afford to lose it. It is a period which in women has often been anticipated with exaggerated fear.

Prepsychotic Personality

In a significant number of cases of the involutional depressive reaction, there is found a certain general type of personality make-up and of habits of life. Usually the patient was an anxious child with a background of early fundamental insecurity. A review of the patient's previous personality and temperament often shows that she has been a compulsive, inhibited type of individual with a tendency to be quiet, unobtrusive, serious, chronically worrisome, intolerant, reticent, sensitive, scrupulously honest, frugal and even penurious. Usually, too, she has been of exacting and inflexible standards, lacking in humor, overconscientious, and given to self-punishment. Such persons have been mild, submissive, and sensitive to the moods and feelings of others. They have never been boastful but have depreciated their own worth which often has actually been high. Not rarely they have been exploited by the selfish. The prepsychotic personality was marked by a rigidity that represented a neurotic defense and the patient has been perfectionistic, prudish and prone to feelings of guilt. The personality has been superego-dominated. Many involutional patients have been self-effacing and self-sacrificing and have had an exaggerated need for and dependency upon the approval of others. Undoubtedly involutional depression not rarely evolves out of a masked neurosis of earlier life. In some instances hostile and aggressive impulses have been repressed with difficulty. Many psychiatrists consider, in fact, that the prepsychotic personality of the involutional depressive has been developed as a reaction-formation against aggression. Not rarely the patient's sex life has been suppressed or unsatisfactory. Often her interests have been narrow, her habits stereotyped, she has cared little for recreation, has not sought pleasure and has had but few close friends. Frequently the patient has been a loyal subordinate, meticulous as to detail rather than an aggressive, confident leader. Many have been fidgety, fretful, apprehensive persons. Others have been characterized by caution or indecision.

The age at which the psychosis develops is one when adjustments to new situations and circumstances are no longer easily made. Perhaps life has not brought either the success or satisfaction that hope had cherished. At this period there is a more or less conscious recognition that early dreams and desires cannot now be fulfilled, that the zenith of life has been passed and that ambition and life's forces are waning. The fact that opportunity no longer exists for repairing old errors or achieving new success creates a sense of frustration and increases the feeling of insecurity. In women, loneliness or fear of a loss of physical attractiveness may be a contributing factor. The high value placed upon youth, beauty and sex in our culture contributes to the drastic reorientation that must be made. The patient may feel that she is no longer attractive and feminine. At this period of life some women have a deeply seated resentment which may be expressed in depression and self-hate. A rebellion against aging may also tend to promote depression. The transition to another stage of life with its new and difficult problems, both psychological and biological, is not easy. Regrets and a sense of failure contribute to the prevailing mood. Perhaps friends are beginning to die, or children to whom the patient has devoted her life are leaving home and becoming preoccupied with their own lives and families. The patient may feel that she is no longer needed. In some cases, aged parents who formerly represented security but are now dependent on the patient constitute a problem. An ebbing potency in the male and the realization of the woman that her most highly prized biological possession, that of childbearing, perhaps long frustrated, is now a lost capacity, is for the patient more than the loss of one of the most fundamental of functions—it is a symbol that both the sources and ends of energy have failed. Sometimes sexual desires which have previously been suppressed are perturbingly aroused. Previous reaction-formations prove inadequate and acquired compensations and other protective mechanisms begin to fail. As the flush of maturity fades, thoughts of death are suggested and contribute to the anxiety so common in the disorder. With the decrease of physical strength, unconscious forces and old conflicts become relatively stronger and return to threaten and torment. This threat to the ego is ceaseless and since the source of the danger is hidden and within, any escape from it is impossible. As a result the apprehension, tension and unrest of anxiety are intensified. In a certain number of cases retirement from business means the renunciation of long-cherished interests and a withdrawal of psychic energy. Sometimes a real economic stress or the possibility of becoming dependent upon someone is added to other problems. It is not surprising, therefore, that in the event of some disturbing experience, such as the breaking-up of the home or other threatening change in the life situation, the loss of position, or the death of one upon whom dependence was felt, that the psychosis with its pathological depression, apprehension, ideas of death, and nihilistic and hypochondriacal delusions should be precipitated.

Symptoms

The manifest symptoms of the psychosis are often preceded by a period of several weeks or a few months during which the patient exhibits hypochondriacal trends, becomes irritable, peevish, pessimistic, suffers from insomnia, is perhaps suspicious, shows a disinclination for effort and may be given to spells of weeping. She is unable to concentrate and shows doubt and indecision. Frequently there is a narrowing of interests and a shrinking from the environment. The patient complains of distressing sensations in the head, eats poorly, loses weight, worries about health or finance and becomes apprehensive and restless. In a more or less typical case the most conspicuous symptoms are profound depression, anxiety, agitation, hypochondriasis, delusions of sin, unworthiness, disease and of impending death. The patient's appearance becomes one of extreme emotional pain and misery. The fear, apprehension and agitation increase; the patient wrings her hands, paces back and forth, weeps, may beat her head against the wall, picks at her face, bites her nails and tears at handkerchief or clothing. She moans, and in a whining voice constantly repeats, "Why did I do it!" "Oh, God, what will become of me!," or some other stereotyped expression indicating hopelessness and affective distress. The patient may constantly besiege doctors and nurses with inquiries, complaints or requests for reassurance. Some patients present a morose depression or a depressive hostility. Misinterpretations and delusions are almost constantly present. Feelings of guilt explain in part both the great emotional depression and many of the delusions. Trifling indiscretions of youth or unformulated sins become the "unpardonable sin." The patient holds herself responsible for the fate of others. She has infected, disgraced or harmed her family. She is about to be horribly butchered, a fate that she says she deserves, but awaits with intense fear and with pleas for mercy—indicating her ambivalent desire both for death and for life. The delusion that she is about to be destroyed may be the patient's rationalization of her sense that life forces are declining. Inner distresses and dissatisfactions are rationalized as physical disease thus producing the hypochondriasis so frequently observed. In this way the patient comes to believe that her intestines are obstructed, that she has no stomach, or that her brain is "dried up." Hallucinations, while less frequent than illusions, may occur. She hears preparations for her torture. Consciousness remains clear and the patient is oriented although in some cases the subjective absorption of attention is so great that she may appear to be confused and not thoroughly in touch with her environment. Some patients are perplexed and bewildered. Depersonalization with feelings of unreality may exist. Food is often refused, sometimes because of a desire for death; at other times when, because of self-accusatory ideas, the patient believes she does not deserve food; again refusal may be because of a belief that the food is poisoned, or to nihilistic ideas that she has no stomach or no intestines. There is no other mental disorder in which suicidal attempts are so common. There is great danger that previous unsuccessful suicidal attempts will be repeated.

While the patient never has a discriminating insight, she nevertheless usually realizes that matters are not as usual with her mentally. Early in the disorder the poorly understood sense of apprehension and the affective distress are so great and are recognized as constituting such a contrast to her previous feeling-state that the patient often expresses the fear she is going to lose her mind. She remains, nevertheless, thoroughly convinced as to the correctness of the ideas she expresses. Most patients lose weight and in severe cases become seriously dehydrated. The hand are usually cold and cyanotic. The pulse is rapid and the respirations are shallow. The bowels are constipated and the urine scanty.

The following summary illustrates many of the common features of involutional melancholia:

> E. M., a single woman of the early fifties, was admitted to a hospital following a suicidal attempt. She was described as having been a shy, sensitive and affectionate child. Although in early life she attended dances she was never known to have had any male friends. She always said she wished to "live alone and not be bothered by a man's company." After coming to America from Ireland at twenty-three she secured employment as a domestic. She seems to have been well regarded by her employers to whom she became quite attached and with whom she usually remained for many years of continuous service. She was described as always employing all her spare time in "doing little things about the house, darning stockings, cleaning something and doing ironing." She was conscientious, likable, ambitious and affectionate, but stubborn and difficult to convince. She was carefully observant of what she considered to be her religious duties and attended church regularly.
>
> On arrival at the hospital her facies denoted fear and apprehension. Although agitated she supplied the usual admission data and when asked if she were married she at first replied in the affirmative, but a moment later stated that she was not married. Shortly afterward when seen in the ward the patient repeatedly inquired if the place were a jail. Upon being asked the reason for such a question she replied, "Because jail is the safest place. I hope I don't be killed." She became increasingly anxious, agitated and apprehensive, and on the day following her admission the patient attempted to thrust her head through a closed window. Whenever a physician entered the ward she approached him and with but little variation constantly repeated: "I am afraid, Doctor, Oh, my God! I am afraid of those men upstairs!" (There were no men in that section of the building.) "Look at those big snakes! Look at those big dogs." The patient had always lived frugally and had methodically deposited her savings in a bank where she had accumulated several thousand dollars. She maintained, however, that her money was all lost and that she was destitute. Several days after her admission the patient was brought before the staff for diagnosis. At that time she showed the same anxious depression and agitation that had characterized her entire hospital residence. Soon after entering the staff room she asked if the door leading to an anteroom where patients of both sexes were awaiting were locked. When asked the occasion for the question, she replied, "I am afraid of the men."

Many of the factors that resulted in this woman's psychosis are comparatively simple and evident. The rigid environment in which she had been reared discouraged a normal interest in those of the opposite sex. That she had repressed any instinctive interest in men was betrayed by her statement that she did not want to be "bothered by a man's company." She became a faithful, conscientious servant, scrupulous as to detail but with an increasing limitation of external interests. Matters continued in this simple but hardly satisfying manner until physical capacity began to decline. The fact that life had not brought all that was desired became more or less vaguely realized, as well as the thought that strength was waning and that whatever life had not already brought could never be attained. As physical energy declined with the involutional changes, the repression of material that had formerly been maintained, although with difficulty, began to fail. With their repression weakened, instinctive tendencies which had always been scrupulously denied any conscious recognition, began to threaten from within. With no escape possible, anxiety, depression, fear and apprehension followed. This fear was projected as one of men since it was the patient's repressed interest in them of which she stood in fear. This sense of danger was rationalized as one of threat to life while affective and subjective material came to possess the vividness the patient had always associated with sensory experiences with the result that she heard voices saying she was to be killed. Doubtless the patient's anxiety and depression represented much more than a weakening in the repression of instinctive tendencies of a psychosexual nature; the approach of an age when physical vigor and means of livelihood were declining, a sense of isolation, vague feelings of disappointment and failure and perhaps of guilt, all contributed to a sense of insecurity that added to the affective tension and apprehension.

It will thus be seen that we must not think of the involutional-depressive reaction as a circumscribed disease entity resulting from clearly defined bodily changes, but rather, an individual is being dealt with who usually has long attempted by neurotic defenses to cope with perturbing problems, gnawing conflicts and resulting threats to security.

Prognosis

Before the introduction of electric shock treatment, about 40 per cent of involutional melancholia patients recovered. Convalescence, however, was slow and those who recovered were frequently ill for two or three years. With the use of electric shock more than 50 per cent of the involutional melancholia patients show prompt recovery. The more nearly the general manifestations of the reaction approach those usually seen in the depressive phase of manic-depressive psychosis, the better the prognosis. The greater the deterioration of personal habits, the more grotesque the delusions or the hypochondriacal ideas, the greater the occurrence of hallucinations, the more marked the poverty of thought and the tendency to aversion, depersonalization or to rut-formation with its meager affect reaction, the worse is the prognosis. Whining, surliness and seclusiveness are not favorable symptoms. The more narrow and rigid the prepsychotic personality the poorer the prognosis.

Diagnosis

Psychiatric disorders that may present features requiring a consideration of differential diagnosis from involutional melancholia are manic-depressive psychosis, cerebral arteriosclerosis and anxiety states occurring in the psychoneuroses. In *manic-depressive psychosis,* the question of involutional melancholia need not be considered unless the age of the patient is compatible with the latter diagnosis. In that case, there is usually a history of previous attacks either of excitement or of depression. Frequently the manic-depressive has been of a cyclothymic temperament whereas the involutional-depressive has not rarely been of compulsive type of personality. In the depression of a purely affective psychosis, there is typically a retardation in the flow of thought and in activity. The presence of anxiety, agitation, hypochondriacal and nihilistic ideas, peevishness and hallucinations point toward an involutional depressive reaction. In this, fear, apprehension and ideas of impending destruction are more marked. Stereotypies of behavior or speech and admixtures of other schizophrenic symptoms are more consistent with involutional melancholia.

Occasionally the *arteriosclerotic* patient is apprehensive and agitated but he lacks profound and sustained fear. If the involvement is principally in the smaller vessels, the headaches and unpleasant cephalic sensations may suggest the hypochondriacal ideas of involutional melancholia, but the easy mental fatigability, occurrence of confused periods, slight delay in comprehension, a lessening of initiative rather than a preoccupation and a slight memory loss should indicate the organic source of the mental disorder.

While there is often a sustained anxiety of a mild type in *anxiety neurosis,* there is little or no fear except during acute paroxysms. Even then there is no genuine affective depression and during the inter-paroxysmal period affective lability is well retained. In the psycho-neuroses, there are no hallucinations or true delusions, and interest in the outer world is comparatively well maintained. In the anxiety of the psychoneuroses, the essential mechanism is a displacement of anxiety from its connection with some emotional dissatisfaction, or from some wish that is not admitted to awareness because of its threat to conscious ideals, to an indifferent idea or situation. In involutional depression, the patient's sense of security is threatened, fear is more intense, the continued striv-ing in the face of frustration and of prospective danger is greater, it is accompanied by pathological depression, and relations with reality may be disturbed. It is quite possible that the foundation of this, as in other depressive reactions, is to be found in a turning inward against the self of aggressive tendencies which can find no other outlet.

Treatment

The patient suffering from an involutional-depressive reaction should usually be cared for in an institution for mental disorders, particularly since there is no other type of mental disorder in which so large a per-centage of patients attempt suicide. The general lines of treatment are the same as those employed in the depressive phase of manic-depressive psychosis but with particular stress on improving the physical state of the patient which frequently becomes weakened and impaired. On arrival at the hospital, many patients are badly dehydrated and nearly always undernourished. There must be assurance, therefore, that the patient receives an abundance of liquid and of food. If the patient is under-nourished, it is often helpful to give her 20 units of insulin thirty minutes before meals. Because of their fear and apprehension, the purpose of any procedure or change from routine should be carefully explained to these patients.

Electroshock therapy is the most effective measure in the treatment of involutional depression. The technique of its application is discussed in Chapter XXXV. While there are usually few contraindications to its use the patient should first receive a careful physical examination. It should not be employed in case of cardiac decompensation. Except for recent fractures, bone disease is not a frequent contraindication. The patient should usually receive from twelve to twenty treatments. Most physicians find it desirable to "soften" the seizure by means of succinylcholine dichloride (Anectine). If the patient is greatly agitated chlorpromazine may be used for its tranquilizing effect.

While estrogenic hormones help to relieve menopausal symptoms such as hot flashes, sweats, tensions, uneasiness and headaches, they are of little or no value in true involutional melancholia. The convalescent patient will frequently be deeply grateful for reassurance and support.

Involutional Paranoid Reaction

A certain number of persons develop a paranoid psychosis during the involutional period. Although never previously psychotic, nearly all such patients will be found to have been persons whose prepsychotic personality was characterized by defensive patterns. Like the person who develops melancholia at the involutional period, the life pattern of the one who develops an involutional paranoid reaction has long betrayed an underlying sense of insecurity which she has striven to meet through certain personality traits. Usually it will be found that she has been critical, inclined to blame others for her failures and has seen slights where none were intended. By her associates she was probably regarded as obstinate in opinion, jealous, unforgiving, secretive, unhappy, dissatisfied, given to nursing of grievances, resentful and suspicious. These defensive character traits prove sufficient support for the personality until the involutional period when, with the added physiological and psychological burdens previously mentioned, they are no longer adequate and resort is made to the more extreme defensive and compensatory measures provided by the paranoid psychosis with its delusions and misinterpretations. The psychosis seems to merge out of the personality. The delusions usually revolve around ideas of persecution and are well organized but lack the fantastic content observed in schizophrenia. Many patients show much bitterness and hostility. The prognosis is less favorable than in melancholia. Electroshock treatment is of limited benefit. The aggressive and disturbed patient may be helped by chlorpromazine.

The following case illustrates many of the features often seen in a paranoid involutional psychosis:

A. S. was admitted to the Norristown State Hospital in September, 1946, at the age of 59. The patient was born in Latvia. Little is known concerning her childhood experiences and the emotional climate of the home. She came to the United States in 1906 at the age of 19 to marry a man who had preceded her to this country. She and her husband returned to Latvia in 1913 to visit his parents but because of World War I could not return to America as planned. During that war the couple was driven into Russia where they endured intense hardship. Finally they returned to Latvia where the husband took over his father's farm and attained considerable success and status. At this point the farm buildings were destroyed by fire and the patient so seriously burned that she required hospital care for three months. In 1924 they returned to America and her husband established an upholstering business in which the patient assisted until the financial depression of the early '30's. The husband then began to drink and in 1934 committed suicide by hanging, a casualty discovered by the patient.

Following the patient's admission to the hospital, her daughter, in describing her mother's personality pattern, reported that she had always been a meticulous, hard-working person who was critical, suspicious, stubborn, uncompromising and domineering. The daughter described her mother as an immaculate housekeeper who also did "beautiful sewing."

About 1940, at approximately 54 years of age, the patient began to complain that people were talking about her, that her son-in-law was maritally unfaithful, that nearly all persons, especially the clergy of a different religious faith were sexually immoral. She expressed a fear that she would be "signed away for experimental purposes." She stated that a physician who had treated her at the menopause had given her cancer. Finally, after having complained to the police on several occasions that her food was being drugged and that a "society of science" was plotting against her, she was committed.

On arrival at the hospital her sensorium was clear and she was fully oriented. She was suspicious and when her abdominal reflexes were tested she asked if the physician was going to operate on her. At times she became quite agitated, hostile and insistent that she be permitted to leave. Someone, she said, was trying to secure possession of her home and to kill her; she must therefore appeal to the police to help her. She complained that the nurses were trying to compel her to perform unpleasant tasks because they were members of a religious organization which was persecuting her. Because of an electrocardiogram suggestive of coronary involvement and myocardial damage, it was decided not to give the patient electroshock treatment. After seven months of hospital residence, the patient became much less tense, was pleasant and cooperative and was regarded as one of the most faithful and capable workers in the hospital cafeteria. Within a year after her admission she was given freedom of the hospital grounds and permitted to spend week-ends with friends. Unless questioned, she expressed no delusional ideas. Upon inquiry, however, it was found that there had been no fundamental change in her paranoid ideation. Fifteen months after her admission the patient was permitted to leave the hospital. A year later her employer wrote: "Mrs. S. is cheerful and pleasant and I am very satisfied with her work."

So little is known about this woman's emotional relations with parents and siblings during childhood and any early traumatizing experiences that it is not easy to construct a desirably complete genetic-dynamic formulation of her psychotic personality disturbance. Her daughter's report that the patient was a meticulous, critical, suspicious, stubborn, dominating and uncompromising person suggests that because of a basic feeling of insecurity she had developed these personality characteristics to serve as defenses. In spite of a long series of threats, these defenses proved adequate for many years. Among these stresses and threats were the drowning of a sibling during the patient's childhood (we do not know what feelings this death may have aroused in the patient), an almost fatal burn with its permanent scarring of the body, the enforced expulsion to Russia with the accompanying exposure to hardship and near-starvation, the destruction of the re-established home in Latvia, the return to America with the poverty that accompanied the financial depression, the unknown fate of relatives in World War II, the suicide of her husband with its probable but unknown psychological reverberations, the elopement of her daughter and the development of mild diabetes. The rigid personality traits proved to be adequate defenses until the involutional period with its various accompanying psychological factors became so menacing that life-long traits were no longer able to control anxiety-producing threats. As a further defense, therefore, the patient resorted to projection to a reality-sacrificing, or psychotic, degree.

While the problems which the patient had found too difficult to meet must remain a matter of speculation one suspects, in view of the nature of her personality traits and the character of her delusions, that a deeply seated hostility, the fear of economic insecurity and a weakening in the repression of instinctive sex drives may have been important ones.

BIBLIOGRAPHY

Davidoff, Eugene: The Involutional Psychoses. Chap. VIII in *Mental Disorders in Later Life*. O. J. Kaplan, Ed., Stanford University, 1944.

Freeman, Walter, and Watts, J. W.: Psychosurgery, 2nd ed. Springfield, Illinois, Charles C Thomas, 1951.

Kalinowsky, L. B., and Hoch, P. H.: Shock Treatments, Psychosurgery and Other Somatic Treatments in Psychiatry, 2nd ed. New York, Grune & Stratton, 1952.

Malzberg, Benjamin: A statistical study of first admissions with involutional psychoses to hospitals for mental diseases in New York. Psychiatric Quart., *22:* Part 1, 141–155, 1948.

Palmer, H. D., and Sherman, S. H.: The involutional melancholia process. Arch. Neurol. & Psychiat., *40:*762–768, 1938.

Rogers, Joseph: The menopause. New England J. Med., *254:*697–703, 1956.

Tait, C. D., and Burns, G. C.: Involutional illnesses. Am. J. Psychiat., *108:*27, 1951.

Titley, W. B.: Prepsychotic personality of patients with involutional melancholia. Arch. Neurol. & Psychiat., *36:*19–33, 1936.

CHAPTER XXV

Psychotic Disorders (*Continued*)

Affective Reactions

In all phases of the group of psychoses to be considered in this chapter, idea and action seem to be so constellated by a dominant affect that the various types are often spoken of as affective psychoses. It had long been recognized that the contrasting affective states, elation and depression, might at different periods characterize the same patient, and it had even been suggested that they might be different stages of the same disorder. The present clinical conception of what, in 1896, he designated as manic-depressive insanity is a result of the remarkable ability for describing, grouping and correlating data possessed by the German psychiatrist, Emil Kraepelin (1856–1926). After having noticed the periodicity and the favorable outcome of the seemingly opposite states of disordered affect, he concluded they were variations of a single morbid process which he believed was the result of some basic physiological or organic disturbance. It seems, however, that Kraepelin overlooked the personality of the patient in its inner totality and content and his psychological adaptation as a person.

Causes

The not uncommon occurrence of manic-depressive psychoses in the same family suggests that a biogenetic factor may be at least a contributory cause but this can scarcely be proven or denied. Rüdin has stated that the incidence of manic-depressive psychosis is twenty-five times as high among the siblings of manic-depressive patients as in the average population. If it occurs in monozygotic twins, both of them will be affected in more than one half of the cases. In a German psychiatric clinic to which patients are admitted irrespective of social position, Luxemberger found manic-depressive psychoses to be nearly three times as frequent in the highest social class and four times as frequent in the professional classes as in the general population. This distribution of incidence seems to be similar to that observed by American psychiatrists. In World War II manic-depressive psychoses were three times as frequent among officers of the American army as among enlisted men. They occur about twice as frequently in women as in men, and the age of onset in women averages to be younger. The aggressive woman with masculine strivings seems to be especially predisposed.

Even if constitutional factors exist mentally dynamic ones are probably rarely, if ever, absent. It is estimated that definite, disturbing life situations exist in about four fifths of the attacks. In many instances, for example, particularly among persons of middle life or later, one finds that difficulties in adjusting to changes in environment or threats to social, economic or physical security may serve as precipitating factors in a depressive attack. Some psychiatrists suggest that the disease is caused by disturbances in the chemical, vegetative or regulatory processes of the body, while others believe that these derangements so often seen in this disorder are but part of the total psychobiological reaction of the organism. No histological, biochemical or biophysical correlates have ever been demonstrated in the brain. The electroencephalogram does not change as the patient shifts from one affective phase to the other.

Frequency

Statistics as to the frequency of manic-depressive psychoses show wide variations. Some institutions for mental disorders report nearly 15 per cent of admissions as suffering from this form of psychosis, while others report 5 per cent only. The smaller figure is probably more nearly correct if those cases are excluded, even though episodic, which are characterized by a disturbance in the integration of thought, feeling and behavior and by falsification of perception and of reality in response to internal needs, and should therefore be regarded as schizophrenic in nature. The experience of psychiatrists in private practice seems to show that many cases are not recognized if they are of mild form or of brief duration. This is particularly true if they assume the form of a period of fatigue or of brief periods of depression lasting perhaps from a few hours to a few days. In such cases the attention of both physician and patient may become focused on alleged or attendant somatic disorders.

Symptoms

There are two well-defined types or phases of the manic-depressive psychoses: a manic or hyperactive phase, and a depressive phase.

While the disorder typically assumes the form of psychotic episodes separated by intervals of mental health, it may happen that a person may never suffer from more than one episode, or again the disorder may become continuous. These episodes may be in the nature of a manic or of a depressive reaction but there is no constant sequence or alternation of these reactions. The swings from one phase to another seem to prove the homogeneity of the manic-depressive psychoses.

MANIC PHASE. In his personality make-up the patient whose episodes are of a manic type has usually been a self-satisfied, confident, aggressive, effervescing extravert at ease with other people. He has been inclined to scatter his energy over a wide field of interests. His affective attitude has been one of emotional expression and responsiveness. The manic phase or reaction is usually preceded by a simple depression. This depression is of brief duration and mild in degree, often lasting for only a few days and either not noted by the patient's family or not considered significant. This brief period is followed by exhilaration or mild excitement. Sometimes the attack remains in this attenuated form known as *hypomania*. In this hypomanic state there is an emotionally unstable, increased assertiveness, an air of self-assurance, careless gaiety, breezy affability, self-satisfaction, buoyant self-confidence and boundless energy. No matter how inhibited the patient may normally have been he is now irrepressible, demanding, uninhibited, effusive and often astonishingly unconventional in speech and manner. He is narcissistic, childishly proud and quite intolerant of criticism. Glib of tongue and genial of hand the patient is socially aggressive, witty, boastful, flippant, argumentative, spends his money extravagantly, pawns his belongings, is full of ambitious schemes and starts enterprises which soon fail or which he soon abandons. His excuses and arguments contain a superficial but specious plausibility. His disregard for the truth may carry great conviction to those not previously acquainted with him. The patient is bored with routine, lacks a sustained interest in any activity and is too busy to submit his impressions to critical examination. Attention is often easily distracted, thought processes are accelerated and the stream of thought is prone to wander. His manner of speaking has an undertone of emphasis and exaggeration.

Many hypomanic patients are mischievous, boisterous, full of pranks, and they indulge in risqué remarks, coarse and unseemly jokes, and make facetious comments about some object, or especially some person in the environment. They are superficial in their relationships with other persons and insensitive to their needs and feelings. Some hypomanic individuals delight in joking efforts to tease the physician. Unbridled criticism and bluntness of speech, even to the point of impudence, are common. Without constraint, the manic patient blurts out what he has doubtless long wished to say but has previously been afraid to express. The usual good humor, which is often infectious in nature, frequently continues as long as every whim of the patient is gratified but tends to be replaced with anger, caustic speech and verbal abuse if anyone questions his opinion or thwarts his wishes. In place of this good humor, one occasionally meets with a sustained anger, argumentativeness, irritability, haughtiness, arrogance, sarcasm and querulousness. Open hostility to members of the family is common. After her recovery, one woman whose hypomanic attacks were characterized by a great outburst of hostility described her psychotic episodes as seeming "like a prolonged spell of anger." In her normal periods she was a friendly person, anxious to help others, and took great pride in her love for them. (One suspects that this desirable personality characteristic was a reaction formation that served as a defense against a deep-seated hostility.) Sudden oscillations of emotion are common. In the midst of an exuberance of manner and spirits, the patient may suddenly burst into tears and give expression to some depressive idea, but after a moment be as cheerful as ever. He may likewise change rapidly from irritability to affability. The hypomanic patient may work with great, but capricious, enthusiasm and energy but his stimulation and expansiveness impair his judgment. He is often so officious and meddlesome that he becomes an annoyance to those about him. He declares that he needs no rest. Although under a constant pressure of activity he feels no sense of fatigue. He writes numerous letters in which he underscores many words and passages and introduces various parenthetical remarks. The style of composition may be flowery and witty and the script large, flowing and perhaps graceful. No sooner, perhaps, has he posted a letter than he decides that the mail is too slow for his urgent business so he dispatches a telegram to his correspondent. He discusses with strangers and without reserve matters of an intimate, private nature. The hypomanic is often erotic and, if a man, may indulge in sexual excesses, while a previously chaste and modest young woman may become sexually promiscuous or marry a man far below her social level. While from custom and convenience the symptoms just described are designated as hypomanic, any attempt to divide the imperceptible gradations of hyperactivity occurring in manic-depressive psychosis into clinical groups is entirely arbitrary.

Before describing a more pronounced form of mania, reference should be made to the fact that it has been customary to speak of the basic symptoms of manic-depressive psychosis, whether of the manic or of the depressive type, as resulting from disturbances in the fields of affectivity, of stream of thought and of psychomotor activity. Although, as will have been already recognized from the description of hypomania just given, one constantly finds changes in affect, associations and activity, yet manic-depressive psychosis must not be looked upon as a disturbance of so-called "faculties," or of circumscribed psychological fields, but rather as a psychobiological reaction occurring when the usual resources of the personality have been unable to deal successfully with the particular strivings and stresses with which the individual is beset—frequently problems which have sprung from deep within his emotional and instinctive life.

In a well developed picture of mania the *affective tonality* is one of eagerness, exaltation and joyous excitement. The tempo of the whole personality is quickened. The patient's patterns of thinking and behavior reflect his mood. He sings, dances about, whistles and may be exhilarated to the point of noisy hilarity. He shows an unrestrained playfulness and mischievousness. His elation stimulates ideas of grandeur and perhaps fleeting delusions of wealth and power. The exhilaration may be punctuated with anger, irritability and even with combativeness if the patient is denied some request or privilege, a granting of which his disturbed state forbids. Again, a well-developed paranoid trend may exist and the patient be verbally abusive to the person toward whom, for the moment, he may feel most resentful. Patients with this impure affect are often haughty, demanding, revengeful, sarcastic and arrogant. They may seem to delight in an unbounded expression of aggressiveness and hostility.

The *stream of thought* is characterized by loquaciousness and rapid association of ideas. Frequently the patient speaks with a crispness and vigor of articulation, with emphatic accents and frequent changes of pitch. His style of phrasing may be pompous and his speech assume the character of theatrical declamation. As the hypomanic state passes into acute mania the pressure of speech develops into a flight of ideas with rhyming, play upon words and "clang" associations of words having similar sounds but no relation in meaning. Superficially the therapist receives the impression of a great variety of ideas but if he carefully observes the manic patient's associational products, he discovers that their range is really limited. As a matter of fact, the manic individual evades thinking and is occupied with phonetics rather than meaning. Associations that remind the patient of some overvalued idea or egocentric interest are particularly apt to divert the stream of thought. Although the patient's racing flow of ideas appears illogical and directed by such stimuli as similarity of sound and environmental objects and events, yet beneath these superficial associations may often be discovered an underlying but limited range of topics toward which associations tend to flow. Without realizing their significance, the patient often makes remarks that afford a hint as to the unconscious motivation of his ideas, since although apparently devoid of motivation they are not so in fact. In both sequence and significance, they approach the character of free associations and therefore, like them, are prompted by unconscious and instinctive agencies.

The third of the mental fields in which it has been customary to describe disturbances as taking place is that of *psychomotor activity*. There is an overactivity ranging from the pressure of occupation described in hypomania to the violent motor excitement of acute mania. In the hospital the patient meddles with ward activities and with other patients; he has numerous suggestions as to how the institution should be conducted. He decorates himself with trinkets and improvised badges and medals. In more excited states, he tears his clothing into ribbons with which he decorates himself in a grotesque manner. He sings, shouts and assumes dramatic attitudes. He may destroy bed and personal clothing, an activity usually not prompted by malice but by an urge to be busy. A woman ordinarily refined and modest may disregard all former sense of propriety, make indecent sexual proposals and be obscene in speech. The overactive manic sleeps but little and yet does not appear fatigued. He sustains cuts and abrasions to which he pays no attention and for which he will permit no treatment. Infections may occur and complicate the clinical picture. Rarely the patient shows such a pressure of activity that he does not eat and requires tube feeding, although in the usual degree of excitement the patient may bolt large quantities of food with complete disregard of manners.

The attention of the manic is usually much disturbed, the disorder being caused not by any defect in vigility but by lack of tenacity, as a result of which attention is easily distracted. Environmental noises and activities constantly divert his attention. Not rarely he misidentifies persons, being particularly prone to identify a stranger as a former acquaintance, because of the fact that he discovers some slight point of similarity but fails to scrutinize the points of dissimilarity. The patient usually remains well oriented but at times his grasp of his environment may be faulty because of an absence of sustained and discriminating attention.

Hallucinations may occur in manic excitement but are not common and are usually more in the nature of illusions.

While delusions are not conspicuous symptoms, they often occur, are usually expansive or wish-fulfilling in nature, are fleeting and not systematized. Ideas of persecution are not rare.

Physically the milder cases appear in excellent health. The eyes are bright, the face flushed, the head erect, the step quick and weight may be gained. In extreme excitement the patient may lose weight because of great expenditure of energy. In greatly overactive states, the patient is usually dehydrated. Pneumonia, acute nephritis and other infections may be unrecognized because of the difficulty in making a physical examination of a patient so extremely excited. In such cases, the real nature of a superimposed delirioid state may escape recognition. Any real clouding of consciousness in a patient who has been greatly excited should suggest the possibility of a complicating infection.

The following taken from the records of a man who first entered a public institution for mental diseases when fifty-four years of age illustrates many of the typical behavior reactions of manic excitement:

At thirty-five, forty-one and forty-seven the patient suffered from depressed episodes, each attack being from four to six months in duration. In January he became restless and talkative. Early in February he began to send checks to friends, sometimes even to strangers who, he said, might be in need. Ten days later he was sent home from the office where he was employed with the explanation that he was becoming overwrought. A few days after his suspension from work he was admitted to a private institution for mental disorders where he pretended to commit suicide by mercury poisoning. He then drew a skull and cross bones on the wall of his room. After three weeks he was taken home but a few days later he was committed to a public institution where he bustled about the ward giving the impression that he had important business to which he must attend. Occasionally he would be seen lying on a bench pretending to sleep but in a few minutes resumed his usual activity. He talked quickly, loudly and nearly constantly. He was interested in everything and everyone around him. He talked familiarly to patients, attendants, nurses and physicians. He took a fancy to the woman physician on duty in the admission building, calling her by her first name and annoying her with letters and with his familiar, ill-mannered and obtrusive attentions. On his arrival he gave five dollars to one patient and one dollar to another. He made many comments and asked many questions about other patients and promised that he would secure their discharge. He interfered with their affairs and soon received a blow on the jaw from one patient and a black eye from another. He wrote letters demanding his release, also letters to friends describing in a circumstantial, inaccurate and facetious way conditions in the hospital. His letters were interlarded with trite Latin phrases. He drew caricatures of the physicians and the nurses and wrote music on toilet paper. He drew pictures on his arms; on one occasion he secured a bottle of mercurochrome and painted the face of another manic patient. When permitted to play the ward piano he would play piece after piece without stopping, improvising a great deal. A doctor rarely passed through the ward without being called by the patient who would slap the physician on the back or shake hands effusively and talk until the door closed. At times during an interview his voice would become tremulous, tears would come to his eyes and he would sob audibly with his face buried in his arms. A moment later, however, he would be laughing—a manifestation of the bipolarity of emotion so markedly illustrated in this disease.

Depressive Phase. While a larger percentage of the episodic depressions of this disorder occur in persons who have also a history of manic episodes, yet in not a few manic-depressives the psychotic episodes are confined to those of a depressive type. In such cases one often finds a rather characteristic type of prepsychotic personality. Many of these individuals whose psychotic episodes are limited to depressive reactions have always been friendly, unobstrusive, timid persons with an underlying sense of insecurity and overdependency. Not a few have manifested sensitive and appreciative emotional responses. Many have been scrupulous persons of rigid ethical and moral standards, meticulous, self-demanding, perfectionistic, self-depreciatory, prudish, given to self-reproach, and sensitive to criticism. Their obsessive-compulsive tendencies have doubtless been defensive mechanisms for handling hostility which characteristically they cannot express externally. Frequently they have had fixed opinions and set ways of doing things and are habitually apprehensive and fearful. Many have been hesitant and without courage, yet have sought and achieved worthwhile accomplishments. Frequently their greatest emotional need seems to have been that of being loved, accepted and of belonging.

Just as in the manic type of manic-depressive psychosis all degrees of overactivity are found, so in the depressive type one meets with varying degrees of depression. If arbitrarily we describe three degrees of manic activity—hypomania, acute mania and delirious mania, in the excited phase, so mild depression, acute depression and stupor may be said to represent the different degrees of depression. One should remember, however, that these arbitrary divisions merge imperceptibly one into the other.

Because of the absence of striking disturbances, the real nature of *mild depression* is frequently not recognized. In fact, it should be borne in mind that various moods which are called normal pass imperceptibly into the different forms of manic-depressive psychosis. Mild depressive phases tend, roughly speaking, to assume one of two general forms: either a period of fatigue, staleness and inertia, or one during which the patient has physical complaints for which no organic basis can be discovered. Affective depression exists in both forms but does not constitute the chief complaint and consists in a mild downheartedness. Occasionally the onset is characterized by obsessive features. If the depression stands a bit to the fore, the patient's friends may speak of his episodes as "blue spells." The patient lacks confidence in himself, loses his zest for living, feels inadequate, tired, shows a growing aversion to activity, likes to be left alone and finds it difficult to perform his ordinary duties. Color and joy are gone out of life. Every task seems a burden and in many cases the patient gives up any attempt to continue his employment. The patient has doubts and fears, is frequently over-anxious about his family, states he has not provided amply for their future welfare and has mild ideas of unworthiness. Thinking may be difficult, ideational content becomes confined to a few topics, spontaneous speech is limited, replies to questions are delayed and condensed as much as possible, and the patient is disinclined to reveal his private thoughts. Social contacts are not sought and the patient may even show an obstinate unwillingness to meet people. Many show a marked indecisiveness, probably indicative of their apprehension of further failure, rejection and retaliation. Those with an "impure" depression tend to be gloomily irritable, sensitive and morose rather than sad. They are often stubborn, peevish, inconsiderate of others and are inclined to project in the form of dissatisfaction and fault-finding.

In the second group of mild depressions, physical complaints are among the most conspicuous symptoms and may mask the depression. There is not merely the loss of weight, coated tongue, disturbed and unrefreshing sleep and poor appetite observed in depressive states but the patient has various hypochondriacal ideas. He feels weak and fatigued, worries over trifles, suffers from insomnia, from headache and debility and perhaps from precordial or epigastric distress. Any bodily sensations that may arise on a physical, tension, or anxiety basis become the principal object of the patient's attention. He therefore believes, as often do his friends, that the real disorder is physical and that his downheartedness is the natural result of ill health, whereas the physical complaints are really but the rationalization of a primary affective distress. To the inexperienced practitioner, these depressive episodes may appear to be neurasthenic. Occasionally there is a history of laparotomy or of pelvic surgery without a discoverable pathologic condition having been revealed.

The onset of a *severe depression* may resemble the mild depressive states just described but the initial downheartedness soon passes into a profound affective distress. Posture, muscle tensions and various physical signs and symptoms present a composite picture indicating depression. The body is stooped, the head flexed, the facies immobile, the forehead is furrowed, and the patient looks fixedly downward. Deep vertical wrinkles appear between the eyebrows, the nasolabial folds are marked, and the down-turned angles of the mouth constitute a picture of dejection. The face may have a troubled, perplexed expression. The patient loses weight and appears ill. Perspiration and other secretions are decreased. Muscle tone is decreased, the bowels are constipated, sexual desire is decreased and the male patient is usually impotent. The patient sleeps poorly and awakes early. The depression becomes more profound and everything is interpreted in terms of hopelessness and despondency.

Occasionally a patient will say he has no feeling. Others complain that things seem strange and unnatural—feelings of unreality. They usually recognize that the change, caused by the influence of depressed feeling-tone on perceptions, by the loss of interest in external phenomena and by the change in affective relationship to them, is in themselves and not in the fundamental nature of environmental objects. Many patients have an indefinite dread or a sense of impending disaster, frequently accompanied by an attitude of submission to their fate. Efforts at reassurance make no impression and the patient shows no response to appreciative and sympathetic counsel. Some patients manifest a hostile bitterness. A sense of fear is not uncommon and, if intense, consciousness may be clouded and the patient be confused.

The purest type of depression is a *retarded depression.* In this there is an inhibition of the stream of thought and of psychomotor activity. The retarded patient speaks slowly, he seems at a loss for words, his replies are brief, frequently monosyllabic, and expressed in a low tone. Not rarely he begins but never completes the reply to some inquiry, or else finishes it only as the examiner moves away. Perhaps he may merely move his lips but fail to utter any intelligible response. Efforts to make decisions result in vacillation or perplexity.

In the psychomotor field externally directed behavior becomes progressively retarded and inhibited. There is slowness both in initiation and in execution. The patient complains of an inability to carry out suggested activities and every attempt requires great exertion. Retardation may be so pronounced as to amount to stupor.

In depressive states the patient's ideas tend to represent a projected expression of his inner feelings and a rationalization of his affects. The delusions both of manic and of depressive patients seem to be more the reflections of their mood than true delusional experiences, as in schizophrenia. The delusional content of the depressive patient is therefore characterized by self-depreciation, ideas of guilt, remorse, self-accusation and hypochondriasis. Not infrequently there is a suspicious, paranoid, complaining and persecutory trend to the patient's ideas. This is particularly the case when the patient's prepsychotic personality was characterized by sensitiveness and feelings of inferiority. Some depressive patients are sullen and morose. Hate is a not uncommon, although at times concealed, constituent of depression. Sometimes the patient may present a hostile, punitive attitude. Resentment and aversion to treatment may be associated. Aversion reactions should not be confused with negativism.

Hallucinations are not conspicuous symptoms in the depression of manic-depressive psychosis, and while they may occur, a persistent falsification of reality in this way should raise the question of a more malignant psychosis, particularly if the hallucinations do not clearly represent the projection of affective distress. Illusionary misinterpretations are frequent—a pounding in the basement is that of workmen constructing the patient's coffin.

The patient usually remains well oriented unless from his affective distress he becomes so preoccupied that attention is impaired. As already indicated, he may be confused if his fear is intense. Depressed patients usually have little or no appetite and some would starve if not encouraged or forced to eat. Spoon or tube feeding is often necessary. This failure to eat may be the result of the profound psychomotor inhibition, or of the patient's belief that he is unworthy to receive the food, or to a desire to die. This feeling of unworthiness and of desire for self-punishment often leads to suicidal attempts and occasionally to mutilation of self.

The most intense form of the depressive phase is depressive *stupor.* It was probably this type of stupor to which Esquirol gave the name "acute dementia." In this profoundly inhibited state, there is practically no spontaneous motor activity. There is a complete, or almost complete, immobility with a minimal response to external stimuli. The patient is mute, his sensorium is clouded and he is intensely preoccupied, often with ideas of death and with dream-like hallucinations. The face is either masklike or rigidly anxious. Many have to be tube-fed while some soil and wet themselves.

Elderly depressed patients may manifest organic mental symptoms such as confusion, disorientation and memory defects which are alleviated or may even disappear with recovery from depression. Not rarely, a depression terminates with a brief hypomanic reaction.

The possibility that crimes of violence may occur with the manic-depressive psychoses is usually considered. Such crimes are not unknown, however, and are more frequent in depressed than in manic states probably because of the fact that depression may be a result of a weakening in the repression of hate and aggressive strivings. It is reported that of ninety patients confined to the Broadmoor, England, "Criminal Lunatic Asylum" because of murder committed during affective psychoses, sixty-two were suffering from depression and twenty-eight from mania at the time the homicides took place. More homicides are committed by depressed women than by depressed men. Usually the victim is not only a member of the patient's family but the one who has apparently been the most loved. It has been suggested that the homicide may be regarded as an extension of the suicidal impulse. If suicide is considered as an act of aggression against self, then the homicide (in depressive patients) might be considered as an extension of aggression to include not only the self but those things which are nearest the self, the victim being almost a part of the self. Perhaps this is the psychopathology manifested when a depressed mother kills both herself and her child.

The following case represents a fairly typical picture of the depressive phase:

E. D., aged sixty, was admitted to the hospital because he was depressed, ate insufficiently, and believed that his stomach was "rotting away." The patient was described as a friendly, sociable individual, not quarrelsome, jealous or critical and with a sense of humor. He was considered even-tempered, slow to anger, tenderhearted and emotional.

At fifty-one the patient suffered from a depression when he was obliged to resign his position. This depression continued for about nine months, after which he apparently fully recovered. He resumed his work but after two years suffered from a second depression. Again he recovered after several months and returned to a similar position which he held until two months before his admission. At this time he began to worry lest he was not doing his work well, talked much of his lack of fitness for his duties and finally resigned. He spent Thanksgiving Day at his son's in a neighboring city but while there he was sure that the water pipes in his own house would freeze during his absence and that he and his family would be "turned out into the street." A few days later he was found standing by a pond, evidently contemplating suicide. He soon began to remain in bed and would sometimes wrap his head in the bed clothing to shut out the external world. He declared that he was "rotting away inside," and that if he ate, the food would kill him. He urged the family not to touch the glasses or towels he used lest they become contaminated.

On arrival at the hospital he appeared older than his years. He was pale, poorly nourished, dehydrated, with his lips dry, cracked and covered with sordes. His facial expression and general bearing suggested a feeling of utter hopelessness. He was self-absorbed and manifested no interest in his environment. When urged to answer questions there would be a long delay before attempting to reply but he would finally speak briefly, hesitatingly, and in a low tone. He occasionally became agitated and would repeatedly say, "Oh, doctor, why did I ever get into anything like this? Doctor, I am all filled up! I can't get anything through me—what am I going to do? Oh, dear! Oh, dear!" In explaining his presence in the hospital he said he realized he had been sent by his family because they believed he would be benefited by the treatment, but added, "I don't know how they sent me here when they had not the means. My wife cannot pay for me and by this time she must have been put out of the house."

After several months the patient began to improve although hypochondriacal ideas persisted for a considerable period. Finally when the matter of freedom of the hospital grounds was considered he seemed in a normal mood and indicated that he was beginning to think somewhat differently concerning his gastrointestinal tract. At that time he commented, "There's a good deal of life in the old horse yet." A month later he passed into a mildly hypomanic state. He became alert, animated, talkative, exuberant in spirits and confident in manner. This mildly excited state continued for about two months when he settled down into what seemed to be his normal mood and state of activity. After a few weeks he was discharged, but several months later he again showed signs of depression and hanged himself before arrangements for readmission had been made.

Cyclic Type. While the episodes suffered by some patients are always manic or always depressive those of others may be of irregular sequence in respect to the mood disturbance. Again the episodes of still other patients may be characterized by an alternation of manic and depressive reactions. In some patients there may be no appreciable interval of normality between the alternations while in other cases there may be variable periods free from symptoms.

The following case illustrates the tendency to cycles and how the frequency of recurring mood swings may prevent successful adjustment during a large part of the patient's adult life:

M. M. was first admitted to a state hospital at the age of 38 although since childhood she had been characterized by swings of mood some of which had been so extreme that they had been psychotic in degree. At 17 she suffered from a depression which rendered her unable to work for several months although she was not hospitalized. At 33, shortly before the birth of her first child, the patient was greatly depressed. "For a period of four days she was in a coma." About a month after the birth of the baby she "became excited" and was entered as a patient in an institution for neurotic and mildly psychotic patients. As she began to improve, she was sent to a shore hotel for a brief vacation. The patient remained at the hotel for one night and on the following day signed a year's lease on an apartment, bought furniture and became heavily involved in debt. Shortly thereafter Mrs. M. became depressed and returned to the hospital in which she had previously been a patient. After several months she recovered and except for relatively mild fluctuations of mood remained well for approximately two years. She then became overactive, exuberant in spirits and visited her friends to whom she outlined her plans for re-establishing different forms of lucrative business. The patient purchased many clothes, bought furniture, pawned her rings and wrote checks without funds. She was then entered in a public mental hospital. Gradually her manic symptoms subsided and after four months she was discharged. For a period thereafter she was mildly depressed. In a little less than a year Mrs. M. again became overactive, played her radio until late in the night, smoked excessively, took out insurance on a car which she had not yet bought, contrary to her usual habits she swore frequently and loudly, created a disturbance in a club to which she did not belong, and instituted divorce proceedings. On the day prior to her second admission to the hospital she purchased fifty-seven hats.

During the past eighteen years this patient has been admitted and dismissed from the hospital on many occasions. At times with the onset of a depressed period she has returned to the hospital seeking admission. At such times she complained that her "brain just won't work." She would say, "I have no energy, am unable to do my housework, I have let my family down; am living from day to day. There is no one to blame but myself." During one of her manic periods she sent the following telegram to a physician with whom she had become much enamored: "To: You; Street and No.: Everywhere; Place: the remains at peace! We did our best, but God's will be done! I am so very sorry for all of us. To brave it through thus far. Yes, Darling—from Hello Handsome. Handsome is as Handsome does, thinks lives and breathes. It takes clear air, Brother of Mine, in a girl's hour of need. All my love to the Best Inspiration one ever had."

For the past year Mrs. M., now 59, has been making an excellent home and community adjustment. Her husband has had several cerebrovascular accidents and has required considerable nursing and assistance. She has efficiently met the various responsibilities and family emergencies that have befallen her and has supplemented her husband's pension by baby-sitting. It is altogether probable, however, that she will experience returns either of excitement or of depression.

MIXED TYPES. Psychomotor activity, flow of thought and affectivity were formerly thought of as independent and more or less separable functions of the mind, which in their positive or negative variations could be combined in various ways as may the letters of the alphabet. Basing his ideas on this conception of a coexistence of manic and depressive elements. Kraepelin described special clinical forms which he designated as the "mixed" types of manic-depressive psychosis. He conceived of these positive or negative unitary faculties as being capable of arrangement and rearrangement in various combinations. It should be remembered, however, that behavior is a unitary, purposive process and that it is not the result of a haphazard union of component elements. Kraepelin described such "mixed" forms as agitated depression, manic stupor, unproductive mania, depressive mania, depression with flight and inhibited mania. The present tendency is to discontinue such artificial classifications.

Of these groups *agitated depression* most nearly deserves a special recognition, yet this group is really a depressive reaction in which the agitation is simply an expression of anxiety—a persistent expression of the apprehension, tension and feeling of prospective harm arising from threatening factors deep in the mental life. The great internal uneasiness produces a psychomotor agitation.

Psychopathology of Manic-Depressive States

Various theories have been offered to explain the psychological dynamics of the two contrasting affective reactions observed in these states. At the present time there seems to be much to suggest that depression should be regarded as a result of anxiety in a person who experienced severe loss, real or fancied, at an early stage of development. The loss is perceived as rejection which precipitates anger. Since the feeling of anger cannot be tolerated it is repressed and turned inward on the self. Although these feelings of anger and hostility are repressed they cause the individual to feel guilty, unworthy and depressed.

It well may be, too, that the shift from depression to elation takes place in association with vacillating processes of identification with parental figures. During depression the patient identifies with the maternal figure in a submissive role. At the initiation of the period of elation he denies the submissive, maternal identification and acts out an intense, acquisitive, sadistic drive with fantasies of strength in which he becomes emancipated, elated and overaggressive toward the paternal figure with whom he is now identified. With the failure of his aggressiveness to accomplish the fantasied aim of revenge, the patient again has to renounce the paternal identification, to deny his aggressiveness and so become depressed and helpless.

Some psychiatrists look upon the manic's behavior as essentially a defense reaction. Although he may appear confident and occupy the role of a leader he is basically overdependent. Although he appears out-going and friendly he is self-centered, actively controlling and manipulating, based on an emotional need for dependency relationship. When his demands are frustrated, hostility is generated which must be repressed so that it does not further imperil the dependency relationship. The imperfectly repressed hostility may, in turn, produce depression.

Sometimes an important source of conflict for the manic-depressive patient seems to be that of strong hostility connected with envy which is repressed and avoided. He is often the best endowed member of the family and has been expected to provide the prestige for the group. This position places great responsibility on him, yet exposes him to the envy of his siblings, or even to envious competition with his parents. The future manic-depressive grew sensitive to envy and competition and to counteract them unconsciously developed the pattern of disparaging himself in order to conceal his full capacity.

Various dynamics other than those already discussed are sometimes mentioned as operative in the production of depression. It is suggested, for example, that depression may be a reaction to painful but unrecognized material which threatens to invade consciousness. Affects are transferred from the unconscious to elements in consciousness the contents of which take on values derived from the unconscious. The affect should be connected with this unconscious mentation but rationalization connects it with experiences accompanied by awareness. The easiest and most natural way, for example, by which an ill-defined sense of guilt or of remorse may be rationalized and thereby find the required sense of reality in the consciousness of the patient, is by linking it up with some trifling indiscretion of earlier life. This indiscretion will usually be found to have really been trivial although it never enjoyed full approval of the individual's socially determined conscience. All the energy of the affect tied up with the repudiated wishes and material that have been repressed, usually with difficulty and for a long period, is displaced to this lapse and its ideational representation. It is this idea which receives the displaced affect that both rationalizes and renders concrete the vague feeling of guilt arising from disowned strivings and desires.

Feelings of guilt and reflected depression springing from them may arise in other ways. Some repressed wish, for example, will occasionally be granted by accident, such as by the death of a parent whose continued existence had prevented the fulfillment of a greatly desired wish. In such a case a depression may sometimes result because of the feeling of guilt that follows the gratification of the consciously repudiated desire. In general, as already indicated, feelings of guilt giving rise to depression arise not so much from what one has done as from what one has unconsciously wished to do. In the opinion of some psychiatrists depression represents a penance for repressed hatred, aggressiveness and other repudiated tendencies and impulses that have given rise to feelings of guilt. Guilt, too, may be expressed in terms of self-punishment. There is much to suggest that hostility is the denominator common to both manic and depressive phases. It may be that the depressed patient because of his rigid superego does not permit himself to live out his hostile, aggressive tendencies against others but re-directs them against himself or expresses them in projected form. The influence of pathological feelings of guilt and of hostile impulses turned against the self may therefore find expression in bereavement, depression or suicide. The fact that feelings of guilt and of self-accusation may be assuaged by attaching to others the motives that created them may contribute to the paranoid features that may accompany depression. If the release of repressed impulses is particularly threatening the depression may be accompanied by manifest expressions of anxiety.

Meyer suggested that depressive reactions, by withdrawing the individual from an ill-adjusted situation, serve a protective purpose. With this withdrawal occur accompanying manifestations of inhibitions at various levels—vegetative, motor, affective and that of ideational content and its expression.

Differential Diagnosis

As stated in the chapter entitled The Causes and Nature of Mental Disorders (Chapter V), there is an increasing tendency among psychiatrists to look upon mental disturbance less as nosological entities and more as reactions to stresses arising from within and from without, reactions capable of being understood only through a knowledge of the individual, his previous experiences, personality trends and present problems. To facilitate discussion and to correlate important data, some of which have prognostic value, a clinical classification based on syndromes and course continues, nevertheless, to serve a useful purpose. This is particularly true in the case of the reactions that are grouped under the clinical title of manic-depressive psychosis the diagnostic classification of which may be suggested by the manifestation of a dominant mood and by the history of recurring disturbances of affect.

Many hypomanics in whom the emotional exaltation is replaced by anger, resentment, irritability, irascibility, litigious tendencies and perhaps paranoid delusions, were formerly diagnosed as cases of acute paranoia. Such hypomanics lack the solitary and asocial tendency usually exhibited by the true paranoid who presents a more sustained, brooding, sensitive, suspicious reaction pattern. Persons in whom these impure affects replace an exaltation are ones who prior to their psychosis have been characterized by a tendency to defensive projections. Emotional difficulties may be a negligible factor in the development of an organic condition but a major one in recovery.

In early syphilitic meningoencephalitis the presenting symptoms may reflect previous personality trends and therefore suggest a manic-depressive psychosis. Neurological signs and serological tests will at once make a diagnosis possible.

The sense of inadequacy, abnormal fatigability, depressive ideas and apprehension that may accompany mild forms of the depressive or mixed types, particularly in the early stages, are often misinterpreted as symptoms of neurasthenia, of a compulsion neurosis or of an anxiety state. The more important points of differentiation between the manic-depressive psychosis and the psychoneuroses are enumerated in Chapter XXX. In addition to what is there mentioned, it may be remarked that in manic-depressive psychosis, sluggishness of thought and action is more common, the patient is more reticent as to his feelings and he does not show the eagerness to interview the physician usually seen in the psychoneuroses. Psychogenic causes and processes are usually more easily ascertained in psychoneuroses. Mild but often unrecognized forms of the depressive type are of frequent occurrence with the result that the number of manic depressives in extra-institutional life probably exceeds those under treatment in hospitals for mental disorders. Doubtless the classification of depressions into psychotic depressions and neurotic depressions, and then the differentiation of the psychotic depressions into manic-depressive and involutional depression is useful even though the boundaries between these different depressions are by no means clear-cut and secure.

The most difficult problem in the differential diagnosis of manic-depressive psychosis is its distinction from schizophrenia. In the typical case this presents no difficulty but in many cases there is doubt as to how symptoms should be interpreted. In general the disturbance in personality in manic-depressive psychoses seems to be a quantitative one, a matter of "too much" or "too little," rather than a disorganization of personality, as in schizophrenia. There is not, moreover, complete agreement among psychiatrists as to how much temporary disorganization of the personality may be considered consistent with the diagnosis of manic-depressive psychosis, nor as to how much diagnostic weight should be assigned different symptoms. This difficulty may exist in the manic, in the depressive and in the clinically mixed forms. Behavior may be equally disturbed in the manic excitement of an affective psychosis and in the catatonic excitement of schizophrenia. In approaching the problem of differentiation, it is necessary first to secure as full a knowledge as possible as to the prepsychotic personality of the patient, determine whether cyclothmic or schizoid characteristics have predominated, and whether psychobiological energy trends have been directed into extraverted channels and been marked by objectivity and realism, or whether they have been of an introverted nature and characterized by subjectivity. The presence of flight of ideas and of psychomotor activity in the early phases of a mental disorder may not constitute unequivocal diagnostic criteria since both may exist in reactions that eventuate as schizophrenia. In schizophrenia there tends to be more incoherence and greater poverty of ideas. The excitement of the schizophrenic lacks the depth of emotional expression that is usually observed in the excitement of manic depressive, is less influenced by the reality of the environment, is more episodic and impulsive, tends to be undirected, to be stereotyped, confined to a limited space and determined more by hallucinations, delusions and autistic processes. The more grotesque, and therefore the more primitive or highly symbolized the ideas, the more are they to be looked upon as schizophrenia. The mood of the schizophrenic lacks both an infectious element and that component which causes one to feel himself empathically into the position of the patient who in general is less accessible than the manic depressive. The greater the harmony between mood, ideational content and behavior the more is a manic-depressive psychosis suggested, while the less the mental processes remain integrated the more is schizophrenia denoted. Even though it at first be temporary, the greater the disorganization of the personality, as shown by absence or inappropriateness of affect, by hallucinations, soiling and apparent noninterpretability of behavior, the more does one expect an ultimate, and for the most part permanent schizophrenic disorganization. The clinical picture of some young patients initially considered to be suffering from a manic phase of a manic-depressive psychosis changes to one that is clearly schizophrenic in nature. Finally, just as personalities are not cast in standardized molds, so we find there are all sorts of gradations between those reactions which we call schizophrenic and those we call manic depressive. Formerly a favorable outcome of an acute episode was considered presumptive evidence of its affective nature but the present trend of psychiatry is to consider that extensive schizophrenic disorganization of personality may not be irrecoverable.

Prognosis and Course

It has already been indicated that the prognosis for a single affective episode is usually to be regarded as good but that recurrences are not uncommon. Perhaps there has been too great a tendency to stress the frequency of recurrence. Of manic-depressive admissions to state hospitals, 55 per cent are first attacks, about 25 per cent second attacks, 9 per cent third and 5 per cent have had more than three admissions.

Another important feature of manic-depressive psychosis is the fact that even repeated episodes usually leave the mind unchanged in its intellectual, affective and conative aspects, and that a disorganization of the personality does not follow. Not a little of Ruskin's best work was during his hypomanic states. Occasionally after a series of attacks the patient shows impairment of initiative and of judgment and becomes less able to deal with everyday affairs of life.

The most frequent age for the first manic episode is between twenty and twenty-five years. The average age of onset for first depressive attacks is about ten years later. The earlier the onset of either type the worse the prognosis for the occurrence of further episodes. If the first attack be manic in type, it almost certainly will not be the only one; if it be of a depressed type it may be. The more the etiological factors appear to be constitutional and endogenous and the less they are exogenous and related to perturbing experiences the worse the prognosis. The patient's prepsychotic personality traits influence the prognosis both as to duration and outcome. If he has shown himself to be flexible, tolerant, conciliatory, without defensive, compensatory or other signs of a deep sense of insecurity, and has had varied and wholesome interests, the prognosis is more favorable than if his personality patterns have been of opposite type. As age increases, there is some tendency for attacks to be depressive rather than manic, perhaps because of the changing outlook on life. (See discussion of etiological factors in Chapter XXIV entitled Involutional Psychotic Reactions.) The duration of manic-depressive episodes is extremely variable. The average duration of untreated manic attacks may be estimated at six months and of depressive episodes at nine months. There is a tendency for depressions to increase in length with advancing age. Many depressions terminate with a brief hypomanic elation. The duration in individual cases may be either much shorter or much longer. One is never safe in predicting the probable duration of a given episode. In cases of sudden, acute onset, the recovery is quicker and perhaps more complete than in those of insidious onset. Some patients may never have more than a single episode while in others a large part of the time may be occupied with recurring psychotic periods. The more frequent the attacks the poorer the prognosis. The more chronic the illness the less severe the symptoms. Depression is much more likely to become chronic than is mania. Chronic mania is uncommon before the age of forty. The prognosis is considered less favorable in depressions manifesting a nihilistic hypochondriasis, particularly if accompanied by anxiety. Some degree of insight is more common in depressions than in excitement. It is apt to be limited in resentful manics and in melancholic individuals whose mood has been characterized less by true depression than by impure affects such as suspicion.

Treatment

The question as to whether the mild forms of excitement or of depression should be treated in a hospital is not always easy. In the case of the hypomanic, it is often evident to the psychiatrist that prudence requires more control of the patient's activities than is possible in the home. Since, however, there is nothing "unpsychological" in his behavior the patient's relatives frequently fail either to accept the statement that his exuberance of spirits, pressure of activity and volubility are evidence of mental disorder, or to appreciate the embarrassment to themselves and the aggravation of the psychosis that may result from the absence of restraining measures. In depressions, too, it is difficult for the relatives to accept the fact that the danger of suicide always exists in such affective states. For these reasons they are frequently averse to the patient's admission to a mental hospital. They often believe that all that is required for treatment is a change of scenery or that the patient be urged to arouse himself. In nearly every instance the manic-depressive patient, even though the overactivity or the depression be mild, should receive prompt hospital care. This is especially true in view of the beneficial results now usually secured through the employment of drug or physical therapies.

The apparently exhaustless energy of the hypomanic may suggest that an outlet for it should be provided. The physician should remember, however, that fatigue produces not tranquillity but excitement. The usual desire for almost constant activity must therefore be curbed, although with as little irritation as possible. The hypomanic patient must be protected from his tendency to enter into unwise business or financial schemes. Careful supervision of the patient who is not hospitalized may be necessary lest an increase in sex drive lead to regrettable indulgences. Frequently the prepsychotic personality of the manic has been characterized by a sensitive pride. The physician will therefore carefully guard against the contradictions and arguments to which the hypomanic's irritability, unrestrained speech and activity and his resentment at interference with his wishes are prone to lead.

Generally speaking chlorpromazine is the therapeutic measure of choice for the treatment of the overactive manic patient and electroshock therapy for the treatment of the depressed patient. If the manic patient is so overactive and dehydrated that quick results are desired chlorpromazine may be administered intramuscularly but a change to oral administration is soon made. A dose of 50 mg. may be injected deep into the gluteal muscles. Because of the necessity for considerable dilution of the drug, not more than 50 mg. should be injected into one buttock. If it is desired to give more than 50 mg., this dose may be injected into each buttock. Usually, however, the drug is given orally from the beginning of its administration. On the first day of treatment the patient is given a test dose of 50 mg. If no untoward results follow this test dose, the patient receives 50 mg. three times a day on the following day. On the third day he receives 100 mg. three times a day. This dose may be gradually increased to 600 to 800 mg. a day. Usually this amount is not exceeded although some physicians may give as much as 1000 mg. a day. As the patient's overactivity subsides, the dose of chlorpromazine is gradually reduced.

Many physicians prefer electroshock therapy to chlorpromazine in the treatment of the overactive manic patient. Sometimes if the manic patient shows extreme psychomotor activity he may be given electroshock treatments twice a day for three or four days. This results in considerable confusion and the frequency of treatments should soon be reduced to three per week. Episodic recurrences of the manic-depressive psychoses are not prevented by electroshock therapy and the duration of symptom-free intervals is not made shorter by reason of its use.

The treatment of mild depressions may, in certain respects, constitute a greater problem than do the deep depressions. The friends of the patient suffering from a mild episode of a manic-depressive nature often refuse to believe that he is suffering from a major mental disorder and may be unwilling to accept the physician's opinion and advice which should usually include a recommendation for the use of electroshock therapy. While most physicians prefer that the patient be hospitalized during this form of treatment some give treatments either at the patient's home or in the physician's office in the case of mild depressions. If the patient has suicidal inclinations there is danger that he will end his life if treatment is undertaken in the home. If there is little danger of suicide and the family is co-operative, treatment may be attempted at home provided the services of a nurse are constantly available. An attempt on the part of the relatives to care for the patient is generally unwise if for no other reason than that they usually either argue with him concerning his fears, constantly attempt to distract him, or urge the patient to rouse himself. An organized program which fills the patient's day is desirable. This should be of a type which will not require spontaneity, close concentration or strenuous activity. The program may include handicraft, walks, reading, games, social and recreational activities and the encouragement of special aptitudes and interests. While the patient should not be idle lest he become unduly preoccupied with his problems and with self-examination, it should be borne in mind that a depressed patient, prompted by his lifelong rigid requirements of self, may undertake too much and become more depressed when he finds he falls short of expected accomplishment. Many depressed patients complain of fatigue but since this type of fatigue is really an expression of mood it is not relieved by rest. One should remember that the depressed patient's tendency to hypochondriasis has at times led to unnecessary surgical operations. Unless carefully supervised, the depressed patient may not receive sufficient food.

In case of severe depression, treatment in a hospital is certainly wise. In nearly all cases the use of electroshock therapy is accompanied by a gratifying improvement. Treatments are usually given three times a week. Some psychiatrists do not administer more than ten or twelve treatments.

Usually, however, a course should not consist of less than twenty treatments. Approximately 90 per cent of depressed patients recover with this form of treatment.

If the patient is greatly agitated, chlorpromazine may be employed, either alone or in conjunction with electroshock therapy, for its tranquilizing effect. He will not receive reserpine since this drug frequently aggravates depressions.

While the use of Phenergan (promethazine hydrochloride) combined with chlorpromazine is still in an experimental stage, there have been favorable reports of the combined administration of these drugs. Their therapeutic usefulness dose not seem limited to the depression of manic-depressive disorder but includes any psychosis in which depression is a marked symptom. The dose of promethazine is 12.5 mg. given orally twice a day. The dose of chlorpromazine is individualized for each patient but kept as low as possible. Usually the dosage will range from 25 mg. to 100 mg. four times a day. If necessary the treatment may be continued for several months.

It is highly important that the depressed patient receive a diet of high caloric content. Usually it is desirable that he receive milk or additional food between meals. Refusal of food should not be permitted for more than twenty-four hours before resorting to tube-feeding. Sometimes after one feeding by this method the patient will, with a little assistance, eat voluntarily. It would doubtless be better for them if patients who must be tube-fed were to receive nourishment three times in twenty-four hours instead of twice as is the practice in many hospitals. The tube through which the food is introduced may be passed either through the nose or through the mouth. Usually the co-operation of the patient is not sufficient to make the latter route practicable so the feeding is most frequently made through the nose, and a nasal tube employed. Feeding in this manner is not devoid of danger. Occasionally a death from pneumonia or from gangrene of the lung occurs; this may result from a particle of food having passed into the bronchi during tube-feeding. During the feeding the patient may lie on a bed in the supine position, or he may sit upright in a chair. Usually the former position is better. In either case care should be taken to see that the neck is not extended as the tube is liable to enter the larynx when the neck is in that position. If the patient is resistive, two nurses should assist, each holding a forearm to prevent his seizing the tube. The head may be held by a towel folded about it and grasped on either side. The tube is lubricated, introduced into the nares and passed directly backward—not upward. It will often be found that because of a deviated septum one side of the nose offers an easier passage than the other. Sometimes as the tube passes the pharynx it is forced forward and doubled up in the mouth. In such a case it must be nearly withdrawn and again passed. If the tube enters the larynx, choking and coughing are, of course, produced and air is expelled from the tube. After the tube has been introduced to a distance of about 18 inches it is well to let the patient rest a moment and to note if he is breathing freely and normally. A little water is then poured into the funnel. If this flows without obstruction and without disturbing the patient's respirations the food to be given is slowly poured into the funnel and allowed to pass to the stomach by gravity. After the food has all been given it is well to withdraw the tube an inch or two and pour a little water into the funnel to remove any bits of food remaining near the end of the tube. The tube is then pinched to prevent dripping of any food as the end passes over the larynx, at the same time being withdrawn by a quick movement. A feeding may consist of 24 ounces of milk or of malted milk, ½ ounce of butter, ½ ounce of cod liver oil, 1 ounce of orange juice, 2 eggs and 1½ ounces of sugar. Fruit juices, apple sauce, thin cereals, mashed potatoes and thin vegetable soups may be added to the feeding. Sometimes patients attempt to regurgitate the food given. Such patients should be made to lie quietly on their backs for a period after they have been fed.

Occasionally the hospital physician finds that for a considerable period before admission a patient has not been receiving sufficient food or water. His tongue is dry and leathery, his breath is foul, he appears dehydrated and has a slight tendency to acidosis. In these patients special effort must be made to have them receive an abundance of fluid. In depressive stupors attention should be paid to the condition of bladder and bowels.

The danger of suicide must be constantly borne in mind, a fact which should be impressed upon both nurse and family. Suicide is more frequent in patients who have shown tension and anxiety. The history of a suicide in the family increases the possibility that the depressed patient may end his life. It is not unusual for a patient to repeat a previous unsuccessful suicidal attempt.

Among the early signs of recovery is a return of self-confidence and initiative. As convalescence proceeds there should be a gradually increasing participation in occupational and recreational activities. The patient should be relieved of the necessity for making decisions until he is well on the road to recovery. An early resumption of usual duties and responsibilities is to be discouraged. The question as to when the convalescing depressed patient may be dismissed from the hospital is not always easy. The usual opinion is that the patient should remain in an institution with its simple routine until convalescence is well established. It must be remembered, too, that because of the increased danger of suicide during convalescence the patient may require closer supervision during that period than is possible at home. On the other hand, a return home before the depression is entirely cured may sometimes hasten the patient's recovery. He should not resume full duties for several weeks.

Some form of psychotherapy, carefully chosen and suited both to the general situation and to the particular problems of the patient as well as to his ability to understand and to his willingness to co-operate, may usually be employed either to the relief of some symptom or to the improvement of personality adjustment. Both by his manner of approach to the patient and by judicious discussion of the situation and of the patient's behavior the physician may be of assistance in controlling the manic's pressure of activity and in preventing dissatisfaction, resentment and a feeling of injustice on his part. At times, too, the fear and apprehension of the depressed patient may to some degree be relieved. During convalescence, psychotherapeutic discussion of dynamic factors and situations as well as of outstanding personality features and their possible modifiability may be helpful.

Psychiatrists will vary greatly in the extent to which they will employ psychoanalytical principles in their therapy. Those who use them to only a slight extent may, through a biographical review and by asking the patient to associate freely about significant life events and his reactions to them, analyze the patient's emotional development during infancy, childhood and adult life. In this way dynamic factors may be discovered, discussed and an evaluation made of the various factors and situations which may have contributed to the specific organization of the patient's personality. Largely by questions that promote their consideration, the patient is encouraged in a critical examination of definite situations and reactions and their possible underlying factors. The psychiatrist so guides the therapeutic interviews that the patient discovers and recognizes for himself the factors and situations which have contributed to the disturbance of his personality and behavior. He then synthesizes, or builds up into a logical formulation and relationship, the elements and influences which have been operative in producing these disturbances. It is the hope of the therapist that through this formulation and a proper evaluation of these different factors the patient may acquire such a constructive understanding of himself, his assets, shortcomings and handicaps, that a greater inner harmony and a less disturbing environmental adjustment may follow. Where the constitutional factors seem to be important the therapeutic possibilities are often limited, but this fact should not deter the physician from constructive therapeutic efforts. Whatever success can be obtained in preventing further episodes depends on a careful regulation of the patient's life in the light of as complete a knowledge as possible of the social, psychological and medical factors peculiar to the individual. The success of psychotherapy depends to a large extent upon whether or not the patient wishes to get well and is willing to know about his problems and takes an interest in the motives and psychical evolution of his illness.

Many efforts have been made to treat the manic-depressive patient by classical psychoanalytical techniques. It has usually been found that neither the retarded nor the hyperactive patient lends himself to the rigid routine of the customary psychoanalytical process. New efforts have made it evident, however, that modified analytically-oriented psychotherapy is possible for some patients and seems beneficial.

Evidence seems to have shown that it is not advisable that psychotherapeutic interviews with the depressed patient be held four or five times a week as is frequently to be recommended in the case of the schizophrenic or often with the neurotic. Interviews, with their implied insistence that the patient be productive, held more frequently than once or twice a week seem to cause him to exaggerate his shame and guilt. Because of the high personal standards which the depressive requires of himself, and because of his feelings of impotence and incapacity, therapy may be very difficult if the psychiatrist urges productiveness. Because of his feelings of guilt and shame, the patient is unable to express his underlying sadness and rage. Since he is unable to meet the demands which he feels the therapist expects pressure by the latter arouses additional feelings of hatred and shame. The therapist does not, however, adopt the passive role usually followed in a more classical form of psychoanalysis.

Other features of this modified analysis are a constant reassurance of the patient that he will recover, and a certain directness and openness in dealing with his problems. It will be remembered that in his depression the patient is overreacting emotionally to an actual or fantasied loss of a love object. He is therefore seeking another, or substitute, love object. The process of calm reassurance fits this need symbolically. The patient has also a need to escape from the feelings of guilt caused by his repressed rage in his depression. If, therefore, he reports events which seem to be conducive to the production of rage and anger within himself but has not expressed their emotional connotation, the therapist may verbalize such feelings and state their relationship to other persons involved in the patient's situation. In this way the patient is relieved of the burden of stating his rage or anger and is not exposed to subsequent feelings of guilt for expressing the forbidden emotions. With this elastic, nondemanding, and at the same time, active, interpretive approach it is at times possible to abort depressions. Some therapists suggest it is better initially to have the depressed patient focus on an experience of recent loss rather than on the earlier events and interpersonal experiences in his life which determined or reinforced his depressive symptomatology. Dream productions in the depressed patient are often helpful in breaking through to deep-seated associations which give a clearer understanding of his basic longings and conflicts.

Psychotherapy with the hypomanic or manic is difficult. Since such a patient usually identifies with a covertly aggressive, sadistic and successful member of the family, the therapist must constantly guard against the provocation of rejecting a patient whose behavior seems designed for such a purpose, *i.e.*, of embarrassing significant object relations. It is generally agreed that the conversion of manic or hypomanic symptoms to depressive ones is desirable. Sometimes this is effected by the therapist's simply indicating his doubts as to the soundness of the patient's presumption that he has reason to behave as if he were successful or in control of the situation.

Psychotherapeutically the aim of treatment of patients with the manic-depressive syndrome is to bring them to the point where they can consciously face periodic loneliness and separation without resorting either to submissive depression or revengeful overactivity.

BIBLIOGRAPHY

Association for Research in Nervous and Mental Disease, Vol. XI, Manic Depressive Psychosis. Baltimore, Williams & Wilkins Co., 1932.

Barta, J. A., and Kline, Nathan S.: Depression treated with chlorpromazine and promethazine. Am. J. Psychiat., *113:*744–745, 1957.

Batt, J. C.: Homicidal incidence in the depressive psychoses. J. Ment. Sc., *84:*782, 1948.

Bellak, Leopold: Manic-Depressive Psychosis. New York, Grune & Stratton, Inc., 1951.

Cassidy, W. L., et al.: Clinical observations in manic-depressive disease. J.A.M.A., *164:*1535–1546, 1957.

Cohen, M. B., et al.: An intensive study of twelve cases of manic-depressive psychosis. Psychiatry, *17:*103–137, 1954.

Diethelm, Oskar: Treatment in Psychiatry, 2nd ed., Chapters VIII and IX. Springfield, Ill., Charles C Thomas, 1950.

Hendrin, Herbert: Suicide. Psychiatric Quart., *30:*267–282, 1956.

Hoch, A.: Benign Stupors, a Study of a New Manic-Depressive Reaction Type. New York, The Macmillan Company, 1921.

Kalinowsky, L. B., and Hoch, P. H.: Shock Treatments and Other Somatic Procedures in Psychiatry, 2nd ed. New York, Grune & Stratton, 1952.

Kasanin, J.: The affective psychoses in children. Am. J. Psychiat., *10:*897, 1931.

Kolb, L. C.: Psychotherapeutic evolution and its implications. Psychiatric Quart., *30:* 579–597, 1956.

Kraepelin, E.: Manic-Depressive Insanity and Paranoia, Translated by Barclay. Edinburgh, E. and S. Livingstone, 1921.

Lewis, Aubrey: Prognosis in the manic-depressive psychoses. Lancet, *2:*997, 1936.

———, et al.: Manic-depressive psychosis—a symposium. J. Ment. Sc., *82:*488, 1936.

Lorenz, Maria: Language behavior in manic patients. Arch. Neurol. & Psychiat., *69:* 14–26, 1953.

———, and Cobb, Stanley: Language behavior in manic patients. Arch. Neurol. & Psychiat., *67:*763–770, 1952.

McHarg, J. F.: Mania in childhood. Arch. Neurol. & Psychiat., *72:*531–539, 1954.

Parnell, R. W., and Skottowe, Ian: Towards preventing suicide. Lancet, *272:*206–208, 1957.

Rennie, T. A. C.: Prognosis in manic-depressive psychoses. Am. J. Psychiat., *98:*801, 1942.

Smalldon, John L.: Prepsychotic personality of manic-depressive patients. Psychiatric Quart., *8:*129, 1934.

CHAPTER XXVI

Psychotic Disorders (*Continued*)

Psychotic Depressive Reaction

NOT ALL psychotic depressive reactions should be included among those of a manic-depressive type. In the latter type of depressions there is usually the history either of previous, perhaps repeated, depressions or of cyclothymic mood swings in which periods of elation as well as of depression may have been of psychotic degree. The depressions of a manic-depressive nature, too, usually develop without obvious cause and in the absence of any experience such as might seem logically provocative of depression. Occasionally one meets with depressions which lack these distinctive features of a manic-depressive reaction. Such depressions arise when the patient has been confronted with a personal situation of great stress. Environmental factors and personal experiences have been cruelly frustrating, have aroused intense feelings of guilt or remorse or have painfully wounded pride. In the disorders now under discussion, the reaction to the current situation is a definitely pathological depression which may be associated with gross misinterpretation of reality in the form of delusions, frequently but not always somatic, suicidal ruminations or attempts, intense feelings of guilt, and retardation of thought and of psychomotor activity. Such a psychotic reaction is illustrated by the following case:

C. H., a married school teacher, was admitted to a hospital for mental disorders at the age of 30. Her father was a conservative banker of comfortable but not affluent economic status. Her mother was described as neurotic but "possessing considerable social drive." As a child the patient occasionally walked in her sleep and suffered from nightmares. She seems, however, to have been well adjusted in her interpersonal relations both in her family and with playmates. The mother described her as follows: "She was a happy, well behaved, lovely child, a perfect darling, who had a beautiful disposition." After graduation from a private preparatory school of high scholastic standing the patient entered a well known college. Here she became president of the athletic association and her college career seems to have been outstanding both in academic and extracurricular activities. In her senior year the dean wrote her mother, "C. has been a fine influence on the college and I personally have come to depend upon her more than perhaps I have realized. In my long service at T. College there have been few girls who have made so great a contribution to the college community." After completing college, the patient continued graduate work and obtained a master's degree. After the completion of her professional training, Mrs. H. began her career as a teacher. Following the patient's admission to the hospital the superintendent of schools under whom she had worked during the first four years of her teaching wrote the patient's physician as follows: "Mrs. H's work was of superior quality and she showed fine relationships with both children and their parents. She was a wholesome appearing woman of much personal charm, was well liked and showed a great deal of sensitivity toward her work and fellow staff members." It seems apparent that up to this point in her life the patient possessed an unusually well adjusted personality.

At twenty-six the patient married a young man from a prominent but highly unstable family. Although charming in manner and extremely brilliant intellectually he was quite immature emotionally. While still in college he had some neurotic difficulty and came to the attention of the university psychiatrist. Soon after their marriage he spent a period in a private sanitarium. Following his discharge from the sanitarium Mr. H. worked at several jobs as a laborer but at no time during their marriage did he hold a responsible, remunerative position. After the birth of the couple's first child the family's financial situation became difficult and they took up residence in a settlement house. Mr. H. became increasingly alcoholic and lost his unremunerative job. Mrs. H. continued, however, to defend her husband with amazing devotion. The family then returned to Mrs. H's parents where they felt rejected. Later they went to live with Mr. H's mother and the patient sought employment. Her mother-in-law proved to be so alcoholic that Mrs. H. worried for the safety of her small son whom she loved deeply and handled with sensitivity and affection. A relative offered Mr. and Mrs. H. a primitive house which they accepted. It was necessary for Mrs. H. to support the family as her husband was drinking and doing little but odd jobs. Mrs. H. became thin, tense, complained of being forgetful and suffered from a brief period of confusion during which she was unable to work. Soon Mrs. H. became pregnant again. After the birth of the child Mrs. H. returned from the hospital to their house, the structure and furnishings of which were so inadequate that it seemed impossible as a residence. At about this time Mr. H. told the patient that he no longer regarded her as sexually attractive and that he was having relations elsewhere. When the baby was slightly over a month old Mrs. H. secured a position as a waitress, at the same time attempting to care for her two children and her household. An accident to herself and an illness of her husband added to her concern. In March, 1941, when the baby was two months old Mrs. H. wrote to a friend, "I am awfully tired and awfully blue. I feel dizzy, confused and lower than low. I snap out of it momentarily and then back I go. I think my anxiety comes mostly because I am trying to decide something which right now I am incapable of deciding. I think in many ways John and I are no good for each other and in many ways wouldn't be much good without each other, and that all is part of the problem."

Mrs. H. grew increasingly confused and depressed and two weeks later after having intimated suicidal intent she was taken to a private institution for mental disorders. On admission there Mrs. H. was obviously confused, agitated and in great emotional distress. Her speech was retarded and its content confined to the topic of fear of injuring someone and of a wish to harm herself. On several occasions she placed her head in the toilet bowl and pulled the flushing lever. She said she did not deserve to be helped and should be sent to jail. She constantly sought assurance that she had not harmed anyone. At no time was there any evidence that she was hallucinated. She was soon placed on electroshock treatment. After ten treatments the patient seemed somewhat better and the electroshock was discontinued. Soon she relapsed and a course of insulin coma therapy was begun. After fifty coma hours Mrs. H. showed a brief period of moderate improvement but soon became worse. After eight months in the private institution the patient was transferred to a state hospital. On arrival there she was mildly depressed but discussed her situation quite rationally. Three weeks after her admission Mrs. H. suddenly became tense, fearful, perplexed, suspicious and so retarded that she could hardly speak. She constantly sought out her ward physician from whom she wished repeated assurance that she was not the wicked person she felt herself to be. It soon transpired that this relapse had followed the receipt of amorous overtures from a male patient whom she had met in the ward kitchen. A few weeks after this recurrence of acute symptoms Mrs. H was seen at a staff conference. At that time she asked, "Why did you stop giving me shock treatments? Is it because—one minute I think it is because I am feeling so well and because you think I am better, and then I think, 'Well, probably the doctors think they wouldn't make me any different, probably they thought the treatments couldn't help me.' Then I think they probably have people they think could profit more by treatment and probably I won't be any better."

Again Mrs. H. improved and six months after her admission to the state hospital she seemed so well that she was permitted to spend a week end with her parents. On her return she was bewildered and preoccupied with depressive ideas. She sat about the ward worrying about her inadequacies and her inability to solve her problems. With questionable judgment she was permitted to continue work in the ward serving room. There she viewed the various knives and queried in her mind if she should not use one on herself. At this point psychotherapy was begun. Slow but sustained improvement followed and sixteen months after her admission to the private institution she left the state hospital in care of her parents. Follow-up psychotherapy was continued for a period. Now for eight years Mrs. H. has been well. She has divorced her husband and has resumed teaching.

In the case of Mrs. H., the physician is dealing with a woman with a basically sound and well adjusted personality who was subjected to a combination of stressful circumstances that finally proved too formidable to be met successfully. She married a psychopathic, indolent, alcoholic man who failed to support her. A college friend commented that Mrs. H. had, before her marriage, been well aware of her fiancé's problems but, in her opinion, Mrs. H's need to protect and champion the "underdog" had been a factor in her marriage—a characteristic which she had long manifested. A cousin of the husband who for a time had lived near Mr. and Mrs. H. wrote: "I urged C. not to let John drink but she always defended him. When I went to their apartment and was critical of John she would rush across the room, throwing her arms around him as though I intended to hit him." As time went on her husband not only failed to support Mrs. H. but subjected her to many humiliating experiences, compelled her to undergo many hardships and flaunted his marital infidelity. The physiological stress of her second pregnancy and the birth of her baby, the burden of caring for it and her household, the necessity of supporting the family and the prospect of raising her children under such pernicious circumstances undoubtedly enkindled an intolerable anxiety as a reaction to the hostile component in the ambivalence felt toward her husband. Overwhelmed by this hostility which she also turned on herself with resulting suicidal impulses Mrs. H. developed a psychotic depression. It is of interest to note that this depression did not yield to electroshock but that recovery took place under psychotherapy.

Another speculation concerning hostility as a component in Mrs. H's personality is perhaps worthy of mention. It will be remembered that after Mrs. H. had begun to improve she spent a weekend with her parents and that immediately thereafter suffered a relapse with depression, anxiety and confusion. Long before Mrs. H. became ill she told a friend that she had a deep feeling of hostility toward her mother. It may be conjectured that with feelings of hostility still but weakly repressed the presence of her mother reanimated these feelings and that they constituted such an anxiety-producing threat that her depression reappeared.

One may suggest still further that this component of hostility may, through reaction formation, have contributed to certain of Mrs. H's personality characteristics. When the patient entered the hospital the friend mentioned commented on Mrs. H's unusual aptitude for handling hostile parents or children. This quality may well have been a defense against her own hostility.

BIBLIOGRAPHY

Kraines, Samuel A.: Mental Depressions and Their Treatment. New York, The Macmillan Co., 1957.

Speiderman, E. S., and Farberow, N. L.: Clues to Suicide. New York, Blakiston Division, McGraw Book Co., 1957.

CHAPTER XXVII

Psychotic Disorders (*Continued*)

Schizophrenic Reactions

In the "normal," "average" or socially well adjusted individual we find a certain orderliness and harmony in the mental life. The various expressions of the personality blend into a coherent, composite picture. Thought is logical, feeling is congruous, action more or less expedient and fitting and sentiments are characterized by a subtle blending of affect and idea. There is such a synthesis of these different aspects of the personality that they seem to create a harmonious dynamic system of cognitive, affective, conative and constitutional forces. We are so accustomed to this harmonious blending of activity, emotional manifestation, ideational content and other expressions of personality organization on the part of our acquaintances that a serious lack of such agreement seems almost inconceivable to one not familiar with abnormal psychology. As we come to study mental disorders, however, we find a group of psychotic reactions characterized by disturbances in the harmonious fusion and co-ordination of the various elements and aspects of the personality. In this impaired unity of the personality, affect tends to be inappropriate, thought to be disorderly, behavior to be regressive and reality to be falsified in the form of hallucinations and delusions. Contributing to this impoverishment of the personality is a tendency to the development of disorganizing fantasy states and to an autistic withdrawal of self with resulting deterioration of habits.

While it is relatively easy to describe some of the more striking characteristics of schizophrenia, no definition of this mental illness has yet received universal assent. Although one of the commonest of serious mental disorders, its essential nature is probably the least understood. Because of the heterogeneity of the manifestations, it may be more accurate to speak of the group of schizophrenias rather than to think of the disordered reactions as a single disease entity. There is, therefore, an increasing inclination to think of schizophrenia as a term for a number of somewhat similar patterns of psychobiological reactions to life situations which the individual has found too difficult to meet. He is not able to deal effectively with needs, drives and inhibiting factors on an adult level. It is also more fruitful to study the patient and what he does than to investigate a possible impersonal disease process. Perhaps schizophrenia can best be looked upon as a form of adjustment characterized by a withdrawal into an autistic state accompanied by delusional preoccupation. If the individual is not sufficiently integrated to handle his overwhelming anxiety by employing less drastic defense mechanisms he may attempt to find some measure of security and satisfaction in the more primitive narcissistic defenses characteristic of schizophrenia.

History of Schizophrenia

Although not so called, the clinical picture we now know as schizophrenia has long been recognized. In 1849 John Conolly (1794–1866) of Hanwell Asylum in England the champion of "no restraint," stated in his Croonian Lectures: "Young persons not infrequently fall into a state somewhat resembling melancholia, without any discoverable cause of sorrow, and certainly without any specific grief; they become indolent or pursue their usual occupations or recreations mechanically and without interest; the intellect, the affections, the passions, all seem inactive or deadened and the patients become utterly apathetic."

The term dementia praecox (démence précoce) was first used by the Belgian psychiatrist Morel in 1860 in the case of a boy of fourteen who previously had always been "first in his examinations, and that without effort and almost without study. . . . Unconsciously he lost his cheerfulness and became sober, taciturn, and showed a tendency to solitude." The boy showed a "state of melancholy depression and a hatred of his father even with the idea of killing him. . . . The young invalid progressively forgot all that he had learned, and his brilliant intellectual faculties entered into a very disturbing period of arrest. A kind of inactivity bordering on stupidity replaced his former activity and when I saw him again it looked as if a transition into an irrecoverable state of dementia praecox was taking place."

Morel interpreted this disorganization of personality as an arrest of development to be included with mental deficiency as a "variety of intellectual, physical and moral degeneracy" resulting from heredity.

The next step in the history of dementia praecox was Hecker's description in 1871 of *hebephrenia,* although the term had previously been used by Kahlbaum. "The characteristic features of hebephrenia," wrote Hecker, "above all are: its appearance in connection with puberty, the succession or changing appearance of various forms (melancholia, mania and confusion), the very quick termination in a psychic enfeeblement and a characteristic form of final deterioration the evidences of which can be seen in the first stages of the disease." He considered hebephrenia to be a progressive disease of puberty and adolescence.

Another step in the development of the dementia praecox concept was the description of *catatonia,* or "*tension insanity,*" by Kahlbaum in 1874.

He described catatonia as "that condition in which the patient sits quietly or completely mute and motionless, immovable, with a staring countenance, the eyes fixed on a distant point and apparently completely without volition, without any reaction to sensory impressions, sometimes with a full fledged cerea flexibilitas as in catalepsy." Kahlbaum assumed that catatonia was the symptom of a structural brain disease.

In 1896 Emil Kraepelin (1856–1926), professor of psychiatry at Munich, often referred to as the great systematist of psychiatry, offered the proposition that a common denominator exists among such apparently unrelated syndromes as the hebephrenia of Hecker, the catatonia of Kahlbaum and many paranoid psychoses. By defining dementia praecox as a distinct syndrome, he introduced order into what had been a clinical chaos so far as observation and classification had been concerned.

In 1906 Adolf Meyer (1866–1950), the first director of the Henry Phipps Psychiatric Clinic and for many years professor of psychiatry at Johns Hopkins University, began to develop the thesis that dementia praecox is not a disease entity but rather a type of reaction developing in certain personalities as a result of progressive difficulty in adaptation and that the accumulation of faulty habits of reaction lead to a "habit deterioration."

Another landmark in the history of dementia praecox was the introduction by Eugen Bleuler (1857–1939) in 1911 of the term "*schizophrenia*." Bleuler was professor of psychiatry at the University of Zurich and director of the Burghöltzli Clinic, positions now held by his son, Manfred Bleuler. Following Bleuler's suggestion there has been an increasing tendency to supplant the designation *dementia praecox* by the name *schizophrenia* (splitting of the mind), since the disharmony or "split" of the psychobiological expression of the organism which we call mind, and the breaking up of a former normal synthesis of thought, feeling and activity, are now considered more characteristic and distinctive of the reaction than are symptom-complex and outcome as stressed by Kraepelin.

Conceptions of Schizophrenia

Since present conceptions of schizophrenia are largely based upon the formulations of Kraepelin, Bleuler, Meyer and Freud, a brief presentation of their respective formulations is added.

Kraepelin was not interested in the psychological meaning of the symptoms of dementia praecox but through his keen observations gave an excellent clinical description of the disorder and classified it into types (simple, hebephrenic, catatonic and paranoid). Bleuler and Meyer, on the other hand, greatly advanced the psychiatric understanding of schizophrenia by their interpretation in dynamic terms of the symptomatic manifestations observed.

KRAEPELIN'S FORMULATIONS. As previously indicated, Kraepelin brought together varied mental syndromes which he concluded were manifestations of a single disease entity to which he gave the name *dementia praecox*, a term previously having a more limited application.

He thought these clinical syndromes arose from the same disease process since they had in common the following features: a beginning in adolescence or early adulthood; a progression toward a similar state of "dementia"; similar morbid processes were, Kraepelin assumed, the causes of the various clinical features. These causes, he believed, might be either a degenerative disease of the brain or metabolic disturbances that produced autointoxication. He believed, too, that injury to the germ plasm might be of significance in its development. Kraepelin was of the opinion that the clinical results of these processes consisted of a weakening of emotional and volitional reactions and a loss of harmonious connections among emotional, volitional and intellectual reactions. He gave an extremely comprehensive and lucid description of the clinical features of dementia praecox but was critical of any attempt to explain the behavior of the patient on a psychological basis.

Bleuler's Formulations. From 1885 to 1897 Bleuler spent many hours each day at the mental hospital in Rheinau, Switzerland, studying individual patients in an effort to understand what, through their symptoms, they were saying or doing. He came to the conclusion that it was wrong to compare even the extreme deterioration of what Kraepelin called dementia praecox with the state of mind of the mentally defective or with that of organic deterioration caused by severe brain atrophy, that therefore the label "dementia praecox" could no longer be considered satisfactory. He pointed out, too, that the patient's psychological reactions to his environment are very complicated and differentiated, quite different in kind from the elementary, simple reactions of feeble-minded persons and those with organic brain disease. Bleuler believed, therefore, that the disease was not one of *de*-mentia, a state of diminished mind, but a disharmonious state of mind in which most contradictory tendencies, thoughts and potentialities were existing together, so that the harmony of the personality was split. According to this conception, the outcome of the disease was not necessarily one of deterioration, as Kraepelin had maintained, and the diagnosis had nothing to do with the course of the disease. Bleuler was the first to point out that it was not only interesting but extremely important to consider seriously and from a scientific point of view the content of the patient's thoughts, of his trends, of his instincts and of everything which he did. He noticed if the patient's hallucinations and delusions were thoroughly studied they could be brought in connection with his life history, with early hopes and fears and with his early relationships with parents and siblings.

Prior to Bleuler's time it was believed that every mental symptom was caused by an underlying physical disorder. Psychological symptoms, such as delusions, hallucinations, mannerisms and catatonic musculature signs had been looked at in the same way as aphasia, apraxia or reflex disturbances. Influenced by the firm and prevailing belief that all psychoses, and even neuroses, were of somatic origin, Bleuler hesitated to conclude that all the morbid manifestations in schizophrenia, or that schizophrenia itself, was of a functional nature and could be understood psychologically. He therefore distinguished between primary and secondary symptoms.

He designated as primary signs those which he considered were the direct manifestations of a hypothetical somatic morbid process. As primary signs he included a peculiar loosening of the associational links in thinking, a morbid ambitendence and ambivalence which dominated the affective life of the patient and a tendency to replace reality by fantasy which was responsible for the various manifestations of autism. Among the secondary symptoms, or those that he believed were of psychic origin, were delusions which he would explain by the patient's frustrations and hopes, a part of the hallucinations, the mannerisms, the catatonic muscular symptoms and a large part of the complicated attitudes which others had called deterioration or dementia. He believed that the secondary symptoms were attempts at adaptation to the primary disturbance. After Bleuler had become convinced of the importance of psychological influences in the morbid picture of schizophrenia, it became clear to him that the disorder should be treated by psychotherapy. He stressed that a sound, strong and personal relationship between nurse and patient and between physician and patient would exercise beneficial therapeutic influence on the latter.

In 1897 Bleuler left Rheinau and became professor of psychiatry in Zurich and director of the Burghöltzli Clinic. Here Bleuler and his first assistant, Carl Jung, became acquainted with Freud who spent a period at Zurich. As a result, Bleuler developed a great interest in psychoanalysis at a time when few psychiatrists had accepted Freud's teachings. He concluded that to a large extent schizophrenic symptoms could be understood by the same symbolization which Freud had discovered in dreams and in neurotic developments. Bleuler's conceptions of schizophrenia and the descriptions of his observations were published in 1912. An English translation, *Dementia Praecox or the Group of Schizophrenias* was published in 1950. Although Meyer, probably justifiably, criticized Bleuler's conception of schizophrenia as assuming an unwarranted dualism of mind and body, this monograph is nevertheless one of the classics of psychiatry.

MEYER'S FORMULATION. Meyer's more dynamic conception of schizophrenia and his naturalistic behavioral approach in its formulation appeared earlier than Bleuler's work. His views were first presented in a symposium on dementia praecox at a meeting of the British Medical Association at Toronto in 1906. He emphasized the clinical picture of schizophrenia, not as an autonomous disease entity, but as a maladaptation logically understandable in terms of the patient's experiences and life history. He emphasized the concepts of habit deterioration and of reaction types. The schizophrenic reaction, he believed, can best be understood as a habit disorganization resulting from a progressive maladaptation with an increasing use of substitutive reactions instead of effective ones, as "a substitution of inefficient and faulty attempts to avoid difficulties rather than to meet them by decisive action." The result is a disorganization of the personality and a final withdrawal from reality. Many of the clinical symptoms represent abortive and "twisted" attempts at balance and reconstruction. He expressed the opinion that the failure to find any structural or physiological changes in neurons excludes an organic etiology, although he believed that an inferior constitution as well as a great variety of pathologic conditions of a physical nature may add to the individual's load of handicaps. He emphasized disharmonies and deterioration of habit as one of the fundamental characteristics of the reaction. Meyer was one of the first to emphasize that the interest should be not so much in a classificatory diagnosis as in the facts and factors at work in the individual patient and in his assets. While admiring Kraepelin's description of the reaction Meyer did not subscribe to his invariably unfavorable prognosis of a progressive intellectual deterioration. As schizophrenic reactions, Meyer would include "disturbances developing in particular constitutional types and expressed in vague, autistic fancy, projections, passivity, paranoid systemization, formal disorders of language and behavior, incongruity of affect and motivity disturbances." He further described schizophrenic reactions as "twists and fundamental or fancy-born incongruities more or less foreign to average, mature, waking life." Because of the close identification of the term schizophrenia with dementia praecox, Meyer preferred the term "parergasia," meaning thereby distorted or "twisted" behavior, performance, or psychobiologically integrated behavior. While etymologically descriptive, this designation has not been generally adopted. His formulation of schizophrenia has contributed greatly to a dispelling of the artificial dichotomy of mind and body and to the establishment of the proposition that mental disorder is a function of biological behavior.

Through his adaptation of the word-association test (page 626) devised by Galton, Jung contributed much to the theory of the psychogenic origin of schizophrenia. Its use may enable the therapist to ascertain emotional problems to which the patient was unable to adjust successfully. In referring to the apathetic attitude resulting from the withdrawal of interest from the real world as observed in schizophrenia Jung used the term introversion of libido—a centripetal movement of energy.

FREUD'S FORMULATION. The psychoanalysts speak of schizophrenia as a narcissistic withdrawal and regression associated with a weakness of the ego, the strength of which may have been weakened through either psychogenic or somatic factors. From this point of view, the individual goes back to the early narcissistic stages of libidinous development. He sacrifices the ego organization, and the state of mind has a meaning from the point of view of the id only. The superego is pushed aside and is without effective power. In the more severe schizophrenic reactions the regression is to primitive, autoerotic stages and is sufficient to provide satisfaction of the id. Remainders of the ego and of the superego functions are, however, usually present to some degree. The ego is deprived of its powers but is not destroyed. It is so altered, nevertheless, that it permits a break with reality. The ego organization forms and then disintegrates. The psychoanalytical school speaks of schizophrenia not merely as a regression but postulates the theory that there is a destruction of the capacity for transference, a fact which in the opinion of many analysts makes successful psychoanalytical therapy impossible.

At the present time the classical concepts of Kraepelin, Meyer, Bleuler and Freud are all more or less shattered. There is a great divergence in concepts concerning this large group of mental disorders. Psychiatry has not yet progressed beyond working hypotheses concerning them. There tends, however, to be an increasing emphasis on subjective psychological experiences.

Causes

Anthropologically minded psychiatrists have pointed out that certain types of physique, temperament and energy direction appear to be associated with a frequency to be regarded as significant, thereby suggesting that the constitution and vital processes of the organism tend to produce specific, correlated forms of bodily structure and mental reactions. In their opinion the prepsychotic personality characteristics of the schizophrenic patient with his introversion and schizoid temperament are so frequently associated with the leptosome, athletic or dysplastic physique of Kretschmer, or the ectomorphic body form of Sheldon, that a specific relationship must exist between physical constitution and personality organization in schizophrenia. While such a correlation seems at times to be present, it by no means exists in all instances and is now generally doubted. A discussion of the alleged interrelated physical and personality characteristics of the schizoid was presented in Chapter III, Personality Development and Structure, and will therefore not be repeated at this point.

The influence of *genetic factors* in the causation of schizophrenia is controversial. Statistical data compiled by Kallmann of the New York Department of Mental Hygiene indicate that schizophrenia occurs more frequently in families which include a known case of schizophrenia than it does in the general population. He postulates that there is an inherited predisposition to schizophrenia resulting from the presence of a specific recessive genetic factor. Kallmann believes that a true schizophrenic psychosis does not develop under usual life conditions unless there is an inherited predisposition, and it is his opinion that whether or not such a "predisposed" individual develops a psychosis depends upon a complex interplay of constitutional and environmental factors. According to Kallmann's statistics, the average expectancy of schizophrenia in the general population is 0.85 per cent whereas the expectancy in the children of one schizophrenic parent is 16.4 per cent. In his study of schizophrenia in twins, he found that if the disorder exists in one of monozygotic twins it occurs also in the other twin in 85.8 per cent of cases but that the expectancy for the dizygotic twin partner of a schizophrenic person is but 14 per cent. In full siblings of the schizophrenic, the expectancy is also 14 per cent. In calling attention to these statistics it should be borne in mind that in assembling them no consideration was given to all those life situations and intrafamily influences generally recognized to be psychopathologically conducive to the development of schizophrenia.

Frequently the opinion of the psychiatrist is sought as to the influence on eugenics in case of marriage of the relative of a schizophrenic individual. In such an instance, advice should not be based merely on the statistical data mentioned above but also, and perhaps even more, on a complete assessment of, and full consideration for, the personality adjustment and maturity and the many other unique personal factors that characterize the prospective parent.

Although not yet established, many research investigators believe that schizophrenia is not merely a personality deviation or disorganization but rather that there are disturbances in metabolism, endocrine balance and body chemistry that may contribute to the disorder. Various neuropathological changes have been described but none has been sufficiently uniform or typical to enable one to make a diagnosis under the microscope.

Although we cannot dismiss heredity, endocrine imbalance, neuropathological changes and metabolic errors or other constitutional vulnerability as contributing agents, the trend is to relate its origin to the psychodynamics of personality development. Increasing stress is now being placed on the influence of early interpersonal relationships within the family that either fail to meet the child's emotional needs or are emotionally traumatizing to him. As a result he develops attitudes and identifications that so check or distort the development of his personality that he is ill prepared to meet the experiences, stresses and responsibilities of mature personality and social functioning. It will be found with significant frequency that schizophrenic patients have spent their childhood in emotionally unwholesome family settings with their dynamic interactions between the future patient and parent or sibling. There is a high frequency of emotionally disturbing parental or sibling influences. A parent may have been lost by death. One or both parents may have been badly adjusted personalities. The combination of an aggressively domineering, perhaps rejecting, father and an oversolicitous mother is not rare. The child may have had ambivalent feelings toward one or both parents. The preschizophrenic child is often more sensitive, less happy and less social than his healthy sibling. Frequently he has felt rejected. A large percentage of schizophrenic disturbances occur in persons who have been "shut in," have presented a barrier of remoteness, have withheld themselves from spontaneous, satisfying, emotional relationship with others. Sometimes, however, social isolation in early youth is a consequence rather than a cause of schizophrenia. Some preschizophrenic adolescents concentrate on religious or intellectual interests to the exclusion of social or recreational ones. Not rarely such persons may early have created defenses which involved avoidance or restriction of social contacts. The resulting situation has been one of separateness, self-concealment and psychological isolation within which the patient has maintained an autonomous inner emotional life. Many such preschizophrenics have been inclined to indulge in vague, autistic fantasies and empty ambitions. Their emotional and social maladjustments and inadequacies have predisposed to, and have often been forerunners of, frank schizophrenic reactions.

If, as is the present trend of opinion, schizophrenia represents a faulty reaction to life situations, a maladapted way of life manifested by an individual grappling unsuccessfully with environmental stresses and internal difficulties, its causes are to be found in the interpersonal experiences of childhood and the environmental ones of later life, in the limits of his adaptive capacity and in the mental mechanisms and patterns of reactions by which he has attempted to deal with his special problems—faulty methods which constitute the symptoms of the disorder. If the personality has been laden with internal tensions and contradictions, the simple routine of everyday living may have been too difficult with the result that it slowly disintegrated in the form of an insidious schizophrenia.

To understand the etiology of a schizophrenic disorder in a given person and to formulate a diagnosis in psychobiological, dynamic terms it is first necessary to know his particular life history as fully as possible. The therapist will therefore seek to formulate the clinical picture of schizophrenia in terms of the familiar problems and experiences of human life rather than those of an impersonal disease entity. Perhaps, instead of speaking of schizophrenia as if it were an entity, one should speak of a schizophrenic solution of a psychological problem. Only through a careful analysis of the personality and its evolution, of an equally detailed study of the concatenated sequence of life events and subjective experiences of the individual are the causes of the psychosis to be found, its manifestations understood and its psychological connections discovered and formulated. Among these factors are early conditioning experiences, intrapsychic conflicts, insistent but consciously rejected demands of various instinctive drives and urges, feelings of guilt, emotional and sexual insecurity, as well as various other long-standing, troublesome problems and frustrated purposes that have given rise to anxiety. In the adolescent, particularly, there may be a conflict between an artificial and perfectionistic code of morals on the one hand, and intensifying sexual impulses on the other. Again there may be increasing rebellious tendencies or a growing realization of unfavorable comparisons with one's fellows. The patient's system of ideals may be too rigid to permit any reconciliation with gross instinctual impulses or to tolerate an increasing awarness of inferiority in competition. Attempts at solution become symptoms of the mental illness. Attempts to repudiate instinctual impulses may lead to autistic reverie, to withdrawal from interpersonal relationships and perhaps to self-punitive measures.

In addition to such specific factors the psychiatrist often has to deal with a personality, imperfectly organized and inadequately prepared for the life experiences to be confronted, inclined to give up the struggle with reality, manifesting evasive and substitutive ways of meeting problems, reacting to handicaps with oversensitiveness and aloofness, and tending to secure satisfactions, not from the real world, but from a subjective world of the individual's own making. Many have been "solitary, silent and serious." They have felt insecure, unloved, unwanted and perhaps angry. It has been difficult for them to participate in adequate emotional relationships with others. Most persons who develop schizophrenia have failed to advance to mature, adult types of social and personal adaptation and integration. While it is by no means true in all schizophrenics, and the same immaturity is often found underlying other personality disorders, yet in a considerable number of cases it will be found that the patient was of passive-dependent type. It has long been observed that at times the mother of a schizophrenic son has been overprotective and never permitted his emotional emancipation from her. As a result he never attained such maturity of personality as is necessary for successful social and heterosexual adjustment. It is now recognized that the father also may presumably be responsible not only for many emotional maladjustments of childhood but he may also be the source of personality problems that may eventuate in schizophrenia. This seems to be especially the case if the father is either a passive, ineffectual person or a sadistic, tyrannical parent.

Not rarely, the schizophrenic has been given to bizarre beliefs and cults or to neurotic complaints. Long before his manifest psychosis he may have felt that no one understood his lonely, unhappy personality. Underneath he may have been daydreaming, hating, fearing and perhaps despairing. In the opinion of many psychiatrists schizophrenia is so much the product of the personality that they question the propriety of speaking of it as a disease. Finally, it should be said that the causes for each schizophrenic's psychosis are presumably individual and multiple. In spite of the difficulty at times, the therapist seeks to establish a dynamic formulation of a dynamic process, *i.e.*, to discover a psychological train of events in which it will be apparent that complex factors have contributed to form an understandable whole.

Age of Onset

The age of onset is from late childhood to late middle age although the most frequent age is adolescence and early adult life. While uncommon it is not as rare in children (3 to 13 years) as formerly believed. The more fully the previous history is taken the more frequently there will be found a previous manifestation not merely of schizoid traits but even of phenomena that were nearly or quite psychotic in nature. The high incidence during adolescence is not unnatural. There is probably, however, no specific relationship between schizophrenia and the puberty period, which is normally a period of turbulence, of emotional crosscurrents and of struggle to adapt emergent, maturing urges to the demands of a restraining world. At that time, the individual is precipitated into a critical emotional period without preparation or understanding. He is perplexed by new problems, particularly by sex, religious, vocational and social ones. He may be plagued by a desire for independence or crippled by a too prolonged dependence. Self-consciousness, sensitiveness, moodiness, vague yearnings, sudden outbursts, defensive attitudes, the tendency to indulge in strange fancies, to project inadequacies and to be irritable are traits often particularly marked in adolescence and frequently, especially in its early course, similar characteristics are met with in schizophrenia.

Frequency

Schizophrenia is one of the most frequent forms of the major psychoses, constituting from 15 to 20 per cent of the first admissions to public hospitals for mental diseases. Because the disorder tends to chronicity and in many instances does not shorten life it will usually be found that 60 per cent of the population of state hospitals is made up of schizophrenic patients.

Symptoms

While there is a striking contrast between a normal, well integrated individual and the person reacting with a malignant form of schizophrenic psychosis, there is frequently no abrupt transition from the schizoid type of personality to the manifest psychosis. Certain disharmonies of thought, of habits and of interests may have long existed. In adolescence there may have been a tendency to loneliness and perhaps to slight depressions. Colorfulness of personality may seem to have been lost. There may have been a vagueness of thinking, a blandness of affect, a tendency to projection of topics touching a special personal sensitivity and perhaps a tendency to be jealous of those more happily adjusted. As seen in the institution for mental disorders, even the so-called "early" case of schizophrenia has frequently been becoming mentally sick for a considerable period before reaching the mental hospital, although the patient's family has not usually appreciated the nature or significance of any personality change. The *mode of onset*, except in the catatonic type, is often a gradual evolutionary process and there may be a transitional "preschizophrenic" phase of a year or two. At this early stage there may be no single symptom that is pathognomonic of the disease. In some instances the early symptoms are more suggestive of a psychoneurosis than of a psychosis. The impoverished, rigid affect of later stages has not yet appeared. A common early symptom is an aloofness, a withdrawal behind barriers which if they could be penetrated would reveal loneliness, hopelessness, hatred and fear. Frequently the patient seems preoccupied and dreamy; his friends may speak of him as appearing "far away." He does not empathize with the feelings of others and manifests little concern about the realities of his life situation. His plans for his future are often vague and unrealistic.

The schizophrenic suffers from a feeling of rejection and from an intolerable lack of self-respect. The characteristic way from which he protects himself against insult is by withdrawal from emotional involvements with other people. The resultant isolation is a protection against painful human relationships but the loneliness contributes further to his feelings of rejection and hence to further withdrawal. The patient no longer trusts or confides in anyone. Instead of mingling with others he remains at home where he may sulk in his room and show an increasing indifference to members of his family, to accustomed interests and to the demands and opportunities of his environment. It seems as if a fear of interpersonal contact had driven the patient into a state of regression and withdrawal. There may be a seemingly unexplainable deterioration in work. There is a shallowness of affect, a paucity of emotional responsiveness, and an impairment in richness and variety of emotional expression. A loss of appreciation of conventional values is noted. An insidious change in mood and outlook takes place. Acquaintances may attribute the patient's listlessness, loss of spontaneity, of ambition, of interest in competition with his group and of sustained effort in pursuit of former goals to laziness. An irritable discontent is common. The patient easily feels slighted and may begin to believe that others are talking about him. He may become ill at ease, restless, taciturn, unapproachable, and wonder what interpretation others are putting on his behavior. A superficial attitude of superiority is not uncommon. Less heed is paid to social amenities and social requirements while former loyalties and affections become blunted. The patient becomes disregardful of, and even resistant to, conventionality. Frequently he becomes neglectful of personal care and cleanliness. Ruminations on sexual topics are not rare. The patient may feel that something wrong or unusual is going on in his environment. Mysterious meanings are discovered until finally misinterpretations and suspicions may cause him to move from place to place. For a few weeks or months the new environment may be free from any suggestion of hostility, then the patient begins to feel that people are watching him or conspiring against him. Odd mannerisms or ways of acting may appear but they cause the patient no concern. Some patients express undue worry over their physical condition. This is especially suggestive of an approaching schizophrenia when the complaints are unusual or unlikely. The patient may add that he feels he should build himself up by means of dieting and exercise. The early schizophrenic is often preoccupied with abstract speculations or with metaphysical ponderings on such subjects as creation and causality, or with religious doubts, mysticisms and meaningless problems. A young truck driver who had but a seventh grade education wrote an essay entitled, "The Imperative Mind." In the very early stages, usually terminated before they reach a hospital for mental diseases, a few patients recognize that their ideas of reference and other abnormal mental experiences are unnatural; they may wish to know the meaning of their experiences and to understand their problems. Occasionally they may have some appreciation of the causes that have led to their illness. At this time they may be willing to discuss their problems. Later this desire is lost and the patient becomes inaccessible while in many the desire never existed. During these early stages before the construction of an elaborate symbolic system that becomes accepted as reality, the conflicts are much less disguised and it may often be possible to discover the problems which the patient is living out in the drama of his psychotic behavior. Occasionally the patient may show some sensorial confusion during the first few days of an acute episode.

As we pass from this initial, and what might be called premonitory stage, or stage of incubation, to the manifest psychosis, there appears an apparent *poverty and disharmony of feeling tone*. The dulling of finer feelings and an insidious narrowing of interests noted in the incipient stages become progressive. The patient is unable to feel and regulate emotions properly. There is a withdrawal of feeling or affect from external realities back into the self. As the disease progresses and the emotional impoverishment increases, the patient becomes indifferent, not merely to those sentiments and subjective values that make life worth living for the person in mental health, but, apparently existing at a vegetative level, he may be unconcerned as to fundamental comforts and needs. A few patients show, not a burned-out affectivity, but a definite, prevailing one, such as euphoria or depression. These feelings, however, usually lack depth or focus. The persistent mood, or emotional rigidity, has no relation to external circumstances or experiences and little or none to conscious mental content.

Another disturbance of affect is one in which emotional expression is unrelated to reality. This is manifested by an emotional disharmony, often first exhibited by inappropriate smiling or laughing and silly giggling. Frequently the disharmony is between mood and conscious idea; there may, for example, be but little subjective feeling of depression even when ideas of despondency are expressed. At times experiences and ideas that should evoke a certain emotional response will produce its opposite—an emotional disconnection or dissociation. The patient, for example, may with a silly laugh speak of the death of his beloved mother. Whenever there is a display of affect by the schizophrenic it seems superficial, unnatural and stilted, quite lacking in any infectious quality. At times one observes capricious, fitful, apparently causeless changes in affect and mood. This inferior affective capacity, the deterioration and impoverishment of emotional expression and the inadequate and inappropriate emotional responses to situations constitute one of the important ways in which the personality is disorganized or split, and attest the aptness of Bleuler's designation of schizophrenia.

One of the most generally accepted hypotheses advanced as an explanation of this serious disturbance in the affective life of the patient is that the affect, contrary to first impression, is not lost or destroyed but is withdrawn from the conscious, perceptive aspects of the patient's life, from matters of objective reality, and attached to complexes and other material in the unconscious. The affect is hidden, because it is fixed in special, limited constellations of ideas. According to this theory the disorganization or disorderliness of affect appears all the greater because it is associated with and determined not by one constellation of unconscious ideas but by many complexes among which there may be active conflict and discord. Since the affect is attached to and determined by material that is inaccessible the emotions appear out of harmony with the contents and expressions of consciousness, although they are really in harmony with the psychic material to which the affect is attached and by which they are governed. The emotional disturbance in schizophrenia may therefore not be really a deterioration but a displacement.

The emotional apathy of the schizophrenic individual may perhaps be theoretically explained in a somewhat different manner. One way by which the normal person may deal with difficult and threatening situations is by minimizing or ignoring them. It is conceivable, therefore, that the patient defends himself by building a wall of indifference around himself. Although this blunting of feeling may have arisen as a mechanism of defense against a definite troublesome situation in the inner world of the patient it irradiates and becomes a general behavior pattern of the personality.

When interest and affect are withdrawn from the conscious, familiar material with which they were formerly connected and are attached to the content of the unconscious, a state known as *depersonalization* may exist. The patient has feelings of vagueness, of unreality, of detachment, or of being a spectator of life instead of taking part in it. He feels himself changed throughout in comparison with his former state. As a result he no longer acknowledges himself as a personality. His actions seem mechanical and automatic. The patient does not believe he is another personality (transformation of personality) but has rather a sense of loss of the limits of his own personality with its directive ego. The identification of one's own personality may become indistinct or confused. It seems to the patient that he no longer has any internal self to which he can refer forces and influences. In his attempt to rationalize this sense, the patient may come to feel that parts of his body or his mind seem strange and as though not belonging to him. He may develop more nihilistic ideas and believe that he no longer has a body, that there is no world, or that he is dead. In addition to this change of self, the environment may seem unnatural and appear to have lost its character of reality. States of unreality are probably closely related to thought block, feelings of stupidity, fugues, dream states and other involuntary withdrawals.

From what has been said it will be seen that there is rarely a dominant affect in schizophrenia as is the case in manic-depressive psychoses. On the contrary, there are numerous inharmonious affects arising from conflicting desires and complexes, or the affect may be fixed to or absorbed by fantasies, by elaborate symbolic systems and other products of the unconscious. The result is a disorderliness and apparent involvement of affect that contribute to the peculiar disorganization of personality which characterizes the schizophrenic patient.

Among the disturbances of affect in schizophrenia, hypochondria is occasionally met with. Sometimes this depressive preoccupation with subjective bodily feelings seems to have for its purpose the exclusion of a disturbing contact with the problems of reality. Again a sort of vicarious relief is afforded if that which is troublesome within, a sense of guilt, for example, is expressed in terms of distress of the body for the processes of which the patient does not feel responsible. Bodily complaints are mainly present at the beginning of schizophrenia and later disappear. Frequently these complaints are bizarre or peculiar, such as a sense of electric currents in the genitals or the body is becoming smaller. Disturbances in reality and object relationships are always suggestive of schizophrenia.

One result of the schizophrenic's loss of capacity for attachment of energy and interest to external objects and reality and of his autistic preoccupations is a *narrowing of attention*. Interest, and therefore attention, is centered on subjective creations, on matters within and not without the patient. This lack of attention and of concentration gives rise to the misleading impression that the patient is intellectually impaired whereas he is intellectually inert. The replies of the schizophrenic individual are often trivial and uninformative because interests and energy are directed toward material not accessible to ordinary questioning. *Paralogia*, a condition in which the patient's reply shows that the question has been understood, but in which the answer, because of defective reasoning, is erroneous, is caused by the dereistic thinking to which the schizophrenic patient is particularly given.

While active attention—concentration—as just indicated, is often disturbed, yet passive attention is much less affected with the result that while the patient may be living in a world of fantasy he is still able to maintain a contact with reality sufficient for certain practical needs, yet often too inadequate for a socialized adjustment. Schizophrenics may be perplexed but rarely suffer from disturbances of the sensorium and therefore from confusion in the correct sense of the term.

Normally, *associations of ideas* follow one another with a definite logical connection, progressing to an ultimate completeness of thought, but in schizophrenia they may be shortened, fragmented, and otherwise so disturbed as to lack logical relationship. Although the disturbances of associations in schizophrenia do not become particularly marked until serious disorganization of the personality has taken place, yet not rarely one finds that long before any manifest psychosis developed the patient showed a loosening of the associational links in thinking. Later the patient may speak in generalities and abstractions which are difficult to grasp—a dereistic type of verbigeration rather than communicative talk. The use of eccentric, metaphorical expressions is not uncommon. Doubtless the communications of the schizophrenic patient are nearly always self-meaningful although often their significance is not grasped by others. One of the earliest symptoms observed by the psychiatrist may be a certain inconsequence of ideas and a thought sequence that is erratic and confused. There is a slight irrelevancy as if the patient has missed the point. As the disease becomes established there is a tendency for associative connections to become more involved, incongruous and at times so broken or incomplete that the patient's utterances become fragmentary, disconnected, illogical or even unintelligible. The train of thought may not be pursued to its logical goal with the result that thinking becomes diffuse and disorganized. Cause and effect may be interchanged. If aware of his disordered thinking, the patient may say that his thoughts are suddenly taken out of his head. Irrelevance in replies to questions, a feature which when consciousness is clear is particularly suggestive of schizophrenia, may be quite striking. Probably, however, irrelevance is not irrelevant to the patient and would be relevant to the listener if the latter had clues to the semantic significance of the patient's autistic productions. Set phrases may come to be used repeatedly as stereotypes. The thought productions of the schizophrenic person often become characterized by vague and unusual symbolism. It is believed that the disordered thought productions tend to express, by condensation, the various problems which concern the patient. Speech may show a curiously distorted use of language varying from a stilted and formal phraseology without apparent substance to a "word salad" of nouns and verbs having practically no articulated structure or even without apparently meaningful connection. Doubtless there was earlier a significance which became lost. Affectations in manner of speech are often observed. The patient may show a "flight into intellectualism." The following is taken from a schizophrenic production entitled "Equalitized Metabolic Demention Metabolism":

"Improper wave length—wave length changes, later visible death. That is a moving trollysis similar to circulation of life action. Born high focussating action may die through wave length charge and still live until visible death takes place.

"Education comes from radiation of action. Anyone can study all science in a compositive way. It takes a compositive mind to be able to understand. Can tell compositive minds by stromonized conception. The mind at birth takes on a birthification, becomes environmental by the radiation to it. Metabolism to dimension differ in every person is of actions of metabolism and dimension balancing. . . ."

How the thinking of a formerly well trained mind may become disorganized in schizophrenia is illustrated in the following intellectualized rumination taken from a letter written by a man who had had a scholastically brilliant college career and after graduation had spent two years at Oxford as a Rhodes scholar:

"I'm too utterly weary from battling with my financial-religious and general-religious problems to be able to survive any shock of learning that unhintably hard-won progress supposed to have been earned in the fraternal-religious problem is illusory. For that would wreck me—in my critically exhausted condition—with horror lest humanity—contrarily from being faith-imbued joy-multipliers of Revelations All Embracing God or Unfathomably Progressive Universe—are duped victims of God's opposite faith deluding us—with illusions of immortality, a Heavenly Father and of progress—into accommodation as evil-absorbers of His unconvertible and endless agonies and struggle."

There is probably no disturbance in the physical associative apparatus, the explanation for the disorders in the thinking of the schizophrenic being found in the great extent to which associations are directed by unconscious factors. Because of their origin in the unconscious, associations are broken, are led into bypaths, are fragmented, incongruous, do not progress, or are joined through common affects rather than through conscious, logical connection, with the result that various forms of incoherence follow. When the connections appear particularly loose we speak of the schizophrenic's thought as being "scattered." This means that the unconscious connection of ideas is unusually marked. This scattering is comparable to and is to be looked upon as having the same significance as free associations. There seems to be much, too, to suggest that the psychological processes operative in the associations of the schizophrenic patient are closely allied to the condensations, substitutions and other processes of dream-work in the normal person as discussed on page 633.

Many schizophrenics show a poverty of associations and of ideas, presumably because of preoccupation with material having its source largely in the unconscious and also because of the accompanying narrowing of attention. To be ascribed to these two conditions, as well, are the casual and trivial remarks and replies of the schizophrenic so peculiar to the disorder as to have important diagnostic significance.

Elements in repressed constellations of ideas may produce various ellipses, short-circuitings of ideas and even neologisms. These words of his own making are condensations and symbolizations of complexes with affect. Within their concealed meaning are compressed the condensations of words that refer to persons or things intimately related to the individual's particular conflict or psychic experience. The use of neologisms by the mental patient always suggests a schizophrenic psychosis.

In connection with disturbances of associations, mention should be made of the fact that in early schizophrenia a fairly typical flight of ideas may occur, which later tends to develop into incoherence.

Blocking may occur as associations approach painful conflict material. It results, perhaps, from a threat that repressed material is approaching awareness. It tends to arise largely in connection with special topics whereas neutral topics may be handled as usual.

The thinking of the schizophrenic tends to become dereistic; associations and symbols are formed in the unconscious, are molded and directed by affective constellations and instinctive undercurrents. They then rise into consciousness where as dereistic thinking they constitute a type of thought much like that of dreams. It may show a tendency to symbolism, displacement and condensation. Dereistic thinking is a pleasurable thinking that tends to falsify reality, to disregard realistic, logical and scientific thought and become autistic fantasy. It is not corrected by the logic of experiences or by the demands of the external world. Vigotsky, a Russian psychologist, believed that an impairment in the function and formation of concepts is the most important deterioration of thought occurring in schizophrenia. Frequently there is an impairment of abstract thinking as demonstrated by the patient's interpretation of proverbs.

Schizophrenic thinking is much like the prelogical thinking of children and of primitive man, both types tending to be paralogical in nature. In the undisciplined and imaginative thinking of the schizophrenic, the primitive man and the infant there seems, too, to be an absence of distinction between the external and the internal world. Ideas are often indistinctly and inexactly outlined. It has been shown by Rorschach test performances that what has been conceived as fantasy is really distortion, misconstruction and inaccuracy, but not fantasy in the sense of a new creation.

The dominant *ideational content* of the schizophrenic is often delusional in nature. Because the satisfactions sought by his beliefs are so highly disguised by their symbolism and because the needs in response to which the *delusions* have been created are often not apparent, the delusions of the schizophrenic often appear grotesque and meaningless. His delusions are never meaningless, however, but are specific and adapted to the peculiar psychological needs and situation of the individual and are in keeping with his particular life experiences, although conspicuously disregardful of reality. Although it is often difficult to ascertain, there is always a relevance in the schizophrenic's ideas and symbols to the problems and purposes of his personality. In referring to symbols, attention may be called to the fact that if he has artistic ability he may show symbolic condensations in his drawings or paintings.

The tendency of the schizophrenic's delusions to be grotesque, to be loosely organized, to center around themes of persecution, of grandiosity and of sex, to arise from autistic sources and yet to be expressed in a relatively clear setting is shown in the following letter addressed by a patient to one of the male physicians connected with the hospital in which she was under treatment:

"Dear Dr.———

"My Plan," or as mother used to call you, "The Little Plant," or else one little Plant for I was the other Plant, called "Tant." Will you please see that I am taken out of this hospital and returned to the equity court so I can prove to the court who I am and thereby help establish my identity to the world. Possibly you do not remember or care to remember that you married me May 21, 1882, while you were in England and that I made you by that marriage the Prince of Wales, as I was born Albert Edward, Prince of Wales, I am feminine absolutely, not a double person or a hermaphrodite, so please know I am England's feminine king—the king who is a king.

Your first duty is to me, and if you do not intend to do the right thing, helping me to get out of here, stop the thefts of clothing, money, jewelry, papers, letters, etc., etc.; you will please let me know so I can make some absolute change and further demand of the nations my release.

1874 Building was to have been a palace for my mother, father, myself and you, that is, if you are the one I married—so why not get busy and furnish it up as such when I go abroad. Make my trips (our trips?) short and return to America on important matters and have the right place to hold court. You and Dr. Black can take me to the equity court where I prove up my individuality and this must be done.

Sincerely,
"Tant"

Queen of Scotland, Empress of the World, Empress of China, Empress of Russia, Queen of Denmark, Empress of India, Maharajahess of Durban, "Papal authority" as a Protestant.

In the early stages of schizophrenia the delusions may not be fixed and the patient may at times be in doubt as to his ideas of reference or as to the hostility of his environment; later he becomes convinced that his delusions are real facts. At the onset of his psychosis the schizophrenic may have obsessive ideas that prove to be the early stages of a process that later becomes frankly one of externalization and projection.

Delusions in the schizophrenic often serve rather effectually in subjectively reorganizing his life situations and in dealing with such problems as thwarted trends and drives, frustrated hopes, biological inadequacies, feelings of insecurity, disowned qualities, gnawing feelings of guilt and the affective constellations and other contents of the unconscious. In no other type of mental disorder are the patient's problems, wishes and conflicts so thoroughly dramatized and symbolized in fantastic form. This fact and the schizophrenic's impairment of his ability to appreciate and test the reality of his fantasies tends to the creation of extravagant and bizarre delusions. The role of fantasy was well expressed by Macfie Campbell: "Fantasy is called on to supply what real life has denied, but the fantasies are not woven into a structure which is compatible with a normal social adaptation." There is a tendency to a reversion to belief in magical cause and effect. Some patients in their schizoid withdrawal show no evidence of delusional ideation.

In no other form of mental disorder do *hallucinations*, or the projection of impulses and inner experiences into the external world in terms of perceptual images, occur in the presence of clear consciousness so frequently as in schizophrenia. Their mechanism is not unlike that of hallucinations in other abnormal states but they tend to be more highly disguised in nature and to constitute a primitive form of adjustment and therefore of much more serious significance than is their presence in delirium or in dissociative states. It is not difficult to conceive of highly significant material in the schizophrenic's inner life as assuming hallucinatory vividness. It is but a step from the figurative "voice of conscience" to its audible perception. Unconscious material and unadjusted tendencies break through and create sense perceptions, perhaps highly symbolized, in response to psychological needs and problems. Disowned desires and feelings of guilt are projected as auditory hallucinations which, as the voice of conscience, accuse and criticize. The patient, incapable, because of his disorganized ego, of recognizing the origin or significance of his hallucinations, believes in the reality of these projected images, accepts them at face value and reacts in accordance with what he has accepted as reality. He can no longer distinguish between subjective and objective experiences with the result that he tends to alter reality with hallucinations and delusions. Hallucinations are not an early symptom of schizophrenia although in the absence of an adequate history they may appear so. As Freud points out, they are not possible until the patient's ego is so far disintegrated that the testing of reality no longer stands in the way.

The schizophrenic may find his hallucinations so serviceable that he is unwilling to relinquish them with the result that they come to constitute one of his cherished means of adjustment and he becomes occupied, not with a real, but with an hallucinatory world protected from the disturbances of reality. His hallucinations may be said to collaborate with delusions in the development of the same theme, the one by means of image symbols, the other by ideas.

But little need be said in the way of description of hallucinations in schizophrenia. They are more frequently auditory than of any other sense. Visual hallucinations are not particularly frequent and tend to be limited to acute phases of the psychosis. During their early occurrence hallucinations are often accompanied by considerable emotional tension and may have a disturbing and disquieting influence on the patient. As time passes they may cause but little concern and exert less influence upon behavior.

Among important symptoms of schizophrenia are the *disturbances of impulse and conation*, of action-tendencies or the striving aspects of the personality. Many of these odd, unexplained and sudden activities grow out of a lack of harmonious association and integration of strivings, affects and wishes—the existence of incompatible and frequently, also, of changing objectives.

The capricious, impulsive behavior of the schizophrenic is to be looked upon as a result of an ambivalence of impulse, a contradiction of conative tendencies. The concept of ambivalence, or contradictory manifestations of impulse, of idea or of affect, was greatly stressed by Bleuler, and considered by him to be a fundamental symptom of schizophrenia. It rests upon the principle that the true meaning of an idea, impulse or affect is to be found in the exact opposite of that manifestly expressed. Many psychiatrists believe that the conscious rejection and denial of expression of a desire yet its indirect and unrecognized expression through projection in the form of hallucination or delusion is a manifestation of the principle of ambivalence. At any rate, we find in schizophrenia a peculiar association of contradictions in mental or personality expressions. Ordinarily our behavior represents a compromise, a working harmony among diverse desires, a resultant of the contrasting considerations, forces and motives prompting us. In schizophrenia, on the contrary, the two conflicting impulses, one, many believe, of conscious origin, the other of unconscious, control behavior in erratic sequence, or even struggle simultaneously to direct it. There is a failure of integration of motive forces. Ambivalence may be manifested by an unstable blending of love and hate with sudden unaccountable shifts in affection and hostility, leading sometimes to impulsive episodes. Occasionally unpredictable suicidal impulses result in the unexpected death of a patient. Impulsive self-mutilation is not rare, especially in case of an adolescent masturbatory struggle.

At times a schizophrenic may consciously resist a certain impulse but nevertheless carry it through into action. Unconscious and dissociated tendencies acting in this way give the patient a feeling of being forced or controlled. The American psychiatrist, Hohman, expresses the opinion that a feeling of being forced may be a result of the fact that the fantasy world in which the schizophrenic patient lives rejects and disowns the experiences of the world of reality. This feeling of being forced may permit the entertainment of thoughts or the indulgence in behavior which the socially determined standards of the individual would not permit but for which, with his feelings of being forced, the patient no longer recognizes any responsibility.

A common disturbance of activity in the schizophrenic is an avoidance of concrete or spontaneous activity, a loss of initiative and purpose, and the development of a state of inaction sometimes designated as anergia. Energy is withdrawn from externality. This deterioration in habits of activity may perhaps best be considered as a loss of interest in, and a retreat from the world of reality, one of the means adopted by the schizophrenic in renouncing the world with which he cannot cope. Instead of being realistic, his behavior tends to become autistic and regressive. While the normal person secures his satisfaction by expending his energy in relation to the world of reality, such a way gives no satisfaction to the schizophrenic whose interest and strivings are progressively withdrawn from the outer world. The ego weakens and the patient secures his satisfactions through flight into unreality and fantasy and by means of a symbolic gratification of insistent strivings and primitive impulsions. Sexuality may be chaotically organized and manifest an admixture of various tendencies.

Another disturbance of conation is negativism which may manifest itself in a perversity of behavior in the form of antagonism to the environment, opposition to the wishes of those about him, and in more marked cases, in mutism, rejection of food, refusal to swallow or even to void urine. Presumably the patient may feel that negativism is a "safe" way of expressing hostility.

Although quite the opposite of negativism in certain of its objective manifestations, one occasionally meets with a *pathological suggestibility* which seems to have for its object the same purpose as negativism may have—a lessening of disturbing contacts with reality. It is less disturbing for the reality-evading patient blindly and passively to accept and follow whatever the environment suggests than it is actively either to oppose or to initiate contacts with reality. He may, therefore, show an automatic obedience to verbal directions without reference to their appropriateness or significance. Instead of answering a question, he may repeat it in a parrot-like manner—echolalia. Again he may at once imitate the movement of a person in his immediate environment—echopraxia. Obediently to follow the suggestion of the environment involves neither initiative nor substantial contact with reality and does not divert interest or energy to the world outside the patient. The waxy flexibility of the catatonic represents this passive acquiescence to suggestions to a degree that may lead the patient to ignore physical discomfort or pain, accompanied usually by a marked disregard of his environment. Among the disturbances of activity, mannerisms and stereotypies occupy a large place in the clinical picture. Schizophrenia mannerisms are of a wide variety. They may consist of affectations of manner, speech, gait, etc. Others consist of grimaces, sniffing, blowing out the cheeks, wrinkling of the forehead, ticlike movements or elaborate methods of performing certain activities and constituting a sort of ritual. Some patients assume certain postures for years. Sometimes the lips are puckered and held protruded in what is known as "snout cramp." In general, the schizophrenic's attitudes, gestures and actions, like many of his verbal communications, appear unintelligible. The bizarre behavior of the schizophrenic has, however, a meaning for him, although its purpose and value are often obscure to others because of condensation and symbolization.

In schizophrenia there is relatively little impairment of consciousness, orientation or memory, although because of lack of interest it is sometimes difficult to test these functions. One often secures incorrect replies in answer to questions as to orientation but these are because of negativism, the habit of giving casual replies in order to avoid troublesome reality, or are occasionally because of a lack of attention associated with a certain falsification by hallucinations and delusions. Forgetting, inattention, distraction and imaginative thoughts are used by normal persons as expedients to overcome a disappointment; these are used by the schizophrenic patient, not as substitutive reactions, but as if he were in a rut of least resistance.

Because of the disturbance in the integrative functions of the personality leading, as it were, to a disturbance in fusion of cognitive, affective and conative mental elements, the schizophrenic is often described as demented. This, however, is not a correct use of the word as there is no irreparable impairment of cognitive and intellectual functions. The result could be better described as a disintegration or disorganization of personality. This does not mean that judgment, the capacity for making conceptual inferences, is not impaired. The patient not only has no appreciation of the disorganization which his personality has suffered but his concepts as to personal welfare and social relationships and purpose are rendered faulty and unreliable by his introverted tendencies and his distortion both of physical and social reality through delusions and hallucinations.

The performance of Stanford-Binet and similar intelligence tests by disorganized schizophrenics differs both qualitatively and quantitatively from that of subnormal persons of the same mental age level. In normal persons and in the mentally deficient, the age levels at which failures and successes are intermixed are grouped fairly closely around the determined mental age level, but in disorganized schizophrenics as in persons suffering from many other psychoses which have led to deterioration, there is usually a spread of failures and successes at a number of age levels above and below the determined one. This phenomenon is known as "scatter."

Because of its value as a means of revealing basic personality traits and structure, the Rorschach test is often employed as an aid in the study of known or suspected schizophrenic behavior. The detection of distinctive schizophrenic features in a Rorschach performance is a rather complex procedure because of the variations in the schizophrenic syndrome itself. There is no set or definite pattern and a diagnosis of schizophrenic characteristics is largely made from inference. Such things, however, as variation in form of responses, contamination of ideas, bizarreness, withdrawal, environmental rejection and poor affective control are a few of the indications suggesting possible schizophrenic disorders. Each case is an individual problem in itself. The information derived from the Rorschach test is only as reliable as the examiner who administers the technique but in skilled hands it is of value in detecting a preschizophrenic process.

Schizophrenia is not rarely accompanied by certain *physical concomitants.* One of the most frequent of these is a general disequilibrium of the autonomic nervous system. This is shown by cold, bluish hands and feet, blotchy skin and widely dilated pupils which, when tested by a strong light, may contract momentarily but quickly dilate again. Occasionally the cyanosis may be quite marked. Sometimes patients in a catatonic stupor who persist in standing about in an immobile manner develop a striking edema of the lower extremities. Attacks of vertigo and of hysteriform and epileptiform seizures may occur, more frequently in the early stages. Many patients lose weight during the acute phases of the disease. Those who enjoy a favorable outcome of a schizophrenic episode often show a marked increase in weight during convalescence; however, an increase in weight without a coincident mental improvement usually denotes an unfavorable prognosis. Malnutrition, which is not uncommon in chronic schizophrenia, is greatest in the physically inactive, and it is often improved by small doses of insulin. The average expectancy of life among chronic patients is estimated to be approximately three fourths of that of a person of the same age in the normal population. For various reasons, one of them being prolonged contact with carriers, pulmonary tuberculosis is frequently diagnosed in institutionalized schizophrenics. The incidence of this disease in mental hospitals can readily be reduced by more active screening, more effective segregation and the use of chemotherapy.

Types of Schizophrenia

In formulating his concept of dementia praecox, Kraepelin classified his cases into different varieties depending on the predominant symptomatology. While classification according to reaction type is commonly made, more understanding is to be gained by studying the patient and his life history as an individual problem than as a representative of some vague classificatory division.

SIMPLE TYPE. In this type the most marked disturbances are of emotion, interest and activity. If hallucinations occur they are rare and fleeting while delusions never play an important role. The disorder is usually gradual in its onset and assumes the form of an insidious change and impoverishment of personality, the significance of which is not understood by the patient's friends. In adolescence a youth who has perhaps shown much promise begins to lose interest in school or occupation, becomes moody, irritable and indolent. His goals are no longer realistic. Shallowness of emotions, indifference or callousness, absence of will or drive and a progressive meagerness of inner resources betray the withering of personality which constitutes the most prominent feature of this type. Neither criticism by others nor chagrin of parents causes concern. Appreciation of esthetic and moral values is lost. The required period of training or apprenticeship in preparation for profession or skilled occupation is not completed. Many become irresponsible idlers, vagrants, tramps, prostitutes or delinquents. In the milder cases, the social maladaptation is less serious but the patients are considered as neighborhood eccentrics and, although intellectually unimpaired, are capable of performing only some simple routine task under supervision. The patient remains uninterested in his environment and unimpressed by responsibilities.

A. R. was committed to the hospital when twenty-one years of age followlowing his arrest for window-peeping. In describing his childhood characteristics, the patient's family stated that he "was always a little hard to understand," but was a quiet boy who never entered into rough games. His school record was excellent and he always stood high in his class. At seventeen when in the fourth year of high school he was obliged, because of a long illness of his father, to leave school and secure gainful employment. He secured work with a large manufacturing company where he soon came to be considered the second best operative on a certain type of machine. For two years he worked steadily, seemed ambitious and appeared to have a normal and wholesome, but not marked interest in girls. At nineteen he gave up his position, showed no interest in securing another and when asked if he worked would reply, "What do I want to work for? I have a father and sister working and they are enough." He appeared quite self-satisfied and felt that he should have a position of importance. At about this time he was first arrested for peeping into women's bedrooms. Through the influence of his father, the charge was dropped. He became careless of his personal appearance and remained unoccupied except for occasional periods when he set up pins in a bowling alley. A year later he was again arrested but again was released on the intercession of his father. He came to say little unless addressed and grew antagonistic toward his father and sister. He would remain out until midnight and then come home, eat a large meal, read until 2 a.m. and sleep until noon. Finally, after his third arrest for peeping, he was committed to a hospital for mental disorders.

On arrival at the institution, the patient was found to be of asthenic physique and slightly effeminate in appearance. His emotional responses were shallow and inadequate. He showed no concern over his situation, laughed about it in a silly manner and referred to his offense as "Just a foolish idea." His hospital residence was characterized by apathy, preoccupation and inactivity. During the summer he would at times take part in the patient's baseball games but in winter he refused ground privileges. He never expressed any delusions and denied hallucinations. At times he would be seen, apparently much preoccupied, walking alone about the hospital reservation, laughing to himself.

Such a case illustrates how at times an individual, perhaps, as seems true in the present instance, fundamentally deviated psychobiologically, is unable to complete the transition from adolescence to maturity with its adult heterosexual and social adjustments. There seemed to be a certain innate limitation to the personality while environmental circumstances contributed but comparatively little to its disintegration. Interest became largely withdrawn from the actual world, psychobiological energy was absorbed by the subjective life and there was a diminished response to social demands. This does not mean that life situations and events or psychological reactions to mental events were not dynamic factors in the patient's personality disorganization but that, as often happens in the schizophrenic, it is difficult, even by attempts at mental exploration, to discover and evaluate these elements.

Hebephrenic Type. The onset of this type is insidious and usually begins in early adolescence. Occasionally the onset is subacute and characterized by a depression that suggests an affective reaction. Usually, however, affective reactions are shallow and inappropriate. Silliness, giggling and incongruous or inappropriate smiling and laughter are usual. Hallucinations, which are frequent, often represent the projection of repressed instinctive urges. The ideational content tends to take the form of fantasy or of fragmentary bizarre delusions rather than of elaborate or systematized beliefs. Associative processes are loose, speech is incoherent, neologisms are common and posturing and mannerisms are frequent. Regressive features are prominent, wetting and soiling are common and the patient eats in a ravenous, unmannerly fashion. The patient comes to lead a highly autistic life; he becomes baffingly inaccessible and greatly introverted and withdrawn. The final disintegration of personality and habits is perhaps the greatest of any of the types of schizophrenia.

T. B., a single young woman of thirty-two when admitted to the hospital, may serve to illustrate the nature of certain of these unwholesome prepsychotic reactions as well as the symptoms and course of a malignant schizophrenia that may be considered of the hebephrenic type. Of her five children Theresa was her mother's favorite. Greatly petted and babied by her mother she always remained dependent upon her. She was described as having been a pretty child with a rosy complexion. She early became aware of this fact and enjoyed dressing up and strutting about to display her good looks. In spite of these signs of vanity she was timid and shy and would blush in a self-conscious way when she realized that people were noticing her. In childhood she did not play freely with other children; "she thought herself above other children," and is described by her sisters as having in later years "a rather good opinion of herself and her abilities," and by her neighbors as "high hat." Soon after leaving school at sixteen she began to work in a bleachery where she remained until shortly before her commitment. She never had any girl chums and did not participate in the activities of other girls at her place of employment. Her attitude was one of "proud distance." While still in school there were several boys who were quite friendly toward her but her sister said she could not remember any instance when the patient had any male callers or associates after she grew up, although she gave much attention to her clothes and personal appearance, obviously in the sister's opinion, in an effort to attract the attention of young men. Her family described her as devoid of humor, sensitive, jealous, stubborn, willful and easily angered. She became more seclusive, had "melancholy spells," became preoccupied, paid less attention to her environment and when addressed would ask in an indifferent way, "What did you say?" She also became irritable and critical, particularly of the wife of her brother with whose family she lived. About six months before commitment she "began to grow thin and nervous," became careless about her work which deteriorated in quality and quantity. She believed that other girls at her place of employment were circulating slanderous stories concerning her. She complained so indignantly that X., an attractive young man employed in the same industrial plant, had put his arm around her and insulted her that her family demanded that the charge be investigated. This showed not only that the charge was without foundation but that the young man in question had not spoken to her for months. The family, however, had not suspected mental disease until six days before her commitment when she returned from her work. As she entered the house that evening she laughed loudly, watched her sister-in-law suspiciously, refused to answer questions and at sight of her brother began to cry. She refused to go to the bathroom saying that X. was looking in the windows at her. She ate no food and the next day declared that her sisters were "bad women," that everyone was talking about her and that X. had been having sexual relations with her, that although she could not see him he was "always around." In her hallucinatory experiences she heard X. say, "Aren't you going to fire her? I've had her. She don't know it." The patient became resistive, was afraid of being killed, and at times said, "I'm dead." She stated that she was being poisoned, saw her dead mother and heard her speak. As the patient became noisy, did not sleep and ate but little and only then when spoon-fed, she was committed to a private institution. Here she was unco-operative, silly, grimaced and whiningly repeated, "Oh, Mama! Mama! I want to see my father before I die." She heard voices outside her window and at night would come to the door of her room several times saying, "What is it all about? Oh, Mama!" Her associations became loose, she took no interest in the care of her person or in other patients but would stand for hours with her back against the wall, her head thrust forward, fingering her hair and unobservant of her environment.

After a residence of four months in the private institution, the patient was transferred to a public hospital. As she entered the admitting office she laughed loudly and repeatedly screamed in a loud tone, "She cannot stay here; she's got to go home!" She grimaced and performed various stereotyped movements of her hands. When seen on the ward an hour later she paid no attention to questions although she talked to herself in a childish tone. She moved constantly about, walking on her toes in a dancing manner, pointed aimlessly about and put out her tongue and sucked her lips in the manner of an infant. At times she moaned and cried like a child but shed no tears. As the months passed she remained silly, childish, preoccupied, inaccessible, grimacing, gesturing, pointing at objects in a stereotyped way, usually chattering to herself in a peculiar high-pitched voice, little of what she said being understood. At an interview eighteen months after her hospitalization she presented an unkempt appearance, was without shoes, sat stooped far over, smiled in a silly manner and presented a picture of extreme introversion and regression. During the attempted interview, she rarely spoke although she occasionally replied, "I don't know" in an entirely indifferent manner and apparently with no heed to the question. The nurse reported the patient as seclusive, resistive, idle and with no interest either in the activities of the institution or in her relatives who visited her.

CATATONIC TYPE. The catatonic type is characterized by phases of stupor or of excitement in both of which negativism and automatism are prominent features. There may be alternation between little or no movement on the one hand to an explosive overactivity on the other. Frequently, however, a given catatonic episode may present but one phase, either stupor or disorganized overactivity, throughout its course. Again, there may be an admixture of symptoms usually thought of as belonging characteristically to one or the other phase. The most frequent age of appearance is between fifteen and twenty-five. Of the various types of schizophrenia, catatonia most frequently has a somewhat acute onset and is most frequently precipitated or preceded by an emotionally disturbing experience. The prognosis for a recovery with reintegration of personality after a catatonic episode is more favorable than in other types of schizophrenia, although after a period, perhaps after several episodes, there is a tendency for the catatonic type to pass over into states approaching the hebephrenic or paranoid with a permanent disorganization of the personality.

Catatonic stupor, or the stupor phase, is often preceded by depression, discontent, or by emotional fermentation. The patient is inclined to be uncommunicative and his reactions become increasingly characterized by failing interest, inattention, preoccupation, emotional poverty and dreaminess. Mute, stuporous, and with masklike facies the catatonic may occasionally keep his eyes closed but more frequently he stares fixedly and blankly downward. He may stand almost immobile, seldom shifting his position during the whole day. The skin of his feet may become turgid and engorged with swelling of unsupported parts. Another catatonic may spend the day sitting on the edge of a chair or crouching on the floor. With his implicit loss of reality sense, he denies the world and actively resists the environment. He opposes any effort to move him from attitudes and positions, often constrained and peculiar, which he has assumed and may maintain for months. The patient refuses to dress or to eat, although occasionally if he thinks he is unobserved he will eat greedily. Saliva, urine and bowel contents are often retained. He may not only soil clothing but even exhibit an apparent purposefulness in his annoying disregard of all cleanliness in his habits of excretion. Gestures, grimacing and grinning are common. The hands may be held tightly clenched and other muscle tensions be maintained. Occasionally the physical manifestations of catatonia show some points of similarity to parkinsonian akinesia and rigidity. Catalepsy, either flexible or rigid, may be present. In this state the patient initiates no spontaneous movements but maintains the postures into which he is passively impressed. Through automatic obedience, the patient may carry out any verbal instructions, regardless of their absurd or even dangerous nature. He shows no avoiding reaction to feinting motions before the eyes, to pin pricks or to other painful stimuli. Although giving no indication whatsoever that he is at all aware of what is going on about him, the patient really registers the events of his environment and when he begins to speak again he may give a surprisingly full account of incidents occurring in his stupor. In spite of the apparent ideational poverty, there seems every reason to believe that ideas and representations are by no means absent, but rather are centered about a dominant ideo-affective constellation. Perhaps an analogue to catatonic stupor may exist in the unapprehending, impassive response with which profound, overwhelming bereavement or catastrophe may at times be met. Both this reaction and the catatonic stupor of the schizophrenic may serve as methods of meeting situations too difficult to be met by active, resolute measures. The stupor may be thought of as a protective withdrawal from contact with surroundings that seem threatening. Again the stupor may be compared to a retreat into an intense, trance-like preoccupation or reverie.

After a period of extremely variable duration, the patient may slowly, or at times suddenly, emerge from this profound generalized inhibition. Occasionally catatonic rigidity and negativism may terminate in response to affective stimuli. The opposite occurrence, the sudden sinking into a stuporous akinesia, following an apparently trivial physical or mental event is more frequent. Interest, affect and behavior may return more or less closely to normal, or the patient may pass into a state of catatonic excitement.

Catatonic excitement is characterized by an unorganized and aggressive motor activity. It is not accompanied with emotional expression and is not influenced by external stimuli; it is apparently purposeless, stereotyped and usually confined to a limited space. Of all schizophrenics the excited catatonic most frequently shows impulsive and unpredictable behavior. Without warning or apparent cause, he may suddenly attack an inoffensive bystander or break a window. He destroys his clothing, remains nude and disregards all excretory cleanliness. Negativism is usually marked. The flow of speech may vary from mutism to a pressure suggesting a flight of ideas. Attitudinizing, mannerisms, sterotypies and grimaces are frequent. The patient may react to terrifying or ecstatic hallucinations of sight or hearing. Mystical experiences are not uncommon. Hostility and feelings of resentment are common. The patient may be sleepless, appear delirioid, refuse food and become dehydrated and exhausted. There is often a rapid loss of weight. On rare occasions the acutely and extremely excited catatonic may collapse and die. Usually no pathologic condition sufficient to explain the cause of death is found at necropsy. In such cases, therefore, the death is ordinarily said to be a result of "exhaustion syndrome."

Probably acute catatonic excitement is often the same as the reaction which Kempf termed acute homosexual panic. The great activity is often accompanied by fearfulness and auditory hallucinations that accuse the patient of homosexual practices or inclinations. As previously noted he is often assaultive.

Meyer considered that catatonia is a psychobiological reaction. Hohman, his former assistant, quotes him as describing it as "closely related to what is seen in hypnotic states and in mystical fancies, and like stages in religious symbolism and feelings of submission to influence by mystic power." When the problems of life are too great we naturally seek death but are deterred from suicide by the instinct of self-preservation. Many psychiatrists, therefore, look upon catatonic stupor as a profound regression, a dramatization of death. Attention is called to the similarity between catatonia and the instinctive immobility reaction exhibited by certain animals when confronted with a life-threatening situation.

The case of A. C., aged thirty-two, will illustrate many of the features observed both in the excited and the stuporous phases of catatonia:

The patient's father was stubborn and self-willed, his mother was excitable and temperamental. At seven years of age he went to live with his grandparents. The grandfather whose "word was law," who suffered from epileptic seizures and subsequently died in a hospital for mental diseases, had no understanding of the child's point of view. His seizures greatly frightened the boy. The patient was a seclusive, daydreaming, timid, shy and sensitive but stubborn and self-willed child. He still remembers with resentment how his father whipped him before another boy whom he would not thank for an apple. He was uninterested in the play life of other children and spent his time either in the town library or in his own room where he made various toys which he guarded jealously from other children, allowing only his sister, his sole confidante, to share them. At seventeen he graduated from high school where he had learned easily but had taken no part in extracurricular activities. His occupational history was without significance except for the fact that his early promise of success as a draftsman and designer of aeroplanes and motors had not been sustained and that for eight years prior to his commitment he had earned practically nothing. At twenty he married. Two months before commitment the patient began to talk about how he had failed, had "spoiled" his whole life, that it was now "too late." He spoke of hearing someone say, "You must submit." One night his wife was awakened by his talking. He told of having several visions but refused to describe them. He stated that someone was after him and trying to blame him for the death of a certain man. He had been poisoned, he said. Whenever he saw a truck or a fire engine the patient stated that it was looking for him in order to claim his assistance to help save the world. He had periods of laughing and shouting and became so noisy and unmanageable that it became necessary to commit him.

On arrival at the hospital the patient was noted to be an asthenic, poorly nourished man with dilated pupils, hyperactive tendon reflexes and a pulse rate of 120 per minute. In the admission office he showed many mannerisms, lay down on the floor, pulled at his foot, made undirected, violent striking movements, again struck attendants, grimaced, assumed rigid, attitudinized postures, refused to speak and appeared to be having auditory hallucinations. He was at once placed in a continuous bath where, when seen later in the day, he was found in a stuporous state. His face was without expression, he was mute, rigid, and paid no attention to those about him or to their questions. His eyes were closed and the lids could be separated only with effort. There was no response to pinpricks or other painful stimuli. On the following morning an attempt was made to bring him before the medical staff for the routine admission interview. As he was brought into the room supported by two attendants he struggled, grimaced, shouted incoherently and was resistive. For five days he remained mute, negativistic and inaccessible, at times staring vacantly into space, at times with his eyes tightly closed. He ate poorly and gave no response to questions but once was heard to mutter to himself in a greatly preoccupied manner, "I'm going to die—I know it—you know it." On the evening of the sixth day he looked about apparently astonished to find himself in the bath, and asked where he was and how he came there. When asked to tell of his life he related many known events and how he had once worked in an aeroplane factory, but added that he had invented an appliance pertaining to aeroplanes, that this had been stolen, patented through fraud and that as a result he had lost his position. He ate ravenously, then fell asleep and on awaking was in a catatonic stupor, remaining in this state for several days. He gradually became accessible and when asked concerning himself he replied that he had had a "nervous breakdown following the physical breakdown." He referred to his stuporous period as sleep and maintained that he had no recollection of any events occurring during it. He said "When I was in the tub I didn't know anything. Everything seemed to be dark as far as my mind is concerned. Then I began to see a little light, like the shape of a star. Then my head got through the star gradually. I saw more and more light until I saw everything in a perfect form a few days ago." Two days later he admitted that he could remember having seen the examiner while in the bath. He rationalized his former mutism by a statement that he had been afraid he would "say the wrong thing," also that he "didn't know exactly what to talk about." From his obviously inadequate emotional response and his statement that he was "a scientist and an inventor of the most extraordinary genius of the twentieth century," it was plain that he was still far from well.

PARANOID TYPE. The features which tend to be most evident in this type or phase are delusions which are often numerous, illogical and disregardful of reality, hallucinations and the usual schizophrenic disturbance of associations and of affect together with negativism.

Frequently the prepsychotic personality of the paranoid schizophrenic has been characterized by poor interpersonal rapport. Often he has been cold, withdrawn, distrustful, and resentful of other persons. Many have been truculent, had a chip-on-the-shoulder attitude, have been argumentative, scornful, sarcastic, defiant, resentful of suggestions or of authority and given to caustic remarks. Sometimes flippant, facetious responses may have covered an underlying hostility.

The paranoid type tends to have its frank appearance at a somewhat later age than the other forms. It is not common until after adolescence and occurs most frequently after thirty years of age. The patient's previous negative attitudes become more marked and misinterpretations are common. Ideas of reference are often among the first symptoms. Disorders of association appear. Many patients show an unpleasant emotional aggressiveness. Through displacement, the patient may begin to act out his hostile impulses. His grip on reality begins to loosen. At first his delusions are limited but later they become numerous and changeable. In the early stages, too, their character usually indicates more clearly the particular psychological needs or experiences which they are created to meet. Occasional remarks may supply fragmentary disclosures of the patient's preoccupations. Rejected tendencies are ideationally projected instead of undergoing repression. Delusions of persecution are the most prominent in paranoid schizophrenia, but expansive and obviously wish-fulfilling ideas and hypochrondriacal and depressive delusions are not uncommon. With increasing personality disorganization delusional beliefs become less logical. Verbal expressions may be inappropriate and neologistic. The patient is subjected to vague magical forces and his explanations become extremely vague and irrational. Imaginative fantasy may become extreme but take on the value of reality. Repressed aggressive tendencies may be released in a major outburst; some inarticulate paranoids may manifest an unpredictable assaultiveness. Many paranoid schizophrenics are irritable, discontented, resentful, angrily suspicious and show a surly aversion to being interviewed. Some manifest an unapproachable, aggressively hostile attitude and may live in a bitter aloofness. Auditory hallucinations usually occur and the voices are most frequently threatening or accusatory in nature. The patient may show varying degrees of tension and be subject to upsurges of rage which he seems unable to control. As personality disorganization proceeds, affective responses become increasingly flattened. Mannerisms, apathy and incoherence are common. In general, paranoid schizophrenia may be regarded as a projective, regressive, defensive type of reaction.

The following is in many respects a rather typical case of paranoid schizophrenia:

A. B., a physician, 38 years of age, was admitted in 1937 to a public hospital for mental disease following his arrest for disturbing the peace. Specifically, he had frightened his neighbors by hurling objects at imaginary people who, he said, were tormenting him, by his beating the air with ropes and by breaking glass in the apartment which he and his wife occupied.

The patient was born in Ukraine. Little is known of parental characteristics. His mother is described as being "sweet and good-natured as long as things went her way but she would have violent outbursts of temper during which she would throw dishes and break glasses when aroused." The patient, the youngest son, is said to have been "the favorite of the whole family. He was spoiled, given his own way, and invariably the other children would be whipped for the misdemeanors of which he was guilty."

When 16 years of age the patient came to United States where he continued his studies. After graduating from college he entered medical school. His medical course continued satisfactorily until the third year when he failed to pass pathology which until that time had been one of his best subjects. For some reason, not stated in his history, he was dismissed from the first medical school he entered, but later was admitted to a second one where he repeated the third year and was graduated.

Upon his commitment to the hospital his wife described his personality traits as follows: "He has always been a deep thinker. Lately, however, he cannot concentrate. He was rather aggressive and is the type who insists upon imposing his own ideas on everyone else. He thinks that people have to agree with him. He is stubborn and argumentative. This trait was even referred to in his college yearbook. He is an independent thinker and is very bright. He had big plans for the future. He was formerly quite extravertive until the last few years when he refused to go out and mingle with people."

Soon after beginning his internship trouble developed between the young physician and the chief resident. The former was compelled to resign but secured appointment in another hospital and completed an internship. Following this he went to Vienna to pursue graduate work in ophthalmology, otolaryngology and bronchoscopy. After his return to America he entered private practice and was apparently successful for the first four years although because of various difficulties he changed locations on several occasions. For some reason not stated in the history, but presumably because of beginning mental disease, the patient gave up his practice and became a medical officer in a Civilian Conservation Camp. He soon began to complain that the commanding officer was "against" him. He made frequent applications of cocaine to his nasal mucous membrane not, he said, because he was a cocaine addict but in order to neutralize the effects of chloral hydrate which was being sprayed upon him. After a few months he was released from his Camp appointment. He then began practice in another city but as he believed that the spraying of chloral hydrate continued there he remained but two months and then returned to his original place of practice. He met with but little success as the same ideas of persecution persisted. According to his history, too, "He became forgetful and neglected his cases. He had lapses of memory and seemed to be preoccupied with his own thoughts."

The patient's wife described him as having usually preferred the company of men, "but he has quite a history as far as the opposite sex is concerned." While studying in Vienna he became involved with a widow and married her. Two weeks after their marriage he discovered, he alleged, that his wife was unfaithful to him and was "a member of a gang of dope peddlers who tried to involve young medical students in their racket." He then returned to America. The following year he married again but the couple lived together for only three months. Three years later the date was set for his third wedding but he did not appear at a party scheduled to precede the wedding. A quarrel with the expectant bride followed but finally the wedding took place. Soon he began to object to his wife's talking with other men and accused her of infidelity. On two occasions when she had not even been absent from home he insisted he had seen her on the street with other men. Four months before his commitment the patient awoke his wife and told her she must leave the house permanently the following day. He insisted that she was not his wife any longer and the next day asked if she had made her plans to leave. In view of the failure of three marriages, his accusations of infidelity in at least two of them and his preference for the company of men the probability at once suggests itself that at least some of the patient's personality difficulties arose from unrecognized homosexual tendencies. Further support to this assumption is added by the fact that during the psychiatric examination after his hospital admission he remarked that certain physical complaints from which he was suffering suggested sexual perversion. Doubtless, too, the fact that for several years he had consumed a half pint or more of alcohol daily may be of corroborative significance.

As the patient's mental disorder progressed, he developed a great wealth of delusions. He stated that he was "the link between the living and the dead," that he was a "universal medium," that a certain physician called on him by mental telepathy for added strength and skill in surgical operations. He believed that someone was hiding in a trunk in his house so he fired several bullets into the trunk. He accused his brother of spraying him with chloral hydrate from the third floor of his house. He therefore sat behind a closed door waiting for his brother and upon hearing a noise shot through the door. He grew a beard because his face, he said, was being changed in subtle ways by outside influences, adding that if he wore a beard his true identity would be known. Following his admission to the hospital he often spent long hours in his room where he could be heard pacing the floor, moaning or making noise like a dog, striking his head with his fist or pounding the wall of his room. When asked the reason for his behavior he explained that he was suffering tortures because people abused their powers of mental telepathy and were directing those powers toward him. He spent nearly all the day in his room where during the fourth and fifth years of his hospital residence he would frequently be heard shouting, screaming and uttering noises which the attendants described as resembling the howling of a wolf. In explanation of these noises the patient stated that there was a woman spiritualist who in some way through persons in the hospital was exerting a peculiar spell on him and that by making these noises he could drive the spirits away. His thought processes became progressively disorganized. Thirteen years after his admission to the hospital he wrote his ward physician a ten-page letter which he concluded as follows: "In view of the facts and their significance, and in view of the connection of tendencies and the contingent and pertinent effects, and in view of my physical condition brought about by the connected and sustained tendencies and actuating reasons behind them, I shall not consider it a mere negligence, or merely a form of criminal negligence, or merely an ethical vice, but I shall consider your interference with the anatomical and physiological requirements of my health as an outright, deliberate, well accounted for and reasoned out criminal and dastardly endeavor at homicide." As the years passed he was rarely to be seen on his ward but remained in his room where most of his days was spent in writing and reading. When approached he was hostile and resentful in attitude. He was, however, less aggressive and less abusive in speech. As frequently happens in the paranoid schizophrenic his prolonged institutional residence had produced a lessening of tension but little or no modification of thought content.

SCHIZO-AFFECTIVE TYPE. Not particularly infrequent are cases of mental disorder characterized by recurring episodes which continue to show admixtures of schizophrenic and affective symptoms. The mental content, for example, may be so reality-disregarding that it seems schizophrenic, whereas the mood is one of pronounced elation or depression. Again the affective features may stand to the fore but the patient's behavior be so bizarre that it must be regarded as schizophrenic. In some instances the prepsychotic personality may have been strongly schizoid or, on the other hand, outgoing and well socialized yet the clinical features of the psychosis be quite at variance or inconsistent with the early personality pattern. It is not uncommon to see depressions in schizoid individuals who in addition to the depression show a great deal of anxiety and many neurotic patterns. Such patients are usually refractory to treatment.

Stanley Cobb suggests that schizoid and affective psychoses are variants of one general disease. He offers the opinion that, although in typical cases these two types of psychosis are quite different and easily separated as to classification, they are the extremes of a continuous series of variables. If cases with purely manic-depressive symptoms are put at one end of the series and those with purely schizophrenic symptoms at the other, the space between can be filled in with a long series of cases which are mixtures. Near one end will be examples of depression or mania with "schizophrenic coloring"; near the other, schizophrenia with depressive elements or cyclic mood changes. Cases in which the symptoms are entirely schizophrenic but run in cycles are well known. In the mid-zone of this series are those cases that can scarcely be diagnosed as either schizophrenic or cyclothymic and so are called schizo-affective. Perhaps, as has already been suggested, instead of being variables in a "disease" the variations in clinical symptoms represent admixtures of affective and schizoid components in the basic personality structure.

PSEUDONEUROTIC TYPE. Hoch and Polatin have described what they term "*pseudoneurotic schizophrenia,*" a condition not rarely seen in private practice and only occasionally in the public mental hospital. As the name implies the dynamics are psychotic in character although the symptom picture, at least in the early stages, is neurotic. The pseudoneurotic schizophrenic usually shows a mixture of anxiety and of phobic, obsessive, depressive and hypochondriacal symptoms. The underlying schizophrenic disorder is hidden by a facade of neurotic manifestations. Hoch and Polatin speak of the symptomatology as a pan-neurosis. A diffuse anxiety does not leave any life-approach of the patient free from tension. Practically everything he experiences influences this anxiety and although he tries to force pleasurable experiences he does not derive pleasure from anything. The neurotic manifestations constantly shift but are never completely absent. The true neurotic is usually anxious to describe his symptoms in minute detail and presses his physician with his explanations. The pseudoneurotic schizophrenic's explanations are vague, indistinct, often contradictory, and repeated in a stereotyped manner without details. The organization of the patient's sexuality is often chaotic. Some of these patients have brief psychotic episodes. About one third of the patients with this misleading neurotic overlay gradually go on to a frank psychosis although with less regression than the usual schizophrenic. Many of these patients have previously received unsuccessful psychotherapy.

Schizophrenia in Childhood

There has been much controversy as to whether childhood schizophrenia is the same as adult schizophrenia or whether it is a reactive pattern, reactive in particular to a cold emotional climate in the home during the first two years. It must be said that the causes are obscure. Theories of etiology range all the way from a psychogenic cause based on early disturbance in mother-child relationship to a deterministic concept rooted in genetics. Bender, who has had an unusually wide experience with childhood schizophrenia, is impressed with the importance of constitutional or, at least, biological factors. She believes that it results from "a developmental lag of the biological processes from which subsequent behavior evolves by maturation at an embryological level, leading to anxiety and secondarily to neurotic defense mechanisms." In her opinion, the fundamental pathological process is a diffuse encephalopathy for which no confirming anatomical evidence is described. While the etiology is still debatable, there is an increasing belief that schizophrenia is the result of an interaction of constitutional and psychological factors. Perhaps childhood schizophrenia is not a separate and distinct clinical entity but rather a group of related and overlapping clinical syndromes.

The diagnostic criteria specific for childhood schizophrenia are not definitely established. There is undoubtedly a wide variety of clinical pictures. Bender points out that some schizophrenic children are regressive, retarded, blocked, inhibited, mute, autistic, withdrawn, physically asthenic, unsocial and unable to relate. Others develop overfast, have an exaggerated intellectual brilliance, are overactive, precocious in language development and are excessively abstract in their thinking. In her experience, any severe psychoneurotic disorder in a child before puberty, whether it is obsessive-compulsive, so-called hysterical or severe anxiety is a reactive response to a deep, inherent, threatening disorder, most often schizophrenic in nature.

The older the child the more does the clinical picture resemble that seen in adults. In such a child, therefore, we may see not only withdrawal, loss of contact and affect, but also hallucinations and delusions. The last two symptoms do not occur below eight years of age. In the older patient the onset may be insidious or acute, the insidious type being more frequent. It may be difficult to date the beginning although retrospectively it is often remembered that peculiarities may have been noted. It is characterized by a general reduction of interests in play and other activities. There is a gradual loss of affective contact with people accompanied by regressive phenomena. Some patients show a tendency to brooding or to obsessive rumination on some topic ordinarily not of interest to a child. Some patients become aggressive and destructive. Not a few, not actually mentally defective, come to appear to be feebleminded and are committed to an institution for mental deficiency. Any great improvement is unusual. Children having an acute onset have usually not been previously regarded as abnormal. Shortly before the appearance of acute features, there may have been an impairment of ability to concentrate with an accompanying drop in quality of school work. The child may then begin to mumble to himself, to sleep poorly, maintain odd postures, show diminished or rigid affect, become inaccessible, extremely restless and perhaps scream and kick. Usually improvement takes place after several weeks but with a reduction of emotional and ideational expression. Subsequent acute episodes are usual, each one followed by increased personality disorganization.

The psychological problems which the child is attempting to meet with his schizophrenic reaction are those which naturally accompany or are appropriate to childhood are therefore different from those of adolescence or adulthood. They are also appropriate to the particular developmental period within childhood at which the onset of the disorder occurs. The symptom formation will therefore be related to the problem which has created the anxiety. In other words, much of the symptom formation will be determined by the way the child deals with his anxiety. Bender is of the opinion that the principal problems, particularly in the small child, are those of self-identity and therefore of relating to the rest of the world, to body function and of relating to objects; for example to play material, food or clothes. In somewhat older children there may be the problem of relationship to a parent, particularly the mother or siblings, or early childhood sex problems. Mental mechanisms which are normal for early childhood become points of fixation, become exaggerated by repetition, become mingled with other mechanisms and are carried into later periods of personality development where they constitute the psychotic symptoms of the schizophrenic child.

EARLY INFANTILE AUTISM. In 1943 Kanner described a syndrome beginning as early as 2 or 3 years and characterized by an extreme withdrawal and obsessiveness. To this syndrome he gave the name "early infantile autism." Because of its similarities to, and its differences from, childhood schizophrenia, its categorical place presents a challenging problem. The present general belief is, however, that while it can be classified as one of the schizophrenias, its separation from other cases of childhood schizophrenia is clinically justified. The striking disability in interpersonal relations and the severe obsessive-compulsive mechanisms are the pathognomonic features of autism but the peculiarities of language and thought, while somewhat different, share the general features of schizophrenia. This early autism occurs more frequently in boys than in girls. The psychotic nature of the illness becomes apparent before the end of the first, and certainly not later than during the second, year of life.

Affective contacts with mother and other persons and the ability of the child to relate himself in the ordinary way to people and situations should normally be well established by 2 or 3 years of age. In early autism there seems to be an inability to form affective ties with a resulting lack of responsiveness. Almost invariably it is found that the parents of these children are intelligent and successful, often professional persons in good economic circumstances but obsessively preoccupied with abstractions of a scientific, literary or artistic nature. The family life is of a cold, formal type and the child has received extremely little fondling, cuddling or warm, genuine parental affection. The behavior of the mother toward the child is mechanical and does not convey love. When a child with early autism is brought to a psychiatrist his parents have usually assumed that he is severely feeble-minded. The autistic child 3 or 4 years of age usually does not talk, does not respond to people and often has temper tantrums if interfered with. He has little ability to empathize with the feelings of others. His autistic and impenetrable aloneness shuts out anything that comes to the child from outside. If the child attempts to form sentences they are usually for a long time mostly parrot-like repetitions of word combinations which he has overheard, often long previously. He frequently refers to himself as "you" and to the person spoken to as "I." Although the child has no interest in people he has a good relation to objects and may play happily with them for hours. He has an obsessive urge for a maintenance of sameness. Furniture must continue to be arranged in the same manner and the routine of life must be unchanged.

Although the extreme withdrawal and limited responsiveness of the autistic child suggests that he is feeble-minded it will usually be found that he has average or even superior intellectual potentiality. The facial expression is often serious and perhaps tense but is usually strikingly intelligent. Frequently those who speak have an extensive vocabulary and a surprising rote memory.

Many of these children continue to function in an emotional vacuum and for all practical purposes remain feeble-minded all their lives. Some of them, through permissiveness and emotional stimulation, attain a normal intelligence quotient, become able to pay attention to persons and to accept and return affection. They may even participate in environmental activities although they often remain "peculiar."

Perhaps the primary psychopathological mechanism in infantile autism may be described as a disturbance in social perception, analogous to, but more complex than perceptual difficulties at the sensorimotor level. The question has been raised if there may not be, parallel to intellectual inadequacy, a syndrome of affective inadequacy.

Follow-up studies of autistic children show that by 15 years of age one third have achieved a moderate social adjustment. About half of those who possess a meaningful language by the age of 5 show further improvement whereas only rarely does the child without ability to communicate verbally by that age show significant subsequent improvement.

DIAGNOSIS. Childhood schizophrenia must be differentiated from mental deficiency, organic brain disease, from severe neurotic disorders, especially anxiety and obsessive-compulsive states, and from behavior disorders based on disturbance in interpersonal relationships.

Course and Prognosis of Schizophrenia

While schizophrenia can perhaps best be regarded as a special type of maladjustment that usually shows a tendency to be progressive and is therefore to be looked upon with apprehension, yet a permanent disorganization of the personality does not invariably follow. Indeed it is now the opinion of many of the closest students of schizophrenia that acute, rather clearly psychogenic schizophrenia may at times disappear without leaving any injury to the personality. Formerly its incurable nature and progressive course were implied in the definition of the disease and a favorable outcome was considered presumptive evidence of an error in diagnosis. Of course the occurrence of an obviously schizophrenic reaction should make the physician exceedingly careful in predicting that a permanently inferior type of adjustment will not be sustained. In recent years, too, there has been an increasing recognition that the episodic nature of a psychosis and the occurrence of symptom-free intermissions may not exclude its schizophrenic nature. Occasionally one observes a schizophrenic episode of a mild, fleeting nature with no subsequent recurrence. In many instances, however, the favorable outcome should be characterized as "social recovery" rather than as "cured," or as full recovery. By this is meant that the patient is able to return to his previous social environment and to previous or equivalent occupation, but with minor symptoms and signs such as irritability, shyness, or shallowness of affective responses.

From what has been said it is evident that in any given case the effect upon the personality and future adjustment of the appearance of a schizophrenic reaction may be quite uncertain. In some cases the course is continuously progressive; in others it is intermittent. More frequently it is a question of remissions and relapses which, although from the first they insidiously tend to undermine interests and habits, there occur periods of adjustment at a lower level for a considerable period of time. It is estimated that 40 per cent of schizophrenic patients who enter public mental hospitals or clinics recover or improve and the other 60 per cent fail to improve or ultimately suffer that permanent, malignant disorganization of personality somewhat inaccurately designated as deterioration. Of committed patients who improve sufficiently to be released, about 80 per cent leave the mental hospital within the first year of residence. The expectancy of recovery falls with each year of continued illness. Roughly about one third of those patients who are hospitalized during the first year of their illness make a fairly complete recovery, one third get a bit better and become able to return to outside life but remain damaged personalities and may have to return to the hospital from time to time. The remaining one third will require indefinite hospital care. The age of onset is not of prognostic significance except that relatively late age offers a less favorable prognosis. Sex has no prognostic significance. Slowly but steadily more and more treatment methods which influence the schizophrenic process, at least in its early phases, are being introduced.

As highly desirable and important as it is, it is not yet possible, with our limited knowledge concerning the factors and processes involved, for the psychiatrist when confronted with acute schizophrenia definitely to predict what the future course of the particular psychosis will be. In making a prognosis the physician will, among other factors consider the patient's past record of ability to derive satisfaction from occupation, wholesome group and social activities and from his record of constructive interpersonal relationships. There are certain facts, however, which may serve as general guides in suggesting an opinion. It will usually be found true that if the psychosis represents an insidious development and unfolding of a previous schizoid personality, the prognosis is unfavorable. Many such psychoses represent the culmination of a long period of unsatisfactory adaptation. The better adjusted the patient's prepsychotic personality, the more directly and confidently the patient has been accustomed to meet the problems and difficulties of life, the richer his interests, the more definite an external precipitating situation and the more rapid the onset the better the prognosis. The existence of anxiety and of an easily ascertained emotional problem makes the prognosis more favorable. With the presence of features such as those just mentioned "spontaneous" recoveries, *i.e.*, without therapeutic efforts by a physician, are not uncommon. A slow, insidious withdrawal is apt to lead to an irreversible disorganization of the personality. If the ego was not strong enough to withstand routine difficulties, the prognosis is not good. If it broke only after overwhelming stress, the prognosis is good. The prognosis is not influenced by the intelligence or previous education of the patient. An apparently "mild" case need not be an early one nor of favorable prognosis. The presence of a well marked affective element is of hopeful significance although a hypochondriasis is not desirable. The presence of cyclothymic factors in the personality background renders the prognosis more favorable. The persistence of hallucinations after an initial emotional tension has subsided is not a favorable indication. If the psychosis has existed for a year without clear-cut signs of improvement, a favorable outcome is scarcely to be expected although it is by no means unknown. Previous remissions should lead one to expect that a given episode will be followed by improvement. The longer the interval between attacks the better the prognosis. In many cases of schizophrenia regression is an important mechanism, so attempts are often made to base a prognosis on the depth of regression manifested by the patient. Infantile posture and behavior, while often of unfavorable significance, should not outweigh other considerations in forming an opinion as to prognosis. It may be parenthetically commented that the physician whose psychiatric experience has been confined to institutions tends to develop an unwarrantably pessimistic attitude in prognosis. The mortality rate among institutionalized schizophrenic patients is estimated to be twice as high as in the normal, community population.

A word should be said as to the prognosis in the different types. In catatonia the prognosis is relatively good if the onset has been stormy and the episode is still acute. Many of these patients are restored to their prepsychotic level of adjustment for varying periods, at times for several years. The prognosis in the simple form with its insidious marasmus of the personality developing in the absence of unusual environmental and experiential stresses is not at all good. A certain number, sheltered by some normal member of the family, maintain a colorless, uneventful existence while others become paupers, hoboes or petty criminals. The course of the hebephrenic form tends to be one of dereistic regression and of progressive disorganization although occasionally remissions occur before the final disorganization of personality. The question as to whether the paranoid type of schizophrenia ever recovers is sometimes raised. The reply to this depends somewhat on a definition of terms. Undoubtedly remissions occur, and these may be looked upon as social recoveries, but they are rarely to be looked upon as psychological recoveries even though the patient's adjustment during the interval may be well socialized and there be no distortions of reality in response to subjective needs. In general surly and bitter attitudes indicate a malignant process.

Finally, both for the sake of stating the opinion of one of the greatest students of schizophrenia as to the prognosis and for emphasizing the responsibility of the physician who undertakes the care of the early case of schizophrenia, the conclusion of Bleuler must be quoted: "Although a certain number of patients become deteriorated with every treatment, and others improve even in apparently severe cases, the treatment will decide in more than one third of schizophrenic cases whether they can become social men again or not." The more individualized and personalized the care and treatment the greater the recovery rate.

"DETERIORATION." While schizophrenia may become arrested at any phase of its evolutionary course, a word should be said about the nature of the unfavorable outcome so frequently observed. This malignant reaction was formerly spoken of as dementia. Such a characterization does not correctly indicate the personality change or disorganization of the ego that may occur in schizophrenia, the deteriorative signs of which are dynamically determined and may be reversible. Dementia, on the other hand, is an impersonal process, a permanent impairment of intellectual function because of degeneration or destruction of neurons. Psychometric tests indicate that intellectual disturbances in schizophrenia are not similar to those in organic brain disease. In schizophrenia any apparent reduction in intelligence should be explained on the basis of emotional maladjustments. Long-term psychological studies of schizophrenic patients show that this apparent intellectual impairment is capable of recovery even after long periods of time. While there is no dementia in the strict sense of the word, yet there is a disorganization of psychic functions, a reduction of, and subtle change in, intellectual performance because of the long-continued influence on behavior of hallucinations, delusions, disorganizing fantasy states and the patient's autistic withdrawal into self. One part of the ego perceives reality while another part is unaware of it. The mental deterioration is more apparent than real and probably never involves an irremediable loss of higher mental "faculties." There is an impairment of contact between the patient and reality and of his ability to appreciate or respond to environmental demands. Reactions tend to become not merely unrelated but wholly irrelevant to the needs and purposes of normal adult life.

Perhaps the malignant state in which many cases terminate would better be described as a breaking up of personality organization, as a habit deterioration rather than as "mental deterioration." This malignant disorganization is not an invariable characteristic but is seen all too frequently on the "back wards" of mental hospitals. Here are found the chronic, unemployable schizophrenic patients, some mutely vegetating on benches, others oddly attired, standing in a corner or pacing automatically to and fro, grimacing and absorbed in their delusions, bursting forth occasionally into spasms of hostility and aggression. Undoubtedly this "deterioration" is to a considerable degree often a hospital artifact and would not occur if the institution offered a more intensive therapeutically oriented program.

Diagnosis

At times perplexing similarities are observed between schizophrenia and the psychoneuroses, between schizophrenia and other biogenetic major psychoses, particularly manic-depressive and rarely between schizophrenia and organic mental disorders. It is doubtful, too, if there is any definite demarcation between psychoneurotic and schizophrenic reactions. Again the distinction between schizophrenic disturbances of the personality and those of the psychopath or character neurotic may be very difficult. Extreme caution should be exercised in declaring that an isolated symptom is conclusive evidence of schizophrenia and in evaluating a symptom, the clinical setting in which it occurs should be carefully examined. Neither should the eventual outcome be the most important determinant in diagnosis.

Many of the differential points among schizophrenic patients, hysteria and dissociative reactions will be discussed in Chapter XXX. In addition to what will be mentioned there attention should be called to the fact that the onset in hysteria is usually more sudden and that a psychological motive is more apparent. In schizophrenic stupor one does not discover the expression of an emotional state. In dissociative stupor, on the other hand, one may note an expression of perplexity, fear, elation or of some other affective state. The history of an insidious change in interests points toward schizophrenia. Not only are the symptoms of hysteria and of dissociation more sudden in onset, but they are more paroxysmal. The symptoms of hysteria are influenced more by certain persons in the environment. While the hysteric desires attention the schizophrenic is more apt to have periods when he is preoccupied, detached and apathetic. In schizophrenia the normal and psychotic elements exist side by side while in hysteria there is an alternation of normal and neurotic. The hysteric uses conventional, intelligible symbols while the schizophrenic uses individual or archaic ones. One can feel himself into the psychic life of the hysteric and of some dissociative states, but with difficulty, if at all, into that of the schizophrenic.

In the early stage of schizophrenia, the differentiation from obsessive neurosis may be difficult. Sometimes schizophrenic reactions result from the release of primitive impulses that had previously been kept under control by the aid of obsessional symptoms. In schizophrenia there is usually more rumination and less tension than in the obsessive neurosis, as the patient who suffers from the latter has a strong conscious resistance to his obsessions and compulsions, a resistance which is lacking in the schizophrenic since he is not particularly disturbed by them. Not rarely the schizophrenic, in the early phases of the disorder, expresses hypochondriacal complaints. His hypochondria lacks, however, the dramatization seen in the psychoneuroses.

Frequently one of the most difficult differentiations in mental disorders is between schizophrenia and manic-depressive psychosis. Doubtless this is a result, in part at least, of the fact that many people are not pure schizoid or pure syntonic types but rather are personality alloys and are characterized by admixtures in their personality. In addition to what has been said in Chapter XXV on affective reactions, attention may be called to the fact that the onset of schizophrenia tends to be more insidious, that the excitement in schizophrenia is more frequently paroxysmal while that of the manic is more sustained and the mood of the schizophrenic rarely possesses the infectious quality seen in the manic-depressive. The delusions of the depressed schizophrenic are more grotesque than those of the depressed manic and he is less distressed by them. Illogical remarks and incongruous statements suggest schizophrenia. The difficulty in differentiating between these two disorders arises largely in the earlier stages of schizophrenia. With recurring episodes the schizophrenic nature of symptoms previously doubtful becomes more apparent with the result that confusion with manic-depressive symptomatology no longer exists. It rarely happens that a psychosis apparently schizophrenic in its early phases proves subsequently to be of a manic-depressive reaction type. The reverse, however, is common. There are, nevertheless, many cases of mental disorder the recurring episodes of which continue to show a mixture of schizophrenic symptoms and of affective ones, especially depression and anxiety.

There is usually no difficulty in distinguishing schizophrenia from epilepsy. Occasionally, nevertheless, the schizophrenic suffers from epileptiform or syncopal attacks which to the inexperienced observer strongly suggest the seizures of epilepsy. In that case, carefully inquiry should be made as to whether the seizures or the mental symptoms appeared first, and the nature of the seizure should be observed; in schizophrenia it lacks the definiteness in type and the genuine disturbance of consciousness occurring in epilepsy.

In discussing the diagnosis of schizophrenia, mention should be made of what is often spoken of as chronic alcoholic hallucinosis. Attention is called to this condition not so much for pointing out distinctions from schizophrenia as for suggesting a possible identity with the latter disorder. The permanent persistence in the chronic alcoholic of auditory hallucinations in a setting of clear consciousness, frequently with systematized delusions, was formerly considered as a symptom of an alcoholic psychosis. Many psychiatrists now believe that such cases are really schizophrenic reactions. In the discussion of the alcoholic psychoses (Chapter X), attention was called to the fact that there is much to suggest that the so-called "acute" alcoholic hallucinosis has a schizophrenic basis and is not a purely alcoholic psychosis.

Adolescent psychoses do not belong in any special classification of their own yet their capacity for variation in duration, intensity and form frequently cause them to present difficulties in diagnosis. At that period one may alternatively see phases of anxiety, behavior disorder, affective disturbance or schizophrenia. In retrospect it may be found that stealing, truancy and other forms of delinquent behavior have marked the onset of a disorder that is subsequently diagnosed as schizophrenia. The adolescent schizophrenic frequently shows a more lively emotional response than is usual in the adult, also less incongruity of affect. The classical subgroups of adult schizophrenia are less frequently observed. The symptomatic emphasis in adolescent schizophrenia is usually on social withdrawal, disorders of activity, of interest and speech and on peculiarities of manner. It must be acknowledged, however, that it is not always easy to differentiate the emotional disorders of adolescence from incipient schizophrenia. That period is normally one of emotional turmoil and instability. Much that would be regarded as pathological in later life may then be but a temporary exaggeraton of normal tendencies. The adolescent with his self-questioning and perturbing heart-searching may verbalize his disruption of emotion and impulse without being schizophrenic. Adolescent maladjustments among shy, withdrawn personalities with feelings of inadequacy or inferiority, with evident internal conflict and family tensions, particularly with one or other parent, are not uncommon. Poor socialization, lack of motivation and a brooding sense of inferiority may be merely a retarded ability to integrate the new emotional drives and experiences of adolescence. Such symptoms may, however, be those of an incipient schizophrenia. The distinction is in many respects one of degree and not of kind.

Treatment

As previously indicated it is undoubtedly true that disorders at the physiological or vegetative levels may disturb integration at the higher mental level of the organism. It is doubtful, however, if there is always an underlying disturbance at these lower levels in every case of schizophrenic reaction. At any rate it must be said that psychological concepts are more helpful in enabling one to understand schizophrenia than are physiological and physicochemical concepts. For the present, therefore, the preferred method of therapy must be to treat any demonstrable disturbances of organic processes, at the same time applying such psychological, social and physical measures as fit the situation and needs of the individual.

The treatment of schizophrenia, particularly in its early stages, is undertaken with far less pessimism than formerly. Its success depends to no small degree upon the therapeutic initiative, energy and effort of the physician, although the results will be small if the psychotic methods of thinking and feeling have become habits and established forms of adjustment. In early cases the remission rate after treatment is about twice as high as is that of remissions occurring spontaneously.

Since it has been said that schizophrenia becomes manifest for the most part only after a prolonged period of incubation, the question as to whether a disease so disorganizing to the personality can be prevented naturally arises. The goal of the modern mental hygiene movement with its child-guidance clinics and its school and college psychiatrists is not merely to prevent or correct faulty attitudes and the less malignant maladjustments of childhood or adolescence but to promote healthful patterns of feeling and thinking and to prevent the establishment of subterfuges and substitutions that result in imbalances of personality and may finally culminate in the major psychoses of which schizophrenia is the most important. How far the rapidly growing mental hygiene movement will be able to modify the various factors the sequence of which leads to a schizophrenic adjustment to life is as yet entirely unknown and will probably never be susceptible of statistical demonstration. In the light of the knowledge now available, however, the body of principles included in the term mental hygiene seems to constitute the most rational means of preventing the malfunctioning of the personality known as schizophrenia. The shy, retiring, seclusive, unsociable child should receive careful guidance designed to promote socialization and a wholesome adjustment between the growing personality and its environment.

Ideally, treatment of the schizophrenic should have begun before obvious symptoms of a mental disorder were manifest. Unfortunately this rarely occurs. Rarely does the patient seek treatment himself and his family, unable or unwilling to recognize that he is mentally ill, does not refer him to a psychiatrist. Treatment should begin, of course, at as early a stage as possible. A prolonged psychotic state tends in itself to develop or aggravate personality patterns of a deleterious nature. Whether treatment should from its beginning be in a hospital or in the psychiatrist's office is a matter to be determined in the individual case. Much will depend on the home situation. Not rarely patient-parent or other interpersonal relations there are morbific. Too often the attitude of the family has been argumentative, critical and even hostile. Fortunately at times the patient's family is understanding, is a source of emotional support and his illness is amenable to psychotherapy. If his symptoms are acute and his behavior is disturbed, prompt hospitalization is desirable. Broadly speaking, the function of the hospital is to provide a kindly, protective environment where a variety of therapies may be employed. Associated with all of them, whether they be primarily physical or individually psychotherapeutic, there should be an attitude of acceptance, promotion of self-esteem and of warm interpersonal relationship. The patient needs a sustained living experience with people who are kindly and understanding and who do not reject him in spite of what he does.

Every case must be studied and treated individually. Not only should the psychic level of the personality be assessed but also the biochemical, physiological and neurological. Even though physiological or other somatic factors have apparently not acted as contributory ones they should, if possible, be corrected.

In addition to the therapies to be discussed efforts should be directed toward re-education including the development of a wider social consciousness and the promotion of an interest in reality. One attempts to stimulate the patient's interests, redirect them to things outside himself, detach his emotions from subjective material, inculcate healthful, socialized habits and abstract him from his spiritual isolation. Among important aids to these ends and to the gaining of satisfaction from adaptive behavior, are forms of occupational therapy chosen to meet his emotional needs. Recreation, games, music and congenial companionships all have a common objective of promoting interpersonal relationships. Occupational therapy not only helps to re-establish contacts with reality but through personal contact with the therapist frequently brings a therapeutic emotional relationship. Probably, in fact, the most important tool which the occupational or other auxiliary therapist brings to the treatment situation is a genuine warmth, understanding, flexibility and objectivity.

Many psychotherapists believe that the primary problem of the schizophrenic is not his anxiety about others and a consequent narcissistic withdrawal, often dating back to childhood, but fear of his own hostile, destructive tendencies. Although preoccupied, suspicious and anxiety-ridden because of the negative impulses he feels in himself, the schizophrenic can often, at least in the early stages of his illness, be helped to relate himself to people. Frieda Fromm-Reichmann stressed that while the schizophrenic longs for interpersonal contact, he equally fears such a closeness.

While not a few patients become permanently isolated in their own autistic lives in spite of every effort at treatment, the degree of improvement is, broadly speaking, directly proportional to the attention and treatment that they receive. There is usually a tendency to a progressive introversion and habit-deterioration. A constant effort should therefore be made to keep alive or re-establish an affective contact with reality and prevent the patient from drifting into a state of inactivity and indifference. The patient should be encouraged to participate in congenial activity and his environment should provide as many as possible of those things of life that interest and satisfy the person in mental health. The hospital offers a protective environment adapted to the patient's capacity for adjustment. However, treatment in an institution should undoubtedly be socialized to a greater extent than is now the case. In no instance should the patient be lost in the obscurity of a chronic ward. It has been said that the picture seen in chronic and hopeless institutional cases is one third a result of disease, while two thirds is a reaction to an unfavorable and unsuitable environment. Institutions are now adopting a more active and aggressive policy of treatment but are handicapped in their efforts because they do not receive the patient sufficiently early in the course of his disease and because they do not have sufficient personnel to render available the known resources of treatment. One of the unfortunate conditions that still exist widely in public institutions is overcrowding which results in a lack of adequate attention, provides an unnatural environment and promotes neglect. In the ideal institution, the hospital would provide what the home cannot, in addition to the advantages which the patient would have received had he remained in the home.

In 1939 Myerson described what he termed the "total push" method for the treatment of the institutionalized chronic schizophrenic. This did not involve any new principles of treatment but consists of the sustained application of an organized program of diversified and individual activities designed to meet many of the psychological needs of the schizophrenic so frequently neglected and ignored in the psychological vacuum of the "back ward." The patient is approached with stimulating and activating procedures from as many sides as possible. Measures which tend to arouse the patient from his automatized isolation are vigorously employed day by day. An attempt is made not to emphasize the separation created by the patient's illness, but to create as nearly as possible an atmosphere like the general community. Daily, weather permitting, the patient is taken for walks. Sustained, active efforts are made to overcome the inertia of the patient and his resistance to participation in games and exercise. Classes in bowling are organized and a game room is provided. As patients improve they participate in dancing, music, craftsmanship and general occupational therapy. Physiotherapeutic measures, such as showers, douches and massages, are utilized daily. Diet is liberal and small doses of insulin are often employed. Stress is placed on keeping the patient properly dressed in attractive clothing, the male patient is shaved regularly and fingers and hair receive careful attention. Praise in the presence of the group and reward under the same circumstances are liberally utilized as motives. The relationships developed between patient and the worker are of therapeutic value. Also, an effort is made to provide the patient with opportunity for experiencing a sense of belonging. A constructive release of hostility is encouraged, a sense of personal worth is fostered and opportunity for social interaction is facilitated. The participation of the nurse and aide in these highly organized activities improves their morale and promotes a greater interest in the welfare of the patient.

Myerson's "total push" therapy was directed to the chronic "deteriorated" schizophrenic. This "deterioration" is largely the result of rejection by others, by the patient's belief that the world is basically hostile, and the great failure of his environment to meet his emotional needs. All too often his hospital life is spent in idleness or futile routine. His surroundings are drab, his communications are not understood and he feels isolated from those assigned to care for him. He feels chronically frustrated in his search for a way of relating comfortably to the hospital environment and as a result becomes more deeply withdrawn. Stanton and Schwartz have made interesting contributions to the conception of schizophrenic deterioration as a psychosocial adaptive pattern. They found it was possible to discern meaningful patterns in the occurrences in a mental hospital. They studied, for example, the symptom of soiling and wetting so common in chronic deteriorated schizophrenics. They pointed out that the term "incontinence" is a misnomer if by that term we mean loss of sphincter control. The so-called incontinent schizophrenic patient, Stanton and Schwartz discovered, discharges his excreta in a highly controlled manner. There are some situations in which wetting and soiling rarely, if ever, occur. On the other hand, they may take place in a specific constellation of circumstances under the pressure of an emotional need. One patient, for example, who was extremely fearful of human contact found that people left her alone when she had soiled. Another patient who craved the attentions of a mother figure soiled herself to compel attentions from a nurse.

Special Forms of Treatment

Insulin Coma Therapy. The history of the therapy of schizophrenia has been characterized by the use of various methods which temporarily had enthusiastic proponents but failed to stand the test of time. Although insulin coma therapy is not a specific, and has in many respects been a disappointing procedure, yet when given at the right time to the right kind of case it is effective in restoring many patients to their preschizophrenic adjustment. This restoration to health is not accompanied by a permanent correction of the factors that predispose the patient to regress to schizophrenia, and its use has greatly decreased since the introduction of tranquilizing drugs. The details of its application will be discussed in Chapter XXXV.

The percentage of remissions following insulin therapy depends largely on the previous duration of the psychosis. The recovery rate is by far the greatest in patients who have not been ill for more than six months. Patients who have been sick less than one year will, under insulin treatment, do twice as well as those who have been sick more than one year. Full remission in patients who have been ill for more than two years is not common. Recovery after illness of longer duration is not rare if there have been symptom-free periods during the illness. The variations in reports of results secured by insulin therapy are probably caused by several factors. Some psychiatrists require a higher degree of insight as the only satisfactory evidence of complete recovery. Others consider that the persistence of slight personality changes is not inconsistent with recovery. It has been found that psychiatrists who applied longer and deeper comas to the patients reported higher recovery rates than those who applied shorter ones. Often, too, if treatments were not continued over a long period there was not as much success. Best results seem to be secured by physicians who closely followed the technique recommended by Sakel. Many psychiatrists believe that in cases of less than one year's duration treatment is followed by immediate improvement more frequently than in any other form of therapy. The percentage of relapses is high—so high that some psychiatrists believe that after a period of five years the percentage of patients who have remained well is no greater than those whose remissions have been spontaneous. Bond and Rivers found that at the end of treatment 55 per cent of all patients treated were enjoying a remission, after one year of treatment 42 per cent continued the remission, after two years 36 per cent were recovered or in a remission, while after three years 32 per cent had maintained their favorable condition. The best results are secured in those patients in whom the prognosis would, in general, be most favorable, *i.e.*, in cases characterized by acute onset, acute symptomatology, exogenic precipitating factors, catatonic reaction and previous extraversive tendencies. Combined insulin and electroconvulsive therapy may succeed where the two treatments given separately have failed. Insulin therapy in paranoid forms produces better results than in hebephrenic or simple types. Treatment is not followed by any change in the prepsychotic personality.

ELECTRIC CONVULSIVE THERAPY. Because of the simplicity of its application, its fewer hazards and the need for a smaller group of specially trained personnel, there has been a tendency to substitute electric convulsive for insulin therapy if some form of shock therapy is desired. There continues to be some controversy as to the relative results secured in schizophrenia by insulin and shock therapy. It would seem probable that a slightly larger number of full remissions will be secured by insulin therapy, yet many psychiatrists believe that if electric shock treatment is prolonged and intensive, with at least twenty treatments, it is as effective as insulin. Of the subtypes of schizophrenia, catatonic excitements and acute paranoid forms respond best to electroshock treatment. The results are naturally best when affective features are present and the assets of the prepsychotic personality are good. Patients who relapse after each of two successive courses of treatment have been kept on a maintenance treatment regimen of one or two treatments a week. The use of electroshock treatments as a maintenance treatment has been largely discontinued since the introduction of tranquilizing drugs.

Manfred Bleuler, who like his distinguished father, Eugen Bleuler, has been a devoted student of schizophrenia, is doubtful if permanence of improvement after either electroshock or insulin coma is hardly greater than after schizophrenic remissions without them. He adds: "Cures effected by shock treatments will be achieved preferably in the case of schizophrenics who would be expected to improve without them on the basis of a wavelike-acute course, administered in the light of personal history prior to illness and of family relationships. In fact, shock therapies seldom produce lasting cures in schizophrenics whose personal psychodynamics, chronic course, and family constellations would necessitate from the very beginning an unfavorable prognosis. . . . Shock (electric and insulin) are probably not causal treatments. They subdue and improve the patient and accelerate his cure. They facilitate human contact and, thereby, psychotherapeutic accessibility."

TRANQUILIZING DRUGS. (See Chapter XXXVII.) Since their introduction in this country in 1953 certain tranquilizing drugs, notably chlorpromazine and reserpine, have been extensively used in the treatment of schizophrenia. For the most part chlorpromazine and reserpine may be used interchangeably in this disorder although the latter will not be used in the case of patients showing depressive features.

Chlorpromazine has been found to be of great usefulness in both acute and chronic overactive schizophrenics. Its greatest usefulness is with those who show tension, psychomotor overactivity, agitation, impulsiveness, aggressive outbursts, destructiveness and antagonistic, paranoid reactions. When rapid sedation is required, chlorpromazine is to be preferred to reserpine. Administration of chlorpromazine to the acutely ill schizophrenic patient frequently results in the disappearance of hallucinations and delusional ideas within the first two weeks of treatment.

The longer the schizophrenic has been ill the less chance there is that the use of chlorpromazine will be followed by recovery. The best results are secured with patients who have not been ill for more than two years, and among these the results will depend largely on the clinical manifestations, the degree of improvement being much greater in the overactive, disturbed patient who improves to a degree that he becomes amenable to occupational and other activity therapies and, hopefully, to some degree of psychotherapy. While most overactive schizophrenics who have been hospitalized for long periods of time show some improvement, not more than 5 to 10 per cent of those who have been hospitalized for more than five continuous years become well enough to leave the hospital, and an appreciable number of these will have to return at a later time. The problem of the care of the chronic, overactive patient who does not improve sufficiently to leave the hospital will be greatly eased by chlorpromazine, however. Delusions and hallucinations may persist but usually they are no longer disturbing to the patient. The sullen, sarcastic and antagonistic patient is less irritable and frequently becomes quiet, cooperative and accessible; there is a remarkable improvement in the atmosphere of the ward for disturbed patients; and many who have long occupied seclusion rooms because of their assaultive and destructive tendencies may mingle with other patients and participate in occupational and other activities.

There is no standard rule as to the dosage and frequency in the administration of chlorpromazine. Both will be determined by the experience and preference of the physician. However, the following schedule has been found satisfactory in the treatment of mildly overactive schizophrenics: For the first week the patient will receive 50 mg. twice a day given orally. If the patient is acutely disturbed he will not receive any drug orally during the first week but will be given 25 mg. intramuscularly twice a day during that period. After one week he will receive no more intramuscular injections. Beginning with the second week he will be given 100 mg. of chlorpromazine twice a day (orally). This dosage will be increased 100 mg. weekly until the patient is receiving 400 mg. twice a day. This amount may be continued indefinitely until improvement of the patient suggests a gradual reduction or undesirable side effects appear. Many physicians do not hesitate to increase the total daily dosage to 1000 mg. Some give proportionately smaller doses three or four times a day but rarely exceed 800 or 1000 mg. for the total daily dosage.

Tranquilizing effects similar to those produced by the use of chlorpromazine may be obtained by the administration of *reserpine*. Its greatest usefulness in schizophrenia is, therefore, in the case of the tense, overactive, combative, hostile and threatening patient. Its effects, however, are less prompt than those secured by chlorpromazine. Like the latter drug, reserpine may be given intramuscularly or by mouth. The dosage should be individually adjusted. The initial dose may be 1 mg. given intramuscularly twice a day. After three days the intramuscular dose may be increased to 2 mg. At that time the patient may also receive 1 mg. twice a day by mouth. After one week intramuscular administration may be stopped and oral dose increased to 4 mg. twice a day. Usually this dosage is not increased although some physicians increase it to 4 gm. or 5 gm. twice a day if side effects do not appear.

In spite of its greater toxicity, chlorpromazine is more widely used than reserpine. Many psychiatrists are of the opinion that chlorpromazine is more effective than reserpine in the treatment of schizo-affective and paranoid schizophrenias.

Combined reserpine-chlorpromazine therapy may be beneficial in chronic deteriorated schizophrenic or in chronic schizophrenic patients in whom apathy and withdrawal are prominent. Their combined use is often advisable in patients who have failed to respond to chlorpromazine alone or in schizophrenic patients in whom long-term maintenance therapy is anticipated.

Preliminary reports suggest that meprobamate may be of much value in relieving the anxiety and tension manifested by some chronic schizophrenics.

PREFRONTAL LOBOTOMY. This form of treatment will not be employed unless all others have failed, but if it is to be employed it should be used before emotional deterioration is well advanced. If, after eighteen months or two years of active treatment which has included tranquilizing drugs, insulin coma and electroconvulsive therapies, the patient has shown no improvement, frontal lobotomy is usually to be recommended. Best results are secured if the patient's original personality was relatively well organized. Patients who show persistent tension, excessive motor activity, resistiveness, destructiveness or combativeness are the most suitable subjects for this treatment. In such cases one may at least reasonably expect that adaptive behavior in simple situations will be generally improved as well as social and ward behavior. Also, work activity will be increased, mood level will be more desirable and aggressive tendencies will be reduced. However, if the schizophrenic process has progressed to a chronic and general personality disorganization marked by persisting emotional dulling, loss of contact with people, widespread delusions and emotional disintegration, the results of the operation will be disappointing, and the results are progressively poorer with each successive year of the disease. In fact, very few patients are helped if the disease has existed ten years or more. If the illness is relatively recent, the problem of care is often simplified by frontal lobotomy even though the improvement is not sufficient to permit discharge from a hospital. Hebephrenics rarely respond favorably. Catatonic excitement usually responds well to lobotomy if, contrary to the usual result, it has not improved with insulin or electroconvulsive therapy, and paranoid schizophrenic patients are usually helped.

PSYCHOTHERAPY. In recent years there has been an increasing use of psychotherapy either as a supplementary or as an exclusive measure in the treatment of schizophrenia. While psychoanalytical techniques such as are usually employed in the neuroses have never been satisfactorily successful in the treatment of schizophrenia, yet modifications have now been evolved which may successfully maintain many patients at a functioning level of social adjustment.

The establishment of a working relationship with the patient is absolutely essential to successful therapy in the schizophrenic. The relationship of the patient to the therapist is of a different quality than that seen in neuroses. It is exceedingly fragile and is subject to withdrawal on the basis of any suspicion or indication that there is a limitation of interest on the part of the physician. Breaking through to obtain the trust of the suspicious, withdrawn, highly sensitive and perhaps disturbed patient requires infinite patience and tolerance. Rarely can the physician confine his contacts with the patient to set office hours. He must be available whenever periods of great anxiety occur. In the early stages of treatment the patient's verbal communications may be incomprehensible to the physician and some form of communication between the two must be established. At this stage the therapist does not attempt to have the patient, as would be done with the neurotic, associate to the verbalizations he is producing. Rather does the therapist listen and try to relate the patient's verbalizations to the feeling tone of particular interpersonal events that are reported to have preceded the distorted communications or are observed to occur in close temporal relationship. Then, when particular communications are heard, the therapist may interpret the patient's feeling directly and make it possible for him to appreciate that he is understood and will not be hurt. The patient must find in the therapist a sustaining source of security on the emergence of anxiety and hostility.

The therapist must be constantly alert to his own behavior and of its possible meanings to the patient. For this reason the therapy is conducted with the patient facing the therapist. The patient has a continuing need to check his reaction through visualizing the gestures and moves of the therapist. The latter must see himself as an active participant with his patient and must be free to disclose his own feelings and the meanings of his actions in order to clarify the patient's frequent distortions of the situation.

Contrary to the usual custom in the analytical therapy of the neuroses, the analysis of dreams is not advised. Preoccupation with dream analysis perpetuates the schizophrenic's propensity for withdrawal into fantasy living. What he needs is to face continually the emotionally toned events of everyday living and to learn socially adaptive methods of accepting them. Usually, too, the primitive impulses of the schizophrenic are so evident in their overt pathology that dream analysis will provide but little additional information. In contrast with earlier attempts to resolve delusional and hallucinatory experiences through analysis of their content, this is now recognized as unsatisfactory procedure in the therapeutic process. Rather, efforts are made to derive an understanding of the interpersonal situations that precipitate the patient's expressions of delusional and hallucinatory material and the significance of the psychopathology in terms of the affect produced in such situations. Frieda Fromm-Reichmann described this technique in some detail.

It should be remembered that there are limitations in the psychotherapy of the schizophrenic patient. Complete resolution of the schizophrenic process, fixed through indelible traumata of early life, is rarely obtained even by therapists of the greatest experience and patience. If, in an effort to reach the ideal, the enthusiastic psychiatrist presses his patient beyond his capacity, he may do him incalculable harm. The therapist must, of course, continue indefinitely a supportive, though distant, therapeutic relationship when the patient indicates the need.

In not a few schizophrenics a "spontaneous" remission or recovery occurs. In such cases the therapeutic agent usually remains unknown. In many instances it would appear that improvement followed because for some years the patient was able to make contact with some individual—

perhaps a nurse, aide or even some other patient—in his environment and that through this interpersonal relationship the individual became a bridge toward reality.

BIBLIOGRAPHY

Association for Research in Nervous and Mental Disease: Vol. V., Schizophrenia (Dementia Praecox). New York, Paul B. Hoeber, Inc., 1928.

———: Vol. X., Schizophrenia (Dementia Praecox). Baltimore, Williams and Wilkins Co., 1931.

Bender, Lauretta: Childhood schizophrenia. Psychiat. Quart., *27:*663–679, 1953.

———, and Helme, W. H.: A quantitative test of theory and diagnostic indicators of childhood schizophrenia. Arch. Neurol. & Psychiat., *70:*413–427, 1953.

———, and Freedman, A. M.: A study of the first three years in the maturation of schizophrenic children. Quart. J. Child Behavior, *4:*245–272, 1952.

Betz, Barbara: Strategic conditions in the psychotherapy of persons with schizophrenia. Am. J. Psychiat., *107:*203–215, 1950.

Bleuler, E.: Dementia Praecox or the Group of Schizophrenias. Translated by Joseph Zinkin. New York, International Universities Press, Inc., 1950.

———: Textbook of Psychiatry. Translated by A. A. Brill. New York, Dover Publications, 1951.

———: The physiogenic and psychogenic in schizophrenia. Am. J. Psychiat., *10:*203, 1930.

Bleuler, M.: Schizophrenia: review of work of Prof. Eugen Bleuler. Arch. Neurol. & Psychiat., *26:*610, 1931.

———: Eugen Bleuler's conception of schizophrenia—an historical sketch. Bull. of Isaac Ray Med. Library, *1:*47–60, 1953.

———, and Stoll, W. A.: Clinical use of reserpine in psychiatry: comparison with chlorpromazine. Ann. New York Acad. Sc., *61:*167–173, 1955.

Bond, E. D., and Shurley, J. T.: Insulin therapy and its future. Am. J. Psychiat., *103:* 338, 1946.

Brody, E. B., and Redlich, F. C.: Psychotherapy with Schizophrenics. New York, International Universities Press, Inc., 1951.

Campbell, C. M.: Clinical studies in schizophrenia. Am. J. Psychiat., *99:*475, 1943.

Clardy, E. R.: A study of the development and course of schizophrenia in children. Psychiatric Quart., *25:*81–90, 1951.

Despert, J. L.: The early recognition of childhood schizophrenia. M. Clin. North America, *31:*680, 1947.

Eisenberg, Leon: The autistic child in adolescence. Am. J. Psychiat., *112:*607–612, 1956.

———: The course of childhood schizophrenia. Arch. Neurol. & Psychiat., *78:*69–83, 1957.

———, and Kanner, Leo: Early infantile autism. Am. J. Orthopsychiat., *36:*556–566, 1956.

Ellison, E. A., and Hamilton, D. M.: The hospital treatment of dementia praecox: Part II. Am. J. Psychiat., *106:*454–461, 1949.

———: Psychosurgery in the Treatment of Mental Disorders and Intractable Pain, 2nd ed. Springfield, Ill., Charles C Thomas, 1950.

Fish, Barbara: The detection of schizophrenia in childhood. J. Nerv. & Ment. Dis., *125:*1–24, 1957.

Fisher, Seymour: Some observations suggested by the Rorschach test concerning the "ambulatory schizophrenic." Psychiat. Quart. Supplement, *29:*81–89, 1955.

Fromm-Reichmann, Frieda: Principles of Intensive Psychotherapy. Chicago, University of Chicago Press, 1950.

———: Notes on the development of treatment of schizophrenics by psychoanalytic psychotherapy. Psychiatry, *11:*263, 1948.

———: Psychotherapy of schizophrenia. Am. J. Psychiat., *111:*410–419, 1954.

Gerard, D. L., and Siegal, Joseph: The family background of schizophrenia. Psychiatric Quart., *24:*47–73, 1950.

Greenblatt, Milton; Arnot, R., and Solomon, H. C.: Studies in Lobotomy. New York, Grune & Stratton, 1950.
Hamilton, D. M., and Wall, J. H.: The hospital treatment of dementia praecox. Am. J. Psychiat., *105*:346–352, 1948.
Hanfmann, E., and Kasanin, J.: Conceptual Thinking in Schizophrenia. New York, Nervous and Mental Disease Monographs, 1943.
Harms, Ernest, Ed.: Our present knowledge of schizophrenia in childhood. The Nervous Child, *10*:1–178, 1952.
Hecker, Ewald: Die Hebephrenie. Virchow's Archiv f. pathol. Anat., Physiol., und klin. Medizin, *52*:394–431, 1871, Berlin.
Himwich, H. E.: Brain Metabolism and Cerebral Disorders. Baltimore, Williams & Wilkins Co., 1951.
Hoch, P. H., and Polatin, P.: Pseudoneurotic forms of schizophrenia. Psychiatric Quart., *23*:248–276, 1949.
Jenkins, R. L.: The schizophrenic sequence: Withdrawal, disorganization, psychotic reorganization. Am. J. Orthopsychiat., *22*:738–748, 1952.
———: Suturing the schizophrenic split. Arch. Neurol. & Psychiat., *73*:110–117, 1955.
Jung, C. G.: Psychology of Dementia Praecox. Translated by Peterson and Brill. Washington, Nervous and Mental Disease Publishing Co., 1909.
———: On the psychogenesis of schizophrenia. J. Ment. Sc., *85*:999, 1939.
Kahlbaum, Karl: Die Katatonie oder das Spannungsirresein. Berlin, August Hirschwald, 1874.
Kallman, F. J.: The genetic theory of schizophrenia. Am. J. Psychiat., *103*:309–322, 1946.
———, and Roth, Bernard: Genetic aspects of preadolescent schizophrenia. Am. J. Psychiat., *112*:599–606, 1956.
Kanner, Leo: Early infantile autism. J. Pediat., *25*:211–217, 1944.
———: Problems of nosology and psychodynamics in early infantile autism. Am. J. Orthopsychiat., *19*:416–476, 1949.
Kasanin, J.: Language and Thought in Schizophrenia. Berkeley, University of California Press, 1944.
Katzenelbogen, S.: Dementia Praecox, formulation by Kraepelin, Bleuler and Meyer. Psychiatric Quart., *16*:439, 1942.
Knight, R. P.: Borderline states. Bull. of Menninger Clin., *17*:1–12, 1953.
Kolb, L. C.: Psychotherapeutic evolution and its implications. Psychiatric Quart., *30*: 579–597, 1956.
Kraepelin, E.: Dementia Praecox. Translated by Barclay, E. and S. Livingstone, Edinburgh, 1919.
Lidz, R. W., and Lidz, T.: The family environment of schizophrenic patients. Am. J. Psychiat., *106*:332–345, 1949.
Lidz, T., Cornelison, Alice, and Parker, B.: The role of the father in the family environment of the schizophrenic patient. Am. J. Psychiat., *113*:126–132, 1956.
———; ———; Fleck, Stephen, and Terry, Dorothy: The intra-familial environment of schizophrenic patients: II. Marital schism and marital skew. Am. J. Psychiat., *114*: 241–248, 1957.
Malamud, William: The present status of research in dementia praecox. Ment. Hyg., *34*:569–581, 1950.
Meyer, Adolf: An attempt at analysis of the neurotic constitution. Am. J. Psychol., *14*:354–367, 1903.
———: Fundamental conceptions of dementia praecox. Brit. M. J., Part 2, 757, 1906; J. Nerv. & Ment. Dis., *34*:331–336, 1907.
———: Dynamic interpretation of dementia praecox. Am. J. Psychol., *21*:385–403, 1910.
———: The nature and conception of dementia praecox. J. Abnormal Psychol., *5*:274–285, 1910.
———: Constructive formulation of schizophrenia. Am. J. Psychiat., *78*:355–362, 1922. (The five preceding articles will also be found in "The Collected Papers of Adolf Meyer, Vol. II, Edited by Eunce E. Winters. Baltimore, Johns Hopkins Press, 1951.)
Morel, B. A.: Traité des Maladies Mentales. Paris, Victor Masson, 1860.

Myerson, A.: Theory and principles of the "total push" method in the treatment of chronic schizophrenia. Am. J. Psychiat., *95:*1197, 1939.
Planansky, Karel: Heredity in schizophrenia. J. Nerv. & Ment. Dis., *122:*121–142, 1955.
Proceedings of Association for Research in Nervous and Mental Disease: Vol. XXXIV, Neurology and Psychiatry in Children, Part VI: Symposium of juvenile schizophrenia. Baltimore, The Williams & Wilkins Co., 1954.
Sakel, M.: Pharmacological Shock Treatment of Schizophrenia. Washington, Nervous and Mental Disease Publishing Co., 1938.
Sands, Dalton E.: The psychoses of adolescence. J. Ment. Sc., *102:*308–318, 1956.
Silver, Archie A.: Management of children with schizophrenia. Am. J. Psychotherapy, *9:*196–215, 1955.
Stanton, A. H., and Schwartz, M. S.: The Mental Hospital. A Study of Institutional Participation in Psychiatric Illness and Treatment. New York, Basic Books, 1954.
Tucker, Kenneth, and Wilensky, Harold: A clinical evaluation of meprobamate therapy in a chronic schizophrenic population. Am. J. Psychiat., *113:*698–703, 1957.
Wahl, C. W.: Some antecedent factors in the family histories of 568 male schizophrenics of the United States Navy. Am. J. Psychiat., *113:*201–210, 1956.
Whitehorn, John C., and Betz, Barbara J.: A study of psychotherapeutic relationships between physicians and schizophrenic patients. Am. J. Psychiat., *111:*321–331, 1954.
Worthing, H. J.; Brill, Henry, and Wigderson, Henry: Evaluation of immediate and late results of prefrontal lobotomy. Am. J. Psychiat., *108:*328–336, 1951.

CHAPTER XXVIII

Psychotic Disorders (Continued)

Paranoid Reactions (Paranoia and Paranoid Conditions)

PARANOIA is a chronic mental disorder of insidious development and is characterized by persistent, unalterable, systematized, logically reasoned delusions. General demeanor, talk and emotional and behavior reactions remain unaltered except as influenced by delusional beliefs which become the uppermost and guiding theme of the patient's life and may therefore seriously impair discretion and judgment. The term was first used in 1863 by Kahlbaum to designate various persecutory and grandiose states. That the most conspicuous symptom is in the field of thought is indicated by the etymology of the name applied to mental disorders of this type (παρὰ, beside, in the sense of altered or changed, and νοῦς, intellect or reason).

Causes

There seems to be convincing evidence that the causes of paranoia and paranoid conditions are psychological. Among these psychological causes may be ambitious but frustrated strivings, a need for defense of the personality against undesirable tendencies and repudiated impulses, feelings of insecurity, guilt or other anxiety-producing factors; a continued failure to achieve overvalued goals, or a need for enhancing prestige or self-esteem. Specific traumatic life experiences may serve as contributory factors. In a significant number of cases it will be found that the paranoiac comes from a family that has been severely authoritarian, harsh and cruel. Frequently a parent, usually of the same sex, has been a hostile, controlling person who rejects the child and through accusations produces fear, anxiety, feelings of inadequacy and a self-image of the "bad" child which, however, he does not accept. In many, perhaps in most, cases there has been an early overidentification with the parent of the opposite sex. As a result of his emotional experiences and frustrations, patterns of hatred and aggression are frequently established which, however, the child must endeavor to repress because of fear of his parent. As is frequently observed, parents whose personalities were warped through unwholesome attitudes and relationships with their parents may affectively distort those of their own children. Early affective frustrations may lead the child to a withdrawal from social contacts and to a resulting feeling of rejection. This may stimulate resentment and contribute a paranoid element to the developing personality that may finally culminate in the paranoid psychosis. Sometimes self-pity or sibling rivalry seems to facilitate the establishment of paranoid tendencies.

Even as a child the future paranoid individual usually shows troublesome trends that make it difficult for him to participate in congenial play with other children for more than brief periods. He is often a lonely, unhappy, brooding, insecure child lacking friends with whom he can share confidences and exchange perspectives. It will frequently be found that he is suspicious, stubborn, secretive, obstinate and resentful of discipline. When crossed he is apt to be sullen, morose, peevish and irritable. As adult life is approached the early personality characteristics become accentuated. The future patient becomes increasingly sensitive about the attitude and behavior of others, "builds mountains out of molehills," and may believe that others wish to do him injury. He is lacking in a sense of humor, is egotistic, self-confident, self-assertive, sarcastic, derogatory, querulous, embittered and resentful. Usually the paranoid person has always been critical, demanding, inflexible, biased, mistrustful, impatient of conventions and often defiant of them. Characteristically he has been argumentative, uncompromising and aggressive. Interpersonal relationships are difficult. He approaches others with a "chip on the shoulder" attitude. The drive for achievement may be intense and impel him to seek goals that are beyond his capacity. Intolerant of criticism and unable to accept suggestions he readily criticises and belittles others. Meticulous and precise, he is in some respects highly efficient but is jealous and unadaptable. He needs to demonstrate his superiority. If in a position of authority he may be a petty tyrant.

At times one meets persons handicapped by such *paranoid personality* characteristics which, however, never develop further. In others these characteristics become gradually and insidiously intensified until the patient is clearly psychotic. In the same problems and factors are to be found the sources both of the paranoid personality and the paranoid psychosis. The latter represents a progressive, developing continuance of the former. In some instances as in other paranoid reactions repressed homosexual impulses seem to be the source of the psychopathology.

The mental mechanisms and reactions observed in paranoia are but exaggerations of ones noted constantly among persons who are not thought of as psychotic. In everyday life fear and insecurity are expressed in such disguises as pettiness, oversensitiveness, irascibility, never-ending bickering, overcompensation, seclusiveness, selfishness or cynicism. Even caution may develop into suspiciousness. Many people are at times inclined to feel slighted, to think that their merits are unrecognized, to blame their environment for what are really dissatisfactions with self, or perhaps in part to fulfill their wishes in fantasy. Daily we meet those who are unable to recognize and admit their faults and defects. Real or imagined injuries to pride tend to result in feelings of resentment and bitterness of variable duration. The well-defined paranoid personality often seems to display a remarkable genius for detecting in the ordinary run-of-life situations just those tiny slights, inadvertencies or trifling disparagements which others overlook but which he builds up into crucial issues, not altogether imaginary but vastly overemphasized. The paranoid personality may be overaggressive and see an aggressor in everyone around him. This makes him feel that his war against the world is waged in self-defense. A rebellious, superior attitude may serve to bolster self-esteem and prevent a realistic but intolerable self-evaluation. Not rarely the paranoid individual treats others as projections of certain of his own unconscious trends. As a result his statements, manner and behavior alienate friends and create enemies. The fact that he thereby incurs the hostility of others and is therefore often rejected and isolated adds more fuel to the psychopathogenic fire. Affective states may for a time give rise to false references to one's self, lead to rationalization and to the suspension of reflective logic, although the ideas thus affectively determined do not continue to multiply and spread as in paranoia. One must agree with the English psychiatrist, Crichton-Miller: "For every fully developed case of paranoia in our mental hospitals there must be hundreds, if not thousands, who suffer from minor degrees of suspicion and mistrust; whose lives are blighted by this barrier to human harmony; and who poison the springs of social life for the community."

In the paranoid personality we meet with an exaggeration of the common tendency to ascribe responsibility to others, to repudiate aspects of the personality that do not measure up to the standards the individual has set for himself, to obtain satisfaction through compensatory strivings, to maintain self-esteem by constructing emotionally satisfying but irrational explanations for his own failures, and to attribute hostile or aggressive motives to others. Disappointments, humiliation or injuries sustained may accentuate a paranoid tendency and even appear to precipitate a paranoid psychosis. The causes of paranoia are, then, to be sought in the need for protecting particularly vulnerable aspects of the personality, in the craving for a recognition greater than acquirement can command, in the particular mental conflicts of the individual, and in frustrations, vague fears, and in a need for relieving one's own anxiety over guilt by blaming someone else. Many cases of paranoid psychoses seem to derive from the mechanism whereby guilt-inspiring impulses are repudiated by projection to a persecutor. As we study the behavior of individuals and the methods by which they meet conflicts within and blows from without, we often find it difficult to say when the expressions of a paranoid personality become the symptoms of a paranoid psychosis. Anomalies of character become continuous with the psychosis, both, to a large degree, going back to the needs and problems of the personality and to the habitual techniques or patterns which the individual has adopted in attempting to meet them.

Formerly there was a tendency to subdivide the permanent paranoid reactions into definite disease entities. Kraepelin looked upon paranoia as a fixed type of disease resulting exclusively from internal causes and characterized by persistent, systematized delusions, the preservation of clear and orderly thinking and acting and by the absence of hallucinations. Intermediate between paranoia and paranoid schizophrenia he recognized an entity he called paraphrenia, differing principally from paranoia by the fact that the delusions lack the logical systematization of the latter disorder, the delusions are more apt to be extravagant and hallucinations are present at times. Not for many years, if at all, is there any deterioration of general interest or of personality. Kraepelin's paraphrenia corresponds rather closely to the psychoses included in the present official classification under the title, "Paranoid State." It would appear, however, that there is no sharp line of distinction between "Paranoia" and "Paranoid State." Rather do the paranoid-reaction psychoses constitute a continuous transition with imperceptible gradations in respect to the following: as to the extent to which affect is adequately and appropriately responsive to individual experience and environment; the extent to which delusions are systematically organized; the correctness of evaluation of reality; the extent to which subjective mental material is symbolized and projected in terms of such sensory experiences as hallucinations; and finally as to the extent to which psychobiological integration is disturbed and personality disorganized. In all of these respects the disintegrative processes become greatest as the schizophrenic pole of the paranoid series is approached.

True Kraepelinian paranoia is much less frequent than are paranoid reactions having a wide variation of schizophrenic features associated with them. The difference in final outcome of the psychoses in the inclusive paranoid-reaction group is one of degree of preservation of personality. Except for the fact that paranoid reactions accompanied by such markedly schizoid features as to place them among the schizophrenias will not be included in this discussion there will no attempt to draw lines of distinction between so-called "true" paranoia and the other paranoid reactions that through a long course of evolution have come to represent a permanent type of life adjustment. Practically, whether one considers those paranoid reactions which are comparatively free from schizophrenic features as cases of paranoia or of paranoid state is a matter of opinion and not important. The fact that the paranoid reactions, represented at one extreme by paranoia and at the other by paranoid schizophrenia, seem to form a continuum and to merge imperceptibly one into the other is what may be expected since types of personalities do not fall into sharply defined categories, neither are there fixed and exclusive mental methods by which individuals meet their emotional conflicts, their limitations and the experiences of life.

Symptoms

As previously noted, there is no clearly defined point at which the personality marked by the characteristics previously described should be called psychotic. Perhaps the criterion should be the degree to which reality is distorted and adjustment disturbed. The paranoid tendencies rarely become so extreme as to justify a diagnosis of paranoia before the age of thirty. The disorder is more common in men. As already indicated, the presenting symptom of paranoia and of paranoid states is a rigid, persistent system of delusions. At times the patient's delusions may take their origin in some actual fact. On cross section his behavior and thought content may be deceptive and a severe disorder be camouflaged by a seemingly normal surface. On longitudinal section, however, the paranoid theme is discovered. The content of paranoid ideas varies widely and is determined primarily by the particular psychological needs they are created to fulfill, and secondarily by the type of rationalization which will appeal to the ideas and beliefs current in the patient's environment. The patient's own inclinations are mirrored in the particular motives and intentions attributed to others. His rationalizations are vigorously defended and he exhibits a convincing earnestness in his efforts to win others to his delusional beliefs. The patient may rationalize so plausibly that his friends accept his allegation that specific individuals, rather than himself, are responsible for his difficulties. His superior intellectual endowment may remain unimpaired. Some paranoiacs become aware that the credibility of their delusions is questioned and therefore attempt to hide them. The patient's judgment may be defective only in relation to his delusional system which often develops slowly and ultimately becomes intricate and complex. The dominating ideas tend to be those of persecution, of expansive grandiosity or of those containing both themes.

As *persecutory* trends develop, the patient attributes hostile or aggressive motives to others, nurses his grievances and becomes increasingly secretive. In the earlier period of his psychosis he may be hypochondriacal and uneasy. He may become depressed, gloomy, spiteful, vindictive and given to morose rumination. Frequently he manifests a self-righteous resentment against others. Misunderstandings and misinterpretations develop into delusions of persecution. The tendency of the paranoiac to seek for ulterior motives on the part of others or to misinterpret events is illustrated by the case of a woman who soon after graduation from a law school, the faculty of which had awarded her the annual prize for the greatest improvement in scholastic work during her professional course, sued the school for damages, alleging that the awarding of such a prize was for the purpose of representing her as having been more poorly fitted than her associates for the study of law. (Doubtless the same sense of insecurity that led to her psychosis determined also her choice of law as a profession.)

In his effort to control his hostile impulses in which the genesis of his paranoid reaction is often to be found, the patient projects them and experiences them as being directed against himself. Filled with hate he feels and believes that he is the victim of persecutors, who, in fact, are but the objects upon whom he has projected his own hate. The mood of many paranoiacs is one of sustained sullenness. Ideas of reference appear: there is a hidden meaning in what goes on around; cryptic significances are read into casual remarks and events; slights and indignities are imagined; far-reaching significance is attached to trivial details in the behavior of others. Vague feelings of fear tend to increase suspicion and the patient's malevolent trend of thought. Although in the case of the "normal" person incredulity, indignation and anger often help to prevent the individual from becoming aware of qualities, strivings and tendencies that offend self-esteem, yet these defensive reactions are used much more by the paranoiac patient. Delusional ideas extend: the patient believes that people spread lies about him; persons tamper with his mail; accusing remarks are overheard; hostility and jealousy are observed on every hand; business plans are thwarted; he is the victim of a conspiracy and the agents of malevolent social organizations pursue him, persecutors seek to conceal their identity by various disguises. He may become depressed and even suicidal because he feels overwhelmed by an environment with which he cannot cope.

In the persecutory as well as in other forms of paranoia there is a central delusional theme that pervades the whole life of the patient who is quite incapable of criticizing the pseudologic he employs in supporting this dominant idea. His premises are not scrutinized and present events, regardless of their relevancy to the prevailing idea, are interpreted wholly with reference to it. Affect determines the patient's logic. Incidents of the past receive a new interpretation and are fitted into the framework of present persecution—a process known as retrospective falsification. As a result the delusional system constantly extends and the most commonplace incidents, because of their affective interpretation with reference to the prevailing idea, become events of the greatest importance. In all paranoid reactions the patient, always confident that he is right, clings obstinately to his opinions since his inner sense of insecurity cannot permit him to feel otherwise. He maintains his delusional misinterpretations, too, by continually overemphasizing the inferred or implied meaning and by discarding the obvious and real content of a statement or action.

A not uncommon form of paranoia is the *litigious* type. While it will usually be found that this type of paranoiac individual was always stubborn, insistent upon his "rights" and with many defensive mechanisms, yet the litigious activities frequently do not appear until after some legal experience which eventuated less satisfactorily than the patient desired. Because of his dissatisfaction, the patient initiates further but ill-advised legal action. He always fails to see that he has not proved his case. Every new litigation brings further controversies and new grievances for which the patient feels prompted to seek redress; his attempts to secure it, however, result in fresh feelings of injustice. Fundamentally, it is often not a question of law and justice, as the patient insists, but of attempts to put others in the wrong, to show that he was right, that he is superior, in order that thereby his sensitive insecurity may be strengthened and the weak points of his personality be protected.

In the *exalted* type of paranoia the ideas of grandeur may appear after a long preceding stage of persecution, or at times the grandiosity may be present practically from the beginning of the psychosis. Ideas of invention constitute a frequent form of grandiosity. Patients with such beliefs usually neglect their usual method of livelihood, and devote their time to the drawing of plans and the construction of models. At times the patient claims that models are completed but that enemies prevent him from securing a patent; again, he is on the point of perfecting the machine. In either case the patient frequently claims to utilize some force or to attain some objective contrary to the accepted laws of science. In this type, the patient may have a sense of mission and pursue his impracticable goal with more zeal than discretion. Others have expansive ideas of noble birth. Frequently the grandiose patient attempts to play the role which his ideas have assigned him. If, for example, he believes he is a religious leader he may wear long hair and a beard and affect an air of humility—an air that often disguises but poorly a repressed hatred.

The exalted beliefs in some paranoid states are of a religious nature. The patient is the chosen one of God, is Christ, prophesied the war, has supernatural powers. Some establish new religious sects and secure adherents; others proclaim themselves leaders of a new order but are so bizarre in belief and behavior that they fail to secure followers.

Occasionally paranoia assumes an *erotic* form. The patient believes that some woman of title or wealth whom he may have casually seen or met is in love with him. He writes her affectionate letters and perhaps poems. Her failure to reply to them is intended solely to test his love. Items in the newspapers, the flight of the birds and various events are disguised recognitions of her presence and acknowledgments of her love. Such patients may become annoyingly persistent in their attentions and threatening in their manner.

Among common causes for the commitment of paranoid patients are homicidal or suicidal attempts, the writing of anonymous letters to persons in authority, litigation or persistent statements that they are the victims of a conspiracy.

PSYCHOPATHOLOGY. Although disparity between achievement and ambition, early experience heavily loaded with affect, vague or subconscious feelings of dissatisfation or irritation with self, injuries to self-evaluation, as well as various other needs for defense may act as dynamic agents and lead or contribute to a fixed paranoid reaction type, yet there is much to suggest that in some but by no means all cases repressed homosexual impulses may be a genetic factor. An increasing number of psychiatrists, although they are unwilling to accept all of Freud's statements concerning the relation of psychosexual factors to the normal or the abnormal personality, have come to believe that unadjusted psychosexual tendencies may in some instances bear a relation to paranoia. The persistence of homosexual impulses, unrecognized consciously, may doubtless be caused by more than one factor, but, characterized as the homosexual is with his infantile survivals and mother imprint, there seems good reason to believe that if at puberty an inhibitive maternal overpossessiveness impedes the maturation of the psychosexual aspects of her son's personality these may remain fixated and never attain a mature heterosexual development.

Assuming that there is a relation between this fixation, or incomplete evolution of the personality, and homosexuality, how does the latter lead to paranoia? According to Freud, it is through the mechanism of projection by which the original but repressed and therefore consciously rejected affect is reversed and transferred to the homosexual object. Because consciously inadmissible the patient's "I love him" is changed to "I do not love him; I hate him" which to be acceptable requires projection as "He hates me" and is elaborated into "I am persecuted by him."

An abnormally high percentage of paranoids do not marry. This is because of not only a basic homosexual orientation but also the fact that their chronic hostility and anger make them undesirable as partners. If the paranoiac does marry, the marital life is so full of discord that it frequently ends in divorce.

The "true" paranoiac is often a person of superior intellectual endowment but his energy is so largely expended in repudiating desires that do not wish to be recognized as such, in compensatory efforts whereby self-esteem may be enhanced, and in striving for satisfactions that life has not supplied, that social relations become disturbed and constructive achievements are nil. The fact that life has failed to bring the success and satisfactions to which the native intelligence of the patient would ordinarily have entitled him undoubtedly tends to aggravate his defensive reactions. As already indicated, a large percentage of cases of paranoia occur among people of superior intelligence. This is perhaps because the person of superior intellectual endowment finds rationalization and projection to be readily available and satisfactory mechanisms of defense. Regression and other inferior mechanisms are not ones which would naturally be the choice of a person possessing unusual intellectual resources which he may utilize in dealing with repressed tendencies, feelings of guilt, frustrated hopes and wounds of pride. The more promptly and passively the individual gives up the struggle for self-esteem and for recognition the more nearly will the reaction approach the schizophrenic, regardless of the native intelligence, while the more active and sustained the struggle the more likely is the result to approach paranoia.

The following case presents, in some respects, many of the characteristic features of paranoia:

> In 1934 P. G. was committed to a hospital for mental diseases because of his peculiar religious ideas and rites, one of them being the practice of going about nude. The patient's parents were strict in their moral principles and rigid in discipline. All the paternal siblings were teachers except the patient's father who was a farmer and who was always dissatisfied with his lot, often expressing the wish that he could "get away where he could read and study and reform the world." The patient had one sister, also a brother who was older and stronger and who used to "lord it over" the patient. His association with his sister was close and shortly before leaving home as a young man he suggested to her that

if she would not get married he would not do so either and they would live together. As a child he was described as sensitive and fearing criticism. "Because he was not strong he was somewhat of a sissy," the sister stated. At school he was a ready scholar and completed the equivalent of two years of high school work. If he received less than 90 in his grades he felt disgraced. Prior to his marriage at twenty-six he had paid little attention to persons of the opposite sex. At that age he married his landlady, a woman of sixty-six, "as a humane act"; this was his characterization of the match when he entered the hospital. When questioned concerning his sex life he stated that men had aroused him sexually more than women, for whom he had no sexual desire. He took part in homosexual practices on only a few occasions. When asked if he thought his religion had helped him in repressing his homosexual tendencies, he replied, "I do not think so, I know it." He acknowledged that he derived pleasure from exposing himself to other men although he claimed that his practice of going about nude was a health measure permitted by his religion and not for the purpose of satisfying exhibitionistic impulses—doubtless a rationalization of socially prohibited inclinations. When questioned concerning his social life, he had, he said, "a distinct aversion to secret organizations"—perhaps an unconscious defense against his homosexual tendencies, since such organizations, made up as they usually are of individuals of one sex, serve to provide a sublimated and socialized outlet for homosexual trends, although the psychological basis of these bodies is also one of narcissism and compensation.

During his early adult life the patient became interested in various unusual religious cults (probably an effort to obtain a feeling of security), although this striving did not result in such a serious disturbance in thought and behavior as to lead to his being considered psychotic until after he was forty years of age. He described himself as suffering at about that period from "Lack of initiative, inability to concentrate, general weakness, anxiety about the future, irritability, and hypopotency of the heart." Doubtless this represented a stage of subjective analysis often occurring in the disease. He addressed a prayer to the "Deity" asking for aid and threatening to commit suicide if it were not forthcoming. Almost immediately it was "revealed" to him, not through a voice or visible signs but "simply through thought process," that he was to establish a new religion to take the place of Christianity, one that would be more comforting and satisfactory. He called his new religion "Omnivitism" and spent day after day writing "a set of mottoes instead of commandments, a set of actions and ideals, prayers, verse, comment on principles, affirmations and denials, suggestions regarding services and miscellaneous dissertations." When questioned as to the specific teachings of his religion little but vague generalities was to be secured. "It teaches," he said "that all forms and phases of existence are essential factors of one all-sufficient existence which is called 'Omniad.'" He had tracts printed which he distributed widely, setting forth "the rule of Omnivitism which is to teach according to his needs."

About this time he began to go to isolated spots and to walk about nude, explaining that he was taking "sun baths." Gradually he made few attempts to retire from sight when taking his "sun baths," particularly after one occasion when he derived considerable enjoyment from the fact that he was seen by the occupants of two automobiles that passed while he was unclothed. Finally, after having been warned on repeated occasions by the local constable that he must not continue his exhibitionistic practices, the patient was committed to a hospital for mental disorders.

On arrival at the hospital the patient was pleasant and smiling but obviously exalted with an air of self-satisfaction and superiority. He was a small man of rather effeminate physique, his hair reached nearly to his shoulders, and his beard was long, his appearance strongly resembling the traditional picture of Christ. He accepted his detention philosophically, expressing the opinion that it was what one in his position must expect—a sort of martyrdom in a worthy cause. He had, he said, founded a religion "more up to date" than that of Christ and one that would supplant Christianity and dominate the world; it had been revealed to him that by 1940 it would have been substantially established. Further, in 1948, the patient would be elected President of the United States. This, he added, was in accordance with the prophecy of Sir William Hope made on the day of Washington's birth. On that day he foretold how a new nation would arise in America and the part that would be played by Washington, and that finally there would come a ruler whom he characterized as "six plus added six—great, good and wise," at the same time referring to "a star that on his way shall shine." This prophecy, the patient said, referred to him since there were six letters in each of his names, while his sister was the star since it was she who had invited him to come to their old home. In an old novel, too, the patient claimed he had found the following: "There will come in the western continent a greater man than this world has seen since this civilization began. It will not be through the ignorance of the people that this man will be carried into the White House. In some respects this man will be the intellectual and philosophical leader. He will be to the world what Mohammed was to Arabia, Columbus to the New World, Moses to the Jews, Plato to the Greeks, etc.—yet he will be greater than all and more powerful for good." This, the patient said, referred to him.

On psychometric examination, by the Stanford-Binet scale, the patient was found to have an intelligence quotient of 115. It is interesting to note that in ability to see logical relationships, language ability and constructive visual imagery he attained an eighteen-year level but on practical judgment in social situations he graded at a nine-year-and-one-month level. In describing his attitude toward the examination the psychologist recorded that he seemed to enjoy the opportunity of demonstrating his intellectual endowment, that he frequently laughed in a superior and condescending manner, that he exhibited great precision of speech and delighted in showing off his large and unusual vocabulary. On several occasions, in a tolerant and somewhat condescending manner, he criticized the examiner for her use of words.

The patient's paranoid system is associated with too great disorganization of personality and disturbance of reality evaluation to permit the diagnosis of paranoia, but may properly, we believe, be regarded as a paranoid state rather than paranoid schizophrenia. The patient is unable to secure a satisfying adjustment to a sense of biological and social inadequacy, to a fundamental homosexuality and doubtless to other conflicts. However, instead of investing the external world with his own unrecognized but repudiated trends and feelings he organized his emotional constellations into ideational systems that afforded a satisfying but unsocialized adjustment. The compensatory feelings of superiority developed to meet the subconscious feelings of inferiority and doubtless of guilt (arising from an imperfectly repressed homosexuality) were rationalized into grandiose delusions. Other factors, too, presumably contributed to the life pattern of the patient's personality and his desire for high personal value. It may well have been that the dissatisfactions with self and the vaguely defined strivings owe their origin in part to absorption from the early family life, since we learn that his father was dissatisfied with his lot and wished to "study and reform the world." The fact that he was "lorded over" by a stronger brother presumably led to feelings of inadequacy and contributed to the psychological need for the artificially obtained feeling of security and self-esteem. To have been taught that school grades below an unreasonably high standard constituted a disgrace tended to lead the boy to form ambitions which, with his limitations of personality and opportunities for training, inevitably resulted in wounds to pride and vanity. Among the traits of childhood were sensitiveness and fear of criticism. His slightness of physique called for compensation, while a certain degree of biological deviation and the failure to emancipate himself emotionally from his older sister who perhaps served as a mother surrogate served to fix the development of his personality at a homosexual level. His exhibitionistic practices are doubtless also to be explained on the basis of arrest in psychosexual evolution. His egotistic wishes prejudiced his judgment and led it to disregard the usual criteria of reality, thereby both preventing a correct perspective and destroying the capacity for self-criticism.

FOLIE À DEUX. Inasmuch as the clinical features are nearly always paranoid in nature, mention may be made at this point of an induced or communicated form of psychosis described by Lasègue and Falret in 1877 to which they gave the name "*folie à deux*." Identification is usually an important mechanism in its production. This is a mental disorder in which mental symptoms, particularly paranoid delusions, from which one of two persons intimately associated with each other, usually for years, is suffering are communicated to and accepted by the other. Most frequently such a dual psychosis involves mother and daughter, two sisters or husband and wife. The person suffering from the primary psychosis is usually the dominant individual while the one who develops the secondary or induced psychosis is of a submissive and suggestible type dependent upon and having a close emotional attachment to the infector. As misinterpretations, illusions and ideas of persecution increasingly disturb the infector he persuasively relates his convictions and psychotic experiences to the weaker or infectee who comes to accept and react to the systematized delusional ideas of the first. It will often be found that both persons have been poorly adjusted individuals having a narrow range of interests, of the same general background and environment and facing perhaps the same situation. The induced ideas must be acceptable and usually offer some satisfaction to the person infected. In nearly every instance the delusional ideas are dropped by the recipient if he is removed from association with the dominant person. The usual setting of the disorder is one in which the two persons concerned live in comparative seclusion. It is more frequently found among women. This is probably because they tend to be more isolated within the domestic circle; they are, on the whole, more passive, submissive and suggestible and their outside interests and ambitions are more likely to be restricted or frustrated.

Diagnosis

At times psychiatric literature contains references to "acute paranoia." While descriptively this is a good term, it is somewhat misleading since it will be found that the episodes thus classified are fundamentally affective in nature, being hypomanic attacks of manic-depressive psychosis in which the usual emotional exaltation is replaced by irritability and anger. The patient is aggressive, haughty, hostile and complaining. In paranoia there is a greater tendency to project and to rationalize one's affective state than in the usual manic episode. The true paranoiac is more restrained both in behavior and in speech and his ideational content is characterized by a more sustained and dominant idea than is the more excited manic with his fleeting charges. As the affect subsides, the delusional ideas of the acute paranoid episode are dropped but they are not corrected and the patient remains without insight as to the beliefs he formerly expressed with great conviction and feeling.

There is often discussion as to whether a given paranoic syndrome should be classified as one of paranoia, paranoid state or paranoid schizophrenia. The general factors which determine the place of a paranoid reaction in this imperceptibly graded series of paranoid psychoses have already been indicated. In addition to what has already been said concerning the mechanisms and symptoms to be observed in making a diagnosis in this paranoid group, it may be helpful to bear in mind that the greater the logical systematization of delusions and the less the patient's relations with reality are disturbed the more nearly does the psychosis approach traditional paranoia, while the greater the extent to which repressed material comes through to consciousness in the form of hallucinations, and the more bizarre the delusional system, the more regressive and disorganized the form of adjustment the more nearly does it approach paranoid schizophrenia. While anger and hatred are common in all the paranoic disorders yet as time progresses there is an increasing tendency for the schizophrenic patient's affect to "burn out." The paranoid schizophrenic patient lacks the intensive drive for achievement usually seen in paranoia.

Not rarely there is difficulty in deciding whether a person whose behavior is governed by and indicates a thorough contact with reality, who has suffered no dilapidation of affect or of personality and who is not hallucinated but who constantly employs projection and other defensive measures should be considered as suffering from paranoia or as a paranoid, but not psychotic, personality. Here, too, an imperceptibly graded series is dealt with, ranging from a mild and perhaps justifiable sense of injury and a belief that merits are not recognized, at one pole, to the exaggerated delusions of persecution or of grandeur of true paranoia at the other. At one extreme is a reaction which would not, except to the psychopathologist, be regarded as abnormal. When this reaction becomes so intensified as to warrant a diagnosis of paranoia may also be a matter of opinion, since paranoia is essentially an exaggeration of mechanisms observed daily. In general, if the exaggerated reaction is continuous, if the beliefs through which it manifests itself cannot be corrected, if they disclose an inadequacy of logic, and particularly if they tend to spread and to reveal that the affective and conative forces are sustained and have great energy, then the reaction must be looked upon as psychotic. The psychiatrist will not forget that paranoid tendencies may be channeled and expressed in many eccentricities and fanatical ways.

One should bear in mind that deafness facilitates the development of paranoid reactions. Those persons who for some reason already suffer from a sense of insecurity are prone to develop these reactions in the event they become deaf. In addition to sensitiveness, seclusiveness, suspicion and misinterpretations as defenses against a sensory handicap, deafness may at times lead to overcompensating aggressiveness.

Prognosis

It is doubtful if a case of traditional paranoia ever recovers. In those cases in the paranoid series which most nearly approach paranoid schizophrenia, a remission may rarely occur but in these, also, the ultimate prognosis is poor. In true paranoia there is little or no general personality disorganization and the patient's conduct usually remains within the bounds that society will tolerate. For this reason a large proportion of such cases do not enter a hospital for mental disorders. In the community they are often looked upon as "cranks," but as they usually do not act without reflection, show a certain amount of self-control, and limit themselves to legal means of redress, they avoid commitment much more frequently than do those paranoid conditions that approach the schizophrenic pole of the series. The latter are less sociable, less industrious and less restrained by social custom and law.

An analysis of the causes of death in the psychoses shows that a larger percentage of paranoid patients than of any other group of biogenetic psychoses die of degenerative circulatory disease. If this be true, the antecedent hypertension and cardiac hypertrophy followed by the subsequent degeneration and failure when the demands upon the cardiovascular system become too great may represent a compensatory somatosis associated with a compensatory psychosis—an evidence of the dynamic unity of the organism.

Treatment

As already indicated, the more nearly the paranoid psychosis approaches "true paranoia" the less frequently is hospitalization required. Unless his behavior is too disturbing socially, it is well for the patient with this disease to remain in the community since interference and restraint embitter him and lead to an extension of his delusional system and to a stimulation of his hatred. If the paranoiac is considered dangerous, commitment, of course, becomes imperative. To determine when he has actually become dangerous is not always easy. A careful evaluation of the patient's history will usually indicate the extent to which delusions may be expected to control behavior. If delusions have exerted an important influence on behavior and if they are directed toward particular individuals, he should be considered dangerous. The willingness and the degree of objectivity with which the patient will discuss his delusions are important. The character and intensity of his emotional reaction will greatly aid in deciding the questions as to the hazard entailed in the patient's liberty; the greater the overt hostility the more imperative is his removal from society. Many times the patient will discuss the extent to which he believes he is justified in protecting himself or his interests or in securing redress. An indication can thus be obtained as to the probability of acts of violence.

In the institution the more permissive, within discrete limits, the attitude toward the patient the more tranquil will be his hospital adjustment. It is important that the physician avoid a critical attitude and that he gain the confidence of the patient. It is often surprising the extent to which this can be obtained if the physician treats the patient with courtesy, consideration, scrupulous truthfulness and good faith. The physician will pay attention to the patient's delusional system but will not imply agreement. "I can understand how you feel, but it does not seem so to me." In paranoid panic-states relief and improvement with a feeling of security may be afforded merely by entrance into a hospital.

Paranoid states are usually too defensive for successful psychotherapy although psychiatric literature contains a few reports of paranoia alleged to have been cured by this measure. The more extensive one's experience with paranoia the more skeptical, however, does he become as to any radical reconstruction of the fixed cognitive-affective pattern characterizing the disorder. This is not to say that judicious psychotherapy may not at times produce a certain alleviation. Electroconvulsive and other shock therapies have no effect upon true paranoid reactions. If improvement follows their use it is probable that the condition was fundamentally a depression with paranoid features.

The treatment of the other endogenous, biogenic reaction-sets known as paranoid conditions is essentially the same as that of paranoia, although as behavior usually becomes disorganized to a greater extent commitment is more frequently necessary. Rigid rules and habits of ward procedure are constant sources of irritation to the paranoid patient. His comfort and convenience should therefore be respected as far as circumstances will permit. Great care should be exercised both by the patient's family and by the hospital personnel that their attitude toward the patient is not of the kind that stimulates aggressive or revengeful feelings. While true of every patient with clear consciousness, it should be particularly emphasized that the first impression which the paranoid patient receives on entering the hospital may determine whether he will assume an attitude which is co-operative and friendly or whether he will become resentful and hostile. Congenial employment of the paranoid patient is greatly to be encouraged.

BIBLIOGRAPHY

Bleuler, E.: Affectivität, Suggestibiliät, Paranoia. Translated by C. S. Ricksher. New York State Hospitals Bulletin. Utica, State Hospitals Press, Feb. 1912.

Bonner, Hubert: The problem of diagnosis in paranoic disorders. Am. J. Psychiat., *107*:677–683, 1951.

Cameron, N.: The development of paranoiac thinking. Psychol. Rev., *50*:219, 1943.

Dewhurst, Kenneth, and Todd, John: The psychosis of association–folie à deux. J. Nerv. and Ment. Dis., *124*:451–459, 1957.

Freud, Sigmund: Certain neurotic mechanisms in jealousy, paranoia and homosexuality. Internat. J. Psycho-Analysis, *4*:1, 1923.

———: Psychoanalytic Notes upon an Autobiographical Account of a Case of Paranoia. In Collected Papers, Vol. 3, London, Hogarth, 1925.

Gralnick, A.: Folie à deux–the psychosis of association. Psychiat. Quart., *16:*230–263, 1942; 491–520, 1942.
Greenberg, H. P.: Crime and folie à deux; review and case history. J. Ment. Sc., *102:*772–779, 1956.
Kahn, E., and Richter, H. G.: Sensibility. Am. J. Psychiat., *96:*609, 1939.
Kretschmer E.: Der sensitive Beziehungswahn. Berlin, Julius Springer, 1927.
Lasègue, C., and Falret, J.: La folie à deux ou folie communiquée. Ann. méd. psychol., *17:*321, 1877.
Rosen, H., and Kiene, H. E.: Paranoia and paranoiac reaction types. Dis. Nerv. System, 7:330, 1946.
———: The paranoiac officer and the officer paranee. Am. J. Psychiat., *103:*614–621, 1947.
Waelder, R.: The structure of paranoid ideas: a critical survey of various ideas. Internat. J. Psycho-Analysis, *32:*167–177, 1951.
Wolff, S.: Folie à trois: a clinical study. J. Ment. Sc., *103:*355–363, 1957.

CHAPTER XXIX

Psychophysiological Autonomic and Visceral Disorders

"The sorrow which has no vent in tears may make other organs weep." HENRY MAUDSLEY

THE REACTIONS included under the caption of psychophysiological autonomic and visceral disorders comprise those which are more frequently referred to as "psychosomatic disorders." Anxiety leads to disturbances that are predominantly physiological rather than symbolic. The expression of affect being through viscera, its feeling or subjective part is repressed and therefore largely prevented from becoming conscious. Neither is its expression under full voluntary control or perception. The long continued and exaggerated physiological expression of anxiety may eventually lead to structural change in the organ or viscus through which it is expressed. The physiological and the organic are secondary to vascular disturbance, smooth muscle dysfunction and hypersecretion or hyposecretion of glands, innervated largely by the sympathetic and parasympathetic divisions of the autonomic nervous system. The tendency, however, to delineate only such psychosomatic disturbances as those expressed through the pathological mediation of the autonomic nervous system is not in keeping with the structural or functional organization of the organism. Furthermore, it tends to provide a too narrow interpretation of psychosomatic interrelations and their disturbances. The broader concept used here is to classify as psychosomatic all those disturbances involving the organs of internal economy, of instinctual function and of the body image as a whole. Thus are excluded the involvement of organs subserving the human relationship to the external world. It is evident that the internal organ systems located within the body cavities are largely controlled through the connections of the central nervous system and various metabolic and hormonal feedbacks. The organ systems which have direct contact with the external environment are used for the intake and elimination of needed bodily substances and for procreative activity (respiratory, gastrointestinal and genital apparatus) and are controlled in part at their orifices by the voluntary nervous system and also by the autonomic through the integrative activity of the central nervous pathways. Here is seen initiation of the functions by utilization of the voluntary nervous system followed by increasing degrees of automatization through the sympathetic and parasympathetic innervations. In the instances of the body image disturbances, the total organism is involved and not a single organ or series of organs. Excluded, then, from the area of the psychosomatic disorders are dysfunctions of the central nervous system subserving the external relations of the individual, his perceptual and conative activities, communicative systems, orientations in space and time, and his capacity to organize and integrate the information provided him from the outside world. It is clear that the borderline between the disorder subsumed under the body image and those of the integrative functions of the nervous system in contact with the external world may not be sharply delimited and subtly merge with personality growth. Yet it is possible to recognize in the phantom phenomena following the loss of a bodily part the perpetuation of a well established percept of the body image.

The concept of psychosomatic medicine, criticized by many, has provided one of the great contributions of psychiatry to medicine during the past quarter century in its re-emphasis of the human factor in illness, the wider appreciation of the personality-illness relationship and of the influence of psychological factors in the genesis of somatic symptoms, and even of somatic disease. Prior to this re-emphasis, there had been an unfortunately increasing tendency for medicine to look upon the patient as "the uninteresting vehicle of a fascinating disease process." Influenced by psychiatry, medical science has in recent years increasingly adopted a more comprehensive point of view and has to a greater extent come to realize that the pathology of disease is that of the living, integrated organism and not merely of cells and tissue. It is now recognized that there are many factors which cannot be studied by the usual methods of medicine or described in terms of physiology. These factors, nevertheless, may disturb the functioning of the organism as greatly as those agencies which are revealed by the microscope or the test tube. Such factors can be ascertained only through "an intimate understanding of the patient as a whole man or woman with a home and anxieties and economic problems and a past and a future and a job to be held or lost." It has become clear, too, that mechanisms invoked by the human personality to deal with problems of adjustment to its environment may either underlie or modify many disease processes. The physician should therefore focus his attention on the patient himself including his emotional life—not merely on his physical complaints. He should remember that physiological processes and the psychodynamics of emotions are intimately bound up, the one affecting the other. He must aim to discover and understand the interrelation and interaction of psychological and organic factors in the development and course of illness. The physician's concern, then, should not be limited to infections and physicochemical deviations determined in the laboratory. As an editorial writer in The Lancet[1] has pointed out there is danger that the student's perspective may be distorted in the ward atmosphere of intensive, largely mechanical, investigation in which the minutiae and the rarities of disease receive so much attention and its human significance so little. He adds that by the time the student enters private practice his mind is often cast in the mold his teachers have given it and that as a result a cardiac murmur may always seem to him more important than an overpossessive mother who may so warp her child's personality development that his mental health and social adjustment are permanently impaired.

Because chronic emotional states frequently associated with physiological malfunctions are often closely related to the everyday problems of living, the physician or psychiatrist makes a careful and extended look into the whole development and experience of the patient. Home life and its jealousies and frustrations, working conditions frequently involving the boredom of constant repetition or a perpetual striving for security or achievement with the attendant drives for prestige or comradeship in relation to those in authority or to other persons are common problems, yet ones that may lead to a variety of symptoms that have no organic basis. Cumulative problems of interpersonal relationships produce a large share of the tensions and anxieties that beset the human being and upset his physiology. Lack of emotional satisfaction in one's life may act likewise. Anxiety reactions to situational difficulties and crises seem particularly prone to be expressed in psychosomatic symptoms. The psychiatrist inquires, therefore, for personal situations that may give rise to anxiety, hostility, aggression, guilt, bottled-up resentment, smoldering discontent, and other disturbing emotions and unwholesome attitudes that may act as the cause or as an aggravating factor in the production of much ill health manifested at the somatic level. All too often it will be found that the sickness has developed in an effort to find a solution for the difficulties that occur in human relationships. Frequently the nature of a body disorder can be appreciated only when psychological happenings, as well as physical disturbances, are investigated. The patient's feelings, his personal relationships, his life situation and his reactions to his environment should be subject to the same painstaking scrutiny as his physical body and its symptoms. If a good life history is taken much time and expense can often be saved in diagnostic studies. Sometimes a temporal relationship can be established between the onset of the apparently physical symptom and some emotionally disturbing event. Again it may be possible to identify experiences of early life which seem highly relevant to adult attitudes and diseases. Ruesch makes the observation that the psychosomatic disorders as organ

1 The Lancet, 152:413, 1947.

reflections of psychological tension are most common in the middle class with its greater burden of self-required striving, conforming and repressing. There seems, also, to be a greater tendency for emotionally introverted persons to show somatic complaints than for those who are extraverted.

Physical symptoms are the presenting ones and so dominate the clinical picture that their mental source is not superficially recognizable. The neurotic patient rarely complains of his anxiety, depression, resentment or sexual tension but rather of his disorder of bodily functions, such as anorexia, vomiting, backache, headache or palpitation.

Psychosomatic medicine does not, strictly speaking, include psychological reactions which the physically ill patient may develop in response to his illness but these may, in themselves, be of great significance to him and constitute an important disabling factor in his illness.

Psychosomatic medicine will deal with several groups of patients: (1) In the first group, are those who suffer from various physical symptoms but who do not have any bodily disease which may serve as a cause for the symptoms. As the result of the failure to recognize that such illnesses are of emotional origin they have often been called "functional." (2) In another group of psychosomatic disorders, a physical disease exists but the original, causative factors were of an emotional nature. The pathologic condition resulting from the action of the emotional causes reaches a point where it is no longer reversible. (3) In a third group of psychosomatic disorders, the patient does have actual organic disease but certain of his symptoms do not arise from this disease but from mental factors, perhaps from anxiety arising from some situation in relation to other persons. In disorders of this type the disability is often out of proportion to the physical disease. The physician must look further than the organic pathologic condition for an explanation of all the symptoms. Since the same symptom may be a result of structural pathology, of personal pathology ("functional"), or of a fusion of both, the physician must make a thorough investigation of both physical condition and personality. Unless he does so he may overlook any psychosomatic components in organic disease and will make a diagnosis of "functional" by a process of exclusion only. If, moreover, the physician makes a diagnosis by exclusion only, he is in no way prepared to prescribe rational and adequate treatment. This can be outlined only if he has a knowledge of the psychological stresses and situations to which the patient's physical symptoms represent a reaction. Most patients with psychosomatic reactions do not have such frank symptoms of the psychoneurosis as compulsions, phobias and anxiety states.

Types of Reaction to Psychological Stresses

In previous chapters we have observed that life experiences, especially those involving meaningful, anxiety-producing human relationships, may be productive of such emotions as fear, rage, resentment, guilt, grief, sadness and loneliness and that as a consequence a psychosis with its disorganization of personality or its disturbance of reality evaluation may follow. Chapter XXX shows that in some instances such experiences with their resulting psychopathology lead to anxiety states and to various defensive and substitutive reactions known as psychoneuroses. In this chapter we shall attempt to show how in other persons life experiences with their resulting anxieties, hostilities, insecurities, fears and emotional tensions and attitudes are expressed not in neurotic symptoms but in physical symptoms and organ-dysfunctions—in other words, how physical symptoms may develop in reaction to psychological stress. Physiological changes are set up by autonomic nerve impulses generated as a result of emotional conflict or tension.

In previous chapters we have seen how emotional forces may affect perception, thinking, feeling and behavior. In this chapter emphasis will be placed on the influence of emotions on physiology. A simple and familiar illustration of the fact that emotions may influence physiological processes is the flow of tears associated with the emotion of grief; another is the quickened heart action associated with anger. Cannon and others showed that various physiological changes, such as those of secretion, muscle tension and circulation, which are under the control of the vegetative nervous system, may be produced by emotions. The chronic emotional state stimulates a response of the vegetative nervous system with resulting physiological malfunctions which if persistent tend eventually to produce pathological changes. Such an influence of emotional factors on physiological functions was well demonstrated by Wolf and Wolff in their patient with a gastrostomy with herniated gastric mucosa. It was found that pleasurable emotions of appetite led to some increase in secretion and vascularity of the mucosa with increased motility of the stomach wall. Sadness, discouragement and self-reproach led to prolonged pallor of the mucosa and hyposecretion. Anxiety produced hyperemia, hypersecretion and hypermotility. Aggressive feelings, including resentment and hostility, led to a great increase in secretion and vascularity and to some increase in motility.

The same investigators showed also in the case of portions of exposed colons in fistulous patients that situations productive of conflict, resentment and hostility were associated with hypermotility and hypersecretion of the enzyme lysozyme and of mucus. In some patients with sustained hyperfunction during anger and resentment the appearance of petechial hemorrhages was noted. Dejection and fear were associated with hypofunction of most of the large intestine. The fact that emotions may influence physiological functions and dysfunctions is now well established by both clinical and experimental observation. That a patient suffering from physical disorder, especially if it is of a serious and progressive nature, is very prone to develop some psychological response to it is equally well known.

To summarize the preceding ideas and express them more concretely, it may be said that tensions generated on the level of psychological experience may be expressed in one of two ways. If the tensions produce disturbances in the functions of organs innervated by the somatomuscular or somatosensory apparatus, the resulting phenomenon is known as conversion hysteria. If, on the other hand, these tensions produce disturbances of organs innervated by the autonomic nervous system the result is a psychosomatic or psychophysiological symptom.

Processes of Origin and Symptom

The psychophysiological responses may be interpreted as the inappropriate perpetuations of organ reactions adaptive to, or protective against, some stress in human life experience. As has been shown in previous chapters, such reactions include not only those caused by assault by other organisms and physical agents but also those consequent to man's capacity to interpret symbols as indicative of danger derived from his past experiences, including the threats resulting from necessary conformity to family and cultural mores, which in themselves lead to deprivation of certain innately desired satisfactions. In response to the stress imposed by various threats and conflicts, organ reactions, in conjunction with various feelings and attitudes, occur to assist in adaptation or to prepare for emergencies to protect the individual. The perpetuation of the organ reactions beyond the period of stress leads to sustained responses that are inappropriate and may end in tissue damage.

The psychosomatic symptom represents the physiological concomitant of an emotional state. In the acute emotional state of rage, for example, it is a normal vegetative process for the blood pressure to be raised. This rise in blood pressure will subside if the angry man releases his emotional tension by physical or verbal attack on the object of his anger. If, however, a persistent, inhibited aggression (chronic rage) continues, the patient's emotional tension does not subside, his blood pressure does not become less and he suffers from "essential" hypertension. In other words a chronic emotional tension has activated bodily changes resulting in vascular hypertension. The physical symptoms of some cases of hypertension are therefore of psychosomatic origin. If a chronic emotional tension acting through the vegetative nervous system stimulates muscular or secretory activity of the gastrointestinal tract, then the psychosomatic symptom will be referable to that system. The physiological expressions of anxiety may then be interpreted by the patient as "stomach trouble." Through introspection these self-diagnosed conditions may be exaggerated.

There is a difference of opinion among psychiatrists as to whether there is a correlation between type of personality and type and locus of psychosomatic disease, or a correlation between certain emotional constellations and the vegetative innervations and responses. Most psychiatrists now agree that the conception of Dunbar of a personality constellation specific to each psychosomatic disorder has no sound foundation. Alexander and others stress rather the specific nature of the conflict situation. Other psychiatrists are of the opinion that the organ system affected by the emotionally acting influences is determined not by psychological factors, but by an inherited tendency to respond somatically to stress and conflict in a fashion consistent for himself. This view, presented by Wolff, differs from the earlier ideas of inherited or acquired systemic or organic weaknesses.

In Chapter XXX, reference will frequently be made to the assumed fact that many mental symptoms, such as phobia, compulsions and various others, represent defenses at the psychological level against repudiated impulses, hostilities and other psychopathogenetic material. It is, perhaps, a pertinent analogy to think of the "functional," psychosomatic symptom as also a defense, expressed not at the psychological level, but at the physiological level through the mediation of the vegetative nervous system. The psychosomatic symptom alone, however, does not fully account for the patient's distress. More influential is the underlying anxiety which gave rise to the symptom and threatens to break through failing defenses. In a way, therefore, the psychosomatic, "functional" symptom may be considered as an emergency measure to prevent the patient from being overwhelmed by anxiety. He may consciously want relief from his neurotic, defensive symptom. The psychosomatic patient, like the neurotic, has likewise an unconscious resistance to the relinquishing of measures that are largely or in part defensive. In his endeavor to stress a purely somatic origin of his symptoms and to deny even the possibility of psychological causes the patient may seem to protest too much. His conscious negation of such an origin amounts to an unconscious acknowledgment. When a pathologic condition actually exists, it will often be observed that symptoms are disproportionate to the extent of the disease. In such cases it may be found that there is much conflict in the personality, its source, perhaps, being a repressed hostility. A specific, as well as a temporal relationship, will often be found between the onset of the psychosomatic symptoms and a psychic event. Sometimes it can be pointed out to the patient that the intensity of mentally determined symptoms fluctuates as difficult situations and stresses occur and are resolved. One objective in therapy will be to help the patient to understand the relation of his symptoms to the particular personality difficulties and maladjustments which are a source of anxiety.

If the physician fails or refuses to recognize the importance of emotional factors in illness, or by a useless repetition of previously negative examinations he continues to search for an organic pathologic condition, the patient becomes even more convinced that his trouble is organic. The doctor's attitudes may, too, be important factors in perpetuating or provoking illness. By his tone of voice, gestures, etc., his own anxiety may readily be transferred to the patient. If some incidental pathologic condition is found the patient's anxiety becomes fixed on the system in which the pathologic condition, often unimportant, is found. In emotional disorders misidentified and mistreated as organic diseases the patient's troublesome symptoms, instead of improving, tend to become chronic.

Types of Psychophysiological Reactions

It has been pointed out that emotional influences, conflicts and tensions produce anxiety which through prolonged action on the vegetative nervous system may seriously disrupt the autonomic regulation of the body with resulting manifestations of symptoms referable to various visceral vegetative organs. These symptoms tend to be manifested in disturbances of certain systems, particularly the cardiovascular system, the gastrointestinal tract, the endocrine system, the respiratory tract, the skin and the genitourinary system.

In the psychophysiological disorders, affect tends to find predominant expression through the persistent involvement of a single organ system. Clinical experience shows, however, that at times an individual may successively or simultaneously have disorders affecting several organ systems. Because the resulting symptomatology is so definitely referred to viscera, many of these disorders were known as "organ neuroses." If the emotionally generated autonomic impulse produced physiological disturbance of heart action, the disorder was known as a "cardiac neurosis." if the disturbance was of the stomach it was known as "gastric neurosis." As described before, the psychosomatic concept and the associated disorders extend beyond the idea of organ neuroses with the interpretation of conversion of energy leading to dysfunctions. For the purposes of classification the dysfunctions are separated into those of various systems.

CARDIOVASCULAR SYSTEM

For various reasons, perhaps largely because it is generally regarded as the most important bodily organ and because the idea of sudden death is often associated with it, anxiety, under conditions creating prolonged tension, may readily become attached to the heart. It has been demonstrated that stress invoking anxiety tends to increase the heart rate, cardiac output and blood pressure, as well as cause changes in the rhythm and the electrocardiogram. Dejection and despair are associated with a diminution in the rate, cardiac output and lowering of the blood pressure. With anxiety and resentment, exercise tolerance is impaired. Such functional derangements may become the neurotic focus, particularly if associated with injudicious comment or procedure by the examining physician, or if some suggestive but not significant symptom adds contributive influence. The majority of persons who have symptoms referred to the heart region do not have organic heart disease.

Symptoms

Common psychosomatic symptom associated with a cardiac neurosis are pain in the heart region, tachycardia, palpitation, arrhythmia, shortness of breath, fatigue, faintness and insomnia. For the most part these symptoms are somatic manifestations of anxiety. The clinical picture known as *neurocirculatory asthenia*, or effort syndrome, and characterized by breathlessness, easy fatigability, palpitation or heart consciousness, trembling, fainting, giddiness, headache, and fear of effort is not of organic but of psychosomatic origin. The term "effort syndrome" is a misnomer since the symptoms of the syndrome are not confined to effort. The term "effort intolerance" has been suggested as more appropriate. To a varying degree the symptoms of anxiety coexist and assume the form of bad dreams, apprehensiveness, sweating, depression, trembling and a tense restlessness. The disorder was first described by Da Costa during the War Between the States. During World War I it constituted a major problem among English soldiers since, because of its supposedly organic nature, it called for discharge from military service. As a result it became widely induced by suggestion. It is most frequently seen in persons who remain dependent and immature emotionally. Weiss, probably with much justification, emphasizes that there is no constitutional or physiological deficit in the cardiovascular system. The symptoms described above in many instances represent the physiological expression of the hyperventilation syndrome which is precipitated by situations that arouse acute anxiety or fear in the individual. This condition, although not always the physiological source of the "effort syndrome," is readily recognizable and is described later in this chapter under the heading of "Respiratory System."

Vascular hypertension is not, of course, a specific disease but rather a systemic reaction which may be induced by a variety of causes. The cases in which the psychiatrist is primarily interested are those in which a major factor is emotional tension operating through the vegetative nervous system to cause vasoconstriction. Some psychiatrists are of the opinion that the unrealized inner tension which often accompanies hypertension is to be attributed to the mobilization of excessive rage in the face of a threat to the dependent relationship of the hypertensive patient. This emotion is seen as partly repressed and suppressed and inadequately discharged through verbal or motor activities. The personality of many hypertensive patients is one of outward serenity and affability which, however, covers conflicting attitudes of readiness for aggressive hostility with needs to conform in order to maintain often strong dependent attachments. However, hostility is not peculiar to hypertension. Many hypertensives are neurotic with strong perfectionistic and compulsive tendencies. It must not, of course, be assumed that psychodynamic factors are the only ones that contribute to essential hypertension. Some patients with early hypertension suffer also from gastrointestinal symptoms, head discomforts and fatigue. Such symptoms cannot usually be accounted for on the basis of the hypertension itself but are presumably a result of the same emotional factors that contributed to but did not cause the hypertension. With the patient's discovery of the hypertension the "blood pressure phobia" may dominate the clinical picture. No final statement can yet be made concerning the influence of psychological factors in the production of essential hypertension. There is much reason to believe, however, that many of the symptoms attributed to hypertension are of emotional origin. Investigation of the life situation and psychotherapy will often make the patient a more contented and effective person even though the hypertensive disease itself is not significantly influenced by psychotherapy.

GASTROINTESTINAL SYSTEM

It is not surprising that the gastrointestinal functions provide the most frequent focus of psychosomatic syndromes. In life experience the first contact of the infant with another person comes in relation to the nursing process. The infant here experiences his first relief from physical discomfort and tension through the intake of milk. The satisfaction of relief from hunger through this experience becomes strongly associated with feelings of well being in maturity. On the other hand, deprivation of food or its irregular presentation is associated with feelings of tension and rage. Compounded with the somatic disturbance and the attending emotions are the gradually developing perceptual processes in relation to contacts with the mother and mother surrogates. In addition to the growing awareness of the dependent relationship on the mother with its satisfactions and frustrations coming as they do through feeding, there is also the similar interpersonal conditioning that takes place through the eliminative activities of the lower end of the gastrointestinal tract. Here again the infant is brought to eliminate and retain fecal matter in terms of relating to the mother. Thus it is seen that the satisfactions gained through the early sucking process are associated with the emotion of being loved and the development of feelings of security and satisfaction. On the other hand, the bowel training process again provides opportunity for the feelings of approval through cleanliness or of stubborness through retention and constipation. Frustration of the pleasures of feeding mobilizes aggressive activity in the form of biting, taking, greed and envy. Again the process of eating is surrounded both in the family and in the culture with many opportunities for pleasure and conflict in interpersonal reactions. This is less apparent in respect to eliminative processes which are usually solitary.

Thus the symptoms of gastrointestinal disturbance through anxiety may extend from anorexia, nausea, "nervous indigestion," vomiting, belching, distress from gas and epigastric pain to problems of diarrhea and constipation. Many patients complain also of fatigue. Not rarely the abdominal pains and discomforts are attributed to "chronic appendicitis" and the patient is subjected to surgery. This is soon followed by a recurrence of symptoms. In other cases the gall bladder is removed. Spastic or mucous colitis with diarrhea and constipation represent another phenomenon of this disturbance of the gastrointestinal tract. In addition obesity and anorexia nervosa may be considered psychosomatic expressions of this system.

Peptic Ulcer

Not only the clinician but the lay person is aware that functional gastric symptoms are commonly produced by worry, business reverses, family quarrels, and other emotionally disturbing experiences. Similarly it is recognized that psychogenic factors are of importance in the etiology of peptic ulcer. The study of Wolf and Wolff of their patient with permanent gastric fistula tends to support these impressions. It is still unknown whether the physiological disturbance in secretory and motor functions produced by emotionally generated autonomic activity result in the formation of ulcers. It is possible that the motor disturbances result in spasm of the pylorus and therefore cause prolonged retention of the acid content of the stomach. Also the blood supply of the stomach may be affected by the excitation of the autonomic nervous system.

At any rate, the ulcer syndrome is now among the most frequently encountered of psychosomatic conditions. It is of interest that the incidence of peptic ulcer has significantly changed within the past half century in western European societies. At one time it was extremely prevalent in women but now occurs chiefly in men. The change in the sex ratio is unexplained.

Saul has indicated that peptic ulcer may occur under a number of circumstances. It may be seen as an acute transient reaction in the face of unusual stress. Such stresses may be the serious threats of military life or, on the other hand, internal inhibition may lead to frustration, mounting tension, and consequent psychosomatic expression through the gastrointestinal tract. In addition there is a group of individuals in whom dependency longings are so exaggerated that they may not be satisfied or are bound to remain ungratified because of the ordinary demands of living. These are individuals with essentially infantile personalities.

Many psychiatrists, including Alexander, consider that the type of conflict situation has a determining significance on the peptic ulcer psychophysiologic reaction. It is asserted that patients with this condition are basically dependent, that the exaggerated aggressive, ambitious and independent "go-getting" attitudes which are noted superficially are a reaction to the underlying basic dependency needs. On the other hand, this type of conflict is not exclusively associated with the peptic ulcer syndrome. It has been pointed out that the description of the ulcer patient as a self-sufficient, independent, and overly responsible person is not always appropriate and many of them are overtly irresponsible, dependent and inactive. Studies of women with peptic ulcer have recently shown that the onset is often related to surgical procedures or other events which have threatened in reality or in fantasy their sexual functioning. Since threat to the sexual functioning may also simultaneously be seen as a threat to the dependency relationship of the patient the production of ulcer symptoms may well be related to the conflict situation described by Alexander.

From the therapeutic point of view, the psychiatrist or psychoanalyst may seldom function successfully as the therapist for these patients. It may be recommended that the repressed dependency needs of the patient be gratified directly or indirectly without inducing shame, guilt or resistance. This can be done by environmental manipulation, including vacation, enlisting the support of key figures in the patient's environment, or by strengthening the patient-physician contact through regularity and frequency of visits. In those individuals with an infantile personality, the facing of the conflict by psychiatric treatment may well lead to serious depression and a more disturbing personality reaction than that accompanying the primary ulcer symptomatology.

Mucous Colitis

In this disease we meet with a group of symptoms into which anxiety-producing problems are not infrequently translated. Among these symptoms are constipation and the discharge of mucus-containing stools. Shreds of membrane are discharged in masses or mixed with soft or liquid fecal matter. The patient complains of indigestion. The appetite is poor and capricious, and the patient resorts to an increasing restriction of diet in an attempt to find one that will not cause discomfort. Distention of the stomach, belching, flatulence, heaviness or pain after eating, nausea and other gastric symptoms are common. Many patients are asthenic and show diminished output of energy. In many cases this physiological disturbance appears to be in response to anxiety, guilt, sensitivity, overconscientiousness and resentment. It is common for the symptoms to be attributed to various alleged causes varying from chronic prostatitis to gallbladder disease. All too frequently the patient is advised to have colon irrigations or an operation. It is stated that mucous colitis is responsible for the removal of more undiseased appendices than any other cause.

Ulcerative Colitis

A relationship between periods of emotional stress and the onset or exacerbation of symptoms has been recognized in those with ulcerative colitis. Quite frequently the attacks commence three or four weeks after a sudden, unforeseen threat to the patient's security, commonly in the form of bereavement through death, separation, rejection, disillusionment or by loss of a part of one's body, or changes in psychological status such as graduation, failures at school or at work, and other causes of diminished self-esteem. While those patients who have been studied psychiatrically often appear to be highly intelligent, their emotional lives suggest impaired capacity for appropriate affective experiences. Yet they seem keenly perceptive and sensitive to the emotional responsivity of others. With ambivalent human contacts they respond to loss with depression and rage accompanied by disorganization of bowel function. Many patients whose primary affective need was the protective care of a maternal figure were disturbed through their early conditioning in relationship to dominating, hostile or rejecting mothers so that they expected humiliating rejection. Again in the family setting physical symptoms often had signified preferential care. With emerging hostility or rage toward the wanted person such patients frequently responded with guilty fear of retaliation. It has been noticed that both men and women with ulcerative colitis, when referred for psychiatric treatment, have shown considerable evidence of disturbance of psychosexual development.

Treatment of the patient with ulcerative colitis must generally be carried out by the physician or internist. The psychiatrist's contribution initially is that of assisting in or advising the establishment of a solid dependency relationship which will again provide the patient with a feeling of mastery over himself and his environment. Dramatic interruption of attacks of colitis have been obtained by some psychiatrists through assuming a simple supportive and protective role for the patient and demanding little. Margolin goes so far as to establish what is termed an anaclitic therapy in which the patient is regarded as a helpless infant and is encouraged to regressive behavior. Here the therapy is somatically directed. It is generally recognized that intensive psychotherapy or analytic therapy is not possible during the acute phases of the illness. Others have criticized analytic therapy even in later stages of the illness as implying too extensive a commitment of the therapist to the patient's emotional and psychological demands. Some patients are unable to accept extreme solicitude and sympathetic behavior because of their own personality make-up and their expectation of further rejection. On the other hand, the effort of Lindemann to restore the patient's former equilibrium in a dependency relationship through attempting to replace the lost supportive figure may fail if the patient's expectations in such a role are not fulfilled. In general, it would seem that the psychiatrist contributes most in affording the internist and other attending personnel interpretations and supportive help in their management of the difficult emotional problems attendant in the care of this severe illness. While it is frequently possible to assist in bringing about an affective relationship and emotional change in such patients with interruption of acute episodes, extended changes in the personality are possible with only a few patients. If the feeling state characterized by anger, resentment and guilt may be modified, the hyperfunction of the colon, the fragility of the colonic mucosa, submucosal bleeding and ulcer may be ameliorated. There is, however, little evidence that the disease of itself may be modified by such treatment.

Obesity

For many years genetic, endocrinological and constitutional factors have received major attention in the study of obesity and have determined to a considerable extent the management of the overweight patient. Recently, however, particularly through the work of Hilde Bruch, a fuller appreciation of the personality development and emotional influences that contribute to obesity in man has been obtained. For the majority of patients these factors are probably the major determinants in the obese syndrome. Without their recognition and consideration the treatment of the overweight patient often fails and in some occasions leads to serious disruptions of personality functioning.

What constitutes obesity or overweight is not well defined. As Bruch has made clear, the changes and fluctuations in weight measured over a period of time provide a better index of a weight disturbance than the percentage of weight excess computed from the standard height-weight tables. Stability in weight, then, is recognized when the individual maintains a relatively constant poundage without concern over dieting. Some individuals maintain weight curves close to the average but only through a perspective on life which is fixed on maintenance of weight through dieting, a measure which for them is abnormal. The study of the extended temporal weight curve provides important clues for the treatment of the obese person who is seeking help. With evidence of many fluctuations up and down, with or without medical supervision, inference may be made that additional attempts at weight reduction will be unsuccessful as the previous failures and successes have not been comprehended in their fullest meaning. Here a study of the weight changes in relation to the total personality functioning which includes an estimate of the sense of well being and adequacy of performance in the individual's spheres of life action become as important as the weight changes. Stability in weight is a reliable guide to estimate whether the obese person is adapting well to his life experiences. This is particularly so during childhood and adolescence. A degree of overweight in these periods, if stable, becomes disturbing only when the growing person is involved in a ceaseless struggle owing to family and cultural pressure, enhanced in Western society in these times by the insistence on slimness as a desirable bodily trait. In recent years the statistical evidence that overweight contributes significantly to increased death rates resulting from circulatory disturbance has been strongly challenged by new information and analysis. Yet the health emphasis on weight reduction continues. It is accepted in many medical circles that a weight twenty per cent above the standard for a particular age and sex constitutes pathological overweight. The concept, while useful in the clinic in detecting individuals at the extremes of the weight curves and providing clues pertaining to pathological disturbances and their changes, fails to do justification to the genetic and constitutional differences in individuals. It is perhaps wiser to think of a "preferred weight" for the individual as Bruch does.

The development of obesity often occurs in a family setting where the parents compensate for their own life frustrations and disappointments through their attachment to the child. In most instances the mother is the dominant family member and holds the obese child or children by anxious overprotection including a pushing of food. The mother frequently has high expectations for achievement for the child, achievement to compensate for the failures of the parents and those of their children. The child is not cared for as an individual with particular problems which require emotional support and, as the aims of the parents are predominant, the child fails to develop personal independence or self-esteem. Often the mother's attitudes reflect her own early sufferings and hardships coupled with resentments to her family's and her own childhood experiences. Toward herself she appears self-pitying yet intent on saving her children from similar experiences. In many instances the obese child is not a wanted child. He is often one who has passively accepted the indulged role without rebellion because of his own demanding attitude which cannot be met outside the home. On the surface the obese child and adult is most frequently seen as submissive and unaggressive. Yet this is not really the case. His demands are met in the family setting by the balance provided through the food expression of love and satisfaction. When exposed to social frustrations with their consequent arousal of hostility, the overweight person seeks his satisfaction in overeating and by this means symbolically obtains an expression of his aggression as if the food represents to the patient evidence that he is the best loved.

In time the obese body image also comes to have high emotional significance as it often represents the desire to be strong and powerful and actually, in life, provides satisfactions. The child is conspicuous and may receive attention through this source even though denied it by other socially more acceptable means. Loss of weight becomes difficult not only because of inability to face the physical discomfort of hunger but also because of the symbolic loss of love and revenge which eating had provided, and later because of a fear of loss of the power symbolically represented by the obese frame.

With the concept of specialness and power that the obese child develops from the maternal association and later attaches to his size the psychological life becomes filled with grandiose daydreams, particularly in those persons who daily suffer defeat in their major aspirations. These fantasies are usually conscious and not deeply repressed as in many with psychoneuroses. The fantasies differ from those of the psychotic as the obese person has awareness of their unreasonableness. Obesity at a later stage then becomes, in itself, the rationalization for failure. In some the overweight is used as a means of escaping the anxieties requisite for the pursuit of a creative social existence. The overweight person's attitude toward himself is further complicated by his felt rejection by family and friends because of his obesity, particularly since he has a deep need to be accepted as he is.

Sexual maturation is complicated for both the overweight boy and girl. In many fat men there is marked lack of interest in women and failure to establish heterosexual relations. Yet homosexuality seems rare. The clear concept of the man as a masculine personality is often lacking. Overweight women are usually outgoing with men and succeed in establishing marriage relationships.

The term "reactive obesity" has been used by Bruch to separate out those problems of overweight that occur suddenly after a psychologically traumatic incident in persons who have not previously been evidently stout. Yet indications from the study of such persons show they have previously reacted to stress with overeating and the family patterns and personality development are very similar to those with "developmental obesity." Most frequently the incident leading to reactive overeating has been either the death, or the anxiety associated with the possible loss of a close and significant person. Among those who may be considered as reactively obese are individuals who have for periods been deprived by starvation. Obesity has been frequently observed in those who have spent long periods in prison camps, deprived of love, happiness and recognition and have substituted eating for satisfaction.

The satisfactions of overeating appear protective in some with incipient psychoses. Not infrequently such a person develops a full blown psychotic state when undertaking to lose weight by dieting. This is particularly so in the schizophrenic, while in the depressive individual we most frequently encounter anorexia with weight loss. A number of patients overeat and become overweight, sometimes with reversal of depressive mood to manic behavior.

The psychology of the obese person, as discussed, explains the usual failure of medical therapies to effect continuing change in the overweight state. Since simple loss of weight in those with developmental obesity threatens their psychological defenses, symbolized by the satisfactions of eating and the personal concept of strength in size, the failure to obtain gratifications either through fantasy or through becoming slender results in relapse. Before yielding to the wish of the overweight patient or of his parents for treatment it is necessary to determine whether the desired change is likely to threaten the physical and psychological balance of the individual. The threat to physical health in terms of later cardiovascular disease appears to be overemphasized and the physician and psychiatrist should take into account possible serious psychological and emotional disturbances that may result from efforts at weight reduction.

Successful treatment of the obese person requires a knowledge of his total personality, also that the goal of treatment be directed beyond the mere reduction of weight. With young people these aims are not likely to be obtained unless the parent in the parent-child symbiosis that led to the overeating is also willing to participate in the treatment, even in some instances to the point of undertaking simultaneous psychotherapy. When psychotherapy is utilized it is unwise to attempt weight reduction initially and then discontinue therapy at the point the patient has attained an ideal weight. The timing of the dieting, in association with psychotherapy, needs careful consideration. The nature of the diet and its palatability are important. There is again a growing appreciation that exercise, coupled with diet, is important in reducing weight and maintaining a slender figure. Since inactivity, like overeating, is often an essential facet of the personality of many obese individuals, a simple medical authoritarian approach is unlikely to increase the exercise of the sick patient. In individuals in whom eating provides the major satisfaction in life and other gratifications are not available, psychotherapy is often not successful.

Anorexia Nervosa

A somewhat uncommon psychophysiologic gastrointestinal reaction is that known as *anorexia nervosa.* The presenting symptom of this reaction is a persistent lack of appetite, or rather disgust for food, with vomiting if it is forced. The disorder was first described in 1868 by Sir William Gull and given the name anorexia nervosa in 1874. In a classical paper he called attention to its neurotic peculiarities. The reaction occurs largely in young, single women. Most patients are intellectually superior and in personality characteristics are introverted, stubborn, selfish, perfectionistic, overly sensitive, and manifest compulsive and self-punitive behavior. In addition to the loss of appetite there is an extreme emaciation with a remarkable preservation of bodily vigor which, Gull pointed out, cannot be reconciled with inanition caused by constitutional disease. Other symptoms are amenorrhea, constipation, low metabolic rate, dehydration, dryness of skin, falling of hair, and restless activity. Roentgenographical gastrointestinal studies are negative and no evidence of pituitary disease is demonstrable by roentgen ray. There is often a preceding history of obesity and overeating, with a feeling of shame at being fat. Usually there are unhappy home relations, often taking the form of hostility between mother and daughter. There may also be sibling rivalry and jealousy. In a striking number of cases there is a history of frustration in heterosexual adjustment. In some cases a pregnancy fantasy seems to have prompted the patient to begin to diet. Probably, however, the neurosis can have many varied conscious and unconscious psychological roots. Some psychiatrists point out that the patient seems to achieve both a primary and secondary neurotic gain through the reaction. They suggest that through working out her hostilities and by provoking the environment to acts of punishment which alleviate a sense of guilt a primary or internal gain is obtained. The illness brings, too, a secondary, but unconscious, gain in the form of desired attention, affection and sympathy from the family. In some instances it seems to lead to a diversion of family notice from a supposedly more popular sibling.

Care must be taken not to confuse anorexia nervosa with Simmonds' disease, which results from insufficiency of the anterior lobe of the pituitary or Sheehan's acute pituitary neurosis which occurs secondary to pregnancy and parturition. Treatment consists of psychotherapy with an associated effort to improve the total adjustment of the personality. During treatment, reference to the anorexia should usually be avoided. Intimate personal attention at meals, including spoon-feeding, may be effective in getting the patient to eat normally. Small doses of insulin are advisable. Some patients may require tube-feeding. Removal from the family environment may be advisable.

MUSCULOSKELETAL SYSTEM

Rheumatoid Arthritis

Psychiatric interest in rheumatoid arthritis stems from the repeated observation that the onset or exacerbation of the illness has been related to a period of emotional stress. The patient with rheumatoid arthritis has often been described as an individual who is composed emotionally, seldom expresses his feelings overtly, and appears to derive gratification from being of service to others. He is usually active physically and intellectually and inclined to outdoor and competitive sports. His dependence on others is masked. The majority of such persons have been brought up in families where the mother has been the domineering parent, while the father has been gentle and compliant. This has led to a strong dependency with fear of the maternal figure and in girls a competitive relationship toward the father and brothers. Control of the intense hostility is accomplished through neuromuscular activity, domineering position, ability to control the environment, and overevaluation of physical functions.

The precipitating events leading to the arthritis have ranged from the death of the mother and threat of the father to remarry, separation or rejections from husbands or other important figures, to birth of a child, miscarriage, or disappointments in the personal relations of the patient. It is believed that the common factor in these various events has been an unconscious increase in the feelings of resentment, rebellion, and hostility associated with guilt which had been previously handled through self-sacrificing activity and service to others. A number of patients have had exacerbations of rheumatoid arthritis following the suppression of feelings of grief on the loss of an important family member. Sometimes such exacerbations are seen as anniversary reactions to the loss, associated with feelings of depression.

There is a frequent association of rheumatoid arthritis with duodenal ulcer. While it has been stated that individuals with psychoses seldom suffer from rheumatoid arthritis, yet in a study of a number of arthritic patients by psychoanalytical technique, covert psychotic defenses were noted and in the course of treatment several became overtly disturbed.

At the time of onset of rheumatoid arthritis, or during emergencies, the therapy is essentially one of management of acute illness by the internist with restoration of the patient's sense of security. The psychiatrist's assistance at this time is most effective as a consultant and advisor unless the patient has been in psychiatric treatment previously. Here active support without too rigid control of therapeutic needs is important. Patients with rheumatoid arthritis do poorly in classical psychoanalytical treatment. They respond best to activity on the part of the therapist and for a long time accept activity, rather than words, as security. Psychiatric therapy may be of assistance in those in whom tissue damage is extensive and where the extent of disability exceeds the impairment of neuromuscular function. Many patients with this illness deny their need for help yet with the establishment of a regular regimen of therapeutic interview arranged on the authority of a physician they often do well over long periods of time on little more than supportive treatment. Only in occasional instances can the patient be freed from his often unrecognized hostile identifications with lost persons.

RESPIRATORY SYSTEM

Hyperventilation Syndrome

Subjective symptoms which result from overbreathing are frequently not recognized by either the psychiatrist or the internist. Hyperventilation is the common physiological means by which the subjective disturbance noted in the usual acute anxiety attack takes place. It may be induced by any condition producing fear and not uncommonly occurs in the course of other personality disturbances when anxiety becomes manifest. Its recognition is of importance since in the medical clinic the afflicted patient is often considered to have heart disease, angina pectoris, asthma or other respiratory disease, or even painful lesions presumed to be a result of spinal cord disease. In the psychiatric clinic many patients have been exposed to a time-wasting therapy in which efforts are made to interpret the symbolic meaning of the subjective phenomenon produced by overbreathing.

The sufferer usually does not recognize that he is overbreathing. The increase and the depth and rapidity of respiration may be so slight that they go unobserved. It is well known that an irregular respiratory rhythm occurs in anxious individuals and is accompanied by sighing and yawning. Furthermore, these respiratory disturbances, if sufficiently prolonged, lead to reduction in the alveolar air and the arterial blood-carbon dioxide tension with a fall in the blood bicarbonate. Consequently many physiological systems are altered. The acid-base equilibrium is disturbed, the urine composition and volume are affected, circulatory changes take place and neuromuscular and electroencephalographic alterations ensue. It is not surprising that subjective disturbances take place.

The initial subjective feelings resulting from overbreathing are light-headedness or giddiness. If overbreathing continues, the individual has the sensation that he is about to faint, he may perspire profusely and, if walking, his gait may seem unstable. There then follows a sensation of air hunger or shortness of breath and feelings of pressure in the thorax. Some patients speak of palpitation or of pain in the heart while others describe a bandlike feeling about the chest. With mounting anxiety over presumed lack of air, many consciously increase the depth and rate of breathing, thereby exacerbating the initial cause of the subjective symptoms. The more commonly recognized symptoms of hyperventilation consist of tingling paresthesias in the fingertips, perioral region or toes, followed by tetanic contractions. If overbreathing persists over a sufficiently prolonged period, disturbance of awareness may result associated with vasomotor collapse, rapid, irregular and weak pulse, pallor, and ending, in many instances, in loss of consciousness or in convulsions.

In those instances where the psychiatrist sees a patient who complains of attacks of breathlessness, palpitation and dizziness or perspiration, consideration should be given to the symptomatology as representative of episodic attacks of hyperventilation precipitated by acute situational anxiety. Such patients frequently are able to define well the situations in which the attacks occur and provide excellent descriptions of disturbing interpersonal contacts with arousal of unbearable feelings of hostility, resentment or sexuality. Not infrequently the attack of hyperventilation takes place as the consequence of a disturbing dream or nightmare. The diagnosis of a hyperventilation syndrome as the source of the symptoms of the individual patient may be easily determined by requesting the patient to overbreathe for a period of two minutes in a sitting position. In order to carry out this test effectively, it is frequently necessary to provide a brief demonstration of what is required, also strongly to encourage the patient to continue overbreathing, as many will attempt to desist after thirty seconds of hyperventilation. At the end of this test the patient may be asked to describe his subjective symptoms. If he is unable to elaborate them spontaneously, the psychiatrist should inquire as to the presence of giddiness, breathlessness, palpitation, shortness of breath, perspiration, and pins-and-needles sensation. The patient then may be asked if he identifies the subjective sensations of overbreathing as those that he has suffered in the episodic attacks of which he complains. Not infrequently the neurological symptoms that occur in the course of this disturbance are unilateral. In general, the carbon dioxide combining power of the blood and the blood calcium are unchanged. However, in those instances where chronic hyperventilation exists, a venous alkalosis has in some instances been demonstrated. Occasionally with chronic, persistent hyperventilation a compensatory acidosis with reduction in blood carbon dioxide has been reported.

Hyperventilation may result not only from sudden emotional stress and anxiety but also in the course of febrile illnesses, high altitude anoxemia, high external temperatures over a long prolonged period of time, and occasionally in the course of encephalitis.

In some sufferers the reduplication of the characteristic symptom complex by means of requested hyperventilation provides immediate and continuing relief of symptoms. On the other hand, in those individuals who have clear-cut evidence of chronic anxiety usually associated with phobic symptoms or with depressive or schizophrenic personality disorders, the demonstration of the physiological source of the symptomatology is effective only in providing an intellectual interpretation of the acutely disturbing symptoms and not in providing them with continuing relief. In these instances it is recommended that the patient receive psychotherapy. In the course of such treatment a modification of the personality structure that predisposes to the eruption of anxiety precipitated repetitively in particular situations may be brought about. The following case report provides an example of the need for psychotherapy in patients who present the hyperventilation syndrome.

A 57 year old woman who had been under medical care since her menopause at the age of fifty was referred for psychiatric treatment. At the onset of the menopause she had complained of headaches, nausea, tremulousness and cold sweats. Her blood pressure was usually about 180 systolic, 90 diastolic. She made regular visits to her physician who treated her with diet and Theominal. The patient did well for a period of five years until her treatment by this physician was abruptly terminated by her husband.

The patient was brought for psychiatric treatment two years later by her husband who stated in her presence that he could no longer stand her "huffing and puffing." In the intervening two years he had taken her to several other physicians for her increasingly frequent and severe attacks of apparent shortness of breath. The patient described these as occurring only in the morning upon awaking. She would then seem short of breath and soon become dizzy and weak. She next suffered from palpitation, followed by tingling and numbness about the mouth and tips of the extremities. The attacks had increased in frequency to one daily. Each morning they prevented her husband and daughter from going to work and kept her from preparing the breakfast and doing the housework. The patient had been advised to "snap out of it," and had been given sedatives and ammonium chloride without avail.

The only abnormality observed on physical examination was a slight elevation of blood pressure. She was requested to hyperventilate and it was demonstrated to her that her symptoms could be reproduced by this procedure. The patient was considered to have essential hypertension complicated by attacks of hyperventilation resulting from chronic anxiety.

From spontaneous remarks made by the patient at this time, it was learned that during the period of overbreathing she was concerned about dying—not the possibility of her own death—but the death of her husband. She spoke of the recent death of her brother from heart disease and cancer, she went on to state that her children had now grown up and no longer needed her and she commented that the family had threatened to place her in a hospital for mental disorders. Her past history indicated that the patient was a driving, energetic woman who had been completely immersed in her family. It was inferred from her remarks about death that she harbored repressed resentment toward her husband who showed little sympathy with her during the initial interview. It soon seemed apparent that situations which aroused repressed hostility toward her husband and family, feelings which were unacceptable to her as a conscientious person and threats of separation from her family induced the acute anxiety attacks manifested by overbreathing.

It was learned that the patient had married her husband suddenly after having been jilted. At that time, too, she had given up an excellent job. Her own daughter had been jilted some six months prior to the consultation. The patient described her husband as self-centered, buried in his work, disinterested in social life, and as disparaging in his attitude toward her church and recreational activities. He was seen and advised to spend more time with his wife.

In four subsequent visits she was encouraged to ventilate her unacceptable feelings concerning her family and husband. She commented on the fact that she wished to resume typing and playing the piano. She was frank in speaking of her anger toward her husband for his years of indifference, obstinacy and ridicule, culminating when he forbade her to continue to attend the doctor who had helped her so well throughout the menopause. The patient was encouraged to plan activities outside the home which might help to make her less dependent on the family. The patient responded quickly. Within six weeks she was free of overbreathing attacks, did not require medication, and had returned to her house work. She then decided that further treatment was unnecessary since her immediate symptoms had been relieved.

This case illustrates several important factors in the management of the hyperventilation syndrome. First, the patient was made aware of the physiological mechanism underlying the attacks by having her hyperventilate. This test also made her realize that her symptoms were regarded as significant in themselves. Second, a series of simple psychotherapeutic discussions allowed the patient to express herself freely concerning her emotions and attitude toward her family. This discussion of her feelings, interspersed only with a few directional questions related to possible anger and resentment, relieved her of her symptoms. Third, this patient was an excellent choice for brief psychotherapy as she gave a history of previous satisfactory adjustment at home, at work and in marriage.

Asthma

The manifestation of anxiety by disturbances of respiratory rhythm is a commonly observed phenomenon. The existence of neurotic factors in asthma has long been noted, and they are by no means excluded by reason of the present concept of asthma as an allergic disease. The precipitation of attacks by sudden, intense emotions in predisposed persons has been well known to clinicians for many years. The relation between asthma and emotional factors appears to be as follows: A prerequisite to the development of asthma, as in the case of persons prone to the development of other psychophysiological reactions, is the existence of an irritable and excitable autonomic nervous system. In the asthmatic, there is the additional factor of allergic tendency. If to these two factors there is added the third one of emotional stress and tension the stimulating effect of the latter on the vegetative nervous system added to the existing allergic tendency is sufficient to produce a spasm of the bronchioles. In other words a combination of emotional stimuli and allergy will produce an asthmatic attack if the autonomic nervous system is unstable and easily excitable. In many cases an unhappy home atmosphere will be found. In treatment the removal of one of the two coexisting causative factors, either the allergy or the emotional stress, results in relief. Psychoanalysts suggest that the emotional factor may be a conflict centering in an excessive, unresolved dependence on the mother.

The asthmatic adult should be encouraged to discuss his environment at home and at work and to relate emotional incidents to attacks of asthma. In the child the psychiatrist will investigate the attitude of the mother toward the child and the relations between parents and between siblings. In children it often seems as if the asthmatic attacks tend to be precipitated by a situation which threatens separation from the mother.

ENDOCRINE SYSTEM

Diabetes Mellitus

Among the more striking examples of the influence of emotional disturbances on somatic functioning is that observed in certain patients suffering from diabetes mellitus. Personality factors and the consequent emotional responses to the treatment regimen of this condition relate to almost all the issues pertaining to the treatment of diabetes. The psychiatrist may make a major contribution in the treatment and management of those difficult patients with "brittle diabetes." Psychosomatic investigations in recent years have clearly elucidated the disturbances in glucose metabolism and in variations in ketonemia resulting from changes in the emotional state of the individual.

It has been suggested that the onset of diabetes is often related to periods of severe emotional distress after such experiences as disruption of the home, or frustration associated with long periods of grinding work. While the inquiry into the personality structure of the diabetic has failed to demonstrate a uniform personality picture, many psychiatrists have emphasized the passivity and immaturity with which diabetic patients look for attention and affection. Psychoanalytical studies of a few patients suggest that certain diabetics are frustrated when their demands for love and attention cannot be met. Others have stated that the psychological trauma derives from reactivation of dependency needs by new exposure to rejection and deprivation through the loss of another person.

On the physiological side it has been shown that urinary and blood glucose levels are elevated following periods of emotional stress and that the glucose tolerance curves may be modified at such times. In general, the glucose tolerance test has been found to be more diabetic when the individual is feeling more hostile and depressed, and it approaches the healthy curve when the patient feels accepted and cared for. It has been shown that an increase in ketone bodies in the blood stream may occur in similar situations; also that with increasing diuresis, the diabetic may lose sugar, ketones and chlorides with depletion of fixed base and a rapid fall of glycogen in the blood stream. Such physiological changes associated with the metabolic defect lead to acidosis and may precipitate coma, particularly when the anxious patient neglects his diabetic regimen, as frequently takes place. Since the customary regulation of diabetes requires both a control of the diet and the administration of insulin, the management of the disease is often complicated by the fact that the symbolic significance of the feeding process and its relationship to provision of emotional support through love may modify the therapeutic indications. It is particularly true that the giving of food and its deprivation become paramount in those homes where tension exists between parents and a diabetic child. The illness magnifies the difficulty between the child and the parent. Those parents with perfectionistic, aggressive attitudes may bring their children to good control of the diabetes but with the creation of a behavior difficulty. On the other hand, parents who pity themselves or blame the child and reject it may foster poor control of the diabetes. The need to limit food often becomes a battleground between the child and parents and the child and physician. This is particularly so since the giving of candy or of food is often a token of approval in the family. The child has an excellent weapon which he can use against rigid and punitive parents by refusing to eat when he is denied his wishes. Other children, under treatment for diabetes mellitus, finding themselves starved for food or affection express their hostility through eating as they wish and then lying convincingly. Thus the rigid dietary management insisted upon by the physician and the family often leads to rather serious emotional disturbance in the child with concomitant change or modification of the glucose metabolism and probable ketosis, or to psychological conflicts that deter the proper acceptance of the therapeutic needs of the illness. In such instances the psychiatrist is needed as a means of working through the emotional conflict of the child with the parents, in assisting the parents to understand the child's problem and occasionally in providing advice to the internist in regard to the personality reactions of the child and the need to modify the dietary regimen and insulin requirements in conformity with the emotional problem that exists.

Adult diabetics who repeatedly go into acidosis are usually individuals who are seriously disturbed. Such individuals either give up all dietary control or cease taking insulin as a means of expressing their depressive and suicidal drives. While this is the case in the majority of instances, other persons are precipitated into states of acidosis by serious transient emotional disturbances. Sexual difficulties are common in both men and women with diabetes. Diabetic women are concerned over child bearing, while diabetic men are frequently impotent. Childbirth itself may activate regressive cravings for care and affection in diabetics of either sex. The new child may be seen as a rival for the affection of the husband or wife. Thus the dependent cravings of the patient may be magnified with resulting feelings of anxiety and depression that disturb the metabolic balance or lead to despair and diminished motivation for control of diet. Obese diabetics who are addicted to sweets or to overeating are likely to overeat when anxious in spite of threats of physicians concerning their future health if they fail to adhere to the diabetic regimen. Here, again, the need for psychiatric aid becomes important.

Hyperthyroidism

The most important of the endocrine glands as related to psychosomatic medicine is the *thyroid*. Although as early as 1803 reference was made to the occurrence of sudden fright preceding hyperthyroidism yet not until relatively recently has the possibility that emotional troubles may play an important part in the cause and course of the disease received adequate attention in the treatment of thyrotoxic states. This recent knowledge is detailed in Chapter XIII of this book.

Menopausal Syndromes

It is often stated that the menopausal syndrome is a result of endocrine changes but it would seem clear that its more serious features, and especially the neuroses and psychoses that accompany or follow the menopause, have their origin in deeply seated psychological factors rather than in endocrine disturbances *per se*. Those women who develop the more serious personality disturbances of that period have nearly always lived narrow lives and have been worrisome, intolerant, scrupulous and inhibited. Weiss and English describe well the psychological problems that confront such women at that period: "It is small wonder that when the menstrual bleeding, which is the symbol of femininity, motherhood, sexuality, and all the ideas that go with these concepts, is about to disappear, the woman who has led an empty life becomes anxious and panicky. She feels that she is passing into old age without having experienced the things which make life worth living. She is depressed in spirits and irritable at a fate which she believes has cheated her in the past and can promise nothing for the future."

For men, there is no convincing evidence of a menopausal state secondary to diminished secretory action of the sexual glands consequent to aging. Those anxious, depressive and asthenic states ascribed to this cause are usually the result of emotional disturbances precipitated through loss of self-esteem, sense of defeat and failure or deprivation of emotional support through death of family and friends.

SKIN

A recognition of the importance of psychological factors in many dermatoses is by no means recent. Sydenham (1624–1689), for example, writing of the "hysteric diseases," described angioneurotic edema affecting one leg. Since the skin is an organ subject to the direct influences of the autonomic nervous system, and the indirect effect of endocrine activity, as well as subject on the body surface to compulsive contact or self-inflicted damage representing unconscious conflict, the means of expression of the psychological disturbance vary greatly from one type of lesion to another. In the past few years with the increasing recognition of psychological factors in the genesis of somatic diseases, the dermatologists have emphasized a high degree of association between various skin diseases such as pruritus, neurodermatoses, hyperhydrosis and other reactions, and evidences of difficulties in adjustment of personality to stressful life situations. Some dermatology clinics have reported that psychiatric factors were found to be of significance in over 75 per cent of their patients.

In cases of the dry type of neurodermatitis, it has been considered that excoriation of the skin is more fundamental than the pruritus usually complained of by these patients. The itching often represents a voluptuous or tantalizing sensation. Events which produce the emotions of anger with depression and feelings of guilt generally precipitate the exacerbation of the cutaneous eruption. The family constellation is often that of a hostile dependent maternal relationship in which itching and scratching symbolize anger at the mother figure handled masochistically due to guilt. In the exudative type of neurodermatitis of children (atopic dermatitis), there has been found evidence of maternal rejection. Here the emotional disturbance is thought to be expressed primarily through a psychophysiological mechanism which induces vesiculation. In urticaria the psychodynamic explanation is very similar to that of asthma with the lesions precipitated by situations which induce resentment, frustration resulting from a threat to an important dependency relationship. With pruritus of the anogenital area repression of various sexual conflicts has been observed. Dermatitis factitia has been recognized for many years as psychologically determined. Sadomasochistic mechanisms associated with the need to maintain a gratifying passive dependency again underlie the self-infliction of the lesions in many such instances.

Various methods of treatment for the neurodermatoses have been devised. Frequently separation from the significant family members brings about clearing with recurrence noted on return to the family. The following case report represents a trial with a brief psychotherapeutic method of the type recently described by Seitz.

The patient, a 46 year old retired policeman, was seen in September 1956 with the chief complaint of a skin rash. The onset of his dermatitis occurred 25 years previously when, shortly after his marriage, he noted the gradual appearance of a diffuse scaling eruption of the scalp. Some time later he developed redness and scaling in the groin, and a more or less generalized eruption, especially around the sides of his neck and in the creases of the knees and elbows. The rash was intensely pruritic and the patient frequently scratched until he bled. Two years prior to admission, the eruption became generalized. No relief was obtained from steroid therapy and a multitude of other medications. Because of a life-long history of emotional problems he was referred for psychiatric consultation.

The patient was the second of six children. His father was described as a strict disciplinarian who beat the children regularly with a cat-o'-nine-tails. Until 17 years of age the patient was not allowed to stay out in the evening without his father's permission and if he arrived home late he was beaten.

The mother was described as a warm, understanding person who was affectionate with the children but showed little love toward her husband. The patient's older brother was a fireman who had retired ten years previously following an acute psychotic episode. The other four siblings appeared to be in good health. The patient explained their good fortune with the statement, "By the time they arrived my father had mellowed."

The patient's early development was unremarkable and his progress at school was average. He remembered that he was never able to express anger and never disobeyed his father's detailed instructions.

As an adolescent the patient was a shy, sensitive boy who was self-conscious and avoided social relationships with girls. There were exaggerated guilt feelings over masturbation. When confronted with social situations that were threatening he would turn to drinking. He stated, "I had a terrific inferiority complex and liquor helped me to overcome it."

Since a civil service position offered a secure position and pension he joined the police force at the suggestion of his father. When 20 years of age he married in the hope of getting away from home. From the first there was marital difficulty and he began to drink a quart of liquor daily.

Fourteen years before psychiatric consultation the patient, during a riot, was struck on the head and sustained a concussion necessitating a brief hospitalization. Following his discharge he became tremulous and complained of extreme nervousness. He believed he was losing his mind, had recurrent episodes of depersonalization and was unable to function at work. His alcoholic intake increased in an effort to alleviate the pruritus, his anxiety and the constant fear that he was about to die. He was discharged from the police force with a pension and the diagnosis of post-traumatic psychoneurosis.

During the subsequent two years he separated from his wife and child, lost contact with his family and lived with an alcoholic woman who was suffering from cirrhosis. There were several episodes of delirium tremens and he was hospitalized for alcoholic neuropathy, hepatic cirrhosis, and hematemesis.

Eight years prior to this consultation and following the death of his female companion he was warned by a physician that if he continued drinking he would probably not survive another year. He discontinued drinking, was reconciled with his wife and his dermatitis cleared, leaving only a few eczematous patches. He returned to work as a law clerk, attended church regularly and, in his own words, "became a model citizen." He maintained a rigid routine involving difficult hours of work. He dressed meticulously and attempted to do a perfect job at the office.

During the past two years his rash has again become generalized and intensely pruritic. His wife informed him that, while asleep, he scratched as if he were intent on killing himself. He was admitted to a hospital in the hope that separation from his family and job would help in the treatment of his skin condition.

When seen in psychiatric consultation he appeared as a well groomed, neatly attired, middle-aged man, alert and accurate, who spoke of his past experiences with obvious embarrassment. His memory was good and he was well oriented with an average intelligence and a normal fund of knowledge. He seemed anxious to please the interviewer and stated that he needed psychiatric help. During consultation he scratched freely. He volunteered that scratching usually brought him great relief and, at times, a satisfaction not unlike that of sexual pleasure. When psychotherapy was suggested he quickly agreed. It was explained that he would be seen once a week for a period of ten weeks by the psychiatrist in the outpatient department and that immediately preceding the interview he would be seen by the dermatologist for a brief examination.

During the first two interviews an anamnesis was obtained with particular emphasis on his current activity. He discussed the present fear of his father and the avoidance of situations which would bring him in contact with him. His wife frequently accused him of being a coward because of this but he could not admit his fear to her. He described his wife as a stubborn, outspoken woman who was usually the disciplinarian with his 17-year old boy. When he attempted to punish his son his wife became outraged and pointed out to him how good it was of both of them to accept him back eight years ago. He nevertheless denied that there was friction in the household and stated that, in many ways, they were an ideal family. His son had recently been arrested on a minor charge and it was suggested to the patient that perhaps he was failing as a father by not setting limits for the son.

During the third visit it was noted that the scratching had increased and there was no improvement in the skin condition. He stated early in the interview, "I followed your advice and asserted myself with the boy but was careful not to become angry." His wife had been angry with him but he pacified her by taking her out for a drive. He admitted that he dare not express anger toward her for fear she would leave him. Scratching was frequent, especially when his fear of expressing anger was discussed. His wife insisted upon knowing what was going on in therapy. He resented this, but felt he could not refuse to tell her. He was told that it was not necessary to tell her and he appeared to have considerable anxiety over this.

At work he was accused by a colleague of being a perfectionist; he admitted being angry at this criticism. When it was suggested that he deal more directly with the problems confronting him at work and at home, he scratched and talked of his extreme loneliness. When the patient attempted to discuss early experiences and relationships he was referred back to current areas of conflict.

At the fourth interview his skin condition was much worse and he was unable to attend work. He had purchased two suits of clothing without consulting his wife who usually accompanied him. He made some rather feeble attempts to tell his wife that he preferred shopping without her but felt that it was unsuccessful. He turned to the interviewer and asked, "Doc, tell me, what do you do when you become angry?" There was a fantasy of telling off a co-worker and he remarked that recently he felt resentful and angry, wondering if his increased scratching was related to this.

At the time of the sixth interview his skin remained unchanged. He expressed his fear of losing control of his anger and appeared more aware of his current problems. He talked of his helplessness and became angry with the interviewer for not being of more help to him.

With the seventh interview his skin looked considerably better. He had informed his wife that he was the boss around the house and, following a minor altercation with his son, had told him that he was "not yet dry around the ears." He appeared surprised that his wife was "snapping to," and that his son was spending more time around the house.

In the ninth week his skin improved remarkably. He related an incident with pride in which when his wife refused to prepare breakfast for him he had advised her that she had better behave herself, ordered her to the bedroom and had intercourse with her. That evening he took her to the movies and noted that she was affectionate.

He remarked that during the previous week he had been able to tell his employer that too much of the work fell on him and that this should be changed.

Treatment was terminated on December 31, 1956. The patient was seen in dermatology clinic two months later. His skin had cleared completely except for a small area of dermatitis behind the knees. He was feeling well, had no difficulty sleeping, required no medication and was much satisfied with the changes in his relations with his family and employers.

GENITOURINARY SYSTEM

It is not surprising that neuroses and psychosomatic symptoms should frequently exist in a system of such fundamental biological importance and concerned with such an elemental instinct as is the genitourinary. This would presumably not be the case were it not for the fact that during the development of the personality, ideas and emotions concerning its functioning have become heavily charged with feelings of shame, guilt, fear, disgust and even hatred. Often such attitudes are the result of faulty education. In view of this conflictive, often emotionally irreconcilable, state of affairs it is no wonder that in no other system, except perhaps the gastrointestinal, are disturbances of function so common.

Although in recent years gynecologists have become increasingly conscious that emotional disturbances may produce disordered function and distress in the pelvic region, far too many women undergo such operations as suspension of the uterus, curettage, cervical amputation, removal of adnexae, plastic operations, appendectomies and even hysterectomies for gynecological complaints that have a psychic basis. Unfortunately the treatment of psychogenic gynecological disturbances and sexual dysfunctions by operative or other physical procedures is not harmless but nourishes and fixates a consciousness of illness. Among symptoms which arise from psychogenic factors are pelvic pain and parethesia, dysmenorrhea and dyspareunia. Both physiological and psychological factors may contribute to dysmenorrhea. Such terms as "unwell" or "sick" used in reference to menstruation may have a harmfully suggestive significance and contribute to the occurrence of dysmenorrhea and other menstrual difficulties. Such sexual malfunctioning as frigidity and impotence are frequently of psychogenic origin. Finally, it should be remembered that neither marriage nor pregnancy is to be recommended as a cure for neurosis or for the solution of involved emotional problems.

NERVOUS SYSTEM

Disturbances of the Image of the Body

While our modern conceptions of the body image derive from the studies of Schilder, the knowledge of phantom phenomena which demonstrate so strikingly the validity of this concept extend well back into medical antiquity. They were known to Ambroise Paré and surgeons before his time. They were the subject of study by Weir Mitchell over a century ago. It is now recognized that with growth the individual develops a total perception of his own body as well as certain attitudes toward his physical self that many consider the core structure in the development of the ego. The body concept slowly evolves through the multiple sensory experiences of the infant in the discovery of his body parts. The various sensory impressions conveyed by means of kinesthetic, visual and tactile apparatus to the cortex lead to an expanding and growing perception of body awareness presumably organized and integrated in the parieto-temporal cortex of the brain. In addition to this physiological substratum acquired over the years by postural, tactile and visual percepts, each individual attaches to this appreciation of body surface and its various parts attitudes with emotional overtones which derive from his early experiences in the family and as a result of the parental evaluations of his physique. The attitudes are ingrained through verbal remarks, nonverbal indications and the expressions of valuation pertaining to desirable physical traits and attainment. The comparison of his own physique with that of his parents and peers and the emphasis on the differences play a large role in the body image of the growing child. The parents imply that the child's body and its parts are good or bad, pleasing or repulsive, clean or dirty, loved or disliked. Thus, in some families in which physical strength and physical accomplishment are emphasized, a boy's attitude toward his body is determined to a large extent by the parents' feelings and attitudes toward development of his limbs and muscles. In a similar manner, the parents or the culture may overemphasize physical beauty or particular physical attributes in girls. The American cultural overemphases are evident in our advertising and writing. It may be mentioned that certain families and ethical groups tend to derogate various body parts which have sexual significance. This, in turn, reflects in part on both conscious and unconscious conceptions and perceptions of body parts in certain individuals. The loss of a hand, for example, may have a very different meaning to a violinist than to a professor of history, and a resulting disturbance or disorganization of the personality be therefore much more apt to result in the former. Lesions in parts of the body which psychologically represent organs of marked value for the personality—such as eyes, breasts, sexual organs—may be highly disturbing even though the disease, objectively considered, is not serious. Disturbances of the personality rarely follow operations upon the appendix or other organs not invested with deep emotional value. On the contrary, psychiatric complications following operations upon highly valued ones, such as the reproductive organs, are not uncommon. Disabling physical handicaps, such as crippling, blindness and deafness, which put the patient at a disadvantage with his fellows, may have profound effect upon emotional health. The sensitive, even paranoid, reactions of the deaf, at times more disturbing to social adjustment than the deafness itself, are familiar observations. In girls, particularly, a serious physical handicap may produce mental problems that completely overshadow the defect. Because of the high evaluations placed upon their biological functions and because any conditions which adversely affect these functions may seriously jeopardize their personal, economic and social security and happiness, women are particularly subject to fears and emotional conflicts when such functions are disturbed. Lack of attractiveness, or physical defects which preclude offers of marriage, an inability to bear children, the loss of physical charm through age or disease, the presence of conditions that make discontinuance of marital relations necessary, or the approach of the involutional period may constitute problems to which emotional adjustment is difficult or impossible within the limits of mental health.

Body image disturbances classically present evidence of psychosomatic relationships expressed in the activity of the highest integrative organ, the brain, in its perceptive and early cognitive functioning. Disturbances in this function will not fit easily in the concept of psychosomatic disorders if this is confined to expressions of dysfunction mediated through the autonomic nervous system. For the clinical psychiatrist, disturbances of the body image will be observed in association with many of the major psychoneurotic and psychotic disorders. However, there are certain expressions of primary body image disturbance of particular interest that may be recognized as separate entities. Among these are the various phantom phenomena and the efforts on the part of the individual to adapt to these phenomena, as well as such conditions as neurasthenia and hypochondriasis.

Phantom Phenomena

Phantom phenomena are considered the expression of the enduring concept of the individual's body image persisting after loss of a body part. It is significant that phantoms have not been noted in those with absence of a limb resulting from a congenital defect or from infantile amputations. The phantom is not explainable then on the basis of wish fulfillment or "gestalt" psychology. The observation of a phantom limb after amputation occurs in some 98 per cent of amputees. Such phantoms are initially perceived as consisting of the whole extremity. Usually the distal portion of the phantom, such as the hand or foot, is most conspicuous. As time passes the phantom appendage tends to shrink and may eventually disappear into the stump. Movements of the amputation stump may induce the impression of movement of the phantom extremity provided kinesthetic sensation remains in the stump.

Three kinds of sensory phenomena may be noted in the phantom limb. In all patients with a phantom there occurs a mild tingling, the basic phantom phenomenon, which may be regarded as dependent upon the function of the sensory-motor cerebral cortex. A stronger momentary pins-and-needles sensation may occur in the phantom by touching neuromas in the stump; this sensation is dependent upon functional activity of lower spinal centers. Also included under the second type of sensory phenomena are sensations referred into the phantom in the presence of disease of other organs such as referred pain of cardiac origin. Referred sensations into the phantom may be elicited by deep pressure on the amputation stump, less often with algesic skin stimulation and least by tactile stimulation.

The third type of painful sensory disturbance in the phantom is the common cause of the amputee's referral for psychiatric or neurologic consultation. Questioning usually reveals that the patient is concerned about sensations which he describes variously as "twisting," "burning," "pulling," or "itching." In most instances the symptom is intermittent. It is more often annoying than agonizing. The introspective, observant amputee will have noted its aggravation by stimulation of the stump, sometimes by micturition in those who have lost a leg, by changes in weather and in many instances by emotionally disturbing incidents.

While limb phantoms are common, mammary, penile, rectal and nasal phantoms are rare. Phantoms of the bladder and rectum have rarely been observed in paraplegic patients, while those of the flaccid penis and erect penis are more frequent. The existence of phantom images of other internal organs is not generally accepted as occurring although it has been suggested that the occurrence of phantom pain in the abdomen may explain the recurrence of peptic ulcer pain in the patients who initially report the disappearance of such pain after vagotomy.

The admission by an amputee of a limb phantom should be regarded as a healthy psychological response. Subsequent to an amputation, the healthy individual slowly reorganizes his body image by means of the new sensory experiences related to the changed body form. The persistence of a physical defect irritating the afferent nerves from the amputated part will delay this reorganization and may cause pain.

The healthy amputee accepts his defect, resumes his family position, returns to his occupation and, with an adequate stump, makes use of an appropriate prosthesis. On the other hand, those who complain of persistent or intermittent pain in a phantom incapacitating them for a return to life in society, in whom the painful symptom does not conform to the recognized descriptions of the sensations resulting from irritation of known structures and referral into recognized areas of nervous distribution and where there is resistance to the acceptance of a prosthesis or poor family, marital or occupational adaptation, are usually suffering a serious personality disturbance. Such disturbances, though rare, occur as amputation leads to an upsurge of anxiety owing to the distortion of the patient's concept of his body and therefore of himself and his relations with others. This distortion requires readaptation in relation to others and to society. Also, hostile feelings may emerge in the amputee toward those people with whom he identifies, on whom he is dependent and whose rejection he now apprehends. The painful symptom thus may symbolize the need for, and apprehension relative to a possible loss of dependency.

Kolb found that in many instances the amputee with the painful phantom has identified in a hostile way with another amputee significantly related to him in his early life. In those amputees with a hysterical personality make-up and identification with another amputee, the fantasy life often discloses superstitious rationalization to explain the existence of the phantom phenomenon. The rationalizations are concerned with the loss and the fantasied disposal of the amputated part. In association with these fantasies, the amputee attempts to master his grief and mourning over the loss of the amputated part. He desires to have the part disposed of tenderly and respectfully as if the whole body were to be buried.

The neurotically overdetermined painful symptom has been relieved by a variety of psychiatric therapies including suggestion, hypnosis, narcotherapy, electroshock, lobotomy and more recently by the tranquilizing drugs. The therapeutic procedure of choice must be determined on the basis of the over-all personality disturbance observed in the individual patient. The following report illustrates an acute emotional disturbance associated with the phantom phenomenon:

A 14-year old boy came to clinic complaining of a "knot in his leg." He said he had bumped the lower part of his right leg against a step one month previously.

On examination a hard, fixed, tender mass was noted in the middle third of the injured part of leg. Roentgenograms showed a primary malignant tumor involving the anterolateral cortex of the right tibia. Three days later amputation of the right leg was performed through the lower third of the femur. The pathologist reported an osteogenic sarcoma of the tibia. The patient complained of pain in the phantom right leg shortly after recovery from the anesthesia. Within two days after operation, large doses of narcotic agents were being employed in an attempt to relieve him of pain. By the ninth postoperative day the patient was complaining bitterly of a burning pain, was overactive, thrashed about in bed and spoke of jumping out of a window. Special nurses were required at this time and psychiatric consultation was requested. The patient was found to be fearful, disoriented and confused. Administration of all drugs except morphine was discontinued in order to alleviate the mild toxic delirious state.

The next day the patient was rolling about in his bed, with his eyes closed, apparently oblivious to those about him. He cried out repetitiously, "Help me, help me. Do something for the pain." It was believed that frightening rationalizations as to the origin of the phantom contributed in part to the state of painful panic. The boy was therefore asked if he were aware of the feeling of a phantom limb after operation. Surprisingly, the boy immediately become silent, opened his eyes and responded affirmatively. Under questioning he stated that a year previously one of his school teachers had casually discussed amputations with his class. The teacher told the class a story of a man who had undergone an amputation after which a severe stinging pain developed in his phantom limb. The story went that the limb was disinterred and that ants were discovered burrowing into and stinging the amputated part.

When inquiry was made as to what disposition the boy believed had been made of his own amputated extremity he stated that he thought it was being burned. He was reassured and informed otherwise. The complaint of pain and his wild overactivity subsided to a large extent immediately after this interview. It was possible to discontinue the use of all morphine within twenty-four hours and to discharge the patient's special nurse shortly thereafter.

Complete relief of his pain, however, required four additional hours of psychotherapy. It was learned that the boy had been severely upset by his mother's death from cancer of the breast five years previously. The boy never spoke of his mother after her death but was morbidly inquisitive whenever anyone became ill and would inquire of his father if the person were about to die. The mother had undergone amputation of the breast. The latter hours of treatment brought to awareness the boy's repressed hostility toward his mother with whom he identified as an amputee and his ambivalent feelings toward his father.

When he was dismissed from the clinic twenty-five days after operation the boy had no pain, did not require medication, was active on crutches and was eager to have a prosthesis fitted. A year later his stepmother wrote that he was without pain and was wearing a prosthesis. He had returned to school, was doing well in his studies and had been elected to a class office.

Neurasthenia

The concept of neurasthenia has undergone many manifestations, and one might say abuses, since the term was first introduced by Beard in 1867 to describe a condition caused, he believed, by an exhaustion of the nerve cells through depletion of their stored nutriment. Probably the term should be dropped altogether and some of the clinical syndromes formerly included under it be assigned to the anxiety reactions, some to conversion hysteria and some included under the category of psychophysiological asthenic reactions. The present tendency is to assign to the last group most of the symptom complexes formerly classified as neurasthenia.

General fatigue with its feeling of overwhelming exhaustion and of diffuse "nervousness" is the predominating complaint in the reaction which should be regarded as a response to emotional conflicts and their attendant anxiety. The causes therefore are psychological. It is no longer believed that "neurasthenia" is caused by a generally impaired or exhausted physical state as a result of which the nervous system is drained of its energy in the manner of a partially discharged battery of low voltage. Some complaints seem to be disappointment reactions while others appear to be the expression of sexual dissatisfaction or conflicts. Sometimes repressed hostility or other anxiety-exciting factors produce the reaction. In other instances the asthenic reaction seems to arise from constant failure, frustration and disappointment. Boredom, monotony and absence of goals may serve as contributory causes. It will be found that many patients have had a difficult childhood with little interest or affection from their parents. The existence of family or social problems should always be considered.

SYMPTOMS. The premorbid personality of the patient with psychophysiological asthenic reaction has usually been characterized by dissatisfaction and by a sense of being thwarted and rejected. The premorbid characteristics often merge so insidiously into the symptoms of the reaction that no definite time of its onset can be stated. As already indicated the asthenic-reaction patient has a long-continued subjective sensation of overwhelming exhaustion. Any exertion, either mental or physical, seems too great. An exaggerated degree of attention is paid to the bodily organs and their functions. The patient may complain of dizziness, of a feeling of pressure on the head, and perhaps of pain at the nape of the neck. There is an excitability of the special senses (intolerance of noise, bright lights, cold, etc.). Muscae volitantes are common. Associated psychophysiologic gastrointestinal reactions are common. Gastrointestinal complaints are therefore frequent. Indigestion, constipation and diarrhea may occur. Gastric secretions may be altered and motility delayed. Palpitation, extrasystoles and tachycardia, symptoms of an associated anxiety state, increase the alarm of the patient. Vasomotor instability is frequent so that the skin is at times flushed and again sweating or cold. Patients with this vasomotor instability wrap themselves in mufflers and are in constant fear of catching cold. Complaints of "fallen stomach" or "loose kidney" are common. The sexual functions of the male are disturbed; impaired potency, nocturnal emissions and failures at intercourse are common. The significance of these symptoms is magnified and the patient greatly distressed. Women with asthenic reaction often suffer from dysmenorrhea. Paresthesias and hypesthesias are common. The patient may suffer from broken sleep and disturbing dreams. In the morning he awakes with a feeling of exhaustion. As the day progresses the patient feels better and in the evening may be comparatively free from his sense of exhaustion. He complains of poor memory but this defect is a result only of preoccupation and lack of concentration. Many patients are shy, awkward, irritable, lack confidence and exhibit irresolution, indecision and irascibility. They are pessimistic and lack initiative and ambition. Not rarely asthenic patients are critical, whining, dissatisfied, envious and resentful. A tendency to projection is not uncommon. Some patients develop a complaining attitude and may appear to take pleasure in finding fault with and annoying others. Moderate depression is the rule. Varying degrees of anxiety are present.

It would appear as if the diffuse nervousness and sustained tension which result from deep-lying personal maladjustment and emotional cross-currents produce in the asthenic-reaction patient a subjective sense of weakness and exhaustion. An instability and irritability of the vegetative nervous system may occur with resulting disturbances in the vasomotor and cardiac functions. The concern that really belongs to emotional problems, frustrations and conflicts is transferred or displaced to an uneasiness of mind concerning physical organs and processes. Fatigue, perhaps, may be the equivalent of depression, and like depression, arise from weakening of repression, feelings of guilt and the frustration of satisfying personality objectives, or be the projection of a sense of inadequacy. The reaction is usually chronically monotonous in its course and the prognosis poor. Unlike many other psychophysiological autonomic and visceral disorders, the psychophysiologic asthenic reactions do not lead to long continued physiological disturbances and eventually to structural visceral changes.

DIAGNOSIS. The differential diagnosis of a psychophysiologic asthenic reaction from a psychoneurotic reaction is easy when the clinical picture is a typical one. There is a marked tendency, however, for mixed reactions. If much anxiety is obvious the case should be classified as an anxiety reaction. Sometimes the symptomatology of the asthenic reaction yields so much secondary gain that it is basically a conversion reaction. One of the most important differentiations to be made is to distinguish the asthenic reaction from the depressive form of manic-depressive psychosis. Many mild cases of this psychosis do not come to the attention of the psychiatrist and are considered by the general practitioner to be suffering from neurasthenia. Manic-depressive psychosis occurs in more definite episodes with intervals free from symptoms of mental disorder while the asthenic reaction is a more continuous, or at least prolonged, process, and the patient even when comparatively well is solicitous as to his health. The chief complaint of the neurasthenic is of weakness and shifting physical ailments which he is eager to discuss on every occasion, whereas that of the manic-depressive is depression. Although the neurasthenic is apparently depressed, his emotional manifestations and responses are well marked and even excessive, whereas the depression of the affective psychosis remains unchanged by experience or environment. Sometimes it is difficult to distinguish early schizophrenia from the asthenic reaction. The schizophrenic does not usually have so great a variety of physical complaints which sooner or later become obviously delusional. The neurasthenic lacks the listless apathy and the indifference to external circumstances usually manifested by the schizophrenic. The neurasthenic, unlike the schizophrenic, is not given to daydreaming.

Neurasthenic-like symptoms first manifested at middle age should arouse the suspicion of neurosyphilis. Experience suggests that some cases of chronic brucellosis have been diagnosed as neurasthenia. Thiamine deficiency may produce an asthenic reaction syndrome characterized by generalized feelings of weakness, fatigability, poor appetite, poor sleep, various somatic complaints and subjective difficulties in concentration and memory.

TREATMENT. The treatment of the asthenic reaction is, of course, psychotherapeutic. Usually encouraging results are limited to relatively early cases.

Psychophysiological Symptom versus *Conversion Hysteria*

Since both conversion hysteria and psychophysiological symptoms arise from emotional factors and both produce "functional" physical symptoms, it might be suggested that they are essentially the same psychodynamically and physiologically. This, however, is not at all the case. The psychophysiological symptom is produced by the fact that emotions may influence the autonomic nervous system with resulting stimulation or inhibition of the function of a visceral organ. It represents the disturbed physiological response of a vegetative organ to psychological stress and tension acting through the vegetative nervous system. Physiological changes are set up in an organ by autonomic nerve impulses generated as a result of emotional conflict or tension. The effects of the emotions are seen especially in secretion, vascularity and motility of viscera. In some cases the prolonged disturbance in the function of an organ may lead to structural changes which may threaten life. In *conversion hysteria*, the symptom is not produced through the vegetative nervous system but is the symbolic expression, either through the voluntary neuromuscular or through the sensory-perceptive systems, of emotionally charged psychological content. The reaction of these last two is not consciously voluntary and does not follow the traditional pattern of physiological responses in the body. Conversion hysteria is quite effective in alleviating anxiety, hence *la belle indifférence* is often associated with it. The secondary gain obtained by the psychosomatic patient from his symptom is either absent or less conspicuous than in the hysteric patient. Hysteria does not produce visceral changes. Basically the only similarity between hysterical symptoms and psychophysiologic symptoms lies in the fact that both are responses to psychological stimuli. Yet both hysteric symptomatology and psychophysiological disturbance may be observed in the same individual, particularly when the conversion response is removed through treatment or is only partially effective in allaying the anxiety consequent on conflict.

DIAGNOSTIC ERRORS. The patient who is reacting with psychophysiologic symptoms thinks that these constitute his illness and does not understand that the essential difficulties are his conflicts and anxieties and his inability to establish order, peace and security in his personal life. While the patient can scarcely be expected to recognize that mental or personality disorders may manifest themselves in terms of the soma yet the physician must not forget that organs may react to anxiety in many ways. Unless he remembers that psychogenic illness may masquerade under the guise of physical symptoms, also that mental illnesses are not ordinarily secondary to physical disease, he will inevitably make many errors in diagnosis and treatment. As Bennett[2] points out: "The sick man's personality must be judged along with the physical and laboratory data." Because much mental illness is either not recognized or is not treated properly, many maladjusted persons go from doctor to doctor and receive treatment that only aggravates their personality problems. If emotional disorders are misidentified or mistreated as organic diseases the tendency of such disorders will be not toward recovery but toward chronicity. If, too, some incidental organic pathologic condition is found the patient's anxiety is very apt to become fixed on the system involved. It should be remembered, also, that repeated tests and examinations tend to fix the idea in the patient's mind that he must certainly have a "physical" illness, probably a mysterious one. He will then even more resist the idea that emotions may have had any part in the production or perpetuation of his illness. Bennett found that 150 patients who finally came for psychiatric treatment had been diagnosed and treated for a deplorably large number and variety of organic diseases, most of which did not exist. The histories of these patients as a group revealed 496 medical treatments, 244 surgical procedures and 71 miscellaneous therapeutic attempts. Most of these patients were suffering from involutional melancholia or psychophysiological ailments. "After proper psychiatric therapy was instituted the percentage of complete and social recoveries was excellent." Except when symptoms are acute, surgery should be avoided in the neurotic person until emotional factors have been investigated.

Emotional Components of Physical Illness

The preceding part of this chapter has been devoted to a discussion of psychophysiological illnesses. Such illnesses may present a great variety of physical symptoms and complaints referable to the viscera through the action of emotional tension upon the vegetative nervous system. Broadly speaking, emotions may, in such disorders, be regarded as the cause of physical disturbance or distress. Conversely, in a general way, organic physical illness may be provocative of emotions that may greatly complicate the somatic disability. Mental and emotional factors may pathologically influence component organs of the body; disordered organs may induce mental and emotional factors that disturb the function or adjustment of the organism as a whole. Although not strictly relevant to psychophysiological disorders, the remainder of the chapter will deal with emotional factors and problems incident to physical illness. Their importance in medical practice is so great that an awareness of personality-illness relationship should be constantly in the physician's mind.

A knowledge of the personality and its development and structure affords a greater awareness of its role in illness. The manifestations of

---

[2] Bennett, A. E.: Faulty Management of Psychiatric Syndromes Simulating Organic Disease. J.A.M.A., *130:*1203, 1946.

a physical illness are frequently much colored by the patient's personality. Many persons who already have a well defined disease of chronic nature experience exacerbations or complications of it in relation to severe life stress. The course and outcome of the organic process may be greatly influenced by the mental attitude of the patient. Illness, therefore, of a clearly established physical nature is often attended by important psychological concomitants which, because of their importance both in prognosis and treatment, should be recognized by the physician. A patient suffering from serious and progressive physical disorder is very prone to develop some psychological response to it. Among such psychological responses may be repression, denial, or perhaps one of exaggeration of symptoms through a desire for pity and attention. At times the damage suffered by the emotional life and mental health of the patient through somatic illness or disability may be more serious and permanent than are the physical results of the organic lesion. It is therefore not only illness or disability in itself that is of psychiatric importance but also what a particular ailment means to a particular individual. This matter has been discussed earlier under the body image.

Many fears and exaggerations of the importance of disease arise from feelings of guilt, particularly from a sense of guilt concerning early sex activities or indiscretions. A slight indisposition may be attributed to a regretted lapse and be magnified into disabling or fatal illness and regarded as a just desert.

The attitude which the patient manifests toward his disability should be taken into consideration. The patient must adapt himself not only to his disability but also to the idea of his disability. Faced with physical disease the patient may readily accept or even suggest that his disability is of mental origin. He may neglect his symptoms or deceive himself as to their seriousness. On the other hand, the patient whose disability is of psychic origin seeks for a physical basis. Instances in which the patient consciously desires cure from a physical disability but unconsciously wishes that the symptom may continue are not uncommon. The patient sincerely believes that he desires to be cured but unconsciously clings to his disability with a tenacity that may defeat the physician's therapeutic efforts. The motives that delay the recovery may be various—self-punishment, self-importance, revenge or protest. For various psychological motives, too, certain patients may welcome or request surgical operations. With some patients surgery may be an attention-gaining device, with others a means of punishing themselves for feelings of guilt or of escaping responsibility or irksome drudgery. If psychic or emotional components accompany definite physical disease, a failure to treat them also will often tend to prolong convalescence or encourage a reaction of chronic invalidism. If the physician concentrates his attention on symptoms without an adequate attempt to ascertain or remove their causes he may aggravate or permanently fix them.

Factors arising from the patient's social environment or from interactions between the patient and his social setting may be important in the causation of illness and require consideration in its diagnosis and treatment. It is not always easy to determine if his symptoms are to be attributed entirely to his disease or in part or even largely to his personality disturbance or to his environment. A study of an unselected series of patients who consulted the outpatient clinic of a large general hospital showed that in 65 per cent of these patients there were adverse social conditions related to their illnesses. In 35 per cent of these cases there were emotional reactions which were largely responsible for their illnesses. The physician should remember that in the general hospital, conditions and situations may constantly arise which tend to produce various stresses and tensions and thereby promote unhealthy mental reactions or physical complaints, perhaps with visceral disturbance. Among them may be protracted convalescence, awareness of incurable or crippling disease, fear of death, conflicting medical statements or advice, the misinformation and misguided advice of other patients and other factors.

Every specialty is accompanied by procedures or situations heavily weighted with elements potentially disturbing to emotional life or personality. In ophthalmology, for example, the bandaging of both eyes during a prolonged convalescence in a darkened room may precipitate a panic reaction of a delirioid nature. In gynecology there may be problems connected with contraceptive practices, illegitimate pregnancy, or the occurrence of cystoscopy addiction. In urology psychiatric problems connected with impotence, frigidity, dyspareunia or premature ejaculations are common. It would be a happy combination if as much effort were expended in the psychological treatment of preoperative fear and apprehension as there is in the search for a drug to alleviate them. In surgical disorders a fear of mutilation or disfigurement or of loss of vital structure or capacity may threaten the patient's sense of security. While frequently this results merely in an apprehensive preoccupation, it may lead to anxiety, depression, mild panic states or to exaggerations of previous personality tendencies. In many other medical situations, too, the associated psychiatric problems may be more disturbing than the physical symptoms. It is essential that positive evidences of emotional difficulty be followed up just as faithfully as indications of physical damage.

Convalescence from a serious physical illness not rarely constitutes a psychiatric problem. The patient may be reluctant to give up the luxuries of the sick room and the unconscious secondary gain of illness. He may be resentful as the warmth of feeling and interest previously manifested by his family seem to lessen. More frequently the family may insist on continuing to be protective and the patient on being babied with the result that regressive personality characteristics persist. He may even create new symptoms as they are needed. The longer the patient defers his return to his responsibilities, the harder it is to come back and the more firmly are fixed any unwholesome personality reactions that have been established. His convalescence and rehabilitation may be largely dependent on his adjustment to an existing emotional problem.

Frequently the manifestations of the patient's illness are determined more by his personality characteristics than by the nature of the etiological agent producing the disease; he experiences his illness in accordance with his personality make-up and established types of reaction to stress. These patterns are brought particularly into the foreground in the case of chronic disabling illness. Some patients accept their handicap in a spirit of apathy and refuse to make any active effort to overcome their handicap. They may regress to a dependency pattern. In some instances the reaction may be one of depression and anxiety; again there may be a greater feeling of optimism and well-being than may rightly be expected. The patient may attempt to maintain a feeling of health by means of psychological mechanisms. If the patient feels that there is an implication of inferiority, abnormality or incurability associated with his disease he may, through brooding and resentment, develop various compensatory and defensive reactions, perhaps of an aggressive nature.

Among the psychological concomitants of chronic illness, the physician should remember the unwholesome effects that may result from the continued presence in the family of a member suffering from prolonged disability, particularly if the patient reacts to his disease with irritability, aggressiveness or some other unpleasant way, or if the responsibility for his care means the frustration of deeply cherished desires on the part of some other member. At times, too, chronic invalids suffer more from diseased family relationships that have grown out of the disability than from the disease itself.

Whatever the individual's physical disability may be, a certain amount of anxiety is added to the burden imposed by the disease or injury itself. The clinical picture may therefore be directly influenced by this anxiety and the particular reactions of the patient to it.

It is hoped that the discussion presented in this and previous chapters will lead the student to recognize that psychiatry should be integrated with medicine in all its branches and that artificial distinctions between body and mind should be obliterated. Man is a biological organism but one whose life expressions are determined not merely by physical, chemical, physiological and neurological factors but by mental, emotional and social ones. At times one group of factors, again another group, plays the more important role in the etiology, diagnosis, development and management of sickness. At no time can one group be disregarded; frequently a reciprocal relationship exists.

BIBLIOGRAPHY

Abramson, H. A., et al.: Psychodynamics and the Allergic Patient. St. Paul, Bruce Publishing Co., 1948.

Alexander, Franz: Psychosomatic Medicine. New York, W. W. Norton & Co., 1950.

Association for Research in Nervous and Mental Disease: The Interrelationship of Mind and Body. Baltimore, Williams & Wilkins Co., 1939.

Bartemeier, L. H.: The attitude of the physician. J.A.M.A., *145:*1122, 1951.

Bellak, Leopold: Psychology of Physical Illness. New York, Grune & Stratton, Inc., 1952.

Bibring, Grete: Psychiatry and medical practice in a general hospital. New England J. Med., *254:*366–372, 1956.

Binger, Carl: On so-called psychogenic influences in hypertension. Psychosom. Med., *13:*273, 1951.

Brosin, H. W.: The psychiatric aspects of obesity. J.A.M.A., *155:*1238–1239, 1954.

Brown, Jr., E. B.: Physiological effects of hyperventilation. Physiol. Rev., *233*:445–471, 1953.
Bruch, H.: The Importance of Overweight. New York, W. W. Norton & Co., 1957.
Burch, George, and Rey, Thorpe: Cardiovascular system as the effector organ in psychosomatic phenomena. J.A.M.A., *136*:1011, 1948.
Cannon, W. B.: Bodily Changes in Pain, Hunger, Fear and Rage, 2nd ed. New York, D. Appleton Century Co., 1929.
Carryer, H. M.: The role of hyperventilation in functional disorders. Proc. Mayo Clinic, *21*:361, 1946.
Cobb, Stanley: Emotions and Clinical Medicine. New York, W. W. Norton & Co., 1950.
Cohen, S. I., Silvermann, A. J., and Magnuson, F.: New psychophysiologic correlates in women with peptic ulcer. Am. J. Psychiat., *112*:1025–1026, 1956.
DaCosta, J. M.: On irritable heart: A clinical study of a form of functional cardiac disorder and its consequences. Am. J. Med., *61*:17, 1871.
Ebaugh, F. G.: Bodily reactions of anxiety. Postgrad. Med. *4*:208, 1948.
Friedman, A. P., et al.: Tension headache. J.A.M.A., *151*:174–177, 1952.
Grace, W. J., Wolf, Stewart, and Wolff, H. G.: The Human Colon: An Experimental Study Based on Fistulous Subjects. New York, Paul B. Hoeber, Inc., 1951.
Grinker, R. R.: Psychosomatic Research. New York, W. W. Norton & Co., 1953.
———, and Robbins, E. P.: Psychosomatic Case Book. The Blakiston Co., Inc., New York, 1954.
Gull, W. W.: Anorexia nervosa. Lancet, *2*:171, 1868.
Halliday, J. L.: Psychosocial Medicine. New York, W. W. Norton & Co., 1948.
Hinsie, L. E.: The Person in the Body. New York, W. W. Norton & Co., 1945.
Kaplan, Harold I., and Kaplan, Helen S.: The psychosomatic approach in medicine. Ann. Int. Med., *46*:1063–1078, 1957.
———: The psychosomatic aspects of obesity. J. Nerv. & Ment. Dis., *125*:181–201, 1957.
Karush, A., and Daniels, G. E.: Ulcerative colitis. Psychosom. Med., *15*:140–167, 1953.
Kay, O. W. K., and Leigh, Denis: The natural history, treatment and prognosis of anorexia nervosa. J. Ment. Sc., *100*:411–431, 1954.
Kolb, L. C.: The Painful Phantom. Springfield, Illinois, Charles C Thomas, 1954.
Kroger, W. S., and Freed, S. C.: Psychosomatic Gynecology. Philadelphia, W. B. Saunders Co., 1951.
Kubie, L. S.: The central representation of the symbolic process in relation to psychosomatic disorders. Psychosom. Med., 15:*1*–7, 1953.
Lidz, Theodore: Principles and Techniques of Therapy in Psychosomatic Disorders. In Proceedings of Association for Research in Nervous and Mental Disease, Vol. XXXI, pp. 156–159. Baltimore, Williams & Wilkins Co., 1953.
MacLean, P. D.: Psychosomatic disease and the "visceral brain." Psychosom. Med., *11*:338–353, 1949.
Menzer, Doris: The importance of the psychologic factors in gynecology. New England J. Med., *249*:519–522, 1953.
Miles, H. H. W., and Cobb, Stanley: Neurocirculatory asthenia, anxiety and neurosis. New England J. Med., *245*:711, 1951.
Miller, M. H.: The borderline psychotic patient: The importance of diagnosis in medical and surgical practice. Ann. Int. Med., *46*:736–743, 1957.
Problems of Hypertension: Panel Discussion. J. Am. Psychoanalytic Assn., *1*:562, 1953.
Prout, Curtis, T.: Psychiatric aspects of asthma. Psychiatric Quart., *25*:237, 1951.
Rosenbaum, Milton; Reiser, M. F., and Higgins, John: Setting Goals of Treatment in Psychosomatic Medicine. In Proceedings of Association for Research in Nervous and Mental Disease, Vol. XXXI, pp. 160–166. Baltimore, Williams and Wilkins Co., 1953.
Ruesch, Jurgen: Chronic Disease and Psychologic Invalidism. New York, Paul B. Hoeber, 1951.
———, and Bowman, K. M.: Personality and chronic illness. J.A.M.A., *136*:851, 1948.
Saul, L. J.: Psychosomatic aspects of peptic ulcer. Samiksa, *7*:225–235, 1953.
Selye, Hans, and Fortier, Claude: Adaptive Reactions to Stress in Life. In Life, Stress

and Bodily Disease, Proc. Assn. Res. Nerv. & Ment. Dis., Vol. XXIX. Baltimore, Williams & Wilkins Co., 1950.

Sneddon, I. B.: The mind and the skin. Brit. M. J., *4602*:472, 1949.

Squier, R., and Dunbar, F.: Emotional factors in the course of pregnancy. Psychosom. Med., *8*:161, 1946.

Stearns, Samuel: Some emotional aspects of the treatment of diabetes mellitus and the role of the physician. New England J. Med., *249*:471–476, 1953.

Sullivan, A. J., and McKell, T. E.: Personality in Peptic Ulcer. Springfield, Illinois, Charles C Thomas, 1950.

Tegner, William, et al.: Psychogenic rheumatism. Brit. M. J., *4620*:201, 1949.

Wall, J. H.: Anorexia nervosa. Bull. New York Acad. Med., *32*:116–126, 1956.

Weiss, Edward: Emotional Factors in Cardiovascular Disease. Springfield, Illinois, Charles C Thomas, 1951.

———, and English, O. S.: Psychosomatic Medicine, 3rd ed. Philadelphia, W. B. Saunders Co., 1957.

Wheeler, E. O., White, Paul D., et al: Neurocirculatory asthenia. J.A.M.A., *142*:878, 1950.

Wittkower, E., and Cleghorn, R. A.: Recent Developments in Psychosomatic Medicine. Philadelphia, J. B. Lippincott Co., 1954.

Wolff, H. G.: Life Stress and Bodily Disease–A Formulation. Chapter LXIX in Life Stress and Bodily Disease, Proc. Assn. Res. Nerv. & Ment. Dis. Baltimore, Williams & Wilkins Co., 1950.

Ziskind, Eugene: Psychophysiologic Medicine. Philadelphia, Lea & Febiger, 1954.

CHAPTER XXX

Psychoneurotic Disorders

General Considerations

The psychoneuroses comprise a relatively benign group of personality disturbances which are often described as being intermediate, or as forming a connecting link, between the various adaptive devices unconsciously utilized by the average mind on the one hand and the extreme, often disorganizing, methods observed in the psychotic on the other. Hysteria, for example, is often but an exaggeration or caricature of comparable protective mechanisms observed in everyday life.

Psychoneurotic personality disorders arise from an effort to deal with specific, private, internal psychological problems and stressful situations that the patient is unable to master without tension or disturbing psychological devices caused by the anxiety aroused. Many psychiatrists, therefore, regard anxiety as the common dynamic source of the neuroses. The symptoms of these disorders consist either of a manifestation of anxiety as it is directly felt and expressed or of automatic efforts to control it by such defenses as conversion, dissociation, displacement, phobia formation or repetitive thoughts and acts. Ordinarily repression, frequently aided by socially acceptable and useful reaction-formations, enables the individual to deal comfortably with feelings and situations that tend to create anxiety. In the psychoneuroses, however, repression is never complete enough to prevent both the feeling and manifestation of anxiety and the formation of unconscious, repetitive techniques designed to control it. These feelings and manifestations of anxiety or the methods of adaptation (defenses) to it constitute the symptoms of the neurosis. The methods of adaptation utilized by those with a psychoneurosis, in addition to their repetitive and unchanging character, are considered to represent behavioral, affective or psychological traits that proved satisfying at an earlier stage of development. In short they represent either a regression to an earlier, more gratifying type of behavior, or a failure to develop beyond a fixation at a developmental level which proves inappropriate and inadequate in the face of the responsibilities of later life. Neurotic adaptations are never fully satisfying since secondarily they lead to feelings of inadequacy, shame and guilt. In the psychoneuroses, therefore, the symptomatic clinical phenomena are usually not significant in and of themselves but merely indicate that anxiety-producing, meaningful situations are perturbing to the individual. Although symptoms observed in the psychoneuroses will be described in this chapter yet these mental disorders should be studied from a functional rather than from a symptomatic standpoint. Many times, it is true, the symptom may afford a clue to the nature of the underlying problem but the understanding of a neurosis depends on a recognition of the unconscious, neurotic purpose it serves.

The form of the neurosis is determined largely by the type of the defensive measure the patient employs to control anxiety. Relatively few patients confine themselves to a single type of measure. Many psychoneurotics, therefore, show mixed features. The patient's symptoms represent his defense reaction to an anxiety-producing situation which he finds unmanageable by other means. Regardless of the form which they may assume, it is now realized that the neurotic patient's symptoms are intelligible only in psychological, or rather psychobiological, terms. The relationship between his emotional conflicts and perturbing situations, on the one hand, and his disturbed personality functioning on the other is not recognized by the patient. For example, he may, without any apparent reason and without ideational content, develop an attack of anxiety, or without apparent reason develop a panic-like reaction in a crowd or in an open place. Again without any recognition of its face-saving function the patient may develop an invalidism that provides escape from a difficult situation. Another patient may experience the persistent recurrence of an appalling or disgusting thought, or feel an overpowering urge for the repeated, ritualistic-like performance of some act that serves to ward off anxiety. Aggressive, hostile wishes may become so threatening that the patient has to employ some neurotic mechanism for handling them. These defenses are often so ego-hampering that they are quite burdensome to the patient. Many persons presenting a variety of symptoms and known to the laity by such terms as "nervous invalids" are really suffering from psychoneurotic disorders. The term "nervous" is, of course, a euphemistic and evasive term since there is in fact no physiological disturbance of the nervous system. Each case is a problem of emotional dynamics.

Psychoneuroses versus *Psychoses*

For a long time psychiatrists have placed much emphasis on a supposed distinction between psychoses and psychoneuroses. Countless hours have been spent at clinical conferences in discussions as to whether the diagnosis in a particular case should be psychosis or psychoneurosis. If, for purposes of the present discussion, one disregards those mental disorders caused by or associated with impairment of brain tissue function, then the remaining ones are regarded as disorders of psychogenic origin (or without clearly defined physical cause or structural change in the brain). It is increasingly accepted that not only do such disorders as the psychoneuroses but also schizophrenia, manic-depressive psychosis, involutional psychosis and the various paranoid states belong among those in which psychodynamic factors are largely or solely operative. To a constantly greater extent it is felt by psychiatrists that there are no such differences in the fundamental nature of psychogenic disorders as to warrant the present rigid and meticulous distinction between psychoses and psychoneuroses. Many agree with Bowman[1] that the distinction is without scientific proof and has been based on rough descriptive differences in symptomatology, also that precise and universally accepted definitions of the two terms have never been established. There is an unbroken line of continuity from the "normal" through the neurosis to the psychosis.

While it is doubtful if there is any scientific basis for the distinction between "psychoses" and "psychoneuroses," yet classifications of symptom complexes that have become so well established must contain some value. The value in this distinction has been largely legal, social and administrative and based arbitrarily on symptomatology. Since differences in symptomatology readily conduce to the establishment of diagnostic categories, the distinction has also been of value as a teaching aid. The matter of classification, too, may be of importance in selecting the type of therapy.

Many criteria have been suggested to differentiate between psychoses and psychoneuroses. The great variations in those proposed suggest, as Bowman points out, that the distinction is not basic but superficial. Some psychiatrists have designated the psychoses as "major reactions" and the psychoneuroses as "minor reactions," the distinction being made on the extent of the involvement of the personality. Other psychiatrists look upon psychoneurosis and psychosis as successive stages in the same mental process.

While it must probably be conceded that there is very little scientific basis for the distinction between the psychoneuroses and other psychogenic mental disorders, there is nevertheless a sufficient difference in their clinical nature to justify the distinction on pragmatic grounds. In general the diagnosis of psychosis implies a greater severity of personality disturbance than in psychoneuroses. The psychoneurotic's defenses against anxiety are largely substitutive or symbolic; the psychotic's defenses are more extreme, regressive, and disregardful of reality. In many instances there is a difference in their outcome as regards the integrity of the personality. In the psychoses the distortion or disorganization of personality is often great and its social functioning is greatly disturbed, whereas in the psychoneuroses the personality usually remains socially organized. In the psychoneuroses inner experiences do not upset external behavior to the extent or in the abnormal manner that occurs in the psychoses. In the psychotic individual, the capacity for discriminat-

[1] Bowman, Karl M., and Rose, Milton: A criticism of the terms "psychosis," "psychoneurosis," and "neurosis." Am. J. Psychiat., 108:161–166, 1951.

ing between subjective experiences and reality may be greatly impaired. In the psychoneurotic individual, there is no grave interference with reality-testing; that part of the personality which the analysts speak of as the ego remains sound. Any evasion of reality is partial and at comparatively little expense to the personality. "Neurosis does not deny the existence of reality, it merely tries to ignore it; psychosis denies it and tries to substitute something else for it."[2]

The psychotic creates a new environment to which he imputes the forces and properties of reality. He may distort or falsify reality in the form of delusions or hallucinations. The environment of the psychoneurotic remains unchanged although certain elements may be invested with abnormal affective values. The thinking of the psychotic may be dereistic, a type of thinking not occurring in the psychoneurotic. The content of thought in the psychoneurotic may be temporarily restricted by overvalued ideas yet true delusional formation does not occur. Associations are frequently disturbed in the psychotic but remain unimpaired in the psychoneurotic. Desires and motives are often projected in the psychotic, but never so externalized in the psychoneurotic, at least not to the extent of producing delusions. In the psychotic repression may be destroyed, the ego being so changed that it will tolerate repressed impulses or fantasies uncritically, or will fail to recognize that they arise from itself. In the psychoneuroses repression appears to be maintained but nevertheless the repressed material returns, although in such a distorted form that it is acceptable to the ego. Conation may be profoundly disturbed in the psychotic, but only to a slight degree does it suffer in the psychoneuroses. In the psychotic the changes in affect may be great and affective lability is often decreased, while the psychoneurotic affective changes are slight and lability is maintained. Any depression in the psychoneuroses is determined more by evident environmental factors than is the case in psychoses and is accompanied by a greater degree of insight and by an absence of retardation. The psychoneurotic usually retains well his interest in the outer world and, as Devine points out, he retains his "herd sense" and remains sensitive to changes in the social atmosphere; the interest of the psychotic may be lost. The psychoneurotic conforms more nearly to the social norm in his relationships, while the regression of the psychotic may be extreme but it is not an important mechanism in the psychoneurotic who never, if consciousness is clear, regresses to an infantile level with its excretory soiling. Generally speaking, the psychotic does not recognize that he is ill and therefore has no desire for change in his subjective status. The psychoneurotic, on the contrary, usually feels keenly his subjective suffering and consciously wants to get well, although it is known that his more powerful unconscious desire is to the contrary. The psychoneurotic, especially the hysteric, often exploits his symptom for secondary gain whereas the psychotic patient acquires no secondary gain from his illness. Finally, as already stressed, there is no sharp line between the

[2] Freud, S.: The Loss of Reality in Neurosis and Psychosis. Collected Papers, II, p. 278. New York, 1924.

psychoneuroses and the major psychoses. They merge one into the other by intermediate, scarcely perceptible stages. The differences are largely descriptive and ones of degree. Given psychogenic factors may in one individual lead to defenses and reactions characterized as psychoneurotic and in another person to those classified as psychotic. Not rarely a reaction which would be classified as neurotic will later assume a form descriptively classified as psychotic. This does not mean that one type of mental illness is being superseded by another form fundamentally different in nature. It is, in fact, the opinion of some psychiatrists that if the life history of a patient suffering from a psychosis not associated with toxic or organic factors is fully known, evidence will always be found of an untreated or inadequately treated pre-existing neurosis out of which the psychosis grew. In the so-called borderline cases both neurotic and psychotic mechanisms may be noted.

Classification of Psychoneurotic Disorders

The Standard Nomenclature adopted by the American Psychiatric Association classifies the psychoneurotic disorders as follows:

1. Anxiety reaction
2. Dissociative reaction
3. Conversion reaction
4. Phobic reaction
5. Obsessive compulsive reaction
6. Depressive reaction

The so-called "types" are not disease entities in genesis, mechanisms or manifestations. Rather should the psychoneuroses be regarded as a series of varying types of reaction brought about by multiple causative factors which vary from case to case. The more carefully the reactions of the neurotic are examined the more frequently it will be found that there are no sharply defined lines among the various types of neuroses. It is rare, for example, to find a "pure" hysteria or "pure" obsessional neurosis. Frequently the neurotic will, in varying degrees, show hysterical, obsessional, anxiety and even psychosomatic manifestations. Clinically a given case will often show such a confusion of symptoms that its definite assignment to a certain type may be difficult or arbitrary. Overt anxiety, for example, although the most conspicuous and characteristic symptom in anxiety states, is frequently an important picture in other forms. Also, just as there is no sharply defined distinction between the psychoneuroses and the psychoses, so there is none between the psychoneuroses and many character traits of the so-called "normal" person. Far more frequently than is realized, outstanding character traits are really neurotic reaction-formations that serve as defenses. Neurotic syndromes fit into the personality pattern of the individual and are allied to the techniques he has employed all his life in handling situations. As will be pointed out in the following paragraph there is an increasing tendency, not to classify the psychoneurotic states into distinct and definite types, but to divide them clinically according to the nature of the principal mechanism the patient employs as a means of defense or compromise. In conversion reaction (conversion hysteria), for example, the repressed impulse producing the anxiety is "converted" into functional symptoms involving voluntary musculature or special sense organs. In phobic reactions (phobia), the anxiety is handled by detaching it from some specific idea or situation and displacing it in the form of a neurotic fear of some object or situation which serves as a symbol of the idea or situation which had originally given rise to the anxiety. The various forms or mechanisms of anxiety-relieving devices will be discussed as different psychoneurotic reactions are discussed.

Causes

When we seek for the causes of the psychoneuroses we must conclude that emotional, meaningful factors play a predominant and, in a broad sense, perhaps an exclusive role. Usually from early life the psychoneurotic has shown personality traits which are so deeply rooted in the make-up of the individual that some psychiatrists refer to them as constitutional. Probably, however, these traits are not inherited but are acquired early in life during impressionable years through close association with and dependence upon various members of the family. There is an increasing belief that most major neurotic patterns are basically dependent on conflicts and feeling attitudes that arose in childhood and that to understand a patient's neurosis an attempt should be made to connect the patient's present symptoms with some unliquidated childhood situation. There seem to be good reasons for believing that in many instances that is true. One will therefore agree with Freud's statement that the analyst deals more with scars than with bleeding wounds. Presumably this is not always true, yet we not rarely find that the childhood of the psychoneurotic was characterized by such disturbances as sleep walking, crying out in sleep, enuresis, disturbances of speech, food idiosyncrasies, delirium accompanying slight rises in temperature, destructiveness, emotional excitability, temper tantrums, phobias, compulsions, shyness, nail-biting and other disguises looked upon as constituting personality and behavior problems. Probably these manifestations should be regarded as evidence that specific conflicts and situational factors have always produced anxiety and led to neurotic symptoms or character traits. It is necessary, however, not only to examine the childhood background for scars which the special circumstances of early life have left but to be alert for feelings of guilt, conflicts over unconscious needs, meaningful life-events, recurrent, cumulative stresses and tensions of interpersonal relationship difficulties and for the everyday stresses of family living including marital or sexual problems. It is also important not to consider immediate reality factors as always being fundamental etiological ones rather than precipitating causes. Not rarely it will be found that an apparently smooth adjustment has been a cover for stormy problems that have long existed beneath the surface.

Whatever determined their personalities there seem to be individuals who are unusually sensitive to tension and conflicts of life, persons who have never really faced its problems and are especially prone to deal with its tensions, wishes and conflicts by the faulty reactions we designate as neurotic symptoms. While the efficiency of most persons is impaired by psychoneurotic tendencies, yet much of the best work of the world is done as an expression of neurotic illness. This has been particularly true in the case of art and literature.

Of the immediate causes for the development of the psychoneurosis it may be said they are frequently to be found in the necessity to repress, distort or displace emotions of hostility or rage, or the drives of sexuality and dependency as they emerge and conflict with order and peace in the patient's personality. These and similar factors, often of a conflict-producing nature, create *anxiety* which is the commonest and most important source of psychoneurotic disorders. Anxiety, engendered by a too severe and exacting super-ego but perhaps stimulated by an external situation, mobilizes the defenses of the personality. As already indicated, the manner in which the patient adapts to this anxiety, which is sometimes characterized as the most unpleasant of subjective emotional states, and tries to mobilize the defenses of the personality against it, determines the type of the psychoneurotic reaction. If the anxiety is felt and expressed directly, is "free floating," and is not confined to definite situations or objects, the neurosis is spoken of as an anxiety state or anxiety neurosis. If the repressed wish or impulse causing the anxiety is "converted" into functional symptoms in organs or parts of the body, the clinical picture is that of conversion hysteria. If the anxiety overwhelms and temporarily controls the individual the clinical picture is that of hysterical dissociation as in hysterical stupor, fugue or amnesia. In compulsion neurosis, the patient controls his anxiety by a repetitive activity. This activity or ritual protects the patient against the threat of repressed impulses. In phobias, anxiety is controlled by detaching it from some idea or situation and by displacement attaching the fear to some specific object or situation that serves as a symbol. As already said, many neurotics exhibit mixed features with hysterical, obsessional, anxiety and psychosomatic manifestations. One should not too readily accept a suggestion that a single factor in the make-up, environment or experience of an individual produces his neurotic personality or psychoneurosis. Rather the neurosis is the result of a "constellation" of factors which in combination one with another tend to create the neurotic pattern. Even though the more obvious evidences of maladjustment may lie in apparently impersonal fields, it will often be found on close examination that the significant factors in the origin of the psychoneurosis lay in subtle, conflictful attitudes and relations with key figures in the child's environment rather than in a single traumatic childhood experience.

The psychoneuroses are more frequent in women than in men, partly because of the fact that a more rigid repression of basic biological needs and instincts is required of women with the result that anxiety defenses in the form of neurotic symptoms are more frequently required than in men. The psychosexual life with its many taboos and social restrictions is by no means, however, the only factor since any fundamental urge or desire against the expression of which a defensive barrier must be constructed, or the gratification of which must be vicarious, may give rise to neurotic symptoms. Feelings of guilt, social situations or irritating relationships that strain the ability to adjust, or marriage with its new responsibilities are examples of the many factors that may contribute to a neurosis. In a married woman a chronic marital dissatisfaction and disappointment may contribute to the development of a psychoneurosis. The husband may not have proved to be the ideal mate that was expected, desired demonstrations of affection may have been lacking, or marriage have failed to be the sustained romance that she had dreamed it would be. The wife may deny any dissatisfaction which may be consciously acknowledged only if she frankly faces her feelings. Other women, interested in a business or professional career, or hesitant to exhibit any interest in, or behavior toward, the opposite sex that would lead to marriage, may put it off until they reach an age when opportunities for marriage are infrequent. The sense of frustration and of a certain emptiness of life may lead to a neurotic reaction. Again the involutional period with its reluctantly acknowledged psychological implications may be accompanied by an anxiety, depression or irritability that is readily converted into functional symptoms.

At times a psychoneurosis may develop as an indirect result of long continued physical illness. In such a case the prolonged and perhaps severe illness may threaten the patient's sense of security, compel him to give up activities and interests that have been highly prized or may jeopardize his ability to function at his previous level. Such factors may stimulate an anxiety that had previously been handled without difficulty.

Most neuroses of adults develop between late adolescence and thirty-five years of age. This is the period when the individual becomes confronted with the problems of adult adjustments and responsibilities. It is the period when satisfying social, economic and sexual situations should be established. Frustrations in these critically important fields may lead to conflict, anxiety and tension that can be met only by neurotic mechanisms.

Elaborate disguises, including fears, which have no obvious connections with immediate realities and make the neurotic's behavior more or less incomprehensible both to himself and others are among the conspicuous features of neurotic behavior. A rational explanation for the apparently unintelligible behavior will be found, however, when its psychodynamics is studied. It will be observed, too, that neurotic syndromes tend to fit into the established personality pattern of the individual and are allied to the techniques he has employed all his life in handling difficult situations.

In some psychoneurotic reactions, particularly in anxiety states, the patient often fears the existence of some serious physical disease whereas the causes of the symptoms are in fact purely psychogenic. In such cases the patient will usually not accept the psychiatrist's assurance of good physical health unless the physician has first made such a painstaking physical examination and has shown such openmindedness and true interest concerning the possible existence of physical disease as will make the patient willing to accept the physician's statement that he has no organic basis for the symptoms. It should be emphasized, however, that a diagnosis of psychoneurosis cannot be made merely by the exclusion of organic factors. It can be made only on the discovery of positive factors in the psychological sphere sufficiently pertinent to offer a logical explanation for the symptoms. This evidence is to be found in a study of the patient's personality aimed both at an analysis of the present picture and at a reconstruction of the sequences of psychological experiences that have influenced personality development and structure. It will frequently be found that as time passes a neurosis becomes more complex and irradiates into more aspects of life.

Anxiety Reactions

As previously indicated, anxiety may be described as a painful uneasiness of mind, a state of heightened tension accompanied by an inexpressible dread, a feeling of apprehensive expectation. It may arise under any situation that constitutes a threat to the personality. The emergence of repressed material is particularly apt to be anxiety-producing. Anxiety may arise, for example, when self-requirements and the security of the personality are threatened through the fact that the repression of forbidden sexual desires or dependency strivings to ward off loneliness or of unconscious hostile and aggressive feelings is in danger of giving way. Again, anxiety with its obsessive apprehensiveness may arise in association with frustrations or dilemmas occurring in some major life problem related to such topics as vocational, sex or marital adjustment.

In the other psychoneurotic reactions some specific, auxiliary form of psychological defense mechanism is devised to control anxiety. In anxiety reactions, however, there is no such specific method of defense. Repression alone is insufficient to control the anxiety. As a result the anxiety, not being displaced as in phobic reactions, not being "converted" into functional symptoms as in hysteria, not being discharged by some gross personality disorganization such as dissociation, fugue or amnesia, and not being automatically controlled by some repetitive thought or act, remains diffuse and uncontrolled with the result that the patient is in a state of constant anxious expectation. Anxiety reaction is therefore sometimes spoken of as the simplest form of neurosis.

If the diffuse anxiety is not too painful, it may be expressed or controlled through certain personality traits. Individuals who are constantly beset by pervading anxiety are characteristically tense, timid, apprehensive, sensitive to the opinions of others, easily embarrassed and tend to worry. Many persons with such a constant sense of anxiety are self-distant, given to inferiority feelings, experience difficulty in making decisions and are afraid of making mistakes. Usually they are scrupulous, overconscientious, ambitious and feel that they must live up to self-imposed high standards. While such a person suffers moderate distress through apprehension and other tendencies previously noted, yet the tension is not usually intolerable. If, however, the anxiety becomes more disturbing it may be expressed in such symptoms as depression, sleeplessness, irritability, restlessness, a paralyzing indecision, psychosomatic disturbances, outbursts of aggressiveness, attacks of weeping and feelings of inadequacy and inferiority accompanied, perhaps, by a paranoid attitude. Usually the patient with an anxiety reaction feels chronically fatigued and complains of inability to concentrate. Some express the fear that they are "becoming insane."

Anxiety Attacks

In addition to a chronic state of tension and mild anxiety, the patient with anxiety neurosis may be subject to acute, terrifying, panic-like exacerbations lasting from a few moments to an hour. In these acute attacks there is an overstimulation of the autonomic nervous system. The patient suffers therefore from rapid heart, palpitation, precordial discomfort, nausea, diarrhea, desire to urinate, dyspnea and a feeling of choking or suffocation. The pupils are dilated, the face is flushed, the skin perspires, the patient suffers from paresthesias, tremulousness, feels dizzy or faint, and often has a sense of weakness and of impending death. Restlessness is acute and the patient may express beseeching and apprehensive appeals. In Chapter XXIX the psychophysiological mechanism of hyperventilation is described; this is the mechanism that causes these symptoms in perhaps the majority of acute anxiety attacks. Other physiological expressions of acute anxiety perhaps occur through activation of various segments of the autonomic nervous system and the adrenal medulla and its secretions. In an acute reactive anxiety attack, the clinical picture may be colored by a traumatic situation. This is well illustrated in the anxiety attacks of combat neurosis.

The patient who is subject to acute anxiety attacks usually suffers also from a chronic anxiety state. He experiences difficulty in falling asleep, is disturbed by fearful dreams, suffers from coarse tremors or "trembling" and complains of a "band around the head" or of a "quivering in the stomach." He is absentminded and seems worried without knowing about what or why. He complains that his mind is in a constant daze and that he is unable to control his thoughts. He is apprehensive, is afraid to be alone yet does not desire conversation. He feels too tired to attempt anything constructive and continually seeks a physical explanation for his distressing mental state.

Physicians lacking an appreciation of psychological factors in the production of symptoms have at times erred in not recognizing that anxiety attacks are psychological, not physiological, disturbances and have diagnosed them as heart disease, thyrotoxicosis, neurocirculatory asthenia, hyperinsulinism or dysinsulinism.

Treatment

Two phases of an anxiety reaction require attention—one the acute anxiety attack, the other the anxiety neurosis. During the attack the rapid pulse and pounding heart lead the patient to believe that only a heart attack could have produced his distress. After an examination of the heart and other organs has been made and no physical disorder discovered the patient should be confidently assured that he has no heart disease. Frequently the cause of the symptoms may be demonstrated easily by the simple medium of requesting the patient to overbreathe for a period of two minutes as described in Chapter XXIX under the hyperventilation syndrome. Further somatic complaints should be disregarded and the examination of the heart not repeated. Usually a sedative drug should not be given, nor should the patient be advised to call a physician during the attack. The patient should not, through the use of drugs, be led to believe that his pathologic condition is physical rather than emotional, and rest should not be advised nor should personal reassurance be repeated to a degree that the patient constantly feels the need for it.

Treatment of the basic neurosis is psychotherapeutic and requires that attention be directed to an uncovering of the unrecognized sources of anxiety, to the action of psychodynamic factors, to their adjustment and to re-education. Less attention should be paid to the anxiety attacks than to a study of the patient's personality and to attitudes and situations that cause frustration and tension. While a more formal analysis is desirable in severe anxiety neuroses, many milder cases can be helped by a psychotherapy on the conscious level and by a face-to-face discussion. Consideration will be given to the meaning of symptoms, the role of emotions, the stress of present circumstances and the effect of well remembered past experience in molding present attitudes and habits of thinking and feeling. The demonstration of a correlation between the time when anxiety appeared and certain preceding events in the patient's life history may give insight sufficient to produce considerable relief. A desire to violate self-imposed rigid standards may at times be discovered. Troublesome sex problems including any arising from faulty contraceptive technique should be adjusted. The patient should be encouraged to continue physical exercise and recreation. If chronic tension states and associated muscular pains occur in neck and shoulders, physiotherapy is helpful. Meprobamate, the various phenothiazines and the barbiturates may be used to provide symptomatic relief from the chronic symptoms of anxiety. In marked anxiety and tension states, subcoma insulin therapy may be of value. Prolonged and permanently disabling anxiety states may be benefited by prefrontal lobotomy if all other measures have failed.

The anxiety reactions are most frequently associated with phobic defenses that are often overlooked in originally describing the anxiety neuroses. Untreated, the phobic anxiety state may extend with either the development of obsessive ideation and disappearance of the acute anxiety reactions or progressive withdrawal associated with phobic diffusion that leads to a state of helpless isolation simulating a psychotic regression.

A 27-year-old woman entered the hospital complaining of multiple fears. She was too frightened to get on streetcars or buses, to go to the movies, and to go out to supper. She was also afraid that she would not live up to the expectations of her mother, was dubious about her own capabilities, and indicated that her marriage was in difficult straits and that she had previously been separated from her husband for a period of eighteen months. She stated that their only son was a bed wetter. In addition she presented the symptoms of acute anxiety with palpitation, perspiration, dizziness, and shortness of breath caused by the hyperventilation syndrome.

Brief questioning elicited the information that her mother had been a nagging, sadistic person, who unmercifully switched the patient and her brother whenever they failed to obey her command. The father, a mild, subservient individual, had seldom been at home. The patient was a quiet and obedient, though fearful, child, usually timid and retiring, who felt that she must always acquiesce to the wishes of others or be subject to their criticism and withdrawal of affection.

The diagnosis in this case was long standing anxiety neurosis, associated with the hyperventilation syndrome and a phobic state. The anxiety attacks occurred regularly in situations in which the patient's husband or mother or even the doctor did something or said something to arouse her anger. She could not allow herself to express her anger, as she feared that this would lead to further criticism and rejections. Although the majority of anxiety attacks were relieved after several months of psychiatric treatment, she was not entirely free of her symptoms of dizziness and palpitation and of her phobias until a year of regular visits had elapsed.

Freud delineated in detail the physical symptoms of anxiety and their intimate association with phobias. Since anxiety and phobic reactions are so frequently associated, the latter are brought to discussion for clinical reasons at this point.

Phobic Reaction

A phobic reaction is a defensive one in which the patient attempts to deal with his anxiety by detaching it from a specific idea, object or situation in his daily life and displacing it to some symbolic idea, object, or situation in the form of a specific neurotic fear. Although the patient consciously recognizes that no actual danger exists, yet if exposed to the specific phobia-stimulating, symbolic object or situation he is powerless to prevent experiencing an intense sense of fear. The intensely distressing sense of apprehension associated with the consciously feared object or situation is actually derived from other sources—sources of which the patient is unaware. A defense against the anxiety arising from his unrecognized source is provided through the mechanisms of displacement and symbolization. By these means, the anxiety is detached from its real source —unconscious, forbidden tendencies and impulses, for example—and displaced to some situation or object which is usually symbolic of the threatening tendency or wish. A great variety of phobias has been described. Among them are fear of dirt, of bacteria, of certain animals, of travel by a certain type of vehicle, etc. Many of them have Greek names attached to them, as agoraphobia, a fear of open places or claustrophobia, a fear of confined spaces. A claustrophobia might, for example, prevent the occupancy of a Pullman berth. When exposed to the specific situation which evokes his fear the phobic experiences faintness, fatigue, palpitation, perspiration, nausea and tremor. He may be unable to continue with the duty at hand and be overwhelmed with panic. He can control his anxiety if he avoids the phobic object or situation. If the patient were to carry out a phobic activity, it would unconsciously mean to him that he was performing the forbidden activity which arouses the dreaded anxiety. He also constantly punishes himself for his unconscious tendencies and impulses by the distressing restrictions and sufferings imposed by his phobia. Phobias are twice as common among women as among men.

Dissociative Reaction

At times anxiety may so overwhelm and disorganize the personality that certain aspects or functions of it become dissociated from each other. In some instances the personality may be so disorganized that defense mechanisms govern consciousness, memory and temporarily even the total individual, with little or no participation on the part of the conscious personality. In such a case the patient may at times appear psychotic. Formerly the dissociative reactions were classified as a type of conversion hysteria.

One of the commonest anxiety-stimulated and defensive dissociative reactions is *amnesia*. Forgetting is a simple expedient. It is therefore not surprising that amnesias obliterate recollections, particularly for definitely circumscribed periods of time. Dissociative amnesia, is however, not a mere forgetting. It is an active process, a blotting out of awareness of unpleasant features. Periods of stupor or of twilight state may precede such an amnesia which then tends to become selective and limited to the particular element or experience which evoked it. Among experiences that suspend the ability to bring pertinent factual data to consciousness are those involving great terror, as in war, or covering periods and behavior with which shame, guilt, or other intense feeling-tone is connected. How satisfactorily an amnesia exercises its protective and escape purpose is shown by the unperturbed manner in which the patient accepts his loss of memory. While most dissociative amnesias are of brief duration, they sometimes blot out long periods, sometimes even the patient's entire previous life. In some instances there is a reversion to an earlier period of the patient's life, with retrograde amnesia for events subsequent to that period. In differentiating between an organic and a dissociative amnesia it will be found that a sudden return of memory is indicative of its dissociative loss. The onset, also, of the dissociative amnesia will have been sudden.

Dissociative reactions are at times characterized by mental symptoms involving *disturbances of consciousness*. These may be in the form of stupor or of various forms of "twilight state." Frequently the latter suggests delirium. Such psychogenic delirious states are usually preceded by marked emotional experiences or displays and consist of dream states accompanied by more or less confusion, dramatic posturings and activities and an excessive flow of speech appearing nonsensical, but in which occur references to strongly affective experiences. Dissociative delirium often represents the dreamlike realization of a wish or the dramatic reliving in fantasy of an affectively traumatic experience. Its clouding of consciousness, illusions and hallucinations may exclude the reality of the outside world and falsify it in accordance with deep-seated motives and unsatisfied wishes. Occasionally the patient spins fantastic stories. Such instances usually represent an effort to supply romance and drama to a life devoid of emotional satisfactions.

At times a psychic escape may be in the form of a dissociative *fugue* in which there is a sudden change in state of consciousness during which the patient may be impelled by unconscious forces to perform complicated activities, perhaps involving travel over long distances. Throughout this period the patient may appear quite normal to the casual observer. In some instances there is a loss of personal identity. In the fugue the patient indulges in acts of fantasies which are in conflict with his superego and the function of the fugue is to permit the carrying out of these acts or fantasies. A further defense mechanism becomes necessary, however, so the patient attempts to protect his ego by forgetting his name and past history; that is, by losing his identity. In other instances there is not a loss but a change in personal identity. In such a case the patient assumes a false name and identifies himself with the person whose name he takes. The assumption of the false name is associated with the unconscious fantasies responsible for the genesis of the fugue. O. Henry has presented a delightful picture picture of a dissociative fugue in his misnamed short story "A Case of Aphasia." As Fisher[3] points out, the psychological formula is as if the patient says, "I did not commit this crime, because I am not I; I am somebody else."

After the termination of the fugue the patient may have a complete amnesia for his journey until the memory of it is restored by hypnosis or other psychic means. Examination of the patient either by Sodium Amytal narcosis or by other means of ascertaining subconscious mental content will usually reveal the personal, emotional factors which prompted an escape mechanism in the form of an automatic, unconscious, uncontrollable withdrawal. In certain recent studies, it has been found that the fugue state is preceded by depression and may be regarded as an attempt to ward off this affect. The model for a number of fugue states apparently has been supplied by a previous head injury with a resulting amnesia or amnesic states induced through alcohol or identification with others who suffered dissociative reactions.

Ganser Syndrome

The Ganser syndrome with its combination of instinctive, rational, purposeful and deceptive elements and theatrical behavior is an alteration of consciousness allied both to simulation and to dissociative dream states. In this syndome, occurring largely among prisoners under detention awaiting trial, the patient, being in a situation which would be solved or mitigated by irresponsibility, desires, although not consciously so acknowledged, to appear irresponsible, and accordingly without being aware of it actually does develop mental disturbance. The conspicuous features of this disorder consist of a childish, ludicrous performance of simple acts with the correct manner of performing which the patient has been fully familiar. The patient's responses to questions are wrong but

[3] Fisher, Charles: Amnesic states in war neuroses. The psychogenesis of fugues. Psychoanalytic Quart, *14*:460, 1945.

are not far wrong and bear an obvious relation to the question. His replies show that he understood the meaning of the questions but they are beside the point and are in the nature of approximate answers—a phenomenon known as paralogia, or "Vorbeireden." The purpose of the patient's behavior is so obviously to appear irresponsible that he may seem to be malingering. Since the circumstances under which the Ganser syndrome occurs are such that the advantages to be gained by a mental disability are greater than by physical disorders, the reaction takes place in terms of the former rather than of conversion hysteria. As in other dissociative reactions the protection from a full realization of his situation affords the patient a relative freedom from the anxiety which might otherwise be intolerable.

At times dissociation may suggest a schizophrenic reaction. Usually a dissociative reaction is of more sudden onset and is preceded by more conscious or felt anxiety. The pre-illness types of personality are not similar.

Conversion Reactions

The term "conversion reaction" is synonymous with "conversion hysteria," the name by which it is better known. Because of the striking and dramatic manifestations that may accompany this reaction it was the first of the psychoneuroses to receive attention. In a conversion reaction anxiety, instead of being consciously experienced, either diffusely as in anxiety reactions, or displaced as in phobias, is "converted" into functional symptoms in organs or parts of the body innervated by the sensorimotor nervous system. The conversion symptoms serve to prevent or lessen any conscious, felt anxiety and usually symbolize the underlying mental conflict which is productive of anxiety. The reaction usually meets some need of the patient and therefore not merely serves as a defense against anxiety but also provides some more or less obvious "secondary gain," a phenomenon to be discussed later in the chapter. Viewed a little differently, the hysterical symptoms may be regarded as expressing a conflict or an idea in symbolic form. It may, for example, "convert" a mental concept into a significant body symptom, as when a hysterical paralysis of an arm expresses a wish to do a forbidden act, yet ambivalently prevents its accomplishment. The form of the conversion symptom is determined by some feature of the situation it was designed to meet.

If a person were consciously to counterfeit some physical sign or symptom or some mental disturbance for the purpose of attaining a particular objective we would say that he was *malingering*. Conscious recognition of its intent is not necessary, however, in order that behavior may be purposive. In conversion hysteria the symptoms, without awareness on part of the patient, provide some form and extent of solution for his problems and afford him a certain relief from the anxiety involved in the perturbing situation. Nature's methods are not of a sharply defined and delimited character but form imperceptibly graded series, so there are found all degrees of awareness and many types of reaction between simulation, consciously adopted to solve some clearly defined external difficulty of which the individual is clearly aware, and hysteria in which to satisfy unrecognized inner needs similar reactions take place without conscious participation. Some hysterical phenomena are on the borderline between psychoneurotic reactions and simulation and therefore come close to malingering. Just where, as to awareness, the line between simulation and hysteria should be drawn is therefore often arbitrary. In both there is a subtle interweaving of conscious factors. Both are related to some definite purpose, usually protective or wish-fulfilling in nature. It is not surprising that the difference in the hysteric's mind between reality and fantasy is often vague.

Causes

The immediate factor in the production of hysteria is some anxiety-producing situation. With the frequent exception of the traumatic hysterias, we find that the hysterias of civil life tend to develop on a certain personality background characterized by immaturity in the psychosexual and emotional fields. Puberty is a favorite period for the appearance of hysteria. What may be called the normal psychic characteristics of that period will often be found persisting in the mental life of the adult hysteric. Maturing drives, for example, may remain in an arrested or infantile state of development, a state to which a failure to attain an emotional independence from a parent sometimes contributes. Impulses, sentiments and other bases of the personality are not integrated into a harmonious system. Some hysterics, with their immature personality development, are basically hostile and aggressive persons.

Kretschmer divides persons of the infantile, psychobiologically inhibited, hysterical character into two groups. In the first group he places persons of normal intellectual development but whose other psychic characteristics, particularly the emotional ones, are of an immature, pubertal type. They are childishly egocentric, selfish, vain, like to be the center of attention, take pleasure in exhibiting their virtues, are oversensitive, irritable, petulant, exhibit emotional capriciousness, moodiness, histrionic poses and pathos, and fleeting enthusiasms which often represent identifications.

In the second group of persons of hysterical personality Kretschmer places those whom he characterizes as having a stunted psyche. These persons are inferior, immature, emotionally indifferent, shy, fearful, excitable, of rather inferior intelligence and because of their primitive and impulsive reactions may become social defectives, criminals and prostitutes. The grosser varieties of hysteria are more common in these persons of inferior make-up than in those of better endowment.

Kretschmer's suggestion as to the genesis of hysterical symptoms is of theoretical interest. After the initial formation of symptoms there is, in his belief, a period when conscious volition and interference could be effective but after that deeper lying automatic mechanisms take over. These become unconscious and put the process of symptom formation beyond the range of volition of the patient.

In ordinary civil life wishes, struggles and disappointments associated with the sex life form, especially in women, one of the most important groups of experiences that produce the major forms of hysteria. The sexual impulse, although often active, may fail to develop toward a natural goal and be gratified in fantasy and autoerotic habits. A confused admixture of sexual desire and aversion, of erotic feelings and prudish attitudes often exists. Erotic fantasies often contrast with conscious expressions of fear and disgust in regard to sexuality. Among the sex problems which in women may give rise to hysteria are an unsuccessful love affair; jealousy, perhaps arising from the marriage of a sister; an undesired marriage; fear of pregnancy; difficulties in intercourse or an unhappy marriage. Not a few are sexually frigid.

The developmental histories of such women make evident the sources for the disordered psychosexuality. In contrast to the earlier concept that the disorder resulted from disturbances in the Oedipal period, it often commences in the initial maternal relationship. In many instances the mother, hysterical herself, has been rejecting, arousing in the child retaliatory fantasies which have been repressed. The mother often has been recognized as hypocritical about sex, dependent herself and subtly clinging to the child for whom she has special ambitions. The father of such patients is inadequate, either repressing this through alcoholism or passivity and usually derogated by the mother. Yet the child, rejected herself, envies the father or male siblings whom she considers receive preferential treatment from the mother. Fixed to the mother, yet envying the father and brothers, she displays early tomboyishness, enuresis, difficulty with menstruation and later difficulty in acceptance of the feminine role which is shown in frigidity, vomiting in pregnancy or by hostile seductiveness with men in which the hysterical symptoms symbolically express her conflicts and confusion in regard to her sexual identifications.

In men, threats to self-esteem, to economic success or to self-preservation more frequently present situations from which escape is sought through the hysterical symptoms. Many men are of immature personality with a strong, dependent attachment to a mother. Striking forms of hysterical reactions, such as functional incapacities and symptoms with histrionic features, occur largely among young people. Such hysterical states rarely occur during or after middle age by which time more permanent and less dramatic protective mechanisms have been established.

Frequently the factor or event which precipitated a conversion reaction may have been trivial but have had some special meaning to the patient. Sometimes the precipitating situation may have some special similarity to a previous occurrence. It is therefore well to ascertain what the setting was at the time of appearance of the conversion reaction, also what the patient's emotional state was at the time. The nature of the earlier experiences that give special meaning to the precipitating event and the patient's predisposition to respond with selective conversion mechanism may usually only be determined by psychoanalysis although much recall may emerge in hypnotic or narcosynthetic states.

Oversolicitude by the mother following minor painful experience may establish the predisposition to obtain gratification, in the face of conflict, by means of painful complaining in later life. Envious observation of the attention given to another sibling or home member sometimes arouses fantasies of suffering that are repressed until the later conflictful period and then aroused as a substitute means of allaying anxiety. Of most importance are the childhood experiences of pain that lead to masochistic suffering in order to obtain gratifying affectional responses. In some instances parents suffer guilt on punishing the child for misdeeds and then lavish affection following punishment as a means of assuaging their own anxiety. If this is the means by which the patient as a child repetitively obtained emotional satisfaction, a pattern for later masochistic pain and suffering is estabished. Another method, described by Freud, has to do with the guilt suffered by a child after secretly enjoying the punishment offered an envied brother or sister. To assuage this guilt he must then suffer some distress. In all these instances the basic issue is the wish for the affection and acceptance by the parent or parental substitute. With the masochistic expression, pain or distress must be expressed in order to obtain the wished for affection and acceptance denied in reality.

Symptoms

While reference has already been made to the type of individual who seems predisposed to hysteria, further mention may be made of some of the personality characteristics frequently observed in the hysteric. It will often be found that evasions and mechanisms of retreat have been habitual since early life. The narcissism which tends to characterize her arrested personality development gives her a proneness to self-display which is often expressed in childish and dramatic ways. Persons of hysterical type of personality desire an immediate gratification of their wishes but avoid effort to gain their goal. They are self-engrossed, offended by trifles and dependent in attitude; they bid for sympathy and attention and are given to suicidal "gestures." Such acts are without intent to die. The threat or shock of the apparent attempt is used by the hysteric to control her environment, to gain attention, to arouse sympathy or to frighten others into submission. Many seek to rule their environment by being sick, pitiful and appealing. Such persons exaggerate any existing physical symptoms and even precipitately develop those of a critical or unique nature. Attention-getting, secondary-gain complaints are common. Craig called attention to the fact that hysterics with their immature personalities, rarely react with awe, reverence, wonder or pity; that they may exhibit self-depreciation, remorse or grief but if so it is because those emotions are the ones that gain them the greatest attention or best obtain a desired domination over their environment. Her childish egocentricity and inner fantasy poorly fit the hysteric for adult reality.

Hysterical patients are notoriously suggestible and their symptoms tend to follow the fashion of their particular period. One now rarely sees the dramatic posturings that were common in Charcot's clinic or the astasia-abasia of Victorian women. They are frequently, however, imitations of actions or disabilities either seen or read about. If a hysterical patient, confronted with some difficult and unpleasant situation, observes the successful evasion of a similar situation by another person he may develop the same symptoms as a means of escape. Such imitations of symptoms were so frequent in World War I and II that attempts were made to isolate from the observation of his associates the soldier who had escaped combat service through his hysterical disability.

The nature of the hysterical symptoms is often determined by some need or feature of the situation that produced them, by the type of disability that will be most useful in satisfying the subconscious purpose they are designed to meet. As a rule the more turbulent the emotional undercurrents and the greater the disturbance of strong impulsive strivings, the more acute and striking the manifestations, and the greater the evidence of anxiety.

Physical Disturbances

Physical symptoms may be sensory or motor. *Sensory symptoms,* like other physical disturbances, are usually those of functional incapacity. Among the more frequent are anesthesias, paresthesias and disturbance of special sense organs, such as blindness or deafness. Hysterical anesthesia does not follow the distribution of a nerve, but involves an extremity up to a sharply defined line above which sensation is normal. It does not follow the actual distribution of the nerve but what the patient believes it to be, what is represented in the patient's mind as a functional unit. One half of the body may be anesthetic, in which case the special senses—hearing, smell, taste and sight—may be lost on the same side. Hysterical anesthesia may be extended in area by the suggestive and repetitious procedure of the physician in examination. Anesthesia probably cannot be produced *de novo* by the physician's examination although this was believed by Babinski. The area and degree of the anesthesia may vary from one examination to another. Hysterical disturbances of vision are of various forms, the most frequent ones being blindness and narrowing of the visual fields. Hysterical blindness usually has a sudden onset. The pupils continue to react to light and usually, but not always, the patient avoids objects which would injure him if he came into collision with them. The onset is usually either closely related to some distressing visual experience or has a fairly obvious symbolic relation and significance.

The *motor disturbances* in hysteria are various. In all of them function is disturbed without demonstrable physiological or anatomical change. Paralyses may be in the form of monoplegia, hemiplegia or paraplegia and may be either flaccid or spastic. The deep reflexes are not lost in flaccid forms; they may be exaggerated in the spastic forms but there will be no true clonus and no Babinski reaction. In hemiplegia the paralysis of the proximal muscles is greater than of the peripheral, being in this respect the contrary of that existing in organic hemiplegia. The forearm will be extended instead of being somewhat flexed as in organic hemiplegia; the leg will be dragged instead of being swung in circumduction. There is no appreciable wasting of the paralyzed extremities. The maintenance of normal electrical reactions in flaccid paralysis is diagnostic, as is an absence of bladder symptoms or of tendency to bedsores in paraplegia. Contractures are not uncommon. A fairly frequent form is that of a tightly clenched fist. In hysterical paralyses the muscles in question may be used in one voluntary movement and not in another. An attempt to exercise the paralyzed function is accompanied by a display of excessive effort. Tics, tremors, usually coarse in nature, and choreiform and clonic movements occur. Aphonia, in which the patient cannot phonate speech but continues to cough as formerly, is not rare. While in aphonia the patient finds no difficulty in communicating in whispers, the patient with hysterical mutism can utter no word although he communicates freely and correctly in writing–a point of differentiation from aphasia. One patient who developed hysterical mutism in prison dreamed that the institution for mental diseases to which he had been transferred was on fire, whereupon he screamed and thereafter talked normally. The occupational neuroses, such as writer's cramp, usually belong among hysterical reactions. The hysterical tic consists of a spasmodic, co-ordinated twitching movement of a small group of functionally related muscles. It may take the form of twitching of the facial muscles, blinking of the lids, sudden turning of the head or a gesturelike movement of the hands. Such tics may represent dramatization of psychic experiences. Because of the suggestion of defense which they manifest, they may appear purposive. Care must be taken not to confuse hysterical tics with the more complex, co-ordinated ticlike movements observed after epidemic encephalitis and certain other organic diseases of the brain.

Painful complaints are often hysterical in nature and may sometimes be of hallucinatory nature. This conversion symptom is perhaps the commonest expression of the illness at the current time and is frequently misdiagnosed and mistreated. As with other hysterical symptoms, the patient presents a bizarre or unusual account of the symptoms that is not easily recognizable as a result of the usual physical illnesses, or he may exaggerate the pain of a relatively minor physical disturbance. In spite of his insistence on the severity and disabling nature of the symptom and his demands for medication and care, he may be observed frequently to appear indifferent and undisturbed by the symptom. Placebos may relieve the symptom. There is often an intermittent history of its occurrence and exacerbations may be found related to incidents arousing emotional conflict. In taking the history many hysterical patients, apparently indifferent to the symptom, may be induced to complain at the point where the psychiatrist touches upon the emotionally disturbing relationship or incidents in his life. If the psychiatrist is easily dissuaded from the task of history taking in an effort to provide immediate relief of a sudden complaint of pain offered by the patient during the interview, a valuable opportunity and significant clue pertaining to the emotional connotation of the symptom will be missed. Reintroduction of the anxiety-ridden topics or associated themes often gives rise again to painful complaining. The arousal of painful complaining may be regarded as perhaps hallucinatory. It may occur in the course of psychoanalysis when the patient associates pertinent information symbolizing the conflicting needs that underlie the symptom.

Organic Factors and Conversion Reactions

The existence of organic symptoms does not exclude the presence of conversion ones also. Symptoms of organic disease that still exist may be exaggerated or symptoms may persist after the organic basis for them no longer continues. In such cases, the symptoms produced by the disease were found to serve some psychological purpose, to be of value in themselves. Because of their usefulness in providing protection, escape or advantage, they are unconsciously exaggerated or prolonged. Hysterical symptoms of this nature occur particularly in industrial, insurance and traumatic neuroses but are by no means confined to them, since there are many situations in which physical symptoms may serve some useful function. At times the organic disease may impose sufficient additional stress so that emotional problems can no longer be dealt with in a realistic manner. Exhaustion, whether a result of fatigue or of anxiety resulting from prolonged indecision or from emotional conflict, may predispose to a hysterical retreat from a situation which would otherwise have been met with ease. The person already having some organic disease will often, if his situation does not demand some other special symptom, select one related to the organic disorder with which he is already familiar. The organic symptoms may merge imperceptibly into the hysterical one.

Psychopathology of Conversion Reactions

It is not surprising that theories formulated to account for the etiology and nature of a personality disturbance that may manifest itself in symptoms apparently purely physical in nature should be various. As would be expected, these theories have been influenced by the concepts which have prevailed during different periods relative to natural phenomena in general, and human behavior in particular; thus, the teaching of Hippocrates that hysteria is caused by the wandering of the uterus through the body in search of humidity, the belief of the seventeenth century that its striking manifestations seen in that period were a result of witchcraft or demoniacal possession, and the conviction now generally accepted that it is an adjustmental technique to which the personality may resort.

Among those who have contributed most to our understanding of conversion and of dissociative reactions are Charcot, Janet, Bernheim, Babinski, Morton Prince and Freud. Although his point of view was entirely neurological, Charcot was the first to demonstrate that the dramatic manifestations of hysteria could be produced and allayed by hypnotic suggestion. He thus demonstrated that psychological influences could affect bodily mechanisms, although with his lack of aptitude for psychological investigation he assumed that a hereditary degeneration was an essential prerequisite for hypnotic or hysterical phenomena. His discovery did, however, lay the foundation for investigative work by others.

Janet, a pupil of Charcot, in an attempt to account for the phenomena of hysteria, developed the concepts of dissociation, the subconscious, and psychological tension. Janet, it will be remembered, believed that the integration of the organism, whether considered from the standpoint of consciousness or of function, depends upon an energy which he called psychic tension. If this hypothetical psychic tension is adequate, there is a unity of the personality with a synthesis of consciousness and of functional processes. If, however, there is a weakness in this tension or energy, caused particularly, Janet believed, by emotional shocks and traumatic memories, there is a lowering in the level of psychological performance and certain mental processes go on in the subconscious independently of (dissociated from) the main stream of consciousness. According to this view, hysteria would be considered a defect, a negative process, rather than a dynamic, purposeful one.

Bernheim emphasized the importance of suggestion and expressed the opinion that all hysterical symptoms were the result of suggestion. Babinski also believed that in the hysteric there is a particular susceptibility to stimuli which therefore are peculiarly potent in inhibiting or dissociating mental processes. He added the opinion that not only could all hysterical phenomena be produced by suggestion but could be removed by persuasion.

It is now universally agreed that conversion hysteria and dissociative reactions are of psychogenic origin. The greatest influence in creating this point of view is to be found in the contributions of Freud although many psychiatrists prefer modifications of his assumptions. Most psychogenic theories as to the nature of conversion hysteria go back to the concepts of conflict and of repression. According to Freud, the wish or other repressed material, although not permitted frank expression, obtains it in disguised form through the mechanism of conversion by which the psychic conflict is transformed into a physical or mental symptom. Freud explained the hysterical symptoms as caused by a conflict between the superego and some wish which because of its consciously objectionable nature is repressed by the superego. This repression is not, however, entirely successful and the wish therefore obtains disguised expression by its "conversion" or transformation into the symptom. The nature and localization of the symptom thus produced will be such as will symbolize or provide disguised expression of the repressed wish and at the same time provide some degree of its fulfillment or of relief from the emotional conflict. Many psychiatrists who accept the role of repression in the production of the hysterical symptom hesitate to accept Freud's belief that a repressed Oedipus complex is an essential condition for the development of hysteria.

At the present time the most widely accepted explanation of the mechanism known as conversion is that impulses and unadjusted, repressed elements in the personality, highly charged with instinctive and emotional components, are productive of anxiety. The anxiety is then mitigated or dispelled by being "converted" into functional symptoms manifested in the voluntary musculature or in special sense organ systems. The exact process involved in this "conversion" is uncertain.

In conversion hysteria we find an excellent illustration of both primary or neurotic gain and of secondary gain. The conversion mechanism yields a primary or neurotic gain through its anxiety-defense function. It also yields a secondary gain by producing something to the advantage of the patient. A hysterical paralysis, for example, may enable one to evade some situation which he feels incapable of mastering.

Expressed a little differently, hysteria may be defined as a phenomenon in which tensions generated on the level of psychological experience find expression through disturbances of functions of organs innervated by the somatomuscular or somatosensory apparatus. In Chapter XXIX attention was called to the hypothesis that in psychosomatic or psychophysiologic disorders such tensions are expressed largely in disturbance of function or organs innervated not by the sensori-motor nervous system but by the autonomic system.

The manner in which conversion or the transformation of an anxiety-producing emotional conflict into a specific symptom that alleviated the anxiety produced by the patient's conflicting desires and at the same time yielded a secondary gain that enabled the patient to escape from an extremely unpleasant situation is illustrated by the following case:

M., a young man who had been a dancer and acrobat in a circus, enlisted in the army long after World War I. Here he found the discipline rigid, his duties irksome and his experiences monotonous. He longed for travel, excitement, attention, and opportunity for exhibition enjoyed in his former life. The situation became quite intolerable, but to leave meant that he would be treated as a deserter. A hysterical conversion reaction, induced by two conflicting motives, the one to conform to the requirements of military life, the other to secure escape from a hated situation, provided a solution which permitted him to gain his own end, to obtain immunity from unpleasant experiences and tasks, and at the same time alleviated his anxiety and enabled him to maintain his self-respect. On arrival at the mental hospital to which he was transferred he could neither walk nor stand, and his legs were anesthetic to even vigorous prickings by a pin. At the same time he displayed a significant attitude of unconcern (*la belle indifférence*) as to his disabilities although as far as he was consciously aware they were complete and incurable. His absence of concern is to be explained by the fact that the penalty was less than the gain, although one must not conclude that this weighing of advantages and disadvantages was at all a matter of conscious reflection. A few months later the man was discharged from the army on a surgeon's certificate of disability. Soon the suspended motor and sensory functions began to return. Persistent efforts to walk met gradually with success and in another three months he left the hospital practically well.

In the case of this soldier it can be seen how a psychological mechanism "converted" the anxiety stemming from his repressed wish for release from military service into an overt and incapacitating symptom which, however, yielded a definite secondary gain.

The hysterical conversion reaction may provide the patient with a defense against anxiety, enable him to maintain his self-respect and at the same time accomplish some purpose the achievement of which respect for self would otherwise have forbidden. It may make possible an escape from an intolerable situation, it may afford an exoneration for oneself, an excuse for one's failures, enable one to evade some duty, shun a responsibility, express some spite, serve as an attention-getting device, or realize some purpose which would not bear the scrutiny of consciousness. Hysteria has its analogue in many acts of everyday life when many psychological processes considered normal take place without full consciousness of their methods and motives, particularly if there is some reason for hiding the truth from oneself. The hysteric is always desirous never to disclose to himself the real nature of his illness, an effort which is successful since the conscious personality has no access to the cause of the illness. Universal, too, is the tendency to project one's difficulties upon something tangible. Similarly any physical basis for an explanation of the symptom is welcomed and assigned an important place.

In connection with conversion reactions such as the one cited, it should be kept in mind that several factors usually play a role in determining the specific nature of the neurotic reaction. This concurrence and integration of adaptive functions unconsciously served by the symptoms is known as *overdetermination.* Through this process a single symptom or neurotic reaction may be a complex compromise-formation to the production of which several needs have simultaneously and unconsciously contributed. If an overdeterminative process is analyzed, it will be found that in many neuroses there are anxiety-relieving values which have been produced by the symptom together with further advantages that the patient secondarily derives from his illness once it has been established. Two or more birds are killed with one stone, so to speak. As already indicated, these two sets of values derived from the neurosis are the primary and the secondary ones. The primary gain is the defense against anxiety supplied by the symptom. The secondary gain is a material advantage which is contributed by the symptom. In the case of the soldier just mentioned, the conversion symptom (hysterical paralysis) relieved him from the anxiety incident to his ambivalent wishes. It also afforded what was to him a very important secondary gain: it rendered him unable to perform military services and therefore made his discharge necessary. Conversion reactions usually meet some immediate need of the patient and are therefore associated with more less obvious "secondary gain." The secondary gain is not always material but may be emotional or social, *e.g.*, the extraction of love, sympathy or consideration from other people. Usually the element of "secondary gain" secured from the disturbing conversion symptoms seen daily in the general practice of medicine is less apparent than in the case of the soldier. Frequently, in fact, when symptoms of anxiety are also present, the element of secondary gain may be slight.

In the case of the soldier, comment was made concerning the attitude of unconcern manifested toward his disability. This satisfied indifference and pathological tranquility of mild, characterized by Janet as *la belle indifférence*, is of diagnostic significance in a conversion reaction, representing as it does the characteristic use of denial as a means of defense. The conflict having been solved and anxiety having been relieved through conversion of the repressed impulses and wishes into a functional symptom, an outward calm follows even though the symptom produced be so disabling that it would presumably be a source of great concern.

Accident or Compensation Neurosis

Industrial accidents in which a question of indemnification for a real or presumed disability may arise are frequently followed by a definite psychoneurotic reaction. The presenting features of these reactions may be those of anxiety, hypochondriasis, conversion or of mixed types. Frequently the conversion symptoms are sufficiently prominent so that compensation neuroses are often classified among the hysterias. It was formerly considered that a desire for what the patient considered adequate compensation was the principal if not exclusive factor in the production of neuroses following industrial accidents. In recent years closer studies of the patient's personality have shown that other factors also are usually dynamically important. Persons of a paranoid tendency, those who are insecure and those who crave sympathy and attention are predisposed to compensation neurosis. The same is true of the individual who finds himself in an employment situation that is becoming progressively more unbearable. The necessity, because of financial obligations, for continuing work beyond mental or physical capacity, or the failure to derive satisfaction from one's work may predispose to a traumatic or compensation neurosis. Some incidental gain resulting from an injury, such as escape from dreary or wearisome conditions of employment, may be important contributing factors. Oversolicitude on part of the patient's family or an injudicious remark by the physician in the first days or weeks after an injury concerning its severity may create fear in the mind of the patient and predispose to the development of a neurosis. Experience connected with bodily helplessness, disturbance of business resulting from the accident, or worry about cure may conduce to its development. Not only a desire for financial gain but the conviction on part of the patient that he has the right to expect indemnification may be motivating factors. Social custom and public opinion tend to encourage the development of accident neuroses by their attitude toward the question of responsibility. The probability of developing a compensation neurosis following a relatively slight injury is greater than if the injury is so disabling as to be obviously compensative. Mild traumatic residuals may become heavily overlaid with hysterical elaborations. The traumatic or accident neuroses rarely occur when the victim of the injury must bear the brunt of the financial responsibility for the accident, as in the case of injuries sustained in sports. There is usually an incubation period between the injury and the appearance of the mentally determined symptoms. This interval before the development of the chronic disabilities is of value in excluding an organic source. It is usually occupied with vague ruminations which tend to be of an imaginative, affective, resentful, wish-determined and suggestive nature.

Symptoms of Accident Neuroses. The symptoms of the accident neuroses are various but these neuroses differ in no essential feature from others except in the matter of compensation. Frequently the symptoms include irritability, stubbornness, argumentativeness, crying spells, anxiety, depression, sleeplessness, headache and dizziness. The patient is garrulous in describing his symptoms and may complain of poor memory and inability to concentrate. If the foreman, "company doctor," or insurance adjuster questions the genuineness of his symptoms or the validity of his claim that the injury was sustained while at work, the patient frequently reacts with an indignation and resentment that aggravates and prolongs his symptoms. The fact that a hysterical reaction may be superimposed on an organic injury that has escaped attention should not be forgotten. Sometimes the neurotic symptoms do not become seriously troublesome until after the patient has returned to his employment, when they become so aggravated that he gives up work. Tremors, paralyses and other motor and sensory conversion symptoms occur. At times the necessary form of treatment for the original injury may be instrumental in suggesting a disability in a person of a hysterical type. Immobilization by splints of an injured extremity, for example, may be followed by its paralysis. As in other psychoneuroses, symptoms may be firmly fixed by overexamination or by overtreatment based on wrong premises. The development of symptoms through suggestion is, of course, in no way limited to accident neuroses involving the matter of compensation. A repetition of physical examinations may aggravate symptoms when organic disease exists and produce them when no disease exists. The fact that the physician's words and acts may have a suggestive effect upon the patient imposes a special responsibility upon him. In those cases in which indemnification is a participating motive the patient remains unaware of such an influence and denies that he desires compensation, declaring that he would gladly forego any financial satisfaction could he be restored to health. He complains of his symptoms but he rarely asks how he may get rid of them. Underlying feelings of guilt may be overcompensated and experienced as self-pity.

Workmen's compensation acts and industrial accident insurance have greatly increased the incidence of compensation neuroses. The effect on the worker of the general practice of awarding compensation for injury is to create a receptive mental state so that when injury occurs there follows an unconscious wishing for compensation. This does not at all mean that a worker who, following an industrial accident, complains of symptoms without organic basis is a malingerer or that compensation is not merited. The disability, it is true, would not have occurred had the results of the injury not possessed potential benefits in some form. The misfortune was that the injury in the "damage-suit" hysteria occurred in a person who was psychologically predisposed to a neurotic reaction. The existence of litigation tends to maintain the patient's focus on his injury, particularly if legal processes are prolonged. Contrary, however, to a frequent belief the end of litigation does not always terminate the symptoms promptly. A termination does usually, however, have a salutary effect on the symptoms by removing one factor that has tended to keep the patient's attention focused on himself.

Mention should be made of the *occupation neuroses*, a large proportion of which, particularly those characterized by spasms, are to be looked upon as hysterical. In these neuroses the patient on attempting to execute some specialized movement in an occupation requiring the co-ordination of groups of muscles suffers from a spasm of the muscles involved in this act. Their function remains unimpaired when an attempt is made to employ the same muscles for the performance of some other act.

Diagnosis of Conversion Reactions

Except for differentiation from the other neurotic reactions, features of which it often shares, hysteria is to be differentiated from organic disorders, malingering, schizophrenia, and from somatization or psycho-somatization reactions. A conversion reaction may in certain respects simulate an astonishing variety of organic symptoms, in making a differentiation from which certain principles should be held in mind. One should, of course, ascertain if sensory and motor disturbances are consistent with known anatomical facts. Conversion symptoms often change from time to time and with suggestion. Reflex and trophic disturbances do not accompany hysterical disturbances aside from the changes that may come from chronic disuse following a paralysis. Before deciding that a physical sign or somatically expressed symptom is of psychogenic origin, one should carefully attempt to ascertain if a setting of affective dissatisfaction existed before the appearance of the sign or symptom. The patient's attitude of satisfied indifference toward his disability and the circumstances under which the disorder arose are often significant. The coincidence or immediate sequence of an acute emotional state and the appearance of physical phenomena are suggestive, especially if the connection between psychological event and the sign is unrecognized by the patient. In actual physical disease the patient readily accepts or even suggests the statement that his disability is of mental origin. On the other hand, the patient whose disability is psychogenic eagerly seeks for a physical basis. Both, of course, are really attempting to hide the truth. It is always well for the physician to ask himself if the signs and symptoms serve a purpose in the life of the patient (secondary gain) and not let the apparent loss or suffering exclude hysteria from consideration. In making the diagnosis of conversion hysteria, too, one should not rely solely on the presence of conversion symptoms but should also consider whether the patient is an emotionally immature type of person. It must be remembered, too, that organic disability and a conversion reaction are not mutually exclusive. Organic neurological disabilities are not rarely complicated by superimposed conversion phenomena.

The confusion of a conversion reaction with malingering is most apt to be made by persons who consider all hysterics as malingerers and mistakenly believe that the hysteric could control his symptom if he wanted to. Discrepancies, contradictions and exaggerations of symptoms are more frequent in malingering; also, the malingerer usually expresses much concern about his symptoms. In the classical form of major conversion hysteria, the patient manifests little concern about them. Because, however, of the considerable component of anxiety often accompanying a recently established conversion reaction, the patient may show signs of concern. Surprise examinations or observation of which the patient is unaware may reveal the deception in malingering. Malingering and conversion reactions have much in common. The difference is largely one of the relative degree in which consciousness participates in the reaction. In malingering there is a subtle interweaving of conscious and unconscious factors.

Since there may be reactions in schizophrenia strongly resembling hysteria, the diagnosis is not always easy. The native temperament of the patient may be somewhat indicative, that of the hysteric person having been characterized by more easily shifting emotions. In hysteria a dominant affect usually exists, there are no inconsistencies in symptoms and no disturbance of associations, there is a greater response to any emotional reaction on the part of nurse or relative and there is no deterioration in habits of dress or cleanliness. In hysteria there is an apparent desire to be the center of attention and it will usually be found that either parent or mate has been accustomed to exhibit a sympathetic and exaggerated emotional reaction to any illness on the part of the patient. Here, the aid of the clinical psychologist may be most helpful, particularly as the usual diagnostic interviewing with the hysterical patient is distorted through his unwitting use of denial and the force of repression.

Attention was called in Chapter XXIX to the fact that conversion reactions should be distinguished from psychophysiological reactions in which tension and anxiety arising from psychological conflicts and emotional stresses are allayed, not by channelizing them through voluntary muscular and special sense systems (conversion) but through the vegetative nervous system into visceral organ symptoms and complaints. Yet many patients show combinations of both varieties of reaction.

Prognosis

The degree to which conversion mechanisms can be eliminated depends to a considerable degree on the extent to which evasions become habitual in early life and on the maturity and independence of the personality pattern. The prognosis depends, too, upon the strength or weakness of the patient's personality resources in relation to the environmental demands and to the other stresses which he will be called upon to face. If the patient's capacity for social adaptation has been limited, if it has been his habit to deal with minor difficulties by evasive methods or if he has led an aimless existence without drive or ambition, it is probable that further conversion defenses will be employed. Symptomatology alone is a poor guide as to the future. If the patient was formerly well adjusted and the conversion reaction was brought on by unusual stress the prognosis is favorable, provided return to the precipitating situation is not required. The patient who has consciously thought how his difficulties would be solved by the chance appearance of disabling illness may easily and unconsciously permit the thought to become a reality. The presence of felt anxiety with its indication that the conversion reaction is not providing an adequate defense makes the prognosis less favorable. The childish egocentric patient who becomes increasingly dependent on his conversion symptoms has a poor prognosis. His conversion reaction becomes a more or less permanent mode of life and he grows increasingly dependent on his symptoms.

The conversion reaction, in many instances, is engrafted upon a basically schizoid personality structure. With such persons the psychotic reaction eventually becomes apparent. This is particularly so in groups of patients diagnosed as hysterical and followed for years after their initial admission to a mental hospital. On the other hand, similar follow-up studies over a period of a decade on patients who presented in a general hospital or outpatient clinic a monosymptomatic conversion makes it clear that even with treatment by measures designed only to modify the symptoms without restructuring the personality the majority remained well and made excellent social adjustments. The outlook is best in the monosymptomatic hysteria which occurs in adult life rather than adolescence. Presumably here the response takes place in the face of a severe stress.

Treatment

In the treatment of a conversion reaction, the psychiatrist attempts to ascertain the purpose of the symptom, to discover the factors which caused anxiety so great that it could be handled only through the mechanism of conversion with functional physical symptoms. Since the patient's disorder arose through mental causes and through the operation of mental mechanisms the treatment should basically be that of psychotherapy. Through such treatment the patient should develop insight as to the origin of his symptoms and adjust himself in the light of that insight. While in all psychoneuroses it is desirable that the patient acquire insight as to the source of his symptoms, it is especially to be sought in conversion reactions. In other neuroses the treatment must often be supportive and aimed to promote emotional security, but in conversion neuroses, especially if of recent origin, the therapeutic attack should be aimed at the cause and purpose of the disability. In conversion, as in other neuroses, the greater the ego potentialities, *i.e.*, the capacity for adapting realistically and rationally to external conditions and internal needs, and the less the secondary gain from the neurosis the better the result to be expected from psychotherapy.

The nature and energy of the dynamic factors which have led to the patient's symptoms are concealed from his recognition and any explanation of the underlying mechanism is often received with resistance and protest. The patient's conversion reaction may, too, appear so remote from his emotional problem that only a searching analysis can uncover the relationship between the two.

Before beginning psychotherapy, the physician should first make a thorough physical examination. If no evidence is found that there is physical disease no more physical examinations should be made even though new symptoms occur. Continued examinations and long hospitalization may cause new symptoms to appear and old ones to become fixed.

The psychiatrist should remember that he must deal with two distinct although related problems: one, the removal of the symptom, the other, that of enabling the patient to apprehend the source of his anxiety and the significance of his symptom in order that he may form a more constructive method of action for the future. It is much easier to dispel a conversion than to help the patient to achieve further emotional growth. The principal attention, too, should be directed to a discovery of the psychogenic factors and their adjustment. If this objective is attained the symptom will, of itself, disappear. It is important to make a correct estimate of the patient's personality stability and maturity and of his intellectual resources. If the personality limitations are relatively minimal, the treatment may be psychotherapeutic and based on analytical principles with an investigation of the dynamic factors of repression. In a majority of cases, however, an extensive investigation of the whole personality and its development is not esssential. In the person of low intelligence and in the unstable individual who develops a conversion reaction in a relatively uncomplicated situation, the principal therapy will probably have to be limited to suggestion, hypnosis and re-education. In no case must the patient be accused of dishonesty or of a lack of desire to get well. As will be pointed out in Chapter XXXVI, hypnosis or many nonspecific measures may be successful in removing the acute conversion symptom but the basic emotional problem remains unchanged and the return of the symptom is therefore frequent. Generally speaking, one of two forms of psychotherapy is employed to work out with the patient the problem which originally gave rise to his illness. One method is that of psychoanalysis, or the free association techinque of Freud. The other is based on Meyer's teaching of psychobiology and its emphasis upon a study of the total personality. The principles and techniques of these two forms of therapy will be discussed in Chapter XXXVI.

Occasionally, because of its major nature, it is wise to attack the conversion symptom directly and after its removal undertake treatment directed against the personality immaturities and the specific factors that gave rise to the illness. This attack may be made by means of suggestion as described in the chapter mentioned. Great caution must be used before attempting the rapid removal of the hysterical symptom either by suggestion, narcosynthesis or hypnosis. It is most important to ascertain whether the symptoms mask a schizophrenic disturbance. Evidence for such an assumption may be gained by careful assessment of the developmental history. Family history of psychotic disturbance, pre-existing information of a dependent, withdrawn and isolated life with resort to fantasy or other disordered behavioral traits should arouse suspicion. Often, because of denial by the hysteric in presenting his life history initially, valid information is not obtained. Many consider that the aid of psychological tests, particularly the projective methods, should always be sought in such instances before treatment goals are determined and therapy initiated. Furthermore such tests may provide clues as to the potentiality of severe regressions which will require hospital treatment if sudden removal of symptoms appears the method of choice. One of the authors has been impressed with the frequency of such regressions in patients who present numerous pure color reactions in their Rorschach responses.

The symptoms that are seriously disabling and in which early removal may be considered highly desirable are the paralyses, blindness, aphasias and choreiform states and amnesias. The hysterical painful conversion, if acute, also may be treated in this way. Such painful conditions, if allowed to persist, are serious threats to health because of the likelihood of addictions or polysurgical therapies consequent to later misdiagnoses.

In the treatment of *accident neuroses* there are certain factors which require special attention. In case of injury any suggestion that it is serious should be carefully avoided. If possible the injured person should be kept at work, and if his condition does not permit this he should return as promptly as possible. Care should be exercised that the treatment of any physical complication is not prolonged. The attitude of the physician toward a patient suffering from a traumatic neurosis should never be one of suspicion or antagonism. If he approaches the patient in a biased, skeptical attitude, disregards his complaints and makes but a superficial examination, he destroys the possibility of any therapeutic rapport and may even contribute to further psychological elaboration.

A hope for indemnification on part of the injured employee makes it impossible for him to disregard unpleasant sensations or unpleasant subjective experiences or to adjust himself to them. In contrast to an athlete similarly injured, the workman, doubtless unwittingly, is prompted to magnify rather than ignore the discomforts resulting from his injury. The harshness and disregard of complaints by representatives of insurance companies, a ready assumption of intent to swindle, and the delays and technicalities of court procedure tend to stimulate unwholesome patterns of reaction. Such attitudes engender resentment and discouragement and may force the injured person to resort to a primitive (conversion) mode of response. Whether a compensation award granted to the workman suffering from a traumatic neurosis is paid in a single sum or extended through a number of installments makes little difference so far as the neurosis is concerned. It is important, however, that a settlement be made promptly and any litigation be terminated.

Obsessive Compulsive Reaction

In the obsessive compulsive reaction, the patient's anxiety is automatically controlled by associating it with persistently repetitive thoughts and acts. The patient recognizes that his unwanted thoughts and ritualistic acts are unreasonable but he is unable to control them. The obsessive-compulsive reaction may be expressed in three clinical forms: (1) the persistent recurrence of an unwelcome and often distressing thought; (2) a morbid and often irresistible urge to perform a certain repetitive, stereotyped act; and (3) an obsessively recurring thought accompanied by a compulsion to perform a repetitive act. Obsessive ideation may be concerned with various topics. Not rarely the patient must fight against thoughts that are repugnant to his conscious moral and esthetic feelings, such as thoughts of a blasphemous nature or fantasies of killing a beloved member of his family. Although horrified that he should entertain such thoughts the patient is unable to rid himself of them. The intruding and constantly recurring thought may be pointless and absurd, such as the case described by Ireland whose well educated patient persistently wondered why a chair had four legs instead of one leg, or a ruminative preoccupation and speculation on such topics as creation, infinity or other philosophical or religious questions. The condition of being obsessively preoccupied with an apparently indifferent topic with marked exclusion of other interests is sometimes known as an obsessive-ruminative state. At times considerable overt anxiety may be associated with such states. The greater the effort to dispel obsessive thoughts the more stubbornly they return. Ritualistic activities may be performed in an effort to dispel or counteract the thoughts. Practically never do such patients carry out any recurring thoughts suggesting an immoral or violent act although they may become very apprehensive lest they do so. The inability of the patient to free himself from the distressing thought may rarely lead him to suicide.

Some obsessive thinking assumes the form of *folie du doute* characterized by persistent doubting, vacillation and indecision usually with compulsive ruminations that lead to repetitive acts aimed to dispel the irrational doubts. Because of them the patient must check and recheck even the simplest acts. He may, for example, lock the front door at night but no sooner has he reached his bed than he is in doubt about the security of the door. He must therefore return and try the lock. Even then his doubts may recur after he is again in bed and require further visits to verify that the door is locked. Obsessive doubts and indecisions not rarely arise in case of conflict between desire and counterdesire.

Insistent, obsessive thoughts are defensive in purpose. The persistent idea is not to be taken at face value, so to speak. It is a substitute for another idea and thereby serves an anxiety-preventing function. Other affects are concealed behind the apparent content. The real sources may be any impulse, tendency or wish which would be consciously intolerable to the patient. A hidden feeling of guilt is not an uncommon source. The manifest and recurring idea is the result of an effort to keep something else out of the mind and is formed by the mechanisms of displacement, symbolization and condensation. The process is much the same as occurs in a dream where the latent or true content is concealed by these mechanisms so that the idea, wish or impulse appears in the conscious dream in distorted and symbolized form.

A second clinical type of obsessive-compulsive reaction is that of compulsive acts. In this there is the obligatory repetition of a certain act. The forces which produce the compulsive act are, of course, unconscious. Since the symbolic act cannot adequately satisfy the forces that produced it the act is stereotyped and repetitive. When the patient is asked the reason for his behavior, he may either offer some explanation which he knows has no rational basis or he may admit that it is absurd and purposeless. Usually the patient consciously experiences some rejection and resistance to the carrying out of his defensive, compulsive act but tension and anxiety mount until the urge to repeat becomes irresistible.

If the patient is prevented from carrying out his compulsive ritual, overt anxiety appears. One of the most frequent forms of obsessive-compulsive rituals is that of handwashing which has for its purpose the warding off of anxiety.

Most obsessive-compulsive acts consist merely of such simple, useless acts as touching or counting, or excessive ones, such as repeated handwashing. Some, however, become elaborate rituals or ceremonials. They superficially appear as meaningless formalities and are only recognized as neurotic ceremonials when a necessity for renouncing them is accompanied by discomfort and anxiety.

The ritualistic ceremonial described by Freud in one of his earliest papers (1896) entitled "The Defense Neuro-psychoses," is often quoted and is an excellent illustration of the complexity that may be assumed by these compulsive devices designed to protect against anxiety:

"An eleven-year old boy had instituted the following obsessive ceremonial before going to bed. He did not sleep until he had told his mother in the minutest detail all the events of the day; there must be no scraps of paper or other rubbish on the carpet of the bedroom; the bed must be pushed right to the wall; three chairs must stand by it and the pillows must lie in a particular way. In order to get to sleep he must first kick out a certain number of times with both legs and then lie on his side."

The function of compulsive acts is to allay or bind anxiety. They therefore serve a neurotic need. By the mechanism of displacement, and to some degree by symbolization, the anxiety aroused by unconscious impulses, wishes, hostilities and aggressive or other threatening tendencies, is "displaced" and expressed, and therefore alleviated, through the compulsive, repetitive act. At the same time the anxiety is still further allayed by the mechanism known as "undoing." By this mechanism the patient makes an additional effort to protect himself against danger. The compulsive act which the patient performs has, it will be found, a symbolic significance. This symbolic act serves as a sort of magic ritual by which he undoes or annuls the possible effect of his unrecognized impulses and achieves a distorted satisfaction, self-punishment and atonement. The compulsive act serves as a sort of magic ritual which temporarily dispels the dangerous situation; as long as it can be carried out, the intensity of the anxiety is reduced. If the performance of the ritualistic substitutive act is resisted or impossible, the effectiveness of the protective obsessive-compulsive defense is eliminated and the forbidden wishes and impulses arouse anxiety. The need for ritualized behavior increases since the unconscious striving threatens to erupt into consciousness; more and more symptoms must be constructed to provide defenses against the forbidden tendencies. In many respects the defensive patterns of the compulsions resemble penances, atonements and punishments or serve as precautions, prohibitions and restrictions. In many respects they are closely allied psychologically to the ceremonies and taboos which primitive people devise as protections against demonological and other supernatural forces.

Compulsive acts are not uncommon in children and adolescents in whom they originate as expiatory ceremonials or as means whereby, through attributing a certain magic-like power to an act, a particularly desired wish may be attained. The acts then become established through habit but normally disappear as repressed tensions subside and more adequate social adjustments are established.

The third type of obsessive-compulsive reaction is that in which a phobia or obsessively recurring idea is associated with a compulsion to perform a repetitious act. This association occurs when there exists an overpowering fear of intolerable impulses. Usually considerable anxiety is observable. One of the commonest examples of this type of reaction is a repetitive handwashing, the result of an obsessive fear of dirt or uncleanliness. Whatever object the patient touches has, he is confident, left his hands contaminated. Since he can scarcely avoid touching objects he must repeatedly wash his hands. As every object is a possible source of contamination the patient may resort to complicated and troublesome means of avoiding the touching of objects. He may open doors with his elbows or handle articles with gloves or other coverings. One patient washed each Saturday the church pew she expected to occupy the following day. Because of this tension, preoccupation and irresistible handwashing the capacity for gainful employment may be destroyed.

Here, too, are found the same mechanisms of displacement and undoing. The real fear is, of course, not of dirt but of intolerable impulses or guilt-laden strivings which have been displaced and symbolized by constant preoccupation with fear of dirt. The anxiety to which they have given rise is temporarily alleviated by the compulsive washing with its symbolically cleansing significance.

Adolf Meyer described a group of persons characterized by difficulty with decisions, by doubts, rituals and fears, and with anticipation of panic should fulfillment fail to be achieved. Anxiety and depression are common accompaniments. He designated these reactions as "obsessive ruminative tension states."

The following case illustrates many of the features of a mixed phobic and compulsive reaction:

S. K. was admitted to a public mental hospital in 1949 at the age of 29. The family history revealed no significant history. During the second and third grades of school "he was a problem to the nuns because of his stuttering. They would ask him to read a paragraph over two or three times." For a considerable period at this age "he felt he had to bless himself a certain number of times in the evening." When in the fourth grade and after an illness "he was afraid to go to sleep at night for fear he might die. He would call his mother two or three times before going to sleep. He would not go to sleep unless she reassured him that he would not die. This lasted for two or three months." He bit his nails until he was sixteen years of age.

At the time of his admission the patient's mother and wife were requested to describe his adult personality characteristics. He was, they reported, a quiet, serious, honest, thrifty, saving, stubborn and somewhat worrisome person. "He was ambitious. He wanted to go through college and be more than an ordinary working man. In college he studied very, very hard and was an honor student." When eighteen years of age the patient drank excessively for a period of several months. He then suddenly stopped and became so opposed to liquor that, to quote his wife, "He wouldn't touch a drop and I remember once when we were both young he walked out of a home where liquor was being served because he was so opposed to it."

In 1942 he enlisted in the Marine Corps. When, after his admission to the hospital, he was asked what prompted him to volunteer he replied, "Well, I felt uneasy a little bit with my scrupulosity. I wasn't too uneasy, but I thought somehow the service would take it away." What do you mean by 'scrupulosity'? "I was doubtful about my confessions." You were doubtful that you didn't confess enough? "That's right; I didn't have enough sorrow for my sins." When the admitting physician asked the patient about his duties in the military service he replied, "I had a job cleaning urinals. I probably was very good. I tried to do a thorough job. I saw cigarettes but I always kept on cleaning all the time. It could have been done in two or three hours but I worked eight or nine hours. I volunteered for the job." In April 1944 he wrote his fiancee that he wished to break his engagement as he was going to study for the priesthood after discharge from service. Six months later he wrote again saying he had decided not to become a priest and asked that their engagement be renewed.

After his discharge from military service in January 1946 the patient entered college from which he was graduated in June 1949 although by April 1949 his neurotic reaction had become so disabling that he was unable to continue his studies for the final two months of his senior year. In June 1946 he was married but had no sexual relations with his wife until seventeen months later.

Soon after the patient's admission to the hospital his wife was asked to give a history of the patient's illness. She reported that he had exhibited a compulsive handwashing for several months before November 1948 but that it became more serious at that time. "He used to wash his hands and keep the water running for fifteen minutes at a time. After he had washed them he would turn off the spigot with his elbow. He had to count and wash and rinse his hands a certain number of times. If he had touched the door or door knob he would go back and wash his hands again. One time he began to wash his hands at one o'clock in the morning. After we moved into our own house he refused to use the front door or to turn the knob on the door for fear there might be germs. He used to go to the back window and call me to go to the front door and open it for him. He reached the point where he would climb in and out of windows so he wouldn't have to enter the doors at all." The wife described also the following compulsion: "He also had the idea that when he walked there was something under his shoe. He would stop and look on the sole of his shoe but there would be nothing there. He also worried as to whether or not his shoe laces were tied. He would pick up his foot and look to make sure. He had to do that a certain number of times before he was absolutely sure they were tied. When he walked down a street if he kicked a stone he felt that he should put it back in the same place. If he walked on a line then he would have to walk on all the cracks in the sidewalk."

On arrival at the hospital the patient frankly stated to the admitting physician, "I like to wash my hands many times a day in order to get them good and clean." While talking to the physician he stood with his arms folded in order to avoid touching anything. He readily acknowledged that he was worried about touching objects lest he give others disease. As he seemed somewhat depressed he was asked about suicidal thoughts. He replied that he felt he would be better off dead than be thinking of the things he did but added that he would "not really" commit suicide. He then added, "When I say things they have to be said a certain way. If I don't say them properly I must apologize. I do this all the time. This irritated my wife and was another reason why she couldn't live with me. I would leave my books to apologize to her. It was the apologizing that was bothering her—not being at peace. I thought if I rubbed my hands eighty-eight times, shut the water off and then went back again it would be all right. Then I thought maybe it hadn't been eighty-eight times."

A month after the patient's admission his ward physician entered the following note in the clinical record: "This patient has become extremely disturbed over his obsessive-compulsive ideation during recent days. He stops his physician at every opportunity and repeatedly asks the same questions, which include the following: "Should I wash my hands after I go to the bathroom and just do number one? Should I wash my hands when I go to the bathroom and have a bowel movement? My penis touches the toilet seat. Do you think I should wash it off with soap and water so there won't be a spread of disease? I wouldn't want anyone to get this disease. There's a rash there. Do you want to look at it? I think it is some sort of a disease. I'm afraid everybody will get it. I don't know, doctor, I'm afraid something is going to happen. I have a feeling that I might go crazy or something. Someone asked me if I thought these things were silly and I said 'yes,' but now that I think of it they don't seem silly. I just can't quite explain them. They must not really seem silly to me or I wouldn't have to do them like I do." The patient manifested an interesting inability to make any definite statement or to take any decisive action. When discussing a point he would say such things as the following: "Well, doctor, it's just like this. Well, no it isn't exactly like that. I should say rather that's a little on the order of—Well, that isn't quite right either. Perhaps I should put it this way. It's more of—uh—well, no that isn't it."

Under therapy the patient gradually improved. Two years after his admission he left the hospital for employment in a brick plant. A report received a year later stated that although not entirely well he was successfully employed.

Prognosis

In adults the prognosis in obsessive-compulsive neuroses is not good although a recent study has shown that a large percentage of individuals with this condition suffer episodic attacks and are able to adapt socially. The patient's compulsive needs frequently interfere seriously with his comfort and efficiency. In extreme cases his constant preoccupation with his protective rituals renders him socially impossible. Some psychiatrists characterize the obsessive neuroses as intermediate between neuroses and psychoses. The obsessive-compulsive states of children usually disappear with time if not taken seriously in the presence of the child. Such compulsions grow out of a childhood anxiety, often a single one. The prognosis is much more serious if the onset is during adolescence or early adult life.

Diagnosis

In all the neuroses there are fine gradations between what at one extreme are usually looked upon merely as personality traits to incapacitating distress at the other extreme. One, therefore, may well be in doubt at times whether a given person should be considered within the limits of normality or whether he should be looked upon as a compulsive neurotic. In the fully developed cases with their well marked obsessive thinking, fears or compulsive acts, there is of course no question. Since, however, we all have defensive character traits the decision must often be arbitrary. Perhaps the criterion should be whether there are repressions that require such drastic supporting measures that these defenses seriously disturb the subjective life of the individual. Ordinarily, the exaggerated traits of character, such as stern conscientiousness or over-moral and overascetic scruples are not included, although, like the frankly neurotic symptoms, they are defensive in purpose.

A diagnosis between early schizophrenia and the obsessive-compulsive neuroses is at times exceedingly difficult. The obsessive thinking of the psychoneurotic may not be unlike the subjective rumination of the schizophrenic, while the compulsive ritual of the former may suggest the mannerisms of the latter. The symbolisms seen in the compulsive acts of the neurotic individual, as well as the substitutive nature of the phobias, are close both in resemblance and in relationship to the symbols seen in schizophrenia. It not infrequently happens that what is first thought to be the ruminative and obsessive tension state of a neurotic subsequently becomes an obvious schizophrenic reaction, usually of the paranoid type. In general it may be said that the greater the rumination and the less the tension the nearer does the reaction approach that of the schizophrenic. A failure on the part of the patient to regard his phobias and compulsions as absurd and particularly to refer them to external influences indicates a malignant, schizophrenic origin. The compulsive neurotic never loses the capacity for discrimination between subjective experiences and reality as is the case in schizophrenia. Finally, as Bleuler points out, the compulsive neurotic struggles *against* his obsession whereas the delusional patient struggles *with* his idea.

At times the genuine depressions of manic-depressive psychosis may be accompanied by obsessive ideas. In differentiating such cases from compulsive states one will inquire which appeared first, the depression or the obsessive idea.

Treatment

Fully developed obsessional and compulsive reactions may be even more refractory to treatment than the milder psychoses. It is therefore important that treatment be early. The obsessive-compulsive neuroses usually develop in individuals who have been characterized by compulsive personality traits to be described later. The neurosis is in many ways an exaggeration and caricature of that pattern. Effort is made, therefore, to discover the factors which through their dynamic action led first to the personality make-up and then to the neurosis. Treatment, then, will be psychotherapeutic and consists either of a formal psychoanalysis or be based on analytical principles. Guided by the therapist, the patient's unconscious is explored and his apparently irrational fears and compulsions take on new meaning when understood in terms of chronologically earlier experiences and early life dynamics. In all cases, but particularly in rigid personalities and in those of limited intellectual development, re-educational measures should be employed. The patient should be encouraged to evaluate the relative importance of matters and to learn that indecision and perfectionism should be curbed even at the cost of errors and mediocrity. Such attitudes as excessive guilt and overconscientiousness should be discussed. Cultivation of latent interests may help to reduce the ruminative thinking to which these patients are often addicted. Self-preoccupation and self-analysis are to be discouraged. Prefrontal leukotomy has at times been followed by improvement. It should, however, be confined to cases so severe that the patient is practically confined to his home and incapacitated for any useful activity because of his compulsions. Results are better when there is evidence of persistence and drive and when the obsessional symptoms are accompanied by considerable anxiety.

While not included in the present official classification of psychiatric disorders the term *hypochondria,* or hypochondriacal reaction, is one that was long applied to a group of psychoneurotic symptoms. Patients presenting these symptoms are now usually included in obsessive-compulsive reaction group. The reaction is characterized by an obsessive preoccupation and concern of the individual about the state of his health or the conditions of his organs. Often he expresses a multiplicity of complaints about different organs or body systems which, the patient reiterates, must be incurably diseased. The hypochondriac is not only aware of various sensations which most persons disregard but he also magnifies the intensity of normal sensations of fatigue, etc. In many cases the hypochondriasis seems to be a displacement of anxiety onto the body with the resulting somatic complaints. Some hypochondriacal reactions may become excessively and persistently obsessional and develop associated compulsions.

Care should be exercised to differentiate this syndrome from the different forms of depressive reactions, from psychophysiological reactions and from early schizophrenia.

Catastrophic Neuroses, or Gross Stress Reaction

Combat Neuroses

Following severe threat to life, whether as the consequence of stress in civilian life in the form of catastrophies experienced in accidents, floods, tornadoes or volcanic eruptions, or the stress of warfare and combat, a well defined personality disorder frequently results. This condition, known much earlier in the German literature as fright (*schreck*) neurosis, in the English as a traumatic neurosis, may occur as an isolated disturbance or complicate pre-existing personality disorders. In the United States it probably occurs most commonly, and is most frequently unrecognized, after automobile accidents. Adler differentiates two types of post-traumatic states: those with immediate, and those with delayed onset. In the current nomenclature of the American Psychiatric Association, this syndrome is not listed under the neuroses but under the Transient Situational Personality Disturbances as Gross Stress Reaction. The more profound reactions to catastrophic stress produce long continuing disruption of personality functioning both in previously healthy and in neurotic persons. For this reason they are discussed here as a neurosis. Since the combat neuroses have been most thoroughly studied, they are given extended comment.

Presumably combat neuroses have long been associated with warfare although their real nature and psychopathology were not recognized until relatively recently. During the Civil War DaCosta described the "Irritable Heart of Soldiers." This was undoubtedly a neurosis induced by the stress and anxiety of combat and closely resembled the "Disordered Action of the Heart," 80,000 cases of which, it is said, occurred among British soldiers during World War I. It is of interest that this high incidence did not recur in World War II, presumably because its nature had become recognized so much more fully that it no longer offered the refuge formerly available. In World War I artillery fire reached a new intensity with a fear-producing potentiality probably never before attained by weapons of warfare. It was noticed that with this terrifying shell-fire often combined with fear-inspiring air attacks there appeared a striking variety of symptoms including paralysis, gross tremors, mutism, blindness, confusion or intense anxiety. In apparent absence of other etiological factors it was at first concluded that the brain must in some undetermined manner sustain damage by a blast concussion attending the near-by explosion of a shell. Soldiers readily accepted the opinion of their physicians that their mental disabilities were of an irreparable nature as a result of brain injury. The term "shell shock" was therefore applied to these psychiatric casualties and prolonged hospitalization prescribed for their treatment. Gradually it become recognized that "shell shock" was primarily a psychological problem and that the effect of air blast could not explain the immediate symptoms and subsequent persistent illness. Late in the War it became apparent, too, that prolonged hospitalization merely fostered and fixated the mental symptoms which because they prevented return to combat and even brought a compensation pension provided a considerable secondary gain. Before the end of World War II it became apparent that recovery was much more prompt and lasting if the patient with an acute, battle-induced neurosis was treated near the front lines and returned to duty as soon as possible. It was also noted that the percentage of recoveries was greater if the attitude of the psychiatrist indicated that no organic damage had been sustained and if the name by which the neurosis was known to the soldier implied that the disability was temporary and recoverable and that no actual physical or mental illness existed. In the opinion of many psychiatrists the term "shell shock" used during World War I probably set off more neurotic reactions through its injudicious use than did battle. In 1943, therefore, the U. S. Army adopted the term "combat exhaustion" for the labeling of nearly all types of psychiatric casualties appearing in the forward areas. This term was adopted advisedly because of its implication that the disability is of a temporary and honorable nature, is the logical result of combat and that rest and recuperation lead to recovery.

Extreme and repeated battle fear with a constant threat of death plus intense fatigue are the precipitating factors in the production of combat neurosis. Physical exhaustion alone is not sufficient to produce the neurosis but it does serve to lessen resistance so that psychodynamic forces are more easily released. The greater, however, the element of decreased physical efficiency resulting from fatigue, lack of food and sleep, or intercurrent illness the more easily does emotional breakdown occur and the greater is the possibility of returning the soldier to active duty.

Although, as has been indicated, exhaustion, hardship and fear are the most important and the precipitating factors in the development of war neuroses, other factors are often of significant influence in preparing the soil, so to speak, for the mental breakdown in battle. It is not easy to select the man who will maintain emotional equilibrium in combat and eliminate the one who will prove inadequate for the stress. It is not always the unstable and neurotic man who, as might be supposed, lacks resistance to the terror that accompanies long and intense combat. In general it is the timid and passive person who cannot mobilize and externalize his anger and react aggressively toward the enemy and thus discharge his tension who is prone to develop a combat neurosis.

Most men, while wishing to meet the demands of their country, are inducted into the armed forces without strong, conscious desire for military life or for combat experience. Many at time of induction are still emotionally dependent on their families, perhaps overprotected by their mothers and intimidated by cruel fathers. It has been found, too, that an unduly large number of combat neuroses come from broken or distorted homes unfavorable for the development of a well integrated and mature personality. Induction into military service is accompanied by the abrupt loss of emotional support provided by family and friends, the deprivation of female companionship and the loss of individuality and privacy. Frequently, too, the unseasoned soldier has a feeling that he is not appreciated and nurses resentment resulting from the change from the relatively flexible and permissive civilian pattern of living to one of subjection to strict discipline, regimentation and subordination. The stresses and conflicts to which the soldier is exposed during his training period are relatively mild and are handled by most trainees without the development of protest symptoms in the form of neurotic or psychotic syndromes. Even though the period of training is not accompanied by the hazards of combat, normal gratifications are renounced and destructive goals are substituted for the constructive ones of previous civil life. New relationships which would meet the soldier's emotional needs in the strange and abnormal state of affairs have to be established. Under these circumstances the most constructive relationship is the soldier's identification of himself as an integral part of his unit, and his unit as a part of himself. He should have confidence in his unit and in the character, capability and bravery of his leader. With the formation of deep emotional relationship with his leader and his buddies the soldier's feelings of security and power are increased and his morale, or those attitudes, feelings and beliefs which promote participation in a united effort, is promoted.

In World Wars I and II and in the Korean campaign the American soldier, following a period of overseas training and waiting with its boredom, suspense and inactivity, moved forward to the field of combat warfare. Arrived there, he was precipitated, often without sufficient time for rest, into a situation fraught with constant danger and hardship and intense emotional and physical stress. The particular combat experiences of the soldier depend upon the branch of military service to which he is assigned but in nearly all instances there is the continued threat of injury and death accompanied by feelings of great intensity and wide variety. Common to all experiences is the emotional reaction of fear, the most potent source of emotional tension in combat. Fear, it will be remembered, is an emotion experienced in response to a stimulus having actual reality, one that either constitutes a present threat to the individual or portends real danger. Anxiety, on the other hand, is an expectation of danger, an emotional state of apprehensiveness, uncertainty and insecurity, that may be produced either from situations symbolic of external danger or from internal conflicts and tensions present in the unconscious. Frequently it springs from the threats of repressed hostility, aggression or resentment. While this distinction between fear and anxiety can be made yet in war situations they operate jointly. Their feeling-tones and their accompanying physiological expressions are the same. Although anxiety really arises from internal threats, it is attributed to (projected upon) some real external source. In the war neuroses this projection is upon a dangerous external situation which is also provocative of fear. Both fear and the feeling of apprehension and insecurity characteristic of anxiety may therefore seem to have a common source. To draw the line between the two is not always possible. In the battle situation fear and other powerful external and emotional forces play upon the internal tensions and threats, upon the unconscious sources of anxiety. Of these sources of emotional stress in combat fear is the most potent, its somatic and physiological effects being a source of great strain. Under combat circumstances the various external and internal stresses conspire to produce a conflict that may become intolerable and an anxiety reaction result from its threat. The psychological defenses hitherto effective collapse with a consequent rise of anxiety and the production of the neurotic symptom. Anxiety and its management constitute, therefore, one of the basic problems in war neuroses.

Factors Contributing to War Neuroses. Before describing what may be regarded as the normal battle reaction and the clinical features of combat neurosis, mention will be made both of certain factors that predispose to disabling neuroses and of those that may exercise a protective influence. As already indicated, fear and an impairment of the ability to repress fear reactions are highly provocative of anxiety. A breakdown of group morale or an attitude of defeatism within the combat unit greatly increases the psychological strain. Such a loss of morale is particularly prone to exist in case of bad leadership, of lack of faith in commanding officers, in the absence of identification with one's unit or during a retreat. The quality of leadership is one of the most important factors in the incidence of neurotic breakdown in any given unit. Prolonged periods of enforced inactivity during which men are exposed to danger predispose to an anxiety reaction. So does the loneliness of foxhole fighting with the usual inability to communicate with comrades. Repeated narrow escapes, high combat losses and repeated exposure to the mutilation and death of close friends increase apprehension and stimulate anxiety. Factors, in addition to fear and exhaustion, which contribute to such a reaction are malnutrition, exposure to heat and cold, disease, hunger, a fear of being a coward or of losing one's self-control, a realization of the responsibility for the lives of others and an insufficient understanding of war or a lack of conviction to fight. A sense of guilt over expression of hostility is at times a psychogenetic factor. The regimentation and frustration of service life, separation from home and the existence of domestic difficulties are often of much significance than more dramatic events.

While the necessity that the man "sweat it out" in a continuously hostile environment results almost inevitably in at least some degree of anxiety, there are certain internal as well as external factors that tend to increase anxiety. One of these internal problems is the soldier's handling of his hostilities. During his civilian life he was called upon to inhibit any hostile or aggressive drives. Whereas he formerly had the value of human life constantly impressed upon him, the soldier is expected to kill as many men as possible. His hostility, which through long inhibition had become well repressed, is now to be released to kill men like himself. This release of hostile and aggressive drives in most destructive expression evokes anxiety. The problem of control of aggressive impulses is probably one of the soldier's heaviest psychological burdens. The combat situation releases a considerable amount of hostility, much of it, perhaps, against members of one's own unit. Whatever their origin, any anxieties and tensions which add to the burden of the ego weaken its defensive functions and increase the possibility of a neurosis. Frustrations, such as unfair treatment in regard to promotions, citations or leaves of absence cause resentment, hostility, tension and anxiety.

Feelings of guilt may also provoke anxiety. Such feelings may arise from the soldier's thought that he has been responsible for the death of someone else, perhaps of civilians as well as an enemy. Again the death of a comrade toward whom the patient entertained ambivalent feelings or whom he had identified with a sibling rival may create feelings of guilt with anxiety or depression. An unconscious hostility may lead to a conviction on the part of the patient that he has actually caused the death of a comrade. At times, following the death of a buddy, a man develops a feeling of guilt through a belief that he failed to take care of his friend. Guilt reactions are particularly frequent in flying personnel. Not rarely the loss of a buddy or of a respected officer, by creating the feeling that one is being left alone, helpless and deserted, deprives the soldier of emotional support and leads to an unendurable anxiety.

One important factor, then, in the production of combat neurosis is that the soldier's experiences mobilize emotions which have always been important in the personality but have not previously strained or overwhelmed the forces of control. Combat is not the only stress that mobilizes emotions and leads to war neuroses. Some men tolerate combat but break under restrictions, discipline, separation from home, loss of buddies or unfaithfulness of their wives. What the man cannot stand is largely a matter of what the greatest stresses and threats to his particular personality are. Neurotic anxiety in battle may be rooted in passivity, hostility or aggressiveness and in the character of the personality defenses constructed against them in early life.

The forces, nevertheless, that threaten most the life of the soldier far outweigh all other causative factors in producing combat neuroses. Psychiatric disabilities, therefore, vary directly with the intensity of combat and the battle casualty rate. The longer, too, that the soldier is in combat and the greater the number of scenes of death and mutilation which he witnesses the more disabling does his anxiety become. The state of the soldier's morale is of the utmost importance. Whatever impairs this lessens his resistance to a development of a neurosis.

NEUROSIS-PREVENTING FACTORS. Attention has been called to certain factors that may contribute to neurotic failure of adjustment. There are also factors that serve as defenses in protecting the soldier from a pathological expression of his conflict. One of the most important mechanisms in strengthening the ego against factors productive of anxiety and other neurotic reactions is the soldier's identification with his unit. By this mechanism he transfers a considerable share of his personal self-love to affection and pride in his outfit. His feelings of obligation and loyalty having their source in this mechanism overrule selfish, personal interests and provide one of the strongest motivations for combat and most effective protections against any expression of his conflicts. The group relationship and its emotional bonds are among the most constructive and integrative forces for the individual. Similarly an intense loyalty to each other on the part of the fighting men and their immediate leaders promotes morale and raises the threshold against anxiety. A resolute personal motivation, good morale, sustained by pride in one's organization, good leadership, respect for officers and fellow soldiers, confidence in equipment, the feeling of being properly trained, high quality of food together with recreational outlets are of great importance in preventing war neuroses. Other factors that aid in warding off anxiety are the desire to avoid loss of the esteem of the group by any failure in courage or in other demands of military tradition, also the habit of obedience and of disciplined behavior established by military training.

An additional factor that doubtless serves as an aid in the prevention of war neuroses is a series of lectures concerning the nature of fear. These lectures are given to the soldier during his training period. He is told that fear is a normal emotion of battle and to experience it should not be considered as occasion for censure or self-depreciation. The soldier is given simple information concerning its physiological manifestations and the nature of the nervous reactions it produces. His recognition of fear and his effort to deal with it on a conscious level tend to minimize its anxiety-stimulating influence.

NORMAL BATTLE REACTION. To protect itself from an overwhelming threat to its existence the organism becomes completely and continuously alert. This leads to severe and continuous emotional tension. In spite of the various factors that aid in the prevention of combat neuroses, such stresses as exhaustion, excitement and mortal terror must almost inevitably produce reactions that would be considered abnormal in a civilian setting yet are not so incapacitating as to demand removal from combat. Unless extreme, such reactions must under the circumstances be considered within the range of normal. Many of the reactions represent psychosomatic responses to stress and fear. Among them are sensations of pulling or pressure over the back of the head and neck, muscular tension, shaking and tremor. In some cases the soldier may be transitorily immobilized. Excessive perspiration is common and some soldiers experience anorexia, nausea, vague abdominal distress, mild diarrhea, and urinary frequency. Tachycardia, palpitation, breathlessness, a sense of thoracic oppression and of faintness together with generalized muscular weakness and lassitude often exist. Many soldiers experience difficulty in sleeping and oversensitivity to threatening combat noises. Irritability is normal in the soldier subjected to long-continued battle and resentment is common among those who have lost friends and withstood privations and dangers.

An 18-year-old Navy radioman was admitted to a hospital with symptoms of anxiety and depression.

The patient was the youngest son in a happy family of four children. He was the favored child and throughout his early life gave no indication of instability. At school he was an average student and later was president of his high school class and an outstanding football player. At the outbreak of the war, he enlisted in the naval service with the consent of his parents, and immediately after completing his recruit training was detailed aboard a destroyer where the morale was high. He made many close friends and with the personal assistance of the communications officer, who helped him with the radio work, made a rapid advancement in rate.

The destroyer was part of the screen of an aircraft carrier engaged in the Coral Sea Battle, the raid on the Gilbert and Marshall Islands, and later the Battle of Midway. At the onset of each engagement, the patient felt apprehensive but once firing commenced he became entirely composed and attentive to his duties. While the destroyer was lying alongside a stricken aircraft carrier following a bombing attack during the Battle of Midway, the patient saw "torpedo wakes," approaching the ship, resumed his post, until suddenly he was thrown out of his seat when the torpedo exploded beneath him. He plunged overboard, reached a near-by raft and was later taken aboard another destroyer. He was then cognizant that his best friend, his immediate chief, and the communications officer, had all been killed. On being taken aboard the ship he collapsed. Following his return to the naval base, it was learned that he had suffered blast injury to the chest and abdomen which eventually necessitated intestinal resection. During convalescence from this operation he first had terrifying nightmares in which various scenes related to the sinking of the destroyer were continually repeated, and which wakened him in a state of anxiety. Sudden noises also produced unusual apprehension.

There was no evidence of physical disease but his insomnia, anorexia, constipation, and fatigue were observed and psychiatric study was requested. The patient was listless, dejected, and emotionally labile. Discussion of his battle experiences was distressing to him and he described in detail his sensitivity to sounds and various combat scenes in motion pictures. The latter stimulus invariably led to anxiety. After one month of treatment on the psychiatric service he became more energetic, content, slept well, commenced to eat, gained some weight, and again desired to return to duty. Nightmares were infrequent and sounds were less disturbing to him.

NEUROTIC REACTION. As indicated, such symptoms as those described should, if of moderate degree, be considered normal and as the base line from which pathological reactions should be evaluated. The combat neurosis consists therefore of pathological degrees of the reactions mentioned.

The most frequent form of combat neurosis is the *anxiety state*. This constitutes over 75 per cent of acute war neuroses. In the most severe reactions the onset is acute and sudden. A coarse tremor is not uncommon. It may be difficult or impossible to establish contact with the patient. Even though no longer under fire he may believe himself still in battle and behave accordingly. He may, with expressions of terror, call to his friends to look out for the shells. Some show highly dramatic reactions and excessive startle patterns in response to slight stimuli. In extreme cases, the soldier's behavior is one of panic reaction in which there is apparently a complete disruption of personality organization. His uncontrolled, catastrophic reaction may vary from wild, impulsive flights to "freezing," or primitive protective withdrawal, with stupor, catatonia or mutism. In moderate or mild anxiety states, the patient shows tension, tremor, apprehension, weeping, depression, feelings of guilt, dizziness, tinnitus, urinary frequency, insomnia and battle dreams. Less frequently than in World War I, and usually in men of poor integration, the neurosis may consist of a *conversion reaction* with paralyses, sensory losses, aphonia, deafness, partial or total blindness, speech defects, astasia-abasia, a fixed stooping posture known as camptocormia, and occasionally a persistent amnesia. Such patients exhibit little visible anxiety and may manifest "la belle indifférence."

Some cases of combat neurosis assume the form of *depression*, usually preceded by anxiety. The depression may not be particularly obvious until after the effort to control anxiety has failed. The depression is frequently precipitated by the death of a comrade to whose loss the soldier was unable to reconcile himself. The conscious mental content is dominated by ideas of failure, guilt and of self-condemnation. The patient is convinced that he has let his buddies down or that in some way he has been responsible for their deaths. Frequently such depressions arise in cases in which the patient has had ambivalent feelings directed toward a comrade. Upon the death of his buddy the unconscious hostility which existed in these feelings stimulates the conviction that he actually caused the death of his comrade. This evokes guilt, depression and self-punishment. The clinical symptoms are characterized by a rigid, mask-like face, staring eyes that wink infrequently, by paucity of movement and by ideas of self-accusation and self-depreciation.

A 17-year-old seaman had seven months' active duty prior to admission to the hospital with a tentative diagnosis of intracranial injury.

He was the third of four boys in a family of six. His father was a "shell-shocked" veteran of World War I, now alcoholic and a chronic complainer. The mother was migrainous. The home was kept discordant by parental quarrels; nevertheless, the patient, though of retiring and quiet nature, adjusted well at school, was accepted by his classmates and was not considered temperamentally unstable.

Following his enlistment in the naval service, he received three weeks basic training and was detailed aboard a transport for drill in amphibious operations.

The patient had hoped for duty aboard a combat ship of the line. Three weeks prior to the departure of the convoys for the North African engagement, he was transferred to another ship. There he was barely acquainted with his new shipmates when the engagement opened. His immediate chief was regarded by him with little respect as an "old man." The seaman was extremely apprehensive as his landing boat approached the beach during the opening operations, but quickly regained composure when not exposed to fire. The following day he was frightened to the point of believing his legs were paralyzed when an enemy plane strafed the ship and he threw himself on the deck. The fourth day the ship was suddenly torpedoed. He was blown against the bulkhead and struck his head but was not injured and quickly climbed down a net into a tank lighter below. While throwing out lines to men struggling in the water he was fascinated by their cries and amazed to see some cast aside their life jackets. After helping one man aboard, the patient felt so weak that he lay upon the deck and later had to be assisted ashore. The following day a plane killed a French woman in town and he morbidly examined her body and the leg wounds of a sailor wounded in the same raid. He then realized how tense and anxious he felt, and in the following weeks had difficulty in sleeping, being repeatedly awakened by dreams in which his ship was torpedoed or he was shot in the leg. While aboard the transport returning home he and the men in his division were quartered in a forward compartment. During a prolonged storm the group repeatedly rushed to the boat deck in panic when a loose hatch cover slammed above them. He was given a thirty-day leave after arriving in this country but the change in his personality was so conspicuous to his family that his mother shortly sought medical advice concerning his symptoms.

On return to duty the patient complained of headaches and dizziness, and was transferred to the hospital for study. As there was no evidence of organic disease, psychiatric examination was requested. His extreme restlessness, amounting to agitation, his inattentiveness and irritability were immediately apparent. He was unable to concentrate, expressed death fears, and presented the history of nightmares and sensitivity to sounds reminiscent of combat. His sleep was broken almost nightly by terrifying dreams. With sedation and psychotherapy there was some diminution in the restlessness, in the insomnia and his response to startle. He put on weight, but continued to complain and insisted upon his inability to return to duty. It was evident that he would not again adjust in the service and, accordingly, he was recommended for discharge.

This youthful seaman, who was raised in a discordant home by a neurotic, alcoholic father and a high-strung mother, presented no evidence of emotional instability prior to his traumatic combat experience. He then developed nightmares, a startle reaction and a personality change marked by agitation, anxiety, and preoccupation, with the complaints of headaches and dizziness. The case study illustrates the importance in determining the neurotic reaction of a disturbed home life with possibility of neurotic identification, and the contributing factors of inadequate training, indifference to leadership, and low morale. The repeated panics during the voyage home probably further served to deepen the patient's anxiety by the process of conditioning.

Psychosomatic Symptoms. Physical symptoms often associated with anxiety constitute a frequent form of psychiatric disability in military service. Such symptoms may be referred to any part of the body and may appear in the soldier's training period or be precipitated or aggravated by battle stress. Sometimes they are seen in areas of the body previously the loci of disease, wounds or injuries. The soldier then suffers pain or other discomfort out of all proportion to physical signs. In other cases the emotionally upset soldier reports "sick" with types of disability—rheumatic, asthenic, gastrointestinal—that are acceptable to his group as having originated through no fault of his own but providing, nevertheless, a relatively nonpunishing escape from a psychologically intolerable situation. The somatic manifestations discussed in this paragraph should be regarded more as physical expressions of anxiety than as conversion phenomena. If such cases are subjected to prolonged study and treatment the symptoms may become fixed and the patient a permanent military loss.

Pseudopsychotic States. In some cases the soldier in his anxiety and panic reaction to combat stress is so out of contact with reality, is so confused and dissociated and his behavior so bizarre that he appears psychotic. The onset is usually sudden and the clinical picture suggests schizophrenia. Many patients are disoriented and fail to reply to simple questions. Some cases resemble catatonic stupor while others suggest a catatonic excitement. These psychotic-like pictures occur in individuals who have not been psychotic in their previous reactions or in their basic personality structures. Such short-lived "three-day" psychoses usually disappear when the patients are removed from the traumatic situations. Sometimes sedation or electroconvulsive treatment is advisable.

Prognosis and Treatment. The presentation of this feature of the combat neuroses is based upon the procedure prescribed by the Office of the Surgeon General, U.S. Department of the Army.[4]

In dealing with these neuroses, in the U. S. Army emphasis is placed on preservation of medical discipline, on early and vigorous treatment, the shortening of the period of hospitalization, the avoidance of unnecessary hospital atmosphere and the promotion in the patient of the expectation of return to full duty. In his treatment, care is exercised to preserve the patient's identification with the combat group, to minimize the secondary gain of neurotic illness and to avoid any suggestion of illness and disability. It is a basic principle in the attainment of these objectives that treatment should be as far forward as possible. So far as practicable soldiers who show symptoms of becoming psychiatric casualties on the battlefield receive what may be called psychiatric first aid from members of their own combat unit. Here company officers promote morale by counsel, reassurance, exhortation and leadership. Soldiers with relatively minor complaints may frequently be prevented from entering medical channels where the dissolution of group ties and the factors of secondary gain and suggestion tend to fix their symptoms.

If his motivation has been reasonably good, the combat exhaustion patient responds rather well to proper therapeutic handling. If formal medical treatment is required, the patient is evacuated to the battalion aid station. Here most patients are those suffering from mild to moderate anxiety states complicated by physical exhaustion and the effects of exposure. They are usually wet, cold, dirty and physically worn out. If the anxiety state is no more than moderate, the patient is kept at the aid station for twenty-four hours where he is cleaned up, dried, adequately fed and given sedation in the form of 7½ to 10 grains of Sodium Amytal orally. By his manner and remarks the battalion surgeon indicates that

[4] Ranson, Lt. Col. Stephen W.: Psychiatric treatment in combat areas. United States Armed Forces Medical Journal, *1:* No. 12, December 1950.

he expects an early return to duty of the soldier after he is rested. Many of the patients evacuated to the battalion aid station are simply suffering from normal fear reactions with the somatic and psychological manifestations of that state consisting of palpitation, nausea, tremulousness and other physical manifestations of fear reactions. The patient has usually become alarmed by these symptoms which he has interpreted as those of cardiac, gastrointestinal, or other physical disorder. A careful physical examination is made and if no organ involvement is found the cause of the symptoms is carefully explained to the soldier who is assured that there will be no lasting effects or disability. After twenty-four hours of rest and psychotherapy consisting of reassurance, support and exhortation many patients are completely recovered or so greatly improved that they may be returned directly to duty.

The more severe and the pseudopsychotic reactions are unsuited for management in the battalion aid station and are therefore transferred to the division clearing station. These patients exhibit marked anxiety states, extreme agitation and tension, acute panic states, hysterical manifestations or symptoms of acute psychosis. Upon arrival at the division clearing station, active psychiatric treatment begins. Sedation is given at once to those who have not already received it and they are placed in adequately heated tent wards, sleep on cots, and are given an abundance of hot food.

The psychiatrist combines an attitude of respect and sympathy for the patient yet he is also firm, decisive and realistic. He permits no doubt to arise in the patient's mind that he will not return to full combat duty after a brief rest. If the patient is allowed to ventilate his fears, hopes and resentments, prompt symptomatic relief often follows. Since loyalty and sense of duty to his comrades are among the most important supports of the soldier in combat, an effort is made to strengthen these forces. Motivations for rejoining his outfit and active duty are strengthened. An attempt is made to avoid any suggestion of illness in the organization and atmosphere of treatment stations and in the attitude and action of the psychiatrist. As much care is used to avoid suggestion of serious psychiatric illness as of physical disease.

Both at the battalion aid station and the division clearing station, in order to emphasize the precipitating role of physical exhaustion, to imply a rapid recovery after a brief rest and to avoid giving the impression of incurable mental illness, the term *exhaustion* is used for psychiatric casualities.

At one period in World War II, intravenous barbiturate narcosis was extensively used in severe anxiety states and in hysterical conversion reactions. During the narcosis, strong suggestion was used with resulting emotional release during which the patient relived his battle experiences. Few patients treated by this method recover to a degree that permits return to combat duty and it is now used in selected cases only.

The earliest possible return to duty prevents progress of the neurotic symptoms, minimizes secondary gain from their existence and has a desirable therapeutic value in lessening guilt over separation from the group.

Inasmuch as psychiatric patients in the combat area are easily convinced that they are seriously ill, either physically or psychiatrically, it is important that after proper physical examination they be assured that they have no serious physical illnesses, that the psychiatric disability is temporary, that it is a reaction to the situation in which the soldier has been placed, that it has no relationship to "insanity" and that there should be no permanent after-effects. It is explained to the soldier that his psychological and somatic symptoms are but a frequent and essentially normal result from battle fear.

Since a neurotic illness occurring in battle places the patient in a safe situation with possible permanent removal from combat, it is extremely important that the element of secondary gain be avoided so far as possible. If it is determined that a patient will not be returned to combat duty, he is informed of this decision and given reason to believe that it is final. The tension and pressure accompanying the anticipation of possible return to combat is thus eliminated together with a further unconscious striving for the secondary gains of the illness. Such a soldier should, however, be returned to some type of duty as soon as possible lest prolonged rest and inactivity in comfortable hospital surroundings provide opportunity for brooding, tend to fixate the neurosis and lead to demoralization and invalidism. Such measures should help to prevent permanent neuroses so many of which followed the combat neuroses occurring in World War I. While the psychiatrist must not be punitive the soldier's discharge from military serivce for psychiatric reasons should not be made too easy and attractive lest others become "infected" and develop similar disabilities. It should be remembered, too, that the burden of guilt that a soldier may assume if he is evacuated from combat for less than excellent reasons may be an intolerable thing which he may carry with him for the rest of his life and morbidly influence his personality or result in a neurosis. It should also be borne in mind that it is psychological mistreatment to evacuate a soldier who has not yet performed with the degree of honor required by his superego and by what he conceives to be the demands of his outfit.

BIBLIOGRAPHY

Adler, A.: Two different types of post-traumatic neuroses. Am. J. Psychiat., *102:*237–240, 1945.

Alexander, V. K.: A case study of a multiple personality. J. Abnorm. & Social Psychol., *52:*272–276, 1956.

Bartemeier, Leo, et al: Combat exhaustion. J. Nerv. & Ment. Dis., *104:*358–389; 489–525, 1946.

Beard, G. M.: A Practical Treatise on Nervous Exhaustion. New York, Wm. Wood & Co., 1880.

Berrington, W. P.; Liddell, D. W., and Foulds, G. A.: A re-evaluation of the fugue. J. Ment. Sc., *102:*280–286, 1956.

Bowman, K. M.: Modern concept of the neuroses. J.A.M.A., *132:*555, 1956.

———, and Rose, Milton: A criticism of the terms "psychosis," "psychoneurosis," and "neurosis." Am. J. Psychiat., *108:*161–166, 1951.

Breuer, Joseph, and Freud, Sigmund: Studies in Hysteria, Translated by A. A. Brill. Washington, Nervous and Mental Disease Pub. Co., 1937.
Brill, N. Q., and Beebe, G. W.: A follow-up study of war neuroses. V. A. Medical Monograph, Dept. Med. Surg., Washington, D. C., 1955.
Carter, A. B.: The prognosis of certain hysterical symptoms. Brit. M. J., *10:*76–79, 1949.
Cobb, Stanley: Emotions and Clinical Medicine. New York, W. W. Norton & Co., 1950.
DaCosta, J. M.: On irritable heart; a clinical study of a form of functional cardiac disease and its consequences. Am. J. M. Sc., *131:*2, Jan., 1871.
Darmstadter, M. J.: The superiority attitude and rigidity of ideas. Arch. Neurol. & Psychiat., *61:*621, 1949.
Diethelm, Oskar: Treatment in Psychiatry, 2nd ed. Springfield, Illinois, Charles C Thomas, 1950.
Engle, G. L.: Primary atypical facial neuralgia. Psychosom. Med., *13:*375–396, 1951.
English, O. S., and Pearson, M. J.: Common Neuroses of Children and Adults. New York, W. W. Norton & Co., 1937.
Fenichel, Otto: The Psychoanalytic Theory of Neurosis. New York, W. W. Norton & Co., 1945.
Fitzgerald, O. S. W.: Love deprivation and the hysterical personality. J. Ment. Sc., *94:*701, 1949.
Freud, S.: Collected Papers (4 Vols.). New York, The International Psychoanalytic Press, 1924.
———: The Ego and the Id. London, Hogarth Press, 1927.
———: The Basic Writings of Sigmund Freud. New York, Modern Library, 1938.
———: The Problems of Anxiety. New York, W. W. Norton & Co., 1936.
Glass, A. J.: Combat exhaustion. U. S. Armed Forces Med. J., *2:* No. 10, Oct., 1951.
———: Current problems in military psychiatry. J.A.M.A., *150:*6–9, 1952.
Grinker, R. R.: Treatment of war neuroses. J.A.M.A., *126:*142, 1944.
———, and Spiegel, J. P.: Men under Stress. Philadelphia, The Blakiston Co., 1945.
———: War Neuroses: Philadelphia, The Blakiston Co., 1945.
Huddleson, J. M.: Accidents, Neuroses and Compensation. Baltimore, Williams & Wilkins Co., 1932.
Janet, Pierre: The Major Symptoms of Hysteria, 2nd ed., New York, The Macmillan Company, 1920.
Kamman, G. R.: Traumatic neurosis, compensation neurosis or attitudinal pathosis? Arch. Neurol. & Psychiat., *65:*593, 1951.
Kennedy, Alexander: Recent hysterical states and their treatment. J. Ment. Sc., *86:* 988, 1940.
———, and Neville, Joseph: Sudden loss of memory. Brit. M. J., *5042:*428–433, 1957.
Kubie, L. S., and Margolin, S.: The therapeutic role of drugs in the process of repression, dissociation and synthesis. Psychosom. Med., *7:*147, 1945.
Laughlin, H. P.: The Neuroses in Clinical Practice. Philadelphia, W. B. Saunders Co., 1956.
Masserman, J. M.: The Practice of Dynamic Psychiatry. Philadelphia, W. B. Saunders Co., 1955.
———: Principles of Dynamic Psychiatry. Philadelphia, W. B. Saunders Co., 1946.
Menninger, W. C.: Modern concepts of war neuroses. Bull. Menninger Clin., *10:*196, 1946.
Michael, R. P.: Treatment of a case of compulsive swearing. Brit. M. J., *5034:*1506–1508, 1957.
Murray, J. M.: Psychiatric aspects of aviation medicine. Psychiatry, *7:*1, 1944.
Myerson, A.: Neuroses and neuropsychoses. Am. J. Psychiat., *93:*263, 1938.
Noble, D.: Hysterical manifestations in schizophrenic illness. Psychiatry, *14:*153–160, 1951.
———; Roudebush, M. E., and Price, D.: Studies of Korean war casualties. Am. J. Psychiat., *108:*495–499, 1952.
Ossipov, V. P.: Malingering; the stimulation of psychosis. Bull. Menninger Clin., *8:*39, 1944.

Palmer, H. A.: Psychobiological approach to acute anxiety attacks. J. Ment. Sc., *87:* 208, 1941.
Pollett, J.: Natural history of obsessional states. Brit. M. J., *1:*194–196, 1957.
Prince, Morton: Miss Beauchamp—the theory of the psychogeneses of multiple personality. J. Abnorm. Psychol., *15:*82–135, 1920.
———: The Dissociation of a Personality: A Biographical Study in Abnormal Psychology. New York, Longmans, Green & Co.
Purtell, J. J.; Robins, E., and Cohen, M. E.: Observations on clinical aspects of hysteria. J.A.M.A., *1946:*902–909, 1951.
Raines, G. N., and Kolb, L. C.: Combat fatigue and war neurosis. U. S. Nav. Med. Bull., 923–936 and 1299–1309, July, 1943.
Rennie, T. A. C.: Psychobiological therapy. Am. J. Psychiat., *97:*611, 1940.
Saul, L. J.: Emotional Maturity. Philadelphia, J. B. Lippincott Co., 1947.
Solomon, H. C., and Yakovlev, P. I.: Manual of Military Psychiatry. Philadelphia, W. B. Saunders Co., 1944.
Thigpen, C. B., and Cleckley, H. M.: The Three Faces of Eve. New York, McGraw-Hill Book Company, 1957.
Ulett, P. C., and Gildea, E. F.: Survey of surgical procedures in psychoneurotic women. J.A.M.A., *143:*960, 1950.
U. S. Army Medical Department, Bulletin of: Combat Psychiatry. Washington, U. S. Government Printing Office, 1949.
Ziegler, D. K., and Paul, N.: On the natural history of hysteria in women (a follow-up study twenty years after hospitalization). Dis. Nerv. System, *15:*301–309, 1954

CHAPTER XXXI

Personality Disorders

UNDER THE term *Personality Disorders* the Standard Nomenclature of the America Psychiatric Association includes those cases in which the personality, instead of utilizing symptoms expressed in mental, somatic or emotional terms in its efforts to secure adjustment, makes use of patterns of action or behavior. In some cases the nosological groupings are largely descriptive, in others the groupings are based on the dynamics of personality development. The personality disorders are characterized by defects in the development of the personality or by pathological trends in its structure. In these personality types the individual has little or no subjective sense of anxiety and is without the distress often seen in mental, emotional or psychophysiological reactions.

The personality disorders may be divided into three groups.

1. Disturbances of Personality Pattern. This group includes individuals in whom the personality structure shows a fixed, lifelong, seemingly inherent pattern. Individuals with such patterns lack the flexibility of personality necessary for a maximum of social adjustability.

2. Disturbances of Personality Traits. Persons in this group are characterized by an inability to maintain emotional equilibrium and independence. There seems to have been a disturbance in the development of the emotional component of the personality.

3. Sociopathic Personality Disturbances. In this are included many of the personality disorders formerly included under the term "psychopathic personality." The presenting manifestations are usually either those of social maladjustments or of deviations of sexual impulse.

Disturbances of Personality Pattern

In the first group the Standard Nomenclature recognizes four basic types of patterns.

Inadequate Personality

In spite of average educational and other opportunities and of normal intelligence as measured by psychometric tests, individuals of inadequate personality fail in emotional, economic, occupational and social adjustments. They are often good natured and easy going but are inept, ineffective and unconcerned. Their judgment is defective, they lack ambition and initiative and may be dreamy. They seem to lack physical and emotional stamina. When it is clear that effort would be rewarded they lack sufficient perseverance to achieve the results already in sight. The pleasure of the moment satisfies; they can neither work nor wait for deferred pleasure or reward. As a result they are improvident and shiftless. Many of the ne'er-do-wells belong in this group. They are defective in sense of responsibility to themselves and to society. They may have a certain sentimentality but have no real appreciation of cultural and esthetic values.

Schizoid Personality

The schizoid personality is characterized by certain inherent features, such as "shut-in-ness," emotional detachment and a tendency to autistic thinking. In many cases these characteristics do not interfere seriously with personality functioning but under stress become pathologically exaggerated as manifest schizophrenia. The characteristics of the schizoid personality are described at some length in Chapter III, Personality Development and Structure.

Cyclothymic Personality

The characteristic feature of the cyclothymic personality is a tendency to frequent variations of mood. The alternations of elation and sadness are usually stimulated by internal factors rather than by external events. Some individuals show not a fluctuation of mood, but either a persistent euphoria or a persistent depression. Individuals in whom accentuation of mood is a personality characteristic readily develop manic-depressive reactions. The characteristics of the cyclothymic personality are also described in Chapter III, Personality Development and Structure.

Paranoid Personality

Individuals who show great sensitivity in interpersonal relations and an exaggerated tendency to utilize projection mechanisms expressed in suspiciousness, jealousy, stubbornness and a tendency to misinterpret events are said to possess a paranoid type of personality. Under stress these paranoid propensities may become psychotic in degree. Characteristics of this type of personality are more fully described in Chapter XXVIII, Paranoid Reactions.

Disturbances of Personality Traits

Emotionally Unstable Personality

Individuals of this type of personality are characterized by the explosive intensity of their emotions in reaction to relatively slight external stimuli. Between their outbursts they are usually outgoing and friendly. happy and likable. Their relationship to other persons, however, is constantly subject to fluctuating emotional attitudes because of strong and poorly controlled hostility, guilt and anxiety. Their emotional tension is usually at a rather high pitch and may suddenly and unexpectedly burst out in uncontrolled anger or other disproportionate emotional display. At these times such persons may shout, bluster, threaten or even become destructive and assaultive. In some, the excitability may be manifested in outbursts of despair, sulky irritability or obstinate inaccessibility. Suicidal attempts in response to frustration or as an effort to relieve a situation regarded as intolerable are not rare. Jealousy and quarrels with those of the opposite sex are common. Far from being the desired evidence of vigor and strength of personality the outbursts of the excitable are often poorly concealed attempts to disguise an inherent weakness. Such reactions, characterized by fluctuating emotional attitudes, unstable and explosive feelings and undependable judgment, are to be regarded as expressions of an immaturity of personality.

Passive-Aggressive Personality

This is basically an immaturity reaction in which the failure to attain a mature emotional development of the personality is manifested in one of three ways:

PASSIVE-DEPENDENT TYPE. In this reaction there is a frank expression of an absence of mature self-confidence and self-reliance. The individual is overwhelmed by feelings of helplessness and indecision. He is irresponsible and childish and may cling to others as a dependent child to a supporting parent. He requires approval and assurance. The clinical picture may include anxiety manifestations. The passive-dependent husband may depend on his wife for all major decisions. Individuals of this type shun overt expression of aggression and withdraw from any situation likely to arouse hostility. They are passive, timid and fearful. An underlying hostility, covered by a rigid shell of timidity and passivity, is entirely unconscious.

PASSIVE-AGGRESSIVE TYPE. In this reaction the personality contains a considerable element of aggression, doubtless largely defensive in origin, but it is expressed by passive measures, such as sullenness, stubbornness, procrastination, inefficiency, and passive obstructions. Some persons of this type complain and are dissatisfied. They usually work poorly with others and may have a demoralizing effect on the group. Some have been fearful of or have shown a covert hostility to their fathers who often have been dominant, rigid, unapproachable, demanding and difficult to please.

AGGRESSIVE TYPE. In this type the oustanding manifestation is a persistent reaction to frustration with such immature measures as irritability, temper tantrums and even destructive behavior. Sometimes there is resentment of pathological degree. Many persons of this type are hostile, provocative, antagonistic, competitive and ambitious. They manifest a "chip-on-the-shoulder" attitude. They may be sharp and biting and aggressively resistant. They demand especial attention and assume unwarranted authority. Frequently they attempt to lure those in authority into long argumentative discussion. Grandiose fantasies are common. Earlier in their lives these persons have been openly hostile to their fathers. Below the surface a deep dependency can be discovered. The aggressiveness in this type is a reaction formation in origin.

Compulsive Personality

Individuals of an obsessive or compulsive personality are those whose superego functions are severe. They tend to be punctilious, rigid, fastidious, formal, meticulous, may be in constant doubt what to do and have to go over things again and again. They are overinhibited, perfectionistic, self-doubting, and are unable to carry on their work if under pressure. They lack a normal capacity for relaxation. They show a tendency to literal obedience, have an exaggerated sense of duty, are harrassed by their responsibilities and scrupulosities and cannot make decisions. If circumstances require a decision, regret is expressed for the choice which was made. The person of compulsive character is stubborn in his convictions and manifests a tendency to hair-splitting. In contrast to the suggestible, demonstrative, extraverted personality of the hysteric, he is likely to be of a daydreaming, introverted, self-centered type. The compliance and "correct" behavior of the compulsive personality are frequently defenses against hostile impulses.

If relatively free from anxiety, the existence in the personality of a certain degree of obsessive compulsive drive and persistence adds a desirable quality. Compulsive personality traits are within the range of normal personality variants as distinguished from symptoms of a compulsion neurosis which are pathological exaggerations of such variants. Such traits impart a desire to succeed; the compulsive person, too, is a hard worker. A degree of compulsiveness adds to strength of character. The difference between a compulsive personality and a compulsive neurosis is therefore one of degree, of the amount of anxiety present and of the extent to which the personality habitually defends itself against chronic anxieties by ritualistic devices. The origin of the compulsive personality, like that of the obsessive compulsive neurosis, is to be found in an investigation of childhood factors which played a role in character formation. Frequently the traits are safeguards against hostile impulses, unconscious aggression and accompanying guilt. Not rarely the chronic tension of the compulsive personality may as a result of stress lead to an obsessive compulsive neurosis.

The third group of personality disorders in which the personality disturbances are sociopathic is so large and so important from a social standpoint that a special chapter will be devoted to its discussion.

BIBLIOGRAPHY

Menninger, K. A.: Manual for Psychiatric Case Study. New York, Grune & Stratton, Inc., 1952.

Plazak, D. J.: Dynamic factors in psychiatric discharges of midshipmen. U. S. Armed Forces Jour. *8*:418–426, 1957.

Whitman, R. M.; Trosman, Harry; and Koenig, Richard: Clinical assessment of passive-aggressive personality. Arch. Neurol. & Psychiat., *72*:540–549, 1954.

CHAPTER XXXII

Sociopathic Personality Disturbances

Definition

In this category are included those disorders of personality which have usually been grouped under such terms as "psychopathic personality" or "constitutional psychopathic state." The term can scarcely be defined with scientific accuracy yet it is a useful one to apply to various defects and deviations in the personality structure of individuals who are unable to make acceptable and successful adjustment to the prevailing social and cultural milieu.

Neither the clinical characteristics nor the clinical limits of these personality maldevelopments are sharply defined. The character and behavior disorders displayed by sociopathic personalities lie in the wide zone between mental health and mental disease and are manifested by continuous or repeatedly recurrent maladjustments that lack the symptomatic features traditionally considered distinctive of neuroses or psychoses. Although widely used for this group of personality disorders and having a certain dynamic justification for its employment, the term *neurotic characters* is not, because of its moral connotations, altogether desirable. Psychiatric custom perhaps permits the use of the term "psychopaths" in referring to individuals who persistently show the disturbances of personality under consideration, yet it does not suggest the concept, increasingly accepted, that internal needs evoke their disturbed behavior.

Until relatively recently these personality disorders were considered at a superficial, descriptive level. Now, however, it has been generally accepted that, like the neuroses and those psychoses in which there is no apparent physical cause or structural brain change, they are psychogenetically and dynamically determined. Indeed the borderline between the behavior of the so-called psychopath on the one hand and the deviant behavior interpreted as mental illness on the other is not always clearly defined. Frequently the behavior of the psychopath is antisocial but it must not be concluded that antisocial behavior is *ipso facto* psychopathic, nor should behavior be so regarded merely because it is "different" or delinquent. Most psychiatrists now consider that the basic feature of the behavior manifested by the sociopathic personality is the unconscious psychodynamic process. Some of the presumed, yet speculative, psychopathological processes that lead to the social maladjustments of the psychopath will be discussed later in this chapter.

The clinical manifestations of the pathological personality are usually expressed in social maladjustments or in the psychosexual sphere in the form of deviations of sexual impulse. As has been intimated, however, the term pathological or sociopathic personality should not be applied to all individuals showing habitual delinquency or criminal tendencies. There are many recidivists who are not psychopaths and many pathological personalities who do not come into conflict with the law.

It was formerly believed that the unmodifiable behavior patterns of such persons were matters of inborn disposition, were constitutionally influenced or directed. Such diagnostic terms as constitutional psychopathic inferior were therefore applied to persons showing recurrent patterns of sociopathic behavior. Probably the so-called constitutional factors are really emotional, psychological ones experienced very early in life and their resulting behavior becomes early so structuralized as to appear to be constitutional. Not only has the assumption of a constitutional basis failed to yield any understanding of the behavior of such persons but it is only logical that although their motivations are doubtless complex yet sociopathic behavior disturbances should, nevertheless, be susceptible of explanation by theories which are at least analogous to those that have been so fruitful in rendering other personality disorders intelligible. In the neuroses and psychoses, the psychopathologically dynamic forces find expression in the psychological field; in psychosomatic or psychophysiological disorder they find physiological expression in the somatic symptom; in the sociopathic personality these forces are expressed not in psychological or in somatic but in the social field. Like the sypmtoms of the neurotic or the psychosomatic patient, the behavior of the psychopath presumably has its psychogenesis and its psychopathology. In some instances his behavior may be the result of frustration in his efforts to achieve a satisfaction of such fundamental needs as love, security, recognition, respect and success. The child who was rejected may react by becoming resentful, rebellious and antisocial. In early years he may be the difficult child, in adolescence the delinquent and in later life the criminal. Punishment, instead of improving his condition, often makes him worse by increasing his resentment and sense of grievance. Absence or loss of constructive identifications may collaborate with other factors. In dealing with delinquency of late childhood and adolescence it is often found that one of the most effective corrective measures is a warm, authoritative father figure with whom boys can identify. Being dynamically, and therefore not consciously, determined the behavior of the psychopath appears irrational. While much of his behavior can be included within the framework of the neuroses, in other instances it can perhaps best be regarded as the expression of an arrested or deviated development of personality. In either case, whether the psychopath's behavior represents a character neurosis or a developmental fault in the process of personality maturation it denotes the continuing activity of psychopathological forces set in motion by very early emotional—usually or always interpersonal—experiences. The behavior of the psychopath is therefore not so much a matter of "free will" as criminal law would have us believe. The persisting drive or reaction to deviated sexual impulse, to aggression, anxiety, rejection, frustration or other psychopathology-creating factors presumably accounts for the apparently compulsive chronicity of the psychopath's behavior. It is increasingly accepted that the behavior of the pathological personality is produced by unconscious forces which are never adequately gratified by his act and therefore it becomes stereotyped and repetitive. At any rate the psychopathology becomes organized into behavior and character patterns. The neurosis becomes woven into the character.

General Psychopathic Characteristics

Even in childhood the future pathological personality usually shows signs of emotional maladjustment and unwholesome personality traits. Typically, he is characterized by an emotional immaturity reflected by his impulsive and instant response to his feelings. His personality seems to be dominated by primitive basic drives to the exclusion of rational behavior. Certain lines of conduct, particularly of a socialized nature, are never learned. Some of these children are sensitive, stubborn, given to tantrums or to outbursts of rage, and frequently these preadolescent psychopaths steal, run away, suffer from enuresis, are destructive, quarrelsome, sulky, deceitful, obstinate, defiant, boastful, shameless and erratic. Antagonism or open rebellion against a dominating parent may be shown. The adolescent resists the ideals and mores of his family and tends to socialize at a lower level. With approaching maturity and the weakening of the restraining forces of the home and with the increase of responsibilities and of environmental contacts and demands, the earlier tendencies become outspoken manifestations. The psychopath lacks a conscience, the result, possibly, of an emotional deprivation in childhood which made it impossible to identify himself with any parental figure. Emotional and personality development lags. Many psychopaths while not intellectually deficient seem emotionally such. They therefore lack keenness and delicacy of sentiment. The psychopath is typically affectionless, selfish, ungrateful, narcissistic and exhibitionistic. He is egocentric, demanding much and giving little. His excess of demand is in fact one of the outstanding characteristics. He has no critical awareness of his motives and lacks foresight and discriminating, reflective judgment. He is unable to judge his own behavior from another's standpoint. In spite of the fact that his conduct is so inadequate or so hostile from a social standpoint the psychopath is satisfied with it. He shows few feelings of anxiety, guilt or of remorse and is unable to profit either from experience or punishment. He lacks definiteness of objective, and his usual state of restlessness may result from a search for the unattainable. Occupational application and efficiency are usually faulty; routine is intolerably irksome. The psychopath lacks purpose, aim and foresight, is deficient in sense of responsibility and lives for the moment. He demands immediate and instant gratification of his desires with no concern as to the feelings and interests of others with whom he forms few emotional relationships or stable affectional ties. He does not, either, build up a sense of social values as normally should occur through the process of identification. As a result such a sense is frequently distorted. The demands of instinct are not adjusted to the demands of society. He is often plausible and talkative but absolutely unreliable. Frequently the only environment to which he can adjust is the one which he can dominate. Surprising irregularities of ability and inconsistencies of behavior are constantly demonstrated. A certain number escape from a difficult situation by way of a psychotic episode, while others at the slightest stress resort to alcohol or drugs. Many psychopaths bear alcohol poorly and under its influence become noisy, quarrelsome and destructive. The sociopathic personality lacks regard for the rights of others and is unable empathically to re-experience situations or to feel himself into the social group. He projects his own insecurity by blaming others. Frequently he so rationalizes his behavior that superficially it appears warranted, reasonable and justified. Whether or not it is antisocial it is usually so defective that it prevents a proper psychosocial adjustment, and ranges from "queerness" to criminality, with a large intermediate group made up of cranks, extremists, eccentrics, habitual delinquents and other social misfits.

Sometimes one sibling in a family may manifest the behavior and personality characteristic usually associated with the sociopathic personality while other siblings may present mature and well-adjusted personalities. Presumably this difference in personality characteristics is because of the fact that the effect of a particular emotional experience or social influence in the family was highly specific to the individual.

Classification

A classification of sociopathic personalities can perhaps be best based on a descriptive grouping. When we consider the various factors, biological, psychobiological, emotional, social, innate and experiential, that contribute to the personality structure, and remember the numerous ways in which its development may be arrested or warped, we realize that the resulting sociopathic adjustments may be of various types. Although largely descriptive instead of dynamic, the general clinical manifestations of these adjustments seem at this time to be the most convenient basis of classification. The extent to which aggressive-destructive and other dynamic impulses may be acted out in sociopathic form before labeling the personality as pathological is a matter of individual opinion and not determined by definite criteria. Likewise there are no fixed types determined by cause, dynamic process or result so that any classification depends upon what manifestations one wishes to stress. Mention will be made of only those in whom certain characteristics stand out most clearly. They are not, of course, diagnostic entities.

The Antisocial Personality

These sociopathic individuals show a moral and ethical blunting, a lack of sympathy for their fellow men and a behavior destructive to the welfare of the social order. As children they are often self-willed, play truant, commit petty thefts, are cruel and untruthful, and as they grow older they may be inaccessible, boorish and without sense of responsibility. Their emotional life is superficial and affectively cold. They seem incapable of mature emotional relationships. They cannot organize an acceptable, constructive expression of their aggressions. They lack ambition, application, seriousness of purpose and foresight. They are irritable, arrogant, unyielding, characterized by a brutal egoism and rarely feel remorse for their most serious offenses against person or property. Frequently they show a rebellious attitude toward authority and society. Changes in mood are sudden and often without apparent cause. They are cynical, devoid of a sense of honor or of shame and are lacking in sympathy, affection, gratitude and other social and esthetic sentiments. When frustrated they may be dangerous to others. Their offenses may constitute the whole register of crime—theft, embezzlement, forgery, robbery, brutal sex attacks and other acts of violence. Many take pleasure in their struggle with the law and feel pride in their accomplishments. They are unable to identify themselves with society and its laws. Punishments are considered as expressions of injustice and have no deterrent effect. At times psychopathic, criminal behavior seems to develop out of a sense of guilt. In such a case the individual finds his unconscious guilt feelings so unbearable that he commits a crime to find relief by being punished. Frequently the sociopsychopath possesses a remarkable ability to rationalize his behavior so that it appears warranted, reasonable and justified.

Merely to indicate the wide variety of behavior patterns which the antisocial personality may manifest, a description will be given of a group formerly characterized as pathological liars and swindlers. In this group are egocentric individuals whose social maladaptation consists of extravagant, often apparently purposeless lying, frequently combined with swindling. They exhibit a marked excitability of imagination combined with an instability of purpose. They are usually good-natured, of agreeable manners, optimistic, of a lighthearted geniality, and make social contacts easily. A glibness of tongue, an unusual aptitude for the use of language, a self-confident manner, a frequently assumed dignity and a misleading appearance of knowledge readily enable them to convince the credulous as to their statements. They acquire a smattering of art, literature or technical parlance which they employ to their own profit and to the expense and humiliation of their victims. They spin remarkable tales concerning past experiences and paint their future with a careless disregard for reality. Some are guilty of sex offenses and others obtain large sums of money under promise of marriage. When discovered in their delinquencies, they profess amnesia, and if charged with offense they often stage an emotionally affected exhibition designed to impress observers and arouse sympathy. They are restless and unstable, and are incapable of exertion or responsibility. They never learn to meet the struggle for existence with industry and perseverance but live in a world of imagination and seek to acquire the necessities of life by deceit and fraud. They are unable to accept the limitations of reality. Their theatrical imitation, their tendency to daydream, to boast, to avoid realities and to surround themselves with an imaginary world suggest a childish immaturity of personality, while their wish-fulfilling fabrications have much in common with the fantasy of childhood. Many times their flagrant lying is defensive in purpose. On a less conscious level is the extravagant and often apparently purposeless romancing known as *pseudologia phantastica.* This egregious disregard of the truth seems to result from a pressing need to indulge in extravagant castle-building in order to make up for a reality that appears to be too onerous or prosaic. While the content of the fantasy is generated by unconscious forces, the patient is not entirely aware that his statement is a fabrication. His unusually rich imagination stirred into active expression by acute emotional needs enables the patient to live in a dream world. Psychometric tests usually disclose a normal or superior intellectual capacity, but as with other psychopaths, intelligence has little regulating influence on behavior. At times it would appear that such personality characteristics grow out of a feeling of inferiority, envy or jealousy.

Theoretical discussion concerning the general psychopathology of the sociopathic personality will be presented shortly. Much of this discussion is applicable to the antisocial personality as well as to other sociopathic personality disturbances. It should be remembered that in all such disturbances, including the antisocial personality, the genetic and dynamic determinants are specific to the individual. Generally speaking, the behavior of the antisocial personality represents a fear and rebellion against society or authority which may be traced to unhappiness, hostility or neglect experienced in childhood. Emotional reactions in childhood may have been seriously affected by one or both sadistic and dominating parents. It should not be forgotten, however, that the home and the cultural environment may have been such as not to offer constructive social identifications.

Psychopathology of Sociopathic Personality

It should not be assumed that all delinquents and criminals, even those guilty of repeated offenses, should be looked upon as pathological personalities. Defects of character may be a result of the cultural, economic and social forces of the environment. It may be debatable as to whether or not antisocial behavior resulting from failure or to lack of opportunity for establishing identifications necessary for the creation of a strong and socialized superego should be regarded as that of a pathological personality. The authors would not regard behavior that merely results from defective and inadequate superego formation as evidence of a pathological personality. Usually, it must be said, there is a failure in both ego and superego maturation but the criterion of psychopathic behavior should be its motivation through unconscious forces, evidence of which the psychiatrist constantly observes. He repeatedly discovers such unconscious drives as hostility, guilt, revenge, frustration, feelings of inferiority and infantile fixations as the source of motivations. The projective psychological techniques may yield significant information concerning personality structure and underlying psychopathology as well as reveal the areas around which the patient's major problems revolve.

Perhaps a little clearer conception of the psychopathology of the sociopathic personality can be secured if we examine some of the methods by which unconscious feelings, desires and other unacceptable content are dealt with. In the "normal" person such material is controlled without tension or is successfully repressed. In the neurotic person these feelings, impulses and wishes give rise to anxiety which is handled symbolically by compulsive or other defensive means which are known as neurotic. If the anxiety produced by these feelings and impulses is channeled through the vegetative nervous system, the patient suffers from psychosomatic, psychophysiological symptoms. In the pathological personality his unconscious feelings and drives and even, in some cases, his defenses are built into his character structure and "acted out" in "psychopathic," often sociopathic, behavior. We see therefore that we may conceive of there being several different ways of dealing with the same problem and its associated anxiety.

A comparison of neurotic behavior and psychopathic behavior is perhaps elucidating. One may, for example, contrast *symptom neurosis* versus *character neurosis.* In the latter, one may with a certain justification, speak of the neurotic pattern as being asocial or antisocial; the psychopathology is expressed not in neurotic symptoms but in social behavior. In the psychoneurotic his compulsive or other defensive symptom alleviates an anxiety which would otherwise be distressing, whereas the character neurotic perceives little, if any, anxiety or distress but in an uninhibited manner he irrationally acts out hostility, aggressiveness or other unconscious feelings, desires and impulses. The psychopath acts out impulses of the source of which he is unaware. The neurotic may have similar impulses which have stemmed from the same pathogenetic source or experience but he deals with them by neurotic mechanisms rather than by giving overt expression to them. Much behavior, the reason for which is not obvious, represents the patient's way of dealing with anxiety—perhaps the only way he has learned to deal with it. According to this concept the psychopath's anxiety rises to a certain pitch when he seeks relief through an antisocial act. Another analogy between symptom neurosis and character neurosis is perhaps permissible. It is known that the manifest meaning of the neurotic's symptom is not the real meaning. Likewise the real meaning of the character neurotic's behavior is usually not to be found in its apparent purpose but in some objective stimulated by the scars of an emotional experience in early childhood. Frequently, therefore, his act is a symbolic one motivated by some early traumatic experience. In his behavior the patient may, for example, be acting out his feelings toward a parent or other significant person in his environment.

Many pathological personalities are persons whose emotional conflicts of childhood and youth were left unresolved. Later, therefore, they continue to seek an emotional expression or outlet to them. The psychopath accordingly goes through later life unconsciously creating situations whereby he can act out his earlier unexpressed feelings. Since, too, the emotional factors that have led to his behavior remain unchanged, his behavior is not modified. He accordingly appears to others as not learning by experience. He is impelled by unconscious compulsive drives demanding a gratification that is insatiable.

Another feature to be noted at times in the pathological personality or character neurosis is worthy of attention. We know that in the psychoneurotic his symptom—a compulsion, perhaps—provides a primary gain by relieving the anxiety. This may be the sole gain afforded by the neurosis. In the case of the psychopath, his uninhibited behavior, *e.g.*, a pathological aggressiveness, relieves the threat of any anxiety and thereby provides an internal, neurotic or primary gain. Should, however, the aggressive behavior yield also some material gain (*e.g.*, psychopathic behavior in the form of a compulsive tendency to steal), this gain constitutes also a secondary one. Sometimes, therefore, but not always, the psychopathic behavior yields an important secondary gain. Mixed clinical pictures in which neurotic and psychopathic features are intermingled are not unusual. Another characteristic of psychopathological behavior is the fact that the drive or motivation behind it is intense and forceful. The immediate urges are stronger than any rational considerations. The pathological personality who repeatedly commits some antisocial act appreciates intellectually that he will doubtless be caught and if so will face severe punishment. His need for his customary anxiety-relieving means impels, nevertheless, the compulsive continuance of his behavior. He may make a genuine effort to "go straight" and yet find his efforts futile in the face of strong, unconscious forces. At times this may be the result of a vicious circle. His dynamically motivated aggressiveness, for example, may generate anxiety and his anxiety, in turn, generate antisocial aggressiveness. While from a psychopathological standpoint the sociopathic personality may be looked upon as not responsible for his conduct, from a legal point of view he is regarded in American courts as accountable for any violations of the legal code.

To summarize the preceding statements, it may said that while they are scarcely susceptible of proof, and may be controversial, yet it is fruitful to approach the study of the personality under consideration in the same manner as that of the neurotic, psychotic or psychophysiologic. It seems logical to assume that the socially deviant, maladjusted personality with which we associate the term pathological or sociopathic should be formed through psychopathological processes or dynamisms. It may be that the pathological personality merely expresses his anxiety in a different way and is therefore differently labeled. His behavior has the structure and function of a symptom. It has its origin in conflict and serves as a way of meeting or of covering up a conflict. Like a symptom, its motivation is unconscious, or at best only vaguely sensed by the patient. Approached from this point of view much adolescent delinquency should be regarded as a symptom of an underlying personality disorder, not as a disorder in itself. The psychogenic factor may often be acted out in such insidious and covert ways that their existence is not apparent. Neurotic features, for example, are often hidden behind a wall of hostility. The fact that psychogenic factors are not obvious is in no sense proof of their absence. An endeavor is made, however, to secure a psychological understanding of the processes that result in such sociopathic behavior rather than to attribute it to some inherent constitutional factor or to pathological functioning of the brain.

In this respect concurrent studies of children exhibiting antisocial activity and of their parents provide new insights both into the form of deviant behavior adopted by the child and its impulsion for gratification. Szurek and Johnson have found that the more important parent, usually the mother, has unconsciously encouraged the amoral or antisocial behavior in the child. Although the parent verbally protests such behavior both to the child and to others, yet it is accepted, either unconsciously or with a guilty permissiveness, by the parent. The permissiveness has appeared to gratify vicariously neurotic needs of the parent which derive from her own lack of current satisfactions or unmet needs of childhood, or both. Since the parent's permissiveness is uncertain and incomplete the child, and later the adult, is inconsistent and confused. Healthy discipline is not administered by such a parent—discipline combining firm prohibition with reward for socially acceptable behavior. Through his own overt acts, inconsistencies, innuendoes in speech or by various nonverbal means of communication, the child has been found to recognize the partial permissiveness. But since the child is both partially gratified and encouraged in his action and partially frustrated by the parent, there are associated with the act feelings of hostility toward the parent and perhaps of guilt. In instances where this variety of family interaction exists, the antisocial behavior is fixed unless the several participating persons can be brought to understand and modify their behavior or they are completely separated.

Treatment

One must not oversimplify the factors that have determined the behavior of the sociopathic personality. It should be borne in mind, too, that the dividing line between normal psychology and psychopathology is not at all definitely drawn. Here as elsewhere in nature there are no discontinuities. Frequently environmental factors as well as inner psychic pressures have been operative. Internal ones, too, are frequently multiple and interacting. Pernicious social and cultural influences may contribute to the creation of the sociopathic personality although they do not serve as the basic genetic agents. Often there is an interplay between psychological and social factors. If environmental influences are contributory, either their modification or the patient's removal from them is desirable if possible. Since, however, the psychopath's behavior is presumably the result of psychopathological processes, one seeks to ascertain their origin and their manner of operation, to retrace the psychological steps, often devious, from the behavior manifestation to its antecedents and etiology. The patient himself is almost invariably unable to comprehend the reasons for his actions since he is unaware of the mechanisms responsible for his behavior. It is the hope of the therapist that under his guidance and the use of psychoanalytical principles the patient may become able to discover and relate past conflicts with present recurrent asocial or antisocial patterns of behavior, and that in the light of this knowledge he may construct socialized, flexible and adapted patterns. Many psychiatrists believe that orthodox psychoanalysis is not feasible with the psychopath. They prefer techniques related to psychoanalysis, such as free associations, dream analysis, word associations and the interpretation of Rorschach and thematic apperception tests. Unfortunately psychotherapy is all too often not successful in correcting the neurotic processes that have led to the sociopathic behavior. There are many reasons for the failure. Frequently the patient is not convinced that he needs psychiatric help. He will then not confide in or co-operate with the psychiatrist sufficiently to permit successful therapy. He is often resistant to the interpersonal influence of psychotherapy. This is particularly so when the deviant behavior has its origins in the family interactions described by Szurek and Johnson. For treatment to succeed, in most instances the parent of the patient must be treated as well or, in the case of a child or young adult, separated during the course of psychotherapy. Such separations are resisted by parents whose major gratification comes from their dependent relations with the "scapegoat" child. In some instances separation of the patient from the parent or change in the behavior of the patient during treatment has led to serious behavior disturbance in the symbiotic parent.

Sometimes the patterned response to pathogenetic factors is so fixed that it is not modifiable. Again the patient seems to lack capacity to experience anxiety with its resulting desire for relief. The hostility, too, often shown by the psychopath may generate hostility in others and hamper treatment. Sometimes a secondary gain from his neurotic-like symptom neutralizes any wish for a change in his behavior. A prison environment is a handicap to therapy. If the sociopsychopath's behavior brings him before court, the judge may be aware that ideally the treatment of the prisoner's behavior is by psychotherapy through which its psychogenesis may be traced and its pathology cured. Like the psychiatrist he may realize that punishment without recognition of the prisoner's emotional problems may intensify his social maladjustment. On the other hand a person cannot be sentenced to therapy.

Frequently the psychiatrist is confronted in the case of the sociopsychopath with the question of criminal responsibility. At such a time he must not be preoccupied exclusively with psychopathological criteria. He must, in view of his obligations to society as well as to the patient, consider also clinical and prognostic criteria. As a scientific psychiatrist, he should seek to ascertain if the criminal behavior is susceptible of psychopathological interpretation but he should also remember that it is not easy to prove or disprove such interpretations, that society cannot yet evaluate them and that it cannot yet, and perhaps should not, establish them as criteria of responsibility.

Situation Psychoses

If, according to the view expressed, the maladaptation of the sociopathic personality is fundamentally an attempted solution of the individual's problems rather than the result of unwholesome social influences, we should expect a higher incidence of psychotic reactions among these poorly integrated individuals than among well adjusted persons. This assumption is found to be true. The great majority of such reactions are schizophrenic, affective or paranoid but some, occurring under circumstances involving great emotional distress, represent attempts, through disorders of belief or of sensorium, to escape from the hard and uncompromising reality of some specific, difficult situation and are therefore called "situation psychoses." Frequently situation psychoses are in the nature of confused states, paranoid episodes, or of periods of irritability, excitement or depression.

Prison Psychoses

Since the most difficult situation into which the behavior of the sociopath usually leads him is confinement, which he bears poorly, the most important of the situation psychoses are the prison psychoses. It must not be concluded that all psychoses developing among prisoners belong to this group; in fact but a minority of them belong to the true prison psychoses. In them delusional ideas tend to be ideas of persecution, innocence or pardon. A majority of the psychotic reactions observed among prisoners are of the usual clinical types, especially schizophrenia and paranoid states, the stress of imprisonment acting merely as the releasing agent.

True prison psychoses that begin after the prisoner has received sentence are most likely to occur among long-term prisoners and comparatively early during the period for which they are sentenced. The forms assumed by the psychotic reactions are various. Occasional forms are sudden excitements manifested by intense emotion, violent rage, cursing and destructive attacks on the environment. Such attacks, usually brief, may, psychologically, represent a protest against an intolerable situation. Episodes characterized by delusions of persecution, ideas of strange influences, olfactory hallucinations of gas, or by anxiety, irritability and uneasiness are not uncommon. Manic-depressive reactions rarely develop among persons held under indictment or sentence and some psychiatrists of extensive experience report that they have never seen this form of psychosis in the case of life prisoners.

There are two forms especially typical of true prison psychoses. One, expressing a deep-seated dissatisfaction, is characterized by querulousness. Patients suffering from this form have numerous delusions of ill treatment. They constantly grumble and maintain that all sorts of obstacles are placed in their way and that attempts are being made to annoy them. Frequently their complaints sound plausible.

One of the most frequent forms of true prison psychoses found among long-term prisoners is that characterized by delusions of innocence or of pardon. The patient may experience auditory hallucinations wherein he is told that he has been exonerated from his alleged crime and is now to be liberated. Other, but similar, wish-fulfilling ideas are heard. As the patient believes himself an innocent and unjustly persecuted individual he becomes bitter toward those who fail to set him at liberty.

Most of the acute prison psychoses recover after transfer from prison to hospital where the general attitude is treatment rather than the maintenance of fixed and rigid discipline. Many life prisoners thus transferred fail to recover but gradually deteriorate mentally. One of the most important elements in the treatment of the prison psychoses is to render the patient's points of contact as little irritating as possible. Occupation, games, amusements and a friendly although necessarily firm attitude are helpful.

GANSER SYNDROME. An interesting type of mental disorder sometimes occurring in the case of prisoners under detention awaiting trial was described by Ganser. It develops only after commission of a crime and, therefore, tells nothing about the patient's mental state when he committed the offense. In this syndrome the patient, being under charges from which he would be exonerated were he irresponsible, begins, without being aware of the fact, to appear irresponsible. He appears stupid and unable to comprehend questions or instructions accurately. His replies are vaguely relevant to the query but absurd in content. He performs various uncomplicated, familiar tasks in an absurd manner, or gives approximate replies to simple questions. The patient, for example, may attempt to write with the blunt end of his pencil or will give 11 as the product of 4 x 3. The purpose of the patient's behavior is so obviously to appear irresponsible that the inexperienced observer frequently believes that he is malingering. The dynamics is probably that of a dissociative process. At the conscious level there is an amnesia for the offense yet the nature of the symptoms suggests an unconscious knowledge of it. Bearing in mind its psychological purpose, it will be seen that the appearance of a pseudo dementia in an accused but as yet unconvicted person is equivalent to a confession. It should be distinguished from malingering in which there is a deliberate, consciously motivated and sustained simulation of symptoms. Simulated symptoms are usually of exaggerated intensity.

Sexual Deviation

Persons whose biological sex urges are directed toward a normal heterosexual goal but who, because they are segregated from those of the opposite sex, casually seek sex satisfaction through various perversions are scarcely to be considered as sexual deviates.[1] In the true deviate the offending sexual act is the surface symptom of a more profound personality disturbance.

While some of the current psychiatric theories concerning homosexuality and other nonbiologically directed sex drives will be presented it, must be admitted that established facts concerning sexual psychopathy are few. Although lawmakers and courts look to the psychiatrist for information as to its etiology and for guidance in its treatment, he cannot yet answer these questions to the full satisfaction either of these agencies or of himself. It is a subject now receiving both psychiatric and social research.

In the opinion of many psychiatrists, the term sexual psychopath, or deviate, should be limited to the individual whose sexual impulse through defects in the step-by-step development of personality has either remained immature or has undergone deviation in the course of its maturation. The arrest or deviation in development is not, of course, in the anatomy or physiology of sex organs but in the psychosexual, *i.e.*, the emotional, dispositional aspect of sex expression. Psychosexual maturation may lag behind biological maturation or be so blocked that normal, mature heterosexual impulses are not established. The emotional and instinctive aspects of sex are not harmoniously integrated into the total personality. Satisfaction of the sex impulse is therefore sought through such expressions as voyeurism, exhibitionism, homosexuality, rape, pedophilia, masochism, sadism and other means. It must not be assumed that the biologically and culturally undesirable behavior of the paraphiliac is merely a matter of being "oversexed." Very few psychiatrists, moreover, regard the deviant behavior of the sexual psychopath as "constitutional" in origin. It has already been seen that neurotic, psychotic and other disturbed personality reactions can best be understood if approached from a genetic point of view. Likewise, it seems, the application of the same method will be most fruitful in shedding light on sexual abnormalities and offenses. In Chapter II, Personality Development and Structure, attention was called to the fact that there is a progressive, sequential maturation of the personality including its psychosexual aspect. Certain instinctive sex expressions are therefore normal and to be expected in the earlier stages of the individual's development. Sometimes, however, these infantile or immature expressions instead of being successfully modified or repressed may continue or re-emerge. It is normal, for example, for the small child at one stage of his development to secure pleasure in looking at or exhibiting sexual organs. If such infantile habits continue instead of attaining a normal heterosexual drive and expression, the individual remains or becomes a

[1] "It is said that only a small proportion of males convicted of sex offenses have been involved in behavior which is materially different than that of most males in the population. This small group, which numbers in the neighborhood of 5 to 10 per cent, is that which engages our attention as psychiatrists. They are hereinafter designated as psychiatrically deviated sex offenders." Group for the Advancement of Psychiatry, Report No. 9: Psychiatrically Deviated Sex Offenders.

voyeur or exhibitionist. Again, these or other infantile sexual expressions may have been apparently repressed or outgrown but when in adolescence the physiological forces that normally establish sexual maturity begin to exert their influence, the infantile sexual expressions may be reactivated and overtly manifested. The individual is then regarded as a sex delinquent. Whether or not the psychosexual maturation proceeds in an orderly and uninterrupted manner depends upon the individual's environment and his critical experiences during the formative period of his personality. If environmental conditions are not favorable to a normal psychosexual development or if he is seduced before psychosexual maturity has been reached, the seduction may block the establishment of normal heterosexual impulses. Again, the boy may have been tied to his mother so long and so intimately that early conflicting identifications have been established or the psychosexual developmental process is blocked and his preferred sexual expression is homosexual. It therefore seems that in the delayed and faulty development of instinctual demands, in the fixations and probably in the conditionings that occur in the individual's psychosexual maturation, are to be found the psychodynamics of many of the adult's sexual aberrations. The emotional and instinctive aspects of sex do not attain full and biologically useful integration in the total personality.

In some persons of *homosexual* tendencies it appears as if sex differentiation was never biologically completed. While developing the genitalia peculiar to one or the other sex, physical anomalies, such as body conformation, or hair distribution of a type indicative of the opposite sex, indicate the failure of the organism to attain complete monosexual differentiation. In such persons there seems to be a similar failure of differentiation in the biopsychic sphere resulting in mixed and opposing impulses, the satisfaction of which is sought by homosexual practices. Such perversions may be considered as a result of innate factors, perhaps of unusual heredity combinations leading to a near equilibrium of male and female genes. In most cases, however, there is no suggestion of incomplete anatomical differentiation through endocrine imbalance or other discoverable physical basis. The arrest is not in biological but in psychosexual maturation. On the whole, and perhaps in every respect, homosexuality is of genetic-psychological origin. In many cases there seems to be a reluctance or failure to leave behind the prepubertal homosexual stage of psychosexual development. This is particularly true when defective parent-child relationships interfere with identification mechanisms. For a normal psychosexual development a child should form a wholesome identification with the parent of the same sex. If the identification is with the parent of the opposite sex homosexual tendencies may be established. Such an identification may occur if the parent of the same sex is hated, feared, ineffectual or entirely absent. But even in such instances, overt homosexual behavior will be avoided unless such acting-out is initiated through disguised parental permissiveness or inhibitions are overcome through the use of alcohol, after cerebral lesions or under the stresses of heterosexual deprivation and homosexual license. The statement, sometimes made, that all homosexuality is caused by a failure to resolve the Oedipus complex is, however, probably not justified.

Pedophilia, or a pathological sexual interest in children, is regarded as a variant of homosexuality in which homosexual strivings are directed toward children. It occurs largely in weak and impotent persons. The pedophile acts toward the child as he unconsciously wished his mother to behave toward himself. Another, and perhaps more logical, explanation of the pedophile's behavior is that he functions on an immature psychosexual level because of his fearfulness and doubt concerning himself. As a result of these feelings, he expects rejection and failure in adult, heterosexual advances. His sexual expression is therefore released toward children.

Fetishism is a perversion peculiar to men. The fetishist is unable to love a real person but becomes attached to some material object having a feminine association, such as a lock of hair or an undergarment. This object attains a highly exaggerated value and becomes a special source of erotic gratification, a reliever of both psychic and sexual tension. The fetish always has a genital meaning and in the opinion of some psychiatrists serves the purpose of denying the anatomical difference between the two sexes, a discovery of which caused an overwhelming genital fear.

Another deviation is that of *transvestism,* a morbid impulse to dress in the clothing of the opposite sex. Formulations of the psychopathology of fetishism and of transvestism are still largely speculative. Transvestism occurs more frequently in the male than in the female. Usually the patient's mother wanted a girl and literally raised her son to be one.

Sometimes the fixation in psychosexual development of an immature level is through a conditioned response but in the male deviant more frequently is through the emotional attitude of his mother. Rickles has pointed out, for example, that in *exhibitionism,* which is one of the commonest sexual deviations, one usually finds that the offender is a son of a dominant, aggressive mother who resents her feminine role and tries to live her life through her children, especially the sons. The father is frequently a weak and ineffective person who has exerted but little influence in shaping the son's emotional development. Because of the mother's spoiling and showering the boy with unusual affection, he comes to identify himself with her and perhaps to develop sexual feelings toward her which he is in no way prepared to deal with at the narcissistic level beyond which he has not developed. With a strong taboo against such insistent but consciously forbidden incestuous wishes the boy must build compulsive but unconscious defenses. The symptom of exhibitionism is merely one of them. While a dynamic genesis and sequence such as that outlined is not susceptible of proof, yet the study of many exhibitionists seems to confirm the theory. Certainly the deviation is observed to be so compulsive that it must arise through a neurotic psychopathology.

In some instances the infantile components of the aggressive-destructive instinct, normal at an early stage of personality development, are not outgrown or sublimated but persist into adolescence and seem to become associated with the sex instinct each reinforcing the other and therefore productive of *sadism,* with the result that the individual's sexual behavior is not merely socially unacceptable or disgusting but even mutilative and murderous. Society is then confronted with a potentially dangerous, perhaps criminal, sex offender. In many instances, however, legal codes do not adequately distinguish between sex conduct that is socially distasteful and that which is socially dangerous.

A characteristic common to all forms of sexually psychopathic behavior or perversions is their repetitive, compulsive, patterned nature. Such behavior represents the expression of an uncontrollable urge committed without logic or rationale and apparently for the purpose of securing relief from an unbearable tension. The satisfaction derived from the commission of the sexually deviated and compulsive act is symbolic and substitutive; it is therefore temporary and requires repetition. These characteristics constitute the criteria of the neuroses. There is, in fact, an increasing tendency to regard the true sexual perversions as basically psychoneurotic in their psychopathology and therefore as a kind of mental illness. As in the case of compulsive handwashing, the apparent motive is not the real, or at least not the only motivating factor. The real motive is to satisfy aggressive or various other immature and deviated aspects of the psychosexual component of the personality. We may think of one child, if confronted with an emotional sexual problem, as converting it into a psychosomatic symptom, or into a neurotic anxiety or depression, while another expresses it compulsively in publicly indecent or potentially aggressive-destructive form. A majority of serious sex offenders are unable to comprehend the reasons, the inner compulsion, for their actions. The sexual psychopath's behavior is not a substitute for normal heterosexual relations. It is a form of sexual activity all its own and satisfies some very specific need that normal sexual activity cannot give. The added fact that the offender is usually unable to comprehend the reason for his actions, that their motivations are to a large extent unconscious, gives the sexual psychopath's behavior a neurotic characteristic. In general, sexual psychopaths are people with deep-seated personality disorders of which sex deviation is but one manifestation. The propension and the pattern of the deviation are determined by emotional, environmental and other personality-molding influences during early developmental years.

It should be borne in mind that during puberty and adolescence a sex drive of great intensity but not basically pathological in nature may momentarily gain control of behavior and find outlet in an isolated unnatural act which may be unlawful and punishable. At this age such acts do not always portend a repetitive pattern.

Recent studies in the pathogenesis of sexual deviation have led to speculations worthy of consideration. It would appear that overt antisocial misbehavior may be caused by parental, often unwitting, seduction. In infancy, nudity, fondling and virtual absence of privacy are appropriate and even necessary. If, however, such evidences of kindly parental affection persist until childhood or adolescence, they become pathological.

Under the guise of "motherly" or "fatherly" affection boys and girls may be bathed by parents, often of the opposite sex, until adolescence. Sleeping with children of the opposite sex may be prolonged into the teen-age period. Habitual undressing may occur in the presence of children. Sometimes legitimate parental embraces of affection extend into the sphere of frank bodily petting of adolescent children. Stimulated by parental behavior, the boy finds no outlet for his aroused sexual impulses. Eventually, mounting frustration and anger force him to follow one of two courses. One is regression to the safety of more infantile attitudes of sexual behavior. The other is sexual aggression toward women. Neither course resolves the rage nor dissipates the overstimulated unconscious sexual drives. The result may therefore later be a direct, sexual, destructive acting-out.

In contrast to the direct, hostile acting-out stemming from the repeated seduction and frustration incident to the child's intimate association with the parent of the opposite sex, such sexual aberrations as exhibitionism, voyeurism and transvestism may be traceable to the unconscious tendencies of the parent. In such cases, the instinctual sexual development of the child seems to represent or constitute an acting-out of the unconscious wishes of the parent.

Treatment

If, as is increasingly believed by dynamically minded psychiatrists, the psychopathologic condition that results in the behavior of the paraphiliac is basically related in motivation to that of the neuroses, the treatment of his deviations should be by methods comparable to those employed in the neuroses, *i.e.*, by psychotherapy.

Before considering therapy, a word should perhaps be said concerning the prevention of sex deviation. This requires a knowledge of its origin, also a recognition and emotional acceptance by the public of the fact that true deviation, in contrast to methods of sexual gratification adopted in absence of opportunity for the satisfaction of a biologically normal heterosexual impulse, is a manifestation of a developmental fault in the mental life which had its beginning in the early formative years of childhood. It is increasingly recognized and accepted that, in the course of its development, emotional and other aspects of the personality may be warped, arrested or otherwise deviated and through dynamic mechanisms give rise to neuroses. Likewise there is reason to believe that the psychosexual aspects of personality through specific pathogenic experiences or situations that lie close to the instinctive may suffer a developmental fault and give rise to sexual psychopathy. Any progress in reducing sexually psychopathic behavior must remain exceedingly slow. The most hopeful approach is doubtless through more and proper sex education in childhood, the establishment of identifications consonant with the child's sex and aid in a constructive sublimation of sexual and aggressive impulses which may be misdirected by the vicissitudes of childhood.

While psychotherapy utilizing psychoanalytical principles is theoretically the rational treatment for the sex deviate, yet in disappointingly few cases are the unconscious forces which have laid the foundation of the deviated impulses redirected thereby. This is not to deny that conscious factors have not participated at all in forming the behavior pattern. Probably determinants were derived from both conscious and unconscious sources, past and immediate. Some sexual psychopaths have no conscious desire to be cured of their behavior. Ideal conditions for therapy exist when the deviate has not been guilty of offense against the person, has therefore not committed a serious social offense and has voluntarily sought therapy. If his offense has been so serious that the community must be protected, the deviate must be confined. The prison environment and routine are not, however, conducive to successful therapy. The personality factors and emotional conflicts that led to the crime will not, of course, be worked through by simply spending a certain amount of time in prison. While the results are frequently disheartening, yet if the offender has not been guilty of violence, it is usually desirable that he be confined in a hospital atmosphere in which the therapist may supervise the surroundings in accordance with the needs of the patient as the therapy progresses. Through therapy and subsequent parole, some such offenders, if their desire for improvement is strong, may be enabled to channelize their impulses into constructive activities. Since sex perversions are of psychic origin, their treatment by glandular injections or by castration is, of course, of no avail. The Committee on Forensic Psychiatry of the Group for the Advancement of Psychiatry to whose report reference has been made gave thoughtful consideration both to the psychiatric aspects of sex deviation and to legislation to be recommended for dealing with sex offenders. It suggested that a psychiatric examination be made of any persons convicted of sexual offense and that if the psychiatrists report that the offender suffers from a fundamental personality disorder the judge, if he deems it wise, should, in lieu of sentence, commit him for an indefinite period to an institution equipped to give psychotherapy. Such a law would satisfy the aims of both community protection from the potentially dangerous offender and for treatment under conditions favorable to restoration. "If the offender is curable he can be eventually released to society; if not, he should never be released. . . . . The Committee is unreserved in its opinion that the committed sex offender should be actively treated in a non-penal institution. . . . . The stigma of sex offenses officially attached to the sex offender committed to a penal institution creates a formidable obstacle to treatment. At best consistency demands that if we diagnose the sex offender as mentally disordered he should be treated as a mental case in a facility for that purpose."

Not all persons concerned with the disposition of sex offenders recommend this treatment in state hospitals for mental diseases. They contend that such institutions lack facilities in both housing and personnel, that sex offenders do not mix well with others, that treatment is unsystematized and difficult, and that there are no criteria of recovery.

BIBLIOGRAPHY

Abrahamsen, David: Study of 102 sex offenders at Sing Sing Prison. Federal Probation, *14:*26–52, 1950.

Aichhorn, August: Wayward Youth. Imago Publishing Co., 1951.

Alexander, F.: The neurotic character. Internat. J. Psycho-Analysis, *2:*292, 1930.

Bowman, K. M.: The problem of the sex offender. Am. Psychiat., *108:*150–257, 1951.

Brancale, Ralph, et al.: Psychiatric and psychological investigations of convicted sex offenders, Am. J. Psychiat., *109:*17–21, 1952.

Bromberg, Walter: Dynamic aspects of psychopathic personality. Psychoanalyt. Quart., *17:*58–70, 1948.

———: Emotional immaturity and antisocial behavior. J. Clin. Psychopath., *8:*423–452, 1947.

Cleckley, H. M.: The Mask of Sanity. St. Louis, C. V. Mosby Co., 1941.

Eissler, K., Ed.: Searchlights on Delinquency. New York, International Universities Press, Inc., 1949.

Farnsworth, D. L.: Mental Health in Colleges and Universities. Cambridge, Harvard University Press, 1957.

Ford, C. S., and Beach, F. A.: Patterns of Sexual Behavior. New York, Paul B. Hoeber, Inc., 1951.

Gardner, G. E.: The community and the aggressive child: The expression of the aggressive-destructive impulses in juvenile-delinquent acts. Ment. Hyg., *33:*537–550, 1949.

———: The community and the aggressive child: The aggressive-destructive impulses in the sex offender. Ment. Hyg., *34:*44–63, 1950.

Glueck, Sheldon and Glueck, Eleanor: Unraveling Juvenile Delinquency. New York, The Commonwealth Fund, 1950.

Group for Advancement of Psychiatry. Psychiatrically Deviated Sex Offenders, Report No. 9, Topeka, 1949.

Guttmacher, M. S.: Sex Offenses: The Problem, Causes and Prevention. New York, W. W. Norton & Co., 1951.

———: New Light on Delinquency and Its Treatment. New Haven, Yale University Press, 1936.

———, and Weihofen, Henry: Psychiatry and the Law. New York, W. W. Norton & Co., 1952.

Henderson, D. K.: Psychopathic States. New York, W. W. Norton & Co., 1939.

Hoch, P. H., and Zubin, Joseph: Psychosexual Development in Health and Disease. New York, Grune & Stratton, 1951.

Johnson, A. M., and Robinson, D. B.: The sexual deviant (sexual psychopath)—causes, treatment and prevention. J.A.M.A., *164:*1559–1565, 1957.

———, and Szurek, S. A.: Etiology of antisocial behavior in delinquents and psychopaths. J.A.M.A., *154:*814–817, 1954.

Karpman, Ben: The sexual psychopath. J.A.M.A., *146:*721–726, 1951.

Kennedy, Alexander: Psychopathic personality and social responsibility. J. Ment. Sc., *100:*873–881, 1954.

Kinsey, A. C., et al.: Sexual Behavior in the Human Male. Philadelphia, W. B. Saunders Co., 1948.

Kolb, L. C., and Johnson, A. M.: Etiology and therapy of overt homosexuality. Psychoanalyt. Quart., *24:*506–515, 1955.

Mettler, F. A.: The semi-responsible individual. Psychiatric Quart., *26:*608–625, 1952.

Peabody, G. A.; Rowe, A. T., and Wall, J. H.: Fetishism and transvestism. J. Nerv. & Ment. Dis., *118:*339–350, 1953.

Redlich, F. C., et al.: Narcoanalysis and truth. Am. J. Psychiat., *107:*586–593, 1951.

Rickles, N. K.: Exhibitionism. Philadelphia, J. B. Lippincott Co., 1950.

Roche, Philip Q.: Sexual deviation. Federal Probation, *14:*1–11, 1950.

Schneider, Kurt: Die psychopathischen Persönlichkeiten, ed. 4. Leipzig, Deuticke, 1940.

Szurek, S. A.: Notes on the genesis of psychopathic personality trends. Psychiatry, *5:*1–6, 1942.

White, W. A.: Insanity and the Criminal Law. New York, The Macmillan Co., 1923.

CHAPTER XXXIII

Drug Addiction

DRUG addiction is usually symptomatic of a personality disorder. It might well, therefore, have been included in Chapter XXXII, Sociopathic Personality Disturbances. Since, however, it is so large a subject, a special chapter will be devoted to it.

Opiates and Their Synthetic Equivalents

The World Health Organization's Committee known as the "Expert Committee on Drugs Liable to Produce Addiction" has suggested the following definition of drug addiction: "Drug addiction is a state of periodic or chronic intoxication, detrimental to the individual and to society, produced by the repeated consumption of a drug (natural or synthetic). Its characteristics include: (1) an overpowering desire or need (compulsion) to continue taking the drug and to obtain it by any means, (2) a tendency to increase the dose and (3) a psychic (psychological) and sometimes a physical dependence on the effects of the drug."

Perhaps there should be further explanation of some of the terms contained in this definition as well as certain others relating to addiction. By *habituation*, or habit-formation, is meant a psychological dependence on the use of a drug because of the relief from tension and emotional discomfort which it affords. By *tolerance* is meant a declining effect of the same dose of a drug when it is administered repeatedly over a period of time. As a result, it is necessary to increase the dose in order to obtain the original degree of effect. *Physical dependence* refers to an altered physiological state brought about by repeated ingestion or administration of a drug in order to prevent the appearance of a characteristic illness called an *abstinence syndrome*. Dependence on analgesic drugs is characterized, on their withdrawal, by autonomic dysfunction, such as yawning, lacrimation, rhinorrhea, gooseflesh and symptoms reflecting general irritability of the central nervous system, such as twitching of muscles, insomnia, hypertension and fever. Dependence on hypnotics and alcohol is manifested chiefly by the development of convulsions and delirium following withdrawal. Physical dependence is a self-limited process. The symptoms appear in a definite time sequence following withdrawal of the drug, reach maximum intensity at a definite time and decline at a definite rate. The symptoms which follow withdrawal of drugs with relatively short lengths of action, such as heroin and Dilaudid, appear quickly, become intense in a short time and decline rapidly. Symptoms which follow withdrawal of a drug with a long length of action, such as methadone, appear slowly, are never intense and decline more slowly.

Theories of Tolerance and Physical Dependence

While there is no proven explanation for the phenomena of tolerance and of physical dependence there are now two proffered theories. According to one theory, morphine has diphasic actions—excitation and depression. The excitant effects persist longer than do the depressant effects. For this reason, as doses of morphine are repeated, excitant effects are accumulated, requiring larger and larger doses in order to obtain a sufficient degree of depression to mask the excitant effects. This is the suggested explanation for tolerance. Following a withdrawal of the drug, its excitant effects are released, thus accounting for physical dependence.

A second theory advanced to explain the development of tolerance and physical dependence is that known as the theory of cellular adaptation. According to this hypothesis, the administration of opiates stimulates compensatory homeostatic mechanisms which oppose the depressant effects of the drug. These homeostatic responses become strengthened upon repeated administration of the drug. More and more drug is therefore required to induce the original degree of effect, and when the drug is withdrawn the enhanced homeostatic mechanisms are released from the brake imposed upon them by the continued presence of morphine within the body, thus giving rise to physical dependence. This theory is based largely on the observation that manifestations of abstinence are always opposite in nature to those of the direct effects of opiates. Thus in the nontolerant, nonaddicted person, morphine constricts the pupils, lowers body temperature, reduces blood pressure and causes sedation. Following withdrawal of morphine from the addict, dilation of the pupils is noted, fever, a rise in blood pressure and insomnia.

While the exact nature of the changes responsible for tolerance and physical dependence are not precisely known they must be due to biochemical changes within the cells of the central nervous system.

Extent of Drug Addiction

Vogel of the United States Public Health Service estimates that when the Harrison Narcotic Act was passed in 1914 there were 175,000 narcotic addicts, mostly women, in the United States. He reports that there are now approximately 60,000 addicts, most of whom are men. About 35,000 of these are known to the authorities. While addiction does exist among underprivileged adolescents, it is not as frequent as articles in the public press would indicate.

The large group of addicts is composed of individuals with personality disorders who become addicted to drugs through contact and association with person already addicted. The addict often seeks to recruit new addicts in order that through sales to them he may secure funds in order to obtain a supply for his own needs. Most members of this group are emotionally immature, hostile, aggressive persons who take drugs in order to secure relief from inner tension. They have few healthy resources or interests and are motivated by immature drives for immediate goals. The addict-to-be-finds in the drug a release from tension felt as a restless need for pleasurable or exotic sensations, the satisfaction of a longing for artificial elation or peace. Conscious discomfort is eliminated, repressed drives may be released and responsibility is evaded. Another group consists of frankly neurotic persons with anxiety, obsessive, compulsive or psychophysiologic symptoms which are relieved by drugs. A third group consists of persons who in the course of physical illness have received drugs over an extended period and after the termination of the ailment have continued their use. However, probably all persons who acquire addiction in this manner have some fundamental emotional problem which caused them to continue the use of drugs beyond the period of medical need. Many addicts were intemperate in the use of alcohol before they became addicted to drugs. In practically all addicts their previous adjustment to life was marginal or unsatisfactory.

Opiate Addiction

Morphine, its derivatives, and its synthetic pharmacological substitutes are so allied in their addictive qualities that they will be considered together.

The amount of morphine taken by addicts varies greatly. A few do not take over 2 grains per day. DeQuincey states in his Confessions of an Opium Eater that at one period in the history of his drug addiction he took 500 ml. of laudanum, or approximately 72 grains of morphine, daily. Perhaps the average addict takes from 10 to 20 grains per day. Many addicts will tolerate, without unfavorable symptoms, seven times the dose they are accustomed to receive. This tolerance is destroyed following disappearance of the withdrawal symptoms. Addicts usually do not realize how rapidly they lose their tolerance for opiates. Sometimes during the "cure" addicts have obtained access to an opiate and taken, with fatal results, what was the usual dose before withdrawal was instituted.

After recourse to his drug, the addict feels a sense of relief and perhaps of exhilaration together with an increase in efficiency. The alleviation and sense of well being obtained by the addict through a dose of his drug is so great that as its pleasant effect diminishes the desire for the satisfaction which the drug affords can scarcely be resisted. While the continued administration of small amounts of the drug will prevent the distressing withdrawal symptoms to be described later, yet increasing amounts are necessary to obtain the desired exhilaration and sense of increased capacity. As a result the quantity taken is gradually increased until enormous amounts are required.

The eventual effect of the habit is an impairment of a higher ethical sense. This moral and social deterioration is not a result of the direct effects of narcotics but, rather of social consequences of the life of addiction. When the narcotic is taken in large doses, ambition and physical energy are lessened, lethargy is produced and the pleasurable feeling that all is well makes the addict contented. As a result he pays less attention to work and becomes an idler. Those who depend upon an illegitimate source for their supply of drugs are sometimes unable to work because of discomfort and weakness resulting from inability to secure the usual dose. When such patients, after a short period of deprivation, secure a supply, they often take more than is necessary to keep them comfortable. As a result they alternate between physical and mental instability and physical and mental lethargy. Frequently addicts are compelled to associate with low moral characters in order to continue their addiction. Financial embarrassment resulting from idleness or the high price of peddled narcotics may impel the addict to beg money, to obtain it by subterfuge, or to steal it. He suffers from self-esteem through the public attitude of contempt and through constant fear of arrest or because of a term served in the penitentiary for having narcotics in his possession. This chain of events results in habit deterioration and in a demoralization of character and converts those who might have been fairly useful citizens into outcasts, idlers and dependents. Contrary to popular opinion the prolonged use of morphine, heroin, cocaine and marihuana has comparatively little effect on the physical health of the addict. Morphine addiction rarely produces psychotic reactions.

Diagnosis of Opiate Addiction

Frequently the addict admits that he is addicted to and needs drugs. If he denies the habit, the diagnosis can at times be made by needle marks, indurations and the scars of abscesses. Miosis is suggestive but not definite evidence. Periods of restlessness, irritability and anxiety followed rather suddenly by ones of euphoria, and apparent relief and contentment should be suggestive of drug addiction.

At times the only method of diagnosis may be isolation of the patient from a source of drugs followed by observation for signs of abstinence. The addict may be exceedingly clever in concealing a supply of his drugs. He may enter a hospital for the purpose of being cured of his addiction yet at the same time have a supply craftily concealed in personal articles or even in body cavities.

Recently, a diagnostic test of considerable sensitivity has been developed which depends upon precipitating the abstinence syndrome by the parenteral injections of *N*-allylnormorphine (Nalline), a morphine antagonist. Before conducting such a test, it is advisable to obtain written permission of the patient or his guardian. This test is performed by injecting subcutaneously 3 mg. of *N*-allylnormorphine. In less than twenty minutes after injection clear-cut signs of the abstinence syndrome will be noted in addicts using 60 mg. or more of morphine daily or equivalent amounts of heroin, dihydromorphinone, methadone or Levo-Dromoran. Symptoms of the abstinence syndrome are described in the next section of this chapter. If the response to the first injection is negative or doubtful, a second dose of 5 mg. should be given thirty minutes after the first, and again a third thirty minutes after the second. At this time, if abstinence symptoms have not become apparent and if the signs of the direct effects of the injected drug have appeared, the test may be read as negative. *N*-allylnormorphine directly produces dizziness, pseudoptoses, mioses and reduction in the respiratory rate with a drunken experience. The absence of response to this test may occur in addicts who have been withdrawn from narcotics for as short as a week's period, or in addicts taking scattered doses. It is unreliable for meperidine (Demerol) addiction and contraindicated in the presence of serious organic disease.

Withdrawal Symptoms

Whenever opium or its habit-forming derivatives are abruptly withdrawn, a definite train of symptoms known as abstinence or withdrawal symptoms appears. If, within twelve to fourteen hours after the administration of morphine, the dose is not repeated, the so-called withdrawal signs and symptoms begin to appear. Among the first are yawning, lacrimation, rhinorrhea, sneezing and perspiration. These symptoms become more marked and anorexia, dilated pupils, tremor and gooseflesh are added. About thirty-six hours after the last dose uncontrollable twitching of the muscles appears and cramps develop in legs, abdomen and back. The patient becomes intensely restless, is unable to sleep and both pulse and blood pressure rise. Vomiting and diarrhea are frequent. These acute signs and symptoms reach their height about forty-eight hours after the last dose of morphine and remain at this height for seventy-two hours. They then gradually subside during the next five to ten days. As the withdrawal symptoms develop, the patient becomes restless, pessimistic, surly, fault-finding, irritable and exhibits an unpleasant, increased psychomotor activity. He has a marked subjective feeling of weakness and considerable prostration may occur. He may curse, cry, be impulsively destructive and make suicidal gestures. To quite an extent the intensity of withdrawal symptoms depends on the amount of drug the patient has been receiving. To some degree the extent of the symptoms can be controlled by the patient himself. Any patient who appears comfortable during the period of withdrawal should be suspected of illicit possession of the drug.

Prognosis

It should be remembered that narcotic addiction nearly always results from emotional problems, compounded frequently with a complex system of habit patterns that add to the difficulty of treatment. In general, these emotional problems are the same anxieties, conflicts and neuroses as those with which other emotionally unstable persons are confronted. While probably more addicts than commonly realized are permanently cured, yet they constitute a minority. The United States Public Health Service Hospital, Lexington, Kentucky, an institution for the treatment of addicts, found that only two tenths of 1 per cent of patients who left the hospital in less than thirty days remained off the drug, whereas

24 per cent of those who remained the recommended period were believed to have remained free from addiction. Some habitués, pretending that they no longer have any desire for the drug, really look eagerly forward to an opportunity to return to their habit and devise every imaginable pretext to hasten their release from the hospital. Even those who believe they wish to be cured return to the drug on the slightest pretext, the alleged occasion being actually but a rationalization of their emotional defects and their psychological need for obliterating reality and its problems. They feel lost without the narcotic and the sense of physical comfort it imparts. Many, too, feel that they are not understood, are in a constant state of mild dissatisfaction, and long to return to the accustomed companionship of other addicts by whom they feel they are understood and with whom they feel a sense of security and comradeship. Other addicts, sometimes for the sake of self-justification, sometimes because, as vendors of morphine, they see in their unhappy companion a potential customer, urge the recently "cured" patient to share the alleviating agent. The profits from this "cured" patient will replenish their own diminishing supply of the drug, of course.

Treatment

A step almost invariably essential in the treatment of addiction to opium and its derivatives is removal to an institution where the activities of the patient and the sources of the drug can be controlled. Treatment of the addicted person on a voluntary, out-patient basis is almost never successful. The period of hospital treatment should be four to nine months. The patient must remain long enough to be relieved of any physical ailments, to have opportunity to develop habits of living and working without drugs and to be helped in discovering the source of his emotional difficulty.

It is not humane and it may be even dangerous to withdraw morphine abruptly. It may be withdrawn rapidly over a period of ten days, in which case 30 mg. may be given every six hours for two days with continued reduction thereafter until withdrawal is complete by the end of ten days. It is probably more desirable to begin with the withdrawal of morphine, then shift to methadone which suppresses the withdrawal symptoms in persons addicted to morphine. In this method one should first ascertain the least amount of morphine that will prevent the appearance of withdrawal symptoms. This is termed the stabilization dosage and can usually be determined in two or three days. Once the stabilization dosage is known, 1 mg. of methadone may be substituted for every 3 or 4 mg. of the patient's accustomed dose of morphine. As methadone is a cumulative, slow-acting drug the patient should be given one half his accustomed dose of morphine and one half his calculated dose of methadone during the first day of substitution. During the second day only methadone is given. After substitution of methadone has been effected the calculated dosage should be maintained for two or three days. The total dosage can be adjusted upward or downward depending on the patient's response. Thereafter, methadone should be withdrawn over the course of seven to ten days depending on the patient's response.

While withdrawal symptoms should be expected near the end of treatment, severe manifestations of abstinence are never seen when this method of withdrawal is used. Chlorpromazine is also useful in the tension states occurring in the withdrawal of opium and other narcotics. Great caution should be exercised in withdrawal of drugs from patients with evidence of myocardial insufficiency.

Sometimes the patient, without knowledge of the physician, has also been taking barbiturates before his admission. In that case the patient may develop an abstinence syndrome resulting from barbiturate withdrawal, as well. This will usually be in the form of a severe convulsion in which fractures may occur. The prevention of this additional abstinence syndrome is the continued but gradually decreasing administration of a barbiturate.

An effort should be made to establish rapport and positive transference between the patient and physician during withdrawal. The patient usually has a resistence to gaining insight into the real causes of his addiction. Psychotherapy should, however, be directed toward his motivations, defenses and adaptations. Group psychotherapy is not successful. The usual recognition of drug addiction as a crime rather than as a disease reacts unfavorably on success of therapy. The vocational and social discrimination experienced by the addict following his discharge tends to lead to relapse.

The discharged addict should be required to report regularly for a period of five years to a center staffed with internists, psychiatrists and social workers who are specifically trained to help him meet his problems. If left to solve his problems unaided he usually returns to the use of drugs. It is frequently helpful if he joins the organization known as Narcotics Anonymous.

Other Opium Derivatives

Heroin, taken both hypodermically and by snuffing, has great addiction ability. Its effect in producing deterioration in personality with disregard for social and ethical conventions is unsurpassed. Many consider it the most difficult of all addictions to cure. *Codeine* has a definite, though low-grade, addiction liability. Both *Dilaudid* (dihydromorphinone hydrochloride) and *metopon* (methyldihydromorphinone) have high physical dependence and habituation liabilities. *Demerol* (meperidine hydrochloride) is a synthetic analgesic which is not chemically related to morphine but is nevertheless addicting. It possesses considerable habituation liability and after prolonged administration its addicts develop physical dependence. Any differences in the addiction liability of the new analgesic drugs from that of morphine are differences in degree, not in kind. The general features of the morphine abstinence syndrome are also characteristic of these drugs.

Cocainism

For many years cocaine addiction constituted one of the major drug problems but because of legislation, its use among addicts is much less prevalent than formerly. At the present time, nearly all its habitués have acquired the addiction through other addicts. Strictly speaking, cocaine is not a narcotic. It produces a marked stimulation, a sense of exhilaration, euphoria and self-confidence, an increased flow of ideas and a pressure of speech and of activity. During this period of stimulation and sense of competency there may be an actual increase in capacity for work. As the stimulus of the drug wears off the patient feels weak, depressed, restless, morose and irritable. Other abstinence symptoms are digestive disturbances, tremors, palpitation, specks in front of the eyes, muscular weakness, slight confusion and impotence.

Frankly psychotic symptoms are common among those who continue the use of large doses of cocaine over a prolonged period. Such addicts may experience terrifying visual hallucinations, become suspicious and perhaps show much excitement. Delusions of jealousy and of persecution are common and may lead to violence. A rather characteristic phenomenon is the frequent existence of formicative paresthesias associated with which there may be the delusion that there are actually insects beneath the skin, the presence of which the patient may attempt to demonstrate.

The moral deterioration in the cocaine addict is even greater than in the morphine habitué. The prospects of any permanent cure of the habit are even less favorable than in the case of the morphine addict. Withdrawal of the drug is not accompanied by the painful experiences and tendency to collapse occurring in the withdrawal of opium derivatives.

Barbituric Acid Group

According to reports of the United States Public Health Service, there has been a great increase in recent years not only in acute barbiturate intoxication but also in barbiturate addiction. Acute intoxication with barbiturates accounts for about 25 per cent of all deaths of acute poisoning admitted to general hospitals, and more deaths are caused by barbiturates, either accidenally ingested or taken with suicidal intent, than by any other poison.

As in alcoholism and in narcotic drug addiction, the important factor in barbiturate addiction is an underlying personality difficulty. Many psychoneurotics become addicted to barbiturates through their prescription for insomnia. Persons with character disorders ("psychopaths") begin the use of the drug in order to experience its intoxicating effect. Morphine addicts often use the drug when they are unable to secure morphine or in order to reinforce the effect of that narcotic. Alcoholics may begin the use of barbiturates to relieve the tension following a debauch and continue their use to induce toxic effects. In contradiction to the situation in other narcotic drug addictions, a large proportion of the cases of barbiturate addiction result from administration by physicians. The physician should therefore remember that in prescribing barbiturates he assumes a heavy ethical responsibility. There is a possibility that these drugs may create a dangerous type of addiction. Especial care should be exercised in prescribing them for emotionally unstable persons. Simple insomnia alone is rarely a valid indication for the use of barbiturates.

SYMPTOMS OF ACUTE BARBITURATE INTOXICATION. The clinical symptomatology of acute barbiturate intoxication is strikingly similar to that of acute alcohol intoxication. The person who has taken large doses of barbiturates shows difficulty in thinking, poor judgment, emotional instability, impairment of ego controls, clouding of consciousness, hallucinations and delusions.

SYMPTOMS OF CHRONIC BARBITURATE INTOXICATION. Since the barbiturates depress brain oxidation it is not surprising that in chronic barbiturate intoxication the patient is confused, often drowsy and depressed, shows poor judgment and impaired intellectual functioning and a regression in habits. Frequently he is emotionally unstable, morose, quarrelsome and if irritated by minor incidents or fancied insults may be assaultive. Some addicts become hostile and develop mild paranoid ideas. In extreme cases the patient may regress to an infantile level and have to be waited on, fed and nursed.

Neurological signs in both acute and chronic barbiturate intoxication include nystagmus, dysarthria and ataxia in gait and station.

BARBITURATE ADDICTION AND WITHDRAWAL. Any of the barbiturates when given daily, for periods of three to six months, in amounts approximately eight or more times the usual effective dose produces addiction. Upon withdrawal all patients who have been ingesting as much as 0.8 gm. or more of pentobarbital daily will suffer anxiety, weakness and tremor. Many will develop a psychotic reaction resembling delirium tremens and probably a larger number will have one or more convulsions. The nature of the biochemical and physiological disturbances responsible for the withdrawal symptoms is not yet known.

TREATMENT. Even a gradual reduction of barbiturates carries a certain risk. Patients should therefore be under constant supervision and observation during withdrawal which should be carried out in a hospital. As already indicated, the drug in barbiturate addiction must not be withdrawn abruptly. For the first two days the patient will receive just enough of the barbiturates to maintain a mild degree of intoxication. This will usually be from 0.2 gm. to 0.4 gm. of pentobarbital or an equivalent amount of another barbiturate. Thereafter the drug will be very slowly reduced, the total withdrawal period being extended over two to three weeks. If excessive anxiety, insomnia or tremor appears during withdrawal, reduction of the drug should be stopped and the amount held constant until these symptoms disappear.

It is important to remember that acute barbiturate intoxication is frequently superimposed on barbiturate addiction. After patients who have been acutely poisoned with barbiturates have recovered from coma, it should be ascertained whether they have been taking the drug chronically. In such cases, barbiturate intake should be restored and gradual reduction begun. After withdrawal has been completed, there should be a long period of psychotherapy.

Many believe that addiction to barbiturates is more serious than morphine addiction. Abstinence from morphine is less dangerous than abstinence from barbiturates and morphine addiction causes less mental and emotional disturbance.

Marihuana

Because of its frequent use, marihuana should also be considered. The active principle of this drug is an oil. The flowering tops of the female plant are used, the action being the same as that of cannabis indica. The usual form of taking the drug is by smoking it in the form of cigarettes, often referred to as "reefers." Much misinformation concerning the action of marihuana has created an unjustified alarm relative to its addicts. Unlike opium derivatives, it does not give rise to a biological dependence accompanied by withdrawal symptoms, and its indulgence can be discontinued without great difficulty. It does not lead to any physical, mental or moral degradation even after prolonged use. Following inhalation, the subject has a sense of euphoria and shows increased volubility and psychomotor activity followed subjectively by a feeling of calm and pleasurable relaxation. The individual may sleep for one to six hours and on awakening he no longer feels exhilarated. Marihuana is probably taken by users for the purpose of producing sensations comparable to those produced by alcohol. It is probable that marihuana may precipitate a psychotic reaction in persons of a poorly organized personality. One of the most undesirable results of marihuana addiction is the more serious addiction to opiate-like drugs to which the use of the former drug often leads because of the degrading social contacts with which marihuana addiction seems to be particularly associated. It is a popular misconception that the use of marihuana leads to criminal habits. This opinion is not sustained by actual experience. Bowman has correctly pointed out that alcohol causes infinitely more murders, rapes and crimes of violence than do morphine, heroin, cocaine, marihuana, and all other drugs combined.

BIBLIOGRAPHY

Allentuck, S., and Bowman, K. M.: The psychiatric aspects of marihuana intoxication. Am. J. Psychiat., *99:*248–251, 1942.

Berry, L. H.: Medical counseling clinics for young narcotic addicts. J.A.M.A., *147:* 1120–1131, 1951.

Council on Mental Health: Report on narcotic addiction. J.A.M.A., *165:*1707–1713, 1957.

Felix, R. H.: An appraisal of the personality types of the addict. Am. J. Psychiat., *100:*462–467, 1944.

Friedgood, C. E., and Ripstein, C. B.: Use of chlorpromazine in the withdrawal of addicting drugs. New England J. Med., *252:*230–233, 1955.

Isbell, Harris: Addiction to barbiturates and the barbiturate abstinence syndrome. Ann. Int. Med., *33:*108–121, 1950.

———: Chronic Opium Poisoning. Cecil and Loeb, Textbook of Medicine. Philadelphia, W. B. Saunders Co., 9th ed., p. 574.

———: The newer analgesic drugs; their use and abuse. Ann. Int. Med., *29:*1003–1013, 1948.

———: Medical aspects of opiate addiction. Bull. New York Acad. Med., *31:*886–901, 1955.

———, et al.: Chronic barbiturate intoxication. Arch. Neurol. & Psychiat., *64:*1–28, 1950.

———, and Vogel, V. H.: The addiction liability of methadon and its use in the treatment of the morphine abstinence syndrome. Am. J. Psychiat., *105:*909–914, 1949.

Maas, J. M.: Increasing promiscuity and abuse with the barbiturates. Am. J. Med. Sc., *222:*121–128, 1951.

Nyswander, Marie: The Drug Addict as a Patient. New York, Grune & Stratton, 1956.

Plum, Fred, and Swanson, A. G.: Barbiturate poisoning treated by physiologic methods. J.A.M.A., *163:*827–835, 1957.

Report of Subcommittee on Barbiturates, New York Academy of Medicine. Public Health Reports, *71:*1144–1155, 1956, U. S. Government Printing Office.

Wikler, A.: Mechanisms of action of drugs that modify personality function. Am. J. Psychiat., *108:*590–599, 1952.

———: Opiate Addiction; Psychological and Neurophysiological Aspects in Relation to Clinical Problems. Springfield, Illinois, Charles C Thomas, 1952.

CHAPTER XXXIV

Child Psychiatry

THE FIRST organized psychiatric study of childhood maladjustments was undertaken by Healy, in Chicago, in 1909. Interest in the subject increased slowly at first but moved forward with greater impetus after 1919 when the National Committee for Mental Hygiene, supported by the Commonwealth Fund, initiated the sponsorship of child guidance clinics and provided fellowships for study in child psychiatry.

The treatment of children's psychiatric disorders differs in many respects from that of adult psychiatric problems. In large measure this is because the child is living through the most active phase of the developmental process. His personality is less structured and formed, and from one stage of growth to another he shows rapid modifications in behavior. The psychiatrist who works in the field of child psychiatry must have a knowledge of the ever-changing patterns of healthy behavior at the various age levels as a means of evaluating the existence of disturbance. Again, the environmental pressures leading to disordered personality functioning in the child may usually be discovered in the present or recent past. They contribute a continuing influence in the life of the child. Since at this age the child is dependent upon his parents emotionally and in all aspects of his living, the psychiatrist must deal directly with the parents in the course of arranging the treatment and in determining future management. The child seldom comes to treatment on his own; he is brought in by the parents or referred by community agencies such as schools or courts. Still another difference is evident in the practice of child psychiatry. This has to do with the means of obtaining information and evaluating the problem of the child. Of necessity, much of the history must be obtained from the parents and from others who are related to the child in his school environment or in other aspects of his training. Inferences in regard to his emotional reactions and relations with others, particularly in the younger age periods, are derived from psychological testing and from play therapy wherein the child acts out his fantasies. Because of the necessity of obtaining information from parents and social agencies and through psychological examination of the intellectual and emotional life of the child, it is necessary that the work of the child psychiatrist be actively supplemented by the skills of the clinical psychologist and psychiatric social worker. Furthermore, in prescribing treatment consideration must be given to the significant persons in the child's environment as well as to the child. The outcome of a particular problem depends to a great extent upon the family structure from which the child comes. There will be some symptoms which are fostered by the family. In such circumstances efforts directed toward understanding and modifying the behavior of the child remain unsuccessful unless the significant family members also come into therapy.

While children may suffer from a psychosis, such as schizophrenia (Schizophrenia in Childhood, Chapter XXVII) from manic-depressive reactions, as well as from delirium, epilepsy, and from juvenile paresis and other mental disorders, child psychiatry has by usage become largely limited to the psychiatric consideration of neurotic and emotionally determined maladjustments observed in childhood. These maladjustments may be manifested in behavior difficulties, disturbance of social adaptation, unsatisfactory character traits, psychogenic disturbances of physiological function or in a more traditional form of psychoneurotic reaction seen in adults. Since there is less fixity of the patterns of disturbed behavior because of the plastic personality of the child, there is less unanimity in regard to the diagnostic schemata for the disorders of childhood than those of adulthood. While in recent years the tendency has largely been to consider the majority of behavior disorders as emotionally determined, there is a growing recognition of the great extent of brain injury consequent to childbirth as contributing to many of these disturbances. The specific problems of brain-injured, epileptic and mentally defective children have been discussed earlier in Chapters XI, XVII and XXII. Whatever the type of disturbance or its etiology, it should be recognized that troublesome trends in the child which make it difficult for him to get along comfortably with other people or for others to get along with him are problems of mental health. They should therefore not be dealt with from the standpoint of moralistic disapproval.

Causes of Psychiatric Problems

The child is a changing personality and in order for his emotional growth to proceed in a natural and spontaneous way it is necessary that he receive affection, understanding, security and discipline and be stimulated by achievement and social acceptance. It is necessary, too, that he feel satisfaction in his relation with his parents, that he develop a feeling that he is lovable, that his individuality be respected by his parents and that he have confidence in his own strength and capacity as a person in his own right. The maladjustments of childhood sometimes originate from a single cause but more frequently, they arise from the combined action of several types, particularly emotional and situational ones; also, in some instances, they arise from intellectual and perhaps other constitutional causes. While care must be exercised not to oversimplify the problem and explain it by one formula, yet it is perhaps reasonable to assume that in many maladjustments of childhood it will be discovered that human relationships have, through their influence upon the developing personality, acted as a significant etiological factor. Of all these relationships, that of parent and child is the one in which the problem is most frequently rooted. There are many phases of the parent-child relationship which may be pathogenetic, and there are many forms of personality maladjustment which may result from them. These will be discussed later in the chapter.

According to psychoanalytical theory, the production of the behavior disorders and neurotic traits in children is attributed to an attempt to adjust two opposing forces in the personality—the *id* desires and the *superego* prohibitions. The child's neurotic symptoms, increased anxiety and other clinical signs arise because he has not relinquished his infantile instinctual cravings normally during the growing-up process. He has failed either adequately to channelize them into reality-adjusted and pleasurable functions of the ego or to adjust them to the requirements of reality and of society by repression, reaction-formation, undoing, isolation, reversal or other mental mechanisms.

Others ascribe these manifestations to disturbances and distortions in the normal personality growth process. As a result there is an undeveloped phase in some aspect of the child's personality. The undeveloped phases may have arisen through such factors as the striving of the mother to hold her child as an undifferentiated part of herself. Thus the child does not obtain the natural love, guidance and direction necessary for his development into an independent personality with fulfillment of his individual potentialities and responsibilities. Again, the failure of the personality development with resulting inadequate capacity of the child to deal efficiently and realistically with the business of living may result from the fact that he struggled to protect his dependency status against the demands of growth, against giving up his infantile relationship to the mother and against an independent organization of his own powers and capacities. According to this point of view the child has been delayed or blocked in some aspect of his growth toward a normally functioning self and cannot handle his feelings in a way that permits those growing relationships with others that are essential for his development.

The psychobiological school makes a comprehensive personality study on the assumption that experiences occurring in any phase of the life of the individual may become potent dynamic factors of personality difficulties. They recognize that the child's behavior disorders may have their origin in a single factor or in a mixture of such different factors as constitutional, physical, intellectual and situational ones. An inclusive investigation of an emotional problem or of a behavior disorder would therefore include a social, physical, psychometric and psychiatric examination—a search for dynamic factors in each and all phases of life. Naturally the psychiatrist's therapeutic approach to the child's difficulty will be determined by his theoretical conceptions as to its etiology and dynamics. Discussion as to therapeutic techniques will be considered later.

To return to a consideration of factors and experiences which may be of importance in the production of the behavior disorders of childhood, including those that are neurotic.

AGE. Observation of infants seems to show that the need for mothering, sensory stimuli to skin and mucous surface, and instinctual emotional gratification is present from the time of birth, and that the lack of these may result in evident inhibition of personality development. Perhaps sudden weaning or attempts to establish toilet training at too early a stage of the child's development may pave the way for later emotional and behavior disorders. At about the beginning of the third year the necessity for growing into relationships with other people and accepting their values becomes definitely greater. Confrontation with this problem may stimulate insecurity and anxiety which then create defense reactions in the form of feeding problems, destructiveness or temper tantrums. Puberty, with its social and sexual problems and its urge to effect emancipation from the home, offers many possibilities for friction and inner conflict with resulting emotional and behavior maladjustments.

ENVIRONMENTAL AND INTERPERSONAL FACTORS. It is generally agreed that the influence of the child's environment is the most important factor in the development of neurotic symptoms or behavior problems. To a large extent those environmental factors that are of greatest influence in molding the personality of the child are interpersonal ones, particularly those in the family. In fact, the determining influence of the family circle on the developing personality of the child is one of the cornerstones of child psychiatry. The healthy family is the ideal medium for fulfilling the basic emotional needs of the child. In the family may arise many, perhaps most, of the psychopathological processes that lead to neurotic reactions, personality difficulties or to behavior disorders. Here are such disturbing influences as parental dissensions, parental alcoholism, hostility, cruelty, neglect, overprotection and excessive parental ambition for the child. Even though the mother be highly intellectual, she may be incapable of mature emotional relationships. Other factors that may distort parent-child relationship and disturb personality development are neurosis, psychosis, or psychopathic, antisocial or aggressive tendencies on part of the parent. The psychological fate of the child is to a considerable extent determined by the emotional health of the parents and by the complex forces interacting within the family group. Many faulty parent-child relationships are related to the parents' own personality structure, their emotional conflicts, biases and past experiences. To secure a clear picture of the influences to which the child is subjected one should know how the parents feel unconsciously about the child, what conflicts disturb the parent-child relationship, even what conflicts have existed between the parents and their parents and how these have affected the ability of the parents to relate themselves to the child. The emotional reaction of the parents to the behavior of the child should not be overlooked. Occasionally the behavior of the parents is a result of the child's behavior rather than the cause of it. Early institutional care or other interruptions in the continuity of parent-child relationship are harmful and lead to defects in personality development expressed as emotional apathy or inadequacy in forming relations with others, inability to accept obstructions, failures and separations, as well as perceptual, intellectual and language disturbances. Relations to siblings may be the source of personality problems. Among these are sibling rivalry, jealousy, parental favoritism, and a feeling of being supplanted by the birth of a younger sibling. It should be remembered that it is particularly difficult for some children to share an adult (especially a parent) with another child. The broken home is a common source of personality difficulties. The prolonged deprivation of the young child of maternal care may have warping or inhibitive effects on his personality development. Frequently this gives rise to a sense of insecurity, a frequent cause of neurotic behavior. Parental instability with resulting shifts of attitude on the part of the child may, as may many other factors, prevent identification which is one of the most important mechanisms in shaping character. Death of a parent, or more frequently desertion or divorce, preceded, usually, by a long period of domestic unhappiness, may be important in the production of personality disorders. Attitudes experienced by the stepchild or the foster child may create personality maladjustments. Many school experiences may be important in giving rise to personality problems. Failure in school and the factors which contributed to the failure, such as mental retardation or unhappy home conditions, faulty handling by teachers or difficulties in relations with classmates may be sources of personality difficulties. Sometimes poverty and privation may operate to produce neurotic traits or behavior disorders. In such a case the deprivation has some special meaning to the child.

There are many situations and features in the child's environment that may have a great influence upon the developing pattern of his personality. Anxiety, frustration, deprivation of love, overprotection, lack of consideration of the individual factor and of personality needs unfavorably influence the developing personality. The emotional attitude of the environment, for example, may promote security or it may create anxiety which may evoke various defensive behavior reactions. Hate, fear, worry, rejection, critical, punitive, and other environmental attitudes may exercise distorting effects and prevent the development of a rounded and smoothly functioning personality. An environment that presents constant frustrations or deprivations may stimulate resentment that later takes the forms of a persistent hostility and aggression, or again it may lead to a pattern of withdrawal. Much of the child's behavior is determined by the manner in which he deals with his aggression. Belonging to a social group regarded as inferior or alien to the major environmental one with the resulting conflicts in identification with one's own family group in ideologies and in accepted culture may create many emotional problems. Difficulties in language and lack of social and educational privileges and experiences may also contribute to the problems. The child who feels rejected is often insecure and anxious as a result of which he is hyperactive, emotionally unstable, has difficulty in concentrating, feels resentment toward the person who denies him the love he wants, and expresses his hostile feelings by temper tantrums and disobedience. He may cover up his need for affection by an air of bravado and attack. Students of child delinquency report that generally the delinquent has had an unhappy childhood characterized by feelings of rejection, inadequacy and guilt and by lack of affection. The environment favorable to a wholesome growth of the personality is one in which are to be found the warm human relations of marriage, parenthood and the family. The child should have a feeling of being liked and wanted, of belonging to someone who cares and of being guided with benevolent interest and confidence.

It has already been indicated that the parent-child relationship is one of the most determinative interpersonal relationships in respect to the child's mental health. It is out of this dynamic relationship that many, probably most, of the child's difficulties arise. Disturbances in this field may be reflected in the child's behavior. The attitude of the parents toward the child, their way of handling, caring for and training him, their general attitude toward life and people, and the way in which the child's environment meets his instinctive and developmental needs are the many sources of his emotional experience. Early emotional security is highly essential in the personality development of the child. This is provided largely by the mother whose fondling and cuddling furnish the baby his first feelings of support and assurance. Without this sense of security, attained only through appropriate and adequate emotional nutrition, immaturities will be manifested in various ways.

The attitude of the parents toward the child is greatly influenced by the degree of satisfaction and contentment they have been able to achieve in their own lives. Not rarely the mother carries over into her relationship with her child the unresolved conflicts that arose in her relationships with her own parents. Hostilities and resentments from such a source may enter into a disturbing relationship with her child that has harmful effect on its social and emotional growth and development. Conflict over hostile feelings is common in parents and much of the behavior expressed in troublesome parent-child relationships derives from that source.

Parental oversolicitude is much more frequent than neglect and is equally pernicious in its results. Such overprotection in every phase of the child's life, including dress, health, food, play and association with other children prevents the development of independence, responsibility and maturity of personality essential for successful adaptation. Such children, shielded from all the ordinary hazards of life, are rendered dependent, infantile and frequently hostile. They lack the satisfying pleasures of childhood and are usually whining and deceitful. Oversolicitous parents, in their anxiety to protect the child against imaginary harm, usually nag, scold and constantly admonish him. As he grows older they continue to treat him as a child rather than as a responsible, or at least partially responsible, person.

Maternal overprotection is more frequent than is paternal oversolicitude. It may be manifested in case both of the wanted and the unwanted child and for various reasons. In the case of the unwanted child, the fact that the prospective arrival of the child was unwelcome may have made the mother feel guilty for having entertained such a thought. A smothering oversolicitude may represent the denial and disguise of a hostile rejection of the child—a device for the denial of hate. The defensive reaction to her unconscious hostility to the child may lead her to extravagant measures of protection resembling an obsessional neurosis. Perhaps her marriage proved frustrating and she finds in her child a solution of her own emotional needs. Overprotection may take the form of continuing such activities as feeding, bathing, nursing or dressing the child long past the usual time. It may be shown, too, by the mother's practice of sleeping with the child even in his teens, or by a desire to have the child constantly in her presence. Usually, also, there is oversolicitous protection against physical danger, illness or the "bad influence" of other children. Levy points out that in her training of the child the overprotective mother is either indulgent or dominating. The child of the indulgently overprotective mother continues his infantile demands and expectations long after they should have been outgrown. He is often a disciplinary problem, and his behavior may be characterized by disobedience, impudence, tantrums, an aggressively demanding attitude, and varying degrees of tyrannical behavior. He may be selfish, conceited and a show-off. His bossy and demanding attitude betrays the fact that maternal indulgence has stimulated the development of aggressive components of the child's personality. Feeding problems are common in the child of the indulgent, apprehensive mother. The problems of the dominatingly overprotective mother's child are largely of anxieties, fears, shyness and submissive behavior. In both cases the overprotection operates against outside influences that make for growth in social adaptation. The child may use neurotic symptoms to control the mother and retain the infantile advantages of the emotionally intertwined mother-child relation.

Levy has shown, too, that many instances of the overprotective relationship arise from the mother's insatiable hunger for love, a hunger based on a severe privation of love in her own childhood. To this impoverishment in the child of all those positive feelings implicit in parental love—recognition, security, affection and sympathy—Levy gives the term "affect hunger."

The emotional influences in a particular family are never identical for any two children. Probably, too, a mother's psychology is such that no two children can bear for her the same emotional meaning. Occasionally a mother may entertain a hostility toward a particular child, arising, perhaps, from a hatred which is directed primarily toward her husband and then transmitted to a child who resembles him. Again, disappointment concerning the sex of the child may create a maternal attitude that is traumatic to it. At times the child's problems may be responses to the difficult situations created for him by the tensions within the family. The child who is deprived of love or raised by fear, terror, punishment and other sadistic methods usually responds by aggressive behavior or by mechanisms of escape. There is danger that the child may become either dependent and submissive or else rebellious toward the authority of parents. The overstrict, punitive father may arouse disturbing tensions and such emotional reactions as fear, anxiety, resentment and hostility with consequent personality or behavior disorders. The tension of actively aggressive impulses evoked by the severity of a father who represents an object of frustration and fear may cause the boy to erect defenses against his aggression, perhaps in the form of an obsessional character or an obsessional neurosis.

In Chapter III, Personality Development and Structure, attention was called to the mechanism of identification as one of the most important factors in affecting personality and in shaping character. Emotional deprivation makes it impossible for the child to identify with the parental figures and thereby utilize the constructive influence of that mechanism in personality development. Although identification is largely an unconscious process, it is based on a feeling of love, and without love, without a feeling of respect or admiration for someone or something, without a desire to be like some member of the environment, identification does not take place and the development of the superego is hindered and behavior difficulties result. It should be remembered, too, that through daily association and identification the emotional difficulties of the parent may be transmitted to the child.

One must not forget the emotionally deprived child who appears to be retarded in every field of personality development including even intellectual functioning. Such children are most frequently found among those who were reared in institutions during infancy.

Other Causes

In previous paragraphs much emphasis has properly, we believe, been placed on the personal maladjustments of parents and their overprotective, rejective and other attitudes as causes of childhood maladjustment. As previously noted, however, the problem or its causes should not be oversimplified. While the majority of emotional and behavior disorders arise from situations, interpersonal relations, and environmental constellations that operate against personality development or produce conflicts, tensions and anxieties, yet organic and other factors must not be disregarded. The child, for example, who is so retarded mentally that he cannot compete with his peers, the one who is small for his age but strives to compensate through his readiness to fight, the child who is deaf or who has suffered from a prolonged physical illness or from encephalitis may react with emotional or behavior disturbances. The brain-injured child must not be forgotten, either. Beneath this child's disturbed behavior there may be a rich and troubled inner life marked by anxiety, regression and frustration. Neurological or orthopedic handicaps, obesity or other physical abnormalities that attract attention require special consideration. Other factors that stimulate self-consciousness or an exaggerated feeling of difference in relation to those about the child may act as potentially pathogenic factors. Overambitious educational expectations may evoke emotional and behavior reactions of a neurotic nature.

Some child psychiatrists regard aggressiveness as an inherent instinctual tendency, a fundamentally normal and desirable human trait which, however, may vary greatly in amount and character. Through frustration, emotional deprivation or fear it may become undirected, misdirected, turned against the self or lead to pathological hostility and become a serious behavior problem. Other psychiatrists deny that aggression and hostility are normal and basic qualities of the personality. They believe that aggression in childhood is a symptom resulting from the fact that because of harmful developmental influences constructive drives find inadequate means of satisfaction. The result is that these drives become exaggerated or disorganized into a hostile and destructive aggression. At any rate it seems logical to assume that overaggressiveness is the result of chronic anxiety, frustration and emotional deprivation. If the child has never known love and kindness, a hostile aggressiveness may be persistent and even untreatable.

Forms of Psychiatric Problems

The anxieties of childhood are often expressed as transient symptomatic reactions related to some current situation or emotional conflict. While the child may present a variety of manifestations of anxiety, one or another symptom is seen as most disturbing. When the child suffers from prolonged and definitive disturbances of the psychotic, neurotic or defective type, these are to be discriminated from the forms of psychiatric problem classified under the Adjustment Reactions of Infancy or Childhood.

ADJUSTMENT REACTION OF INFANCY. Those transient disturbances in infancy such as undue apathy, undue excitability, or the disturbances in feeding and sleeping which take place on a psychogenic basis and are unassociated with physical disorder are usually classified under the nosological term mentioned. In most instances it will be found that as a result of the infant's interaction with the mother, or a mother surrogate, or because of a deprivation of such a relationship, these disturbances take place. An example of the types of disorders which one might classify as adjustment reaction to infancy are those symptomatic responses of the infant to separation from the mother. Disturbances of behavior due to isolation or maternal deprivation in children raised in institutional homes during the first two years of life have been known for the past three decades. Schlossman[1] coined the term "hospitalism" in 1926 to designate the condition. Levy[2] defined the genesis of the condition in his paper, "Primary Affect Hunger," in 1933, and Spitz has more recently studied experimentally the withdrawal of the infant, his apprehension on the approach of others, weepiness, sadness, loss of appetite and of weight, and insomnia, which take place in the periods

[1] Schlossman, E. E.: Zur Frage des Hospitalismus in Sauglingsanstalten. Ztschr. f. Kinderheilkunde, *42*:31–38, 1926.

[2] Levy, D. M.: Primary affect hunger. Am. J. Psychiat., *94*:643–652, 1936.

between six and twelve months as a consequence of a separation from the mothering one. The child may show a retardation of development with inability to walk and delayed reaction to external stimuli with slowness of movement and stupor if the separation is continued for a period of time. If the mother returns there is a rapid disappearance of the evidence of disturbance and behavior. Illness, tension, or anxiety in the mother may also lead to similar, though usually less severe, disturbances in the behavior of the infant. Prolonged maternal deprivation is productive of severe personality maldevelopment, as described earlier in this chapter.

ADJUSTMENT REACTIONS OF CHILDHOOD. As mentioned before, these reactions are to be differentiated from the rare psychotic, psychoneurotic or organic disturbances of childhood. They are usually subclassified according to the most prominent manifestations in the following way:

HABIT DISTURBANCE. This is manifested in such simple repetitive activities as nail biting, thumb sucking, enuresis, masturbation and temper tantrums. One group of these disorders concerns the manipulations of certain parts of the body. Here we find such conditions as thumb sucking, nail biting, nose picking, tongue sucking. These conditions are generally differentiated from tics; they are felt to occur at a high level of awareness, are intermittently present, are variable in duration, intensity and course, and the action in itself seems to be pleasurable. If they are interrupted at any stage of a single performance, they are recognized by the patient as actions for which he is responsible and subject to his control.

Thumb sucking, one of the earliest forms of body manipulation, is usually either the consequence of deprivation in the early sucking activities of the infant or in older children is a regressive act during periods of tension or fatigue. Levy, from his observations, concluded that in the majority of the infants thumb sucking is a result of insufficient lip movements or incompleteness of the sucking phases of the feeding act, regardless of the type of feeding. Thumb sucking results not only from difficulties in feeding of the infant, expressions of anxiety in the mother, but also from faulty techniques of nursing. Probably of more concern are those anxieties in the parents related to the presumed effects of thumb sucking. In the past various statements were made to the effect that distortions of personality as well as malformations of the jaws and palate resulted from thumb sucking. The management of this adjustment reaction is to be directed from the parental attitude rather than to the sucking thumb of the infant.

Nail biting is probably the commonest of the forms of habitual body manipulation occurring both in children and adults. It is usually first seen around the fifth year of life and increases in its occurrence up to the tenth or twelfth year when children gradually relinquish the habit. Threatening efforts to prevent the child from carrying out this act are usually unsuccessful. The condition is now recognized as an expression of tension. Its removal may be attempted through understanding and relieving the source of the underlying anxiety.

Masturbation, commonly practised by children, requires treatment only if the parental or adult attitudes toward the act have instilled in the child anxieties and fears that affect his personality development adversely. More frequently the problems of masturbation in a child involves clarifying misconceptions of the ill effects of the procedure in the minds of the parents and preventing radical efforts to prevent the act.

The other varieties of body manipulation, aside from hair pulling (trichotillomania), are relatively of little importance. The latter calls for more careful attention and may be associated with serious problems within the family.

Enuresis, the involuntary passage of urine, is a common disturbance frequently referred to the child psychiatrist. In some psychiatric clinics enuresis is the problem for which the majority of children are referred. At the age of two years some eighty per cent of children have ceased to wet themselves. By the end of three years the average child is usually able to keep his clothes and bed clean and dry. The condition occurs twice as frequently in boys as in girls, it is unrelated to intelligence, and in the majority of instances has been persistent. There is a group of children in whom the habit disappears only to recur at a later date during a period of tension. By far the most frequent variety of enuresis is the nocturnal type although diurnal enuresis and combinations of both have been noticed. In the majority of instances no physical disturbances of the nervous system or genitourinary apparatus are found on examination. Enuresis may occur as a matter of inadequate training resulting either from parental attitudes or because of lack of opportunity for adequate training. In some infants the mother is overprotective and the child's continuing inability to maintain himself dry is accepted by her on the basis that he is too small or weak for training. The child is thus infantilized and retains an infantile lack of control. Lack of opportunity for training as a causative factor occurs only in children raised in rural homes or in crowded urban areas where toilet facilities are inadequate and the child is not expected to visit the bathroom under conditions of cold or crowding. In other instances enuresis occurs as an expression of revenge in which the child wets, a reaction to too rapid and punitive training.

A common type of enuresis is the regressive. In children suffering from this form of enuresis, wetting occurs as a means of again obtaining the gratification of maternal contact. Very frequently regressive enuresis may be seen as a consequence of the birth of a younger child with the loss of the mother's attention. The child now wets in order to obtain the care and personal attention and affection he misses because of the mother's preoccupation with the newborn. In such instances, the proper parental reaction conducive to change is to allow the youngster more attention for a time in order that he may grow beyond his childish needs. Punishment seldom leads to modification of regressive enuresis. The series of studies by Margaret Gerard suggests that two thirds of the enuretic children have failed to identify with the parent of the same sex. The failure of sexual identification seems to take place in families where the parent of the opposite sex has a passive personality while the parent of the same sex is feared as more strict and rigid. Enuretic boys consequently tend to be passive and unassertive youngsters who are unable to compete actively, while girls with the wetting problem are found to be tomboyish and aggressive.

While enuresis occasionally is interrupted by simple suppressive measures, it is well to recognize that it is often symptomatic of anxiety-arousing problems in the family. On the other hand the symptom is often severe, prolonged, and not easily modified by therapy. It leads, if continued, to many additional conflicts in the growing child depending upon the attitudes of people with whom he is in contact. As a result of punishment and shaming, the enuretic child develops secondary feelings of inadequacy. Many suffer from sleeplessness in their attempts to control their bladder. These children have feelings of embarrassment and lack of self-confidence which restrict their capacity to form easy relationships with others as well as feelings of helplessness resulting from their inability to control the habit. They are often told repeatedly that they suffer from "weak bladders" or "weak kidneys," deepening their personal conviction of physical weakness and disability. Exposed to the consequences of teasing when sent to camp or to school with other children, their sense of social inadequacy is again magnified.

A 12½-year-old girl was brought to the pediatric psychiatric clinic by her mother who complained that she wet her bed, was very nervous and restless, bit her nails, and screamed while playing with other children. The mother recounted that her daughter had been enuretic since infancy. Initially, she wet her bed every hour or so during the night; now she wets once or twice a week. The mother wakes her up twice during the night. She stated that if the children got her daughter to laugh in the day time she occasionally wet herself. The mother recounted that the daughter had slept with her for two years in the same bed. She said her daughter always liked exciting things, was admired by everyone around her but did not care for work about the house and wished to be a lady; nor did she wish to learn anything. When asked to help with the housework she argued and became angry.

The daughter is the only child. The mother felt that the pregnancy was quite normal. The child was breast fed for 14 months and walked at one year but was slow in beginning to talk. Her dentition was completed at seven months and bowel control at three years. The mother continued to feed the girl until the age of 8 since she would not take a spoon in her own hand. Her mother bathed her until she was eleven years old and reported that her daughter dressed herself only for the past six months. She first allowed her daughter to cross the street alone within the same period of time. The explanation for this was that the mother had seen another child run over some time before. The girl had had no unusual illnesses but was sick with teething and vomited a great deal at this time. Her school work was good. She began school at six and a half and was regularly promoted with her class. On psychological testing she was found to have an I. Q. of 113.

The mother described the father as a nervous man whose hand shook and who was preoccupied with palpitation of the heart. He was seen as impatient and easily upset. The mother considered herself a fairly healthy person but nervous since an operation for appendicitis the previous year. She spoke of crying quite easily and complained about her marriage stating it had not been happy in the early years as her husband was attached to his mother.

When the daughter was seen she was found to be a tall, gangling, very talkative, "smart alecky" girl, rather restless, walking about uneasily. In discussing the problem of bed wetting she stated that she used to have difficulty in sleeping because "I was afraid I couldn't wake up in time and then I couldn't get to sleep; then I would worry because I couldn't sleep and I wouldn't." She said she had slept better since her parents did not put her to bed so early. In discussing her parents she said, "They have to love me, I'm the only one." She described her mother as "treating me like a baby." "She won't let me go to the movies alone." She volunteered that she would not like to grow up but would prefer to remain the same age as she is now. "It is more fun."

In subsequent treatment hours with the mother and child it was learned that the daughter had been unwanted but always overprotected, the mother believing that some harm would come to her. Initially she was a shy child but later developed many friends, mostly among older children. While she was at first distant with her father she has become quite close to him since the mother became ill and was not available to do everything for her. She stated that her father was a mother to her. The child and her mother were seen only intermittently over the following three years as they lived at a distance. She did better at school but continued enuretic although with diminished frequency. After three years the enuresis disappeared although there was occasionally frequency of urination at night or during the day. In the meantime the child worked out many of her conflicting feelings in regard to her dependent relationship with her mother and her ambivalent attitude toward her father.

Conduct disorder includes those disturbances in behavior or social activity in the child which are of such concern that they are reported in the home, in the school, in the community, or in all three. Such conditions are noticed by parents, teachers or members of social agencies. Among the common conduct disorders are disobedience, lying, stealing, destructiveness, fighting, firesetting, truancy, cruelty, running away, and various sexual activities. Occasionally such disturbances may be secondary to brain damage as as consequence of epilepsy, epidemic encephalitis, or caused by mental deficiency.

Usually the child with such disorders expresses little self-criticism or reproach, feels no guilt and is unresponsive to punishment. He is frequently lacking in the capacity to relate himself emotionally to others or to receive affection. Many of these early behavior disorders represent transformations or reactions to aggression. Aggression may play a part in the very symptoms which at first sight seem to bear no relation to it. Frequently, in fact, the troublesome behavior of the child is not of such a nature as to suggest its real source. The conduct disorder may be an adaptation to submissiveness or be an effort to obtain a substitute or compensatory satisfaction for those not received at home. Again, the conduct disturbance may represent an attempt to bolster up feelings of inadequacy or inferiority, an effort to make himself feel courageous and superior by overemphasizing his independence in the form of aggressive and disturbing behavior. Sometimes it serves as defiance of authority or as a means of controlling the mother or of tyrannizing the household. Some forms of conduct disorder represent efforts to escape from anxiety-ridden situations. In others the behavior disorder arises as a consequence of a desire for punishment created in response to marked feelings of guilt.

In Chapter XXXII, Sociopathic and Personality Disorders, the etiology suggested by Szurek and Johnson for such antisocial conduct disorders as firesetting, truancy, stealing and unacceptable sexuality as it occurs in some children was discussed. Here the source for the antisocial behavior is believed to be in the parent's unwitting sanction or indirect encouragement of the child's behavior. In these instances the child is healthy, not deprived emotionally, nor exposed to cultural patterns that encourage the pattern, but comes from an apparently "good" family. In such instances the parent appears overtly to interdict the act which is the source of complaint. However, study of the parent-child interaction in the course of collaborative treatment has demonstrated that through unconsciously driven behavior the parent or both parents communicate their permissiveness to the child. The approval is often expressed in nonverbal forms by undue attention to the child's disturbing behavior, by the lack of consistent firmness, and in its management through unwitting and sometimes suggestive remarks, smirks or encouragement. In such instances, change in behavior requires treatment of the permissive parent who obtains a vicarious gratification from the child's misbehavior which acts out the parents' repressed impulses.

A seven-year-old boy was referred for psychiatric consultation from the Board of Education because of his inability to make a satisfactory adjustment in his class room. The teacher reported that he was constantly aggressive toward other children and that much of his behavior seemed bizarre. He had been discharged from a class the previous year because of similar disturbances of behavior. The mother reported that she had had difficulty in controlling him at home. To her he seemed very restless, blinked his eyes frequently and masturbated constantly. She summed up her problem in one sentence, "I can't seem to get through to him." She dated the change in his behavior to the age of two and a half when he first was observed to be tense and seemed to joke about everything said to him. When the boy was examined he was found to be pale, stocky but well developed, and with a husky voice. He frequently asked what would happen to him when he would return to the class room. He seemed anxious concerning the possibility of bodily injury and became very apprehensive when feeling the cutting edges of carpentry tools in the play room. He did not talk spontaneously and was evasive in his replies. There was evidence of poor motor co-ordination and little patterning in what he did. Psychological tests showed him to be hesitant, suspicious and interpretive of all remarks as hostile. He frequently evaded by apparent misunderstanding or not hearing what was said to him. It was felt the child needed assistance in a residential hospital setting.

In discussion of the problem with the father it was learned that on many occasions the father had beaten the boy severely. It seemed evident that the father was competing with his son in many ways, and he remarked in regard to games with him, "He can't lose, he wants to win the games we play. I usually win. It's hard for him to beat me. If he loses, he loses legitimately!" The father also indicated his resentment toward the son and spoke of his son's interest as silly. He expressed favoritism for a younger child. The mother was found to be an immature, dependent and self-centered person, limited in her fantasy life and depressed in mood.

When the boy was brought to the hospital he first expressed much concern about "who is boss" on the ward. He frequently insisted that he was "the boss" and often attempted to engage in power struggles with other children and the doctor. He remarked, "Well, if you are strong how come you haven't killed me yet." Frequently he talked of his own strength or expressed desires of being killed. In play sessions he acted as the father and behaved in an impatient, angry and cruel way to a doll. The game often ended with the doll killing all other little dolls and destroying the furniture and the parents. With continuing treatment he became destructive and aggressive in the hospital. This behavior subsided when he was provided an interpretation that apparently it was his wish to provoke the psychiatrist to respond as would have happened at home. He then made efforts to seek closeness to the psychiatrist.

Additional history disclosed that the patient was a planned child and his early development had been quite normal. The mother reported that bowel training had been difficult and that she had had a constant struggle with the child. She stated that she had beaten him if he failed to excrete properly and admitted being constantly frustrated and angry in caring for him.

In the course of the treatment of the child it became apparent that the problem was one of a hateful struggle for control between the boy and his chronically distressed mother. His only conception of existence seemed to be in fighting and attaining the position of "the boss." The father contributed to the child's hostility through his competitive feelings and his hostile aggression toward the child. His behavior slowly but gradually improved in the protective milieu of the residential treatment center and with play therapy sessions in conjunction with special schooling. After eighteen months he was discharged home. By then his parents had received some understanding of their problems through psychotherapeutic treatment.

Another common type of conduct disturbance occurs in children who have learning disturbances at school. As Levy has recently pointed out, the motivational explanation for the conduct disturbance is inappropriate in such instances. The motivational problem is secondary; the primary issue is the capacity of the child to learn. At the present time approximately twelve per cent of all children in the United States fail to learn to read as well as the average. While these children have better than normal intelligence and their social and vocabulary development is excellent, as well as their vision, they suffer from dyslexia, occasionally, but not always, associated with left-handedness and with difficulty converting to right-handed writing. This disability manifests itself in a variety of ways, sometimes as confusion of one consonant with another, such as b's for d's, p's for q's, or t's for f's, or as a reversal of the syllables, words, or entire sentences as mere writing, with a complete failure to recognize words. Another group of children suffers from an inability to learn as a consequence of the newer methods of teaching reading. By these methods children are taught to read whole words, phrases and sentences with an analysis of individual words into phonic sounds and letters undertaken only secondarily. Because of their particular perceptual capacity some children are unable to learn to read or spell by this method of pedagogy. In such children the emotional expressions of fear and anxiety because of failure to meet the standards of the family or class, and to a hostility resulting from feelings of rivalry and jealousy tend to imbue concepts of personal inferiority and encourage behavior disturbance. Many conduct disabilities founded on such a basis disappear rapidly with improvement in the reading. The important element in treatment is recognition of the underlying incapacity to learn. Here the use of a remedial teacher is often the effective technique to bring about a satisfactory modification of the behavior disturbance. The following case illustrates this problem:

O. E. was an eight-and-one-half-year-old boy referred for evaluation and for possible treatment of emotional problems involved in the patient's inability to read. The school teacher and psychologist felt the patient had an emotional block which prevented his learning to read. The child was restless and unruly in school and a difficult problem in management. Physical examination was negative except for confusion in handedness. Past history was free of gross emotional disturbances. He was well liked by his many friends and had many interests. His parents had high academic aspirations for him and were distressed by his poor scholastic performance. He was compared unfavorably with his very bright ten-year-old brother.

During the psychiatric interview he appeared friendly, co-operative and fully understood the reason for his being in the doctor's office. He said, "I can't read and it gets me worried." He handled a pencil very poorly in either hand and in printing reversed several letters and words. He could not read. Psychological tests revealed an average intelligence. He could not be tested in reading achievement since this was so defective. Bender gestalt designs were below his age level but he showed difficulty in integration of the designs. A diagnosis of learning disability was made. It was felt that the problem of anxiety was secondary. A remedial reading teacher was engaged. Parents and teachers were encouraged to let him progress and learn at his own speed. He did well under special instruction, progressing slowly but quite satisfactorily in reading. His restlessness, tension and disobedience subsided quickly.

Neurotic traits are closely related to habit disturbance and the distinction between the two is often difficult. Here are classified tics, habit spasms, somnambulism, stammering, overactivity and phobias. Tics occur as repetitious, involuntary but apparently purposeless, movement of interconnected muscles. They frequently involve the muscles of the eyelids with blinking or squinting. Often, tics are first noticed in childhood; they then disappear, only to recur at a later date at the time of some conflict. Frequently it will be found that the tic was first noticed after a frightening experience leading to a fear of injury and represents a defensive muscular withdrawal response of small muscle groups appropriate to the expected trauma. While initially the defensive muscular contraction may have involved many muscles, the tic represents a rudimentary response of small muscle groups. Because of the persistence of the response beyond the particular time of the injury the tic-like movement becomes inappropriate and involuntary. The use of the small muscle groups develops as a consequence of parental prohibition for the full movement. The tic then represents both the fear of injury and the attempt to maintain gratification by complying to parental wishes. In addition to the tic, the child frequently is restless, self-conscious, sensitive or spoiled, or may be overambitious and overconscientious. Frequently easy excitability and fatigability are observed. There are other children who are shy, seclusive and embarrassed. The tics of psychogenic origin are to be differentiated from those which occur as a result of encephalitic disease affecting the basal ganglia. Treatment of the latter is often difficult.

A six-year-old boy was brought to the clinic by his mother who complained that he jerked his head and blinked his eyes frequently. She stated that he had begun this habit about four or five weeks previously. When the habit spasm began she paid little heed to it but later she slapped him in the face for it. At first she thought it might be caused by disease of his eyes. She became annoyed when he began to open his eyes with his fingers. The boy reported it was his feeling that his eyes were closing on him when the lids were heavy.

The mother went on to describe her son as restless, unable to sit in a chair and as very fidgety. She also reported that he had occasional headaches and had begun to suffer from asthma at his seventeenth month. His last attack had taken place twelve months previously. Early in life he had played with younger children but now he played only with those of his own age. The boy had been breast fed for six months and bottle fed until a year and a half. At five months of age he had been able to sit alone and had stood up and taken some steps at nine months. At the end of the first year he had said a few words. She indicated that his bowel and bladder training had been completed in less than a year. The mother had dressed the boy until a year and a half ago and said that he wished her to dress him even now. It was only at this time that he had begun to wash himself. The story of his schooling showed that he had entered the first grade at six, had done very well and was jumped several classes. He is now the youngest child in his class. It was the mother's impression that he feels uneasy at the present time. The father was described as a happy-go-lucky person who enjoys his children. The mother thought of herself as being well. There are three children, the patient being the eldest. A sister is two and a half years younger and a baby is eighteen months old.

When the boy was seen he was found to blink, roll his eyes and grimace about his mouth. He said that the trouble with his facial muscles came on after he had arrived home from school some weeks before and done his homework. He felt he could not stop the movements once started. He also reported that he had been unable to sleep well and admitted some recent worries about masturbation. He saw himself as a sickly boy and described his fear of playing rough games with others. The matter of the boy's masturbation was discussed with the mother who became overtly anxious in dealing with this subject. On returning home she was able to talk to her son on the subject without threatening him. The mother discontinued bathing him and allowed him to go to bed later. During several additional hours the matter of the sexual interests of the son was brought up for discussion by the mother. The physician worked with her and the boy with gratifying results. The facial tics disappeared following a series of four visits. Treatment for the asthma was continued for several years.

Psychological Tests

Psychological examinations often serve as an aid to the evaluation of the limitations and assets of the child referred for psychiatric study. This is especially true if there are questions involving learning difficulties, mental retardation, the possibility of brain injury or the existence of a psychosis. They may, too, help to obtain a general picture of the child's problem areas and intrapsychic dynamics. In deciding as to whether or not the child should be tested, consideration should be given not only to the amount of meaningful information that can probably be secured by his test performance but also to the degree of emotional trauma the tests may cause him.

Three types of tests are generally used in children's clinics: intelligence tests, achievement tests and projective tests. While intelligence tests have a high degree of validity when used with children of school age or older, the reliability of those designed for infants and pre-school age is comparatively poor in and of themselves exclusive of other studies of the child.

Achievement tests measure the benefits the child has derived from his educational endeavors. Often the lack of correlation between educational achievement and mental ability uncovers the nature of general learning problems or specific ones such as in reading or arithmetic.

The Rorschach Ink-Blot Test is the projective test most likely to reveal nuclear conflicts, basic anxieties and the level of emotional maturation. The validity and meaningfulness of projective test results are very dependent on the skill, experience and the personality of the psychologist. Sometimes they tend to arouse anxiety and hostility on the part of the child.

Therapeutic Measures

The treatment of personality difficulties of the child must vary with the individual and his problems. The principal emphasis, however, is on "the child's needs, strivings, and growth tendencies in a social and cultural background." The fundamental objective is a healthy personality re-organization and an improved emotional adjustment. Many of the child's behavior problems and neurotic difficulties arise from emotional handicaps sustained through earlier relationship experiences which were not conducive to healthy emotional growth. One seeks, therefore, to acquire an understanding of the forces which have been operating in the early life of the child. While the child cannot, of course, develop beyond the limits of his constitutional potentialities, it is the aim of therapeutic measures to remove or reduce his persistent and crippling emotional difficulties and to aid him in reorganizing those emotional attitudes and patterns of reaction that have been governing his personality functioning. In this way growth of the patient's personality toward new and more spontaneous and satisfying patterns is made possible. A growth-promoting relationship must be substituted for the previous ones that produced insecurity, aggression or hostility, that reinforced infantilization and prevented growth in the direction of self-reliance and social maturity.

The details of the therapist's technique of treatment will be determined by his theoretical conceptions of etiology, dynamics and therapy, and by the specific nature of the child's problem. In the older child, psychobiological principles with distributive analysis as the therapeutic technique may be used. Other psychiatrists may prefer to use psychonanalytical principles to a large extent. In either case the physician may wish to make use of "*environmental*" or "*manipulative*" *therapy*, consisting of boy's clubs, camps, dancing classes, boarding schools, or other activities which will enable the patient to make contacts with others and develop interests of his own. In some cases separation for long periods of time from an overprotective mother may be desirable. In younger children play techniques involving psychoanalytical principles are largely used.

One element common, however, to all forms of therapy is the use of the *therapist-patient relationship*. Into this relationship the child brings the resentments, anxiety, fears, guilt and the fantasies which have arisen from such feelings. The first essential is for the psychiatrist to establish a friendly, interesting and satisfactory relationship between the child and himself. He accepts the child as an equal and as a person in his own right. He neither stresses nor ignores the difference in age and maturity but assumes it as a matter of course and does not assume an artificially childish language. In the therapist the child finds someone who can help him as he is. The therapeutic approach must be a gradual one. To hasten it may defeat the relationship and cause the child to withdraw into evasion, indifference or falsification. Any early reference to behavior disorders may stimulate hostility or tension. Early discussions may therefore deal with the child's interests, activities and in direct questioning about neutral matters. With the therapist-child relationship satisfactorily established, the patient may, in this friendly atmosphere, verbalize his conscious conflicts, opinions, ideas and feelings which can then be discussed. In another way, too, the therapist-child relationship may be of value. Through this relationship the child projects his anxiety and hostility onto the personality of the physician. By projection the child may make use of the therapist to symbolize an unacceptable part of himself as he moves toward freeing himself of the unacceptable aspect. The child may also project onto the therapist desirable qualities which he hopes to attain. The therapist will not be critical of the child's behavior and will take his ideas seriously and as worthy of attention and consideration. He will seek to feel and understand just what problems the child is trying to solve when by that very effort he is creating the problems which have brought him to the psychiatrist. His attitude will not be one of condescension. Within the security of the dependent relationship with the emotionally more mature therapist whom he trusts and imitates, the child relives his emotional conflicts. The physician will aim to have the child feel that the therapist is a kindly adult, a helpful, protective father who understands his feelings and is helping him.

Occasionally with older children and adolescents, if the problem is a simple and largely environmental one, talks with the patient concerning situations which are troublesome may be not only a direct but also an important treatment. He may have reacted to a situation with confused apprehension and undesirable behavior because he did not understand the chain of circumstances that produced a given result. One must not, however, be merely attempting to have the child see what is wrong or undesirable about himself, expect him to relinquish his old ways or control them more effectively. Even with simple problems there must usually be a reorganization of emotional attitudes and patterns of reaction. To secure this the patient must not only have wholesome compensations and outlets but, through an acceptable and gratifying, and therefore therapeutic, relationship with the psychiatrist, gain a stimulus toward new ways of feeling, *i.e.*, to change, to grow.

Child-Parent Relationship

Since, as already indicated, the child's problem usually arises from the living relationship between himself and a parent and is interwoven with a parent's attitude, the parental attitudes form part of the examination. Frequently, therefore, it is not so much a symptom as the child-parent relationship that needs treatment. The psychiatric examination consists therefore of interviews with the parents and the examination of the child. Usually a series of interviews either with both parents or with the mother is desirable before the child is examined in order to discuss the problem which the latter presents. Frequently the atmosphere of the home has been one of emotional tension and unrest. The physician, by giving the parents—usually the mother—opportunity to express and relieve her perturbation and anxiety, gains the confidence of the parent, often secures revealing information about personality characteristics of the parents and assists the mother in seeing the child's trouble in a truer perspective. She may like to explain the child's behavior as a result of heredity but the therapist will usually discover that the mother's neurotic conflict has entered the child's handling. Her expressions of guilt, accusations, hostility, anxiety and excuses may betray the nature of interpersonal relations that have been a source of difficulty. Inquiry should be made as to the onset of the child's difficulty, the mode and circumstances of its first appearance and its development. The interview will presumably, too, assist the physician in securing desirable information concerning the child's cultural background, the family's ways of living, its intelligence, its beliefs and problems, the relationships between father and mother, and the child's group relations. Through a knowledge of the parents' past and present attitudes toward the child, the psychiatrist learns much as to what situations the child's behavior is an adjustment. As previously indicated, it will not rarely be found that the mother is carrying over into her relationship with her child the unresolved emotional problems that arose in her relationships with her own parents. The aim is to uncover a dynamic picture of the experiences and emotions of the child in relation to those surrounding him.

The problem may have arisen from the father-child relationship, but more frequently it arises from that of mother-child. If, as is probable, the problem has arisen from the relationship between the child and the mother, both require therapy. They are not, however, interviewed together. In child guidance clinics the psychiatric social worker will usually do case work with the mother at the same periods as the psychiatrist treats the child. In other clinics or private practice the problem of the mother may receive paramount attention from the psychiatrist while the child is seen by the social worker. The psychiatrist and social worker collaborate in helping parents and child to resolve difficulties that have arisen through living together. Through visits with the social worker, the mother acquires a new understanding of her relation to the child and a realization that she has part in the child's therapy. The simultaneity of these appointments, usually held weekly and forty-five minutes in duration, assists mother and child to realize that the problem requiring help does not exist solely in the child or in the mother but in the relationship between them. As previously indicated, the parents' psychological problems are usually one of the most serious obstacles to a resolution of the child's problem. It is the task of the psychiatrist or social worker to assist the mother to a better understanding and an emotional acceptance of herself in her relation to the child. If, as is not rarely the case, the mother's feeling for her child is one of rejection, treatment of the latter's problems is often difficult. The mother, burdened with anxieties and fears, cannot emotionally accept or understand a direct interpretation of her unconscious feelings or her personality patterns. By indirect methods, therefore, the worker helps the mother to objectify the problem and to formulate her thinking, feeling and behavior in relation to the child and to allay her guilt and anxiety. She will assist the mother in establishing a normal and satisfying relationship with the child that will permit a progressive and wholesome growth of her personality. No attempt should be made to make the mother recognize that she is coming to the worker for treatment for herself as a patient. If a favorable rapport is established with the worker, the mother accepts her relationship with the worker as a search for causes for the child's difficulties, and in examining the family life, she may begin to examine herself. The mother's influence and behavior in relation to her child are partially dependent upon her own self-understanding. The worker may help the mother to see family members in their respective relationships and, knowing their life experiences, the parent may begin to find new meaning for their behavior. In this manner her understanding of, and her relation to, the problem child may become clearer. The method of treatment directed toward influencing the parents' modes of managing and training the child as well as helping them with their own problems and attitudes which have caused or contributed to the child's difficulties is known as "attitude therapy." In addition to treatment with the parents, the social worker carries out any necessary manipulation of the environment.

Play Technique in Diagnosis

It is well recognized that free association is a valuable technique in adults for the investigation of significant psychological material below the level of consciousness. In children, however, play is a more normal mode of expression than is one limited to verbal forms. Play technique consists of introducing a child to a group of toys and permitting him to use them freely while the observer looks on. The toys given him represent all the common interests of childhood—animals, blocks with which to build houses, etc. Dolls often represent members of the family. Play being the medium in which the child expresses himself most freely, the use which he makes of the toys reveals his fantasies, offers insight into his mental mechanisms and gives clues regarding his unconscious. In the child, play may be regarded as the speech of the unconscious. He may use the imaginary characters of his play to express his own disturbed feelings. Being a projective technique, it may show human relations and problems arising out of them. It therefore sheds light on the family relationships as no other medium can. It illuminates both the relation of the child to his parents and of the parents to the child. Hiding behind the anonymity of a doll he may tell of death wishes directed toward a parent or sibling. The child should be permitted to choose the toy and use it spontaneously since he will select the medium of expression best suited to himself and therefore best adapted to express his immediate problem or situation. In play, therefore, we find an excellent projective technique for the diagnosis of hidden aspects of the personality and for a study of the emotional life of children. We know that the child's emotional life revolves primarily around his mother, father and siblings. Since play provides a feeling-projecting medium, we find in it a readily available means of investigating the child's emotional attitudes toward the family. These, it will be found, are often ambivalent. We have already seen that the child's problems often arise from the interpersonal relationships in the family. Play, therefore, is often used by the child as a spontaneous projective technique for expressing the nature of the relationship in which his problem is rooted. He brings into his play the reactions and feelings connected with this problem. Drawing and painting may also be used as projective techniques not only for securing clues as to the child's problems and psychic dynamics but also as therapeutic adjuncts. In his art sessions, the child may attribute various imaginary roles to parent or sibling and may use his products as a channel of release.

There are many interesting phenomena in play technique comparable to those observed in psychoanalysis. For example, the child may show an anxious care in excluding some toy from his play, or on approaching some aspect of the play which he seems to find unsafe, not permissible, or unsatisfactory to the point of discomfort, he becomes upset and is unable to go on playing in peace. This is strikingly similar to the signs of emotional disturbance when in free association conflicts and anxieties push too near the surface. In this way the psychiatrist may secure clues to the sources of the child's difficulties. To be able not only to interpret the disruptions or interruptions of play such as just described, but also to interpret the symbolic gestures and words which the child constantly presents is of great aid in ascertaining the source of his difficulties. To do so, however, requires experience, insight and imaginative vision on the part of the psychiatrist.

Pharmacological Therapy

Pharmacological treatment with the phenothiazines, rauwolfia derivatives and other agents is now attempted widely for a number of the disorders of childhood as a means of providing symptomatic relief and reduction in anxiety for both child and parent. The eventual place of such treatment in child psychiatry remains to be established. The use of these agents is described in Chapter XXXVII.

BIBLIOGRAPHY

Ackerman, N. W., and Sobel, Raymond: Family diagnosis: An approach to the preschool child. Am. J. Orthopsychiat., *20*:744–746, 1950.

Allen, F. H.: Psychotherapy with Children. New York, W. W. Norton & Co., 1942.

———: Aggression in relation to emotional development, normal and pathological. Ment. Hyg., *34*:353–363, 1950.

———: Psychopathic behavior–fact or projection. Am. J. Orthopsychiat., *20*:236–240, 1950.

———: Horney's conception of the basic conflict applied to child psychiatry. Am. J. Psychoanalysis, *16:*99–111, 1956.

Baruch, Dorothy: One Little Boy. New York, Julian Press, Inc., 1952.

Bender, Lauretta: Techniques of Child Psychiatry. In *Current Therapies of Personality Disorders.* Bernard Glueck, Ed., New York, Grune & Stratton, 1946.

———: Psychological problems of children with organic brain disease. Am. J. Orthopsychiat., *19:*404–415, 1949.

Bender, Lauretta, and Nichtoni, S.: Chemotherapy in child psychiatry. New York State J. Med., *56:*2791–2795, 1956.

Bornstein, Berta: Emotional barriers in the understanding and treatment of young children. Am. J. Orthopsychiat., *18:*691–697, 1948.

Bowlby, John: Maternal Care and Mental Health. World Health Organization Monograph Series No. 2, Geneva, 1952.

Bruch, Hilda: Psychosomatic approach to childhood disorders. In *Modern Trends in Child Psychiatry,* Lewis, N. D. C., and Pacella, B. L., Eds. New York, International Universities Press, 1945.

Childrens Bureau: Emotional Problems Associated with Handicapping Conditions in Children. Washington, Federal Security Agency, 1952.

Creak, Mildred: Psychoses in childhood. J. Ment. Sc., *97:*545–554, 1951.

Despert, J. L.: Play Analysis in Research and Therapy. In *Modern Trends in Child Psychiatry,* Lewis, N. D. C., and Pacella, B. L., Eds. New York, International Universities Press, 1945.

———: Delusional and hallucinatory experiences in children. Am. J. Psychiat., *104:* 528–537, 1948.

———: Diagnostic criteria of schizophrenia in children. Am. J. Psychotherapy, *6:*148–163, 1942.

Esman, A. H., et al.: School experience in training of the child psychiatrist. Dis. Nerv. System, *13:*266–268, 1952.

Finch, S. M.: Psychosomatic problems in children. Nerv. Child, *9:*261–264, 1952.

Freud, Anna: Introduction to the Technique of Child Analysis. Washington, Nerv. & Ment. Dis. Monographs, 1928.

———, et al.: The Psychoanalytic Study of the Child, II. New York, International Universities Press, 1947.

Gerard, M. W.: Enuresis: A study in etiology. Am. J. Orthopsychiat., *9:*48–58, 1939.

———: The psychogenic tic in ego development. The Psychoanalyst. Study of the Child, *II:*133–162, 1946.

Goldfarb, W.: Effects of psychological deprivation in infancy and subsequent stimulation. Am. J. Psychiat., *102:*18–33, 1945.

Greenwood, E. D.: The role of psychotherapy in residential treatment. Am. J. Orthopsychiat., *25:*692–698, 1955.

Group for Advancement of Psychiatry: The contribution of psychiatry to pediatric training and practice. Quart. J. Child Behavior, *4:*178–195, 1952.

Group for the Advancement of Psychiatry, Report No. 38: The Diagnostic Process in Child Psychiatry. New York, 1790 Broadway, 1957.

Hamilton, Gordon: Psychotherapy in Child Guidance. New York, Columbia University Press, 1947.

Hulse, Wilfred, and Rapoport, Jack: What can pediatrics expect from psychoanalysis? Nerv. Child, *9:*270–277, 1952.

Ingram, T. T. S.: A characteristic form of overactive behavior in brain damaged children. J. Ment. Sc., *102:*550–558, 1956.

Johnson, A. M., and Szurek, S. A.: The genesis of antisocial acting out in children and adults. Psychoanalyt. Quart., *21:*323–343, 1952.

———: Etiology of antisocial behavior in delinquents and psychopaths. J.A.M.A., *154:* 814–817, 1954.

Kanner, Leo: Child Psychiatry, 3rd ed. Springfield, Illinois, Charles C Thomas, 1957.

———: Problems of nosology and psychodynamics of early infantile autism. Am. J. Orthopsychiat., *19:*416–426, 1949.

Klein, Melanie: The psychoanalytic play technique. Am. J. Orthopsychiat., *25:*223–237, 1955.

Levy, D. M.: Maternal Overprotection. New York, Columbia University Press, 1943.
———: Critical evaluation of the present state of child psychiatry. Am. J. Psychiat., *108:* 481–494, 1952.
———: Capacity and motivation. Am. J. Orthopsychiat., *27:*1–8, 1957.
Lewis, N. D. C., and Pacella, B. L., Eds.: Modern Trends in Child Psychiatry. New York, International Universities Press, 1945.
Lippman, H. S.: Treatment of the Child in Emotional Conflict. New York, McGraw Hill Book Co., 1956.
Lorand, Sandor: The psychoanalytic contribution to the treatment of behavior problems in children. Am. J. Psychiat., *105:*357–360, 1948.
Lowrey, L. G.: Personality distortions and early institutional care. Am. J. Orthopsychiat., *10:*576–585, 1940.
———: Therapeutic play technique; a symposium. Am. J. Orthopsychiat., *25:*747–787, 1955.
Mahler, M. S., and Luke, J. A.: Outcome of the tic syndrome. J. Nerv. & Ment. Dis., *103:*433–445, 1946.
Murphy, L. B.: Childhood Experience in relation to personality development. *In Personality and the Behavior Disorders,* Hunt, J. McV., Ed., New York, Ronald Press Co., 1944.
Pasamanick, Benjamin, Rogers, M. E., and Lilienfeld, A. M.: Pregnancy experience and the development of behavior disorders in children. Am. J. Psychiat., *112:* 613–617, 1956.
Pearson, G. H. J.: The chronically aggressive child. Nerv. Child, *9:*261–269, 1952.
———: Emotional Disorders of Children. New York, W. W. Norton & Co., 1949.
Redl, Fritz, and Wineman, D.: Children Who Hate. Glencoe, Free Press, 1951.
———: Controls from Within. Glencoe, Free Press, 1952.
Ribble, Margaret: Infantile Experience in Relation to Personality Development. In *Personality and the Behavior Disorders,* Hunt, J. McV., Ed., New York, Ronald Press Co., 1944.
Shirley, H. F.: Psychiatry for the Pediatrician. New York, The Commonwealth Fund, 1948.
Shugart, George: Casework with parents of psychotic children. Social Casework, *38:* 8–15, 1957.
Slavson, S. R.: Play Group Therapy for Young Children. Nerv. Child, *7:*318–327, 1948.
Spitz, R. A.: Anaclitic depression. The Psychoanalytic Study of the Child, *2:*313–342, 1946.
Szurek, S. A.: Comments on the psychopathology of children with somatic illness. Am. J. Psychiat., *107:*844–859, 1951.
Witmer, H. L., Ed.: Psychiatric Interviews with Children. New York, Commonwealth Fund, 1946.
———: Pediatrics and the Emotional Needs of the Child. New York, Commonwealth Fund, 1948.

CHAPTER XXXV

Shock and Other Physical Therapies

THE EMPLOYMENT of the so-called shock therapies dates from 1933 when Manfred Sakel, then working in the Clinic of the University of Vienna, reported that deep hypoglycemic states produced by large doses of insulin produced a beneficial effect on the course of schizophrenia. With the subsequent introduction of other forms of shock therapy, attempts were made to establish a common denominator of action in them all. Not yet, however, has any theory been presented that satisfactorily explains the therapeutic action in any one of the forms of shock therapy, much less one that applies to all forms. This subject will be discussed more fully later in the chapter. The use of insulin shock treatments and the various psychosurgical operations have been superseded to a large extent in the past few years by the introduction of the new pharmacological agents of the tranquilizing group. There are now available a number of important follow-up studies that describe and delineate the nature of the therapeutic effect of these procedures over long periods of time, a necessity for the understanding of any treatment offered in the field of psychiatric therapy.

Insulin Shock Treatment

In 1928 Sakel, believing that the nervous hyperactivity occurring in morphine addicts during withdrawal of that drug was caused by an excess of epinephrine, expressed the opinion that the excitement might be relieved by large doses of insulin. Later the similarity of the abstinence symptoms to other excited states suggested to Sakel that the latter also might be influenced by the same drug. He accordingly administered insulin to excited schizophrenic patients. After a period of experimental clinical work he published his results in 1933, and in 1936 introduced his technique in this country. The basic features in the technique developed by Sakel are still regarded as most effective. At first Sakel tried to avoid the development of deep hypoglycemic states but soon observed that better results occurred if coma were induced. He then increased the dose with the avowed intention of producing insulin shock.

Neurophysiology

Unlike other organs which can utilize carbohydrates, proteins and fats for energy requirements, the brain is able to oxidize carbohydrates only. Since the rate of oxidization of carbohydrates is determined by the amount of insulin in the blood stream, the injection of a large amount of insulin into the body greatly reduces the sugar content of the blood. With a decrease in the amount of sugar available, the oxidative processes of the brain may be so reduced that the effects are similar to anoxia of that organ, a condition known to lead to coma. The loss of consciousness in hypoglycemia is presumably caused by the fact that the brain cells are being deprived of glucose, their principal fuel, without which the metabolic processes in the brain are progressively depressed.

According to the segmental-suprasegmental concept of evolutionary development of the central nervous system, there are ascending levels of integration both of structure and function. We may therefore think of successively higher levels beginning with the lower medulla and culminating with the cerebral hemispheres. It has been shown that the rate of metabolism in each of the higher levels is greater than in that of the level immediately lower or older. The greatest susceptibility to low blood sugar exists therefore in the more complex and phylogenetically more recent areas of the forebrain. With the injection of large amounts of insulin, therefore, there is a step-like depression of function and the appearance of progressive neurological signs and symptoms corresponding to a phyletic regression or functional disturbance in the successively lower anatomical levels of cerebral cortex, diencephalon, midbrain, upper medulla and lower medulla. There is a progressive dissolution of the functions of the brain, a dissolution that seems to turn back that organ through the path of evolution. As the blood sugar falls following the injection of a "coma dose" of insulin, various deficiency and release phenomena linked with functional patterns of different levels of the neuraxis become manifest in the signs and symptoms which characterize the successive stages of insulin coma. The symptoms and signs are listed in the table on page 602. The therapist must remember that the signs in Stage V are largely those of functional impairment of the cardiac, circulatory and respiratory centers and therefore those of approaching danger.

All patients manifest in a general way the functional groups of signs listed in the table indicated. Each patient, however, presents an individual response and there is often much overlapping of the stages. It is not uncommon, in fact, to see signs of various stages (such as II and IV) occurring simultaneously. This phenomenon is sometimes referred to as "irregular descent" and would seem to indicate that there is a variable resistance to hypoglycemia in various parts of the brain.

Preparation for Treatment

Although insulin shock therapy is a relatively safe procedure in the hands of a skilled therapist most serious complications may occur with patients in whom an organic pathologic condition has been overlooked. In addition to careful and complete psychiatric, physical and neurological examinations, such laboratory examinations should be made as will exclude the possibility of undertaking the treatment of a bad risk. It is generally agreed that there should be roentgenologic studies of the chest and of the lateral thoracic spine, a serological examination, urinalysis, blood count and a determination of the fasting blood sugar. An electrocardiogram, especially in older patients, is highly desirable even though the clinical examination is negative. Some therapists feel that the Rorschach test and an intravenous pentothal interview yield helpful prognostic criteria. It is advisable to discuss results and dangers with a responsible relative, also to secure written permission for treatment.

Contraindications to Treatment

The presence of any organic disease must be individually evaluated and its seriousness weighed against the urgency for treatment. The following disorders, however, are usually considered as contraindications: (1) any active infection, or any chronic or subacute infection which may be "lighted up" by treatment; (2) serious heart, liver or kidney disease; (3) diabetes or other endocrine disorder; (4) skeletal pathology; (5) lack of adequate superficial veins; or (6) age under 16 or over 45 years. Some therapists, however, have successfully treated patients who were pregnant or had epilepsy, myxedema or allergy.

Technique of Treatment

The patient usually receives his dose of insulin at about 7 a.m. while still fasting. He remains under vigilant nursing observation from the time the drug is given until after coma is terminated and consciousness fully regained. Because of the danger of "after-shock" or other complications, the patient should be under competent nursing supervision during the succeeding 24 hours. A physician trained and experienced in insulin therapy should watch him constantly from the time he becomes unconscious until consciousness is fully restored.

The original method of Sakel, still very widely followed, begins with the intramuscular injection of 15 to 25 units of insulin which is increased by 10 to 15 units daily until the desired depth of coma is reached. This is usually not reached until the dosage is between 80 and 275 units and from 7 to 15 treatments have been given. After coma dose has been reached, the dosage may usually be reduced somewhat in the hope that excessively deep reactions may be avoided but it is adjusted daily for the remainder of the course of treatment. The dose of insulin required to produce coma is not related to the degree of hypoglycemia produced.

A technique in which rapidly increasing doses are administered was developed by Shurley and is often used. This method requires closer observation and greater skill than does the original Sakel technique but attempts to follow more closely what is known of the physiological principles of resistance and sensitivity to the drug. It seems, also, to have the advantage of shortening the induction phase, of producing a more rapid amelioration of symptoms, of reducing the amount of insulin required for the course of treatment and of being safer for the patient. With this technique, the procedure begins with the administration to the fasting patient for five successive days of small doses of insulin increasingly graduated from 5 to 25 units. The purpose of this series of injections is to ascertain if the patient has a predisposition to allergic or hypoglycemic reactions. If there is no evidence of undue sensitivity, the course of treatment is begun. The therapist seeks to produce the maximum physiological effect for the longest period of time permissible

HYPOGLYCEMIC SYMPTOMS
(*Modified from Himwich*)

STAGE	PSYCHOLOGICAL	MOTOR	SENSORY	AUTONOMIC
I Depression of cerebral and cerebellar functions	1. Gradually increasing clouding of consciousness with defects in: a. orientation b. attention c. understanding d. perception 2. Wild excitement, with or without psychotic syndromes 3. Sleep	1. Muscular relaxation (hypotonia) 2. Tremors Imperfect voluntary acts (apraxia) 4. Imperfect (incoherent) speech	1. Visual disturbances	1. Parasympathetic overactivity a. Watery sweat b. Watery saliva c. Bradycardia d. Constricted pupil or 2. Sympathetic overactivity a. Viscid sweat b. Viscid saliva c. Tachycardia d. Dilated pupil 3. Vital signs vary within normal limits—temperature dropping
II Release of subcorticodiencephalon	1. Loss of environmental contact, *i.e.*, coma	1. Stereotyped (primitive) movements a. Involuntary grasping b. Involuntary sucking c. Protrusion of tongue d. Kissing e. Snarling f. Grimacing 2. Motor restlessness 3. Choreiform, athetoid, and hemiballistic movements 4. Fine myoclonic twitchings ——→clonic spasms————→ convulsions (release of subcortical motor nuclei)	1. Increased sensitivity to external stimuli (release of the sensory thalamus)	1. Sympathetic overactivity in waves a. Tachycardia b. Dilated pupils (react to light) c. Exophthalmos d. Flushing e. Viscid perspiration f. Viscid salivation g. Increased blood pressure and perspiration (release of hypothalamus)
III Release of the mid-brain	1. Deep coma	1. Loss of primitive movements 2. Increasing hypertonus 3. Spasm a. Tonic (flexion of upper extremities with extension of rest of body) b. Torsion 4. Dissociated eye movements 5. Pathological pyramidal reflexes most easily elicited	1. Decreased sensitivity to external stimuli	1. Parasympathetic signs which are overcome periodically by sympathetic signs with each spasm (dilated pupils do not react to light) 2. Paradoxical pupillary dilation and hippus 3. Vital signs variable
IV Release of upper medulla	1. Deep coma	1. Recurrent extensor spasm in all extremities 2. Magnus and de Kleijn reflex	1. Loss of sensitivity	1. Sympathetic signs with each spasm (pupils dilate but do not react)
V Release of lower medulla	1. Deep coma	1. Muscular flaccidity 2. Depressed reflexes	1. Loss of all sensitivity 2. Loss of corneal reflex	1. Parasympathetic signs a. Pallor b. Pin point pupils (do not react) c. Slow heart rate d. Depressed respiration

by the largest doses of insulin consistent with the patient's safety. Patients possess varying degrees of resistance to insulin. For that reason the initial treatment dose does not exceed 50 units of U 100 ordinary insulin given by deep intramuscular injection. This dose is doubled each day until a clinical response is secured or a maximum dose of 1600 to 2200 units is reached. Some patients are extremely resistive to insulin. If in such cases coma does not occur within the dosage range stated, the maximum dose may be repeated for five or six days or the dose may be "zigzagged." This procedure may be conducted in one of several ways. The most common method is first to give double the dose with which treatment was begun, the next day to give half the maximum dose, and on the third day to repeat the maximum dose. If a patient does not respond to this routine, larger doses may be given or the route of administration may be changed to intravenous. When a clinical response is obtained the rate of dose increase is reduced from a doubling of the amount to one of 10 to 20 per cent. When sensitization occurs as manifested by a deeper coma on the same or a smaller dose, by an earlier onset of coma, or by a somatic crisis or other complication, the dose is reduced rapidly (by halves) until one just sufficient to produce the desired depth of coma is reached. Thereafter the maintenance dose must be determined daily as indicated by the patient's response. The depth and duration of each coma will vary in accordance with the opinion and experience of the individual therapist. Some physicians believe that Stage II is sufficiently deep to produce beneficial effects. Others insist on various combinations of Stages III, IV or even V. Many allow a maximum of two hours of coma per day reckoned from the time of loss of consciousness. The coma should be terminated when Stage V is reached or if some complication develops. It is generally agreed that fifteen minutes of Stage V is the extreme limit of safety. Few therapists permit the patient to reach this depth of coma.

Termination of Coma

Hypoglycemic coma is terminated by giving an adequate amount of carbohydrates by one of three methods: orally, by gavage, or by intravenous administration. In emerging from the coma the patient ordinarily retraverses the phyletic stages through which he passed in developing coma. If he is able to drink the patient is given eight ounces of a 50 per cent sugar solution. If he is unable to drink the coma is terminated by tube-feeding or by glucose given intravenously. Each method has its proponents. Probably, however, a gavage of 500 ml. of a warm 50 per cent glucose solution is preferable, especially if the patient has had a convulsion, has been uncooperative upon waking, has inaccessible veins, or needs a reservoir of glucose during a prolonged coma. The intravenous method is always used in an emergency and routinely by many therapists. When glucose is given intravenously the patient receives from 20 to 50 ml. (sometimes more) of a 33⅓ per cent solution. This method should be used also if the patient is not alert within twenty minutes after having received glucose by mouth. If he is suffering from simple hypoglycemia he should respond to intravenous glucose within five minutes. If the coma is terminated intravenously, it is wise to give additional glucose by mouth lest there be a return of the hypoglycemic state. Following the termination of the coma, the patient should receive a substantial meal. It is important that he receive sodium chloride to replace that lost through perspiration.

Adjuncts to Treatment

Atropine sulfate (grains 1/150 to 1/75) is given routinely with the insulin dose and again before electroshock if that is used in conjunction with insulin therapy, to decrease vagotonia. Vitamins B_1 and C are given to supplement the deficiencies resulting from the intake of large quantities of vitamin-poor carbohydrates. Dilantin,® 4½ grains daily, may be given orally at the same time the patient receives insulin in order to prevent hypoglycemic convulsions. It should be gradually discontinued upon completion of the course of insulin therapy and not used if combined electric convulsive therapy is employed. Postural drainage and the insertion of gauze wicks should be used to prevent aspiration of the excessive amount of saliva. Care must also be exercised to prevent aspiration of vomited material. Airways, oxygen and artificial respiration may aid in preventing serious complications. Some therapists use potassium chloride prophylactically to correct electrolytic balance and to prevent prolonged comas. Its value is still undetermined. Hyaluronidase, in doses of 75 to 150 turbidity reducing units (T.R.U.) added to the insulin has been found of value in reducing the amount of insulin required to produce coma, to increase the effective length of treatment levels and to increase the number of therapeutically valuable reactions (comas). It is also said to diminish the frequency of after-shocks, as well as convulsions, restlessness and exhaustion.

Duration of Treatment

Treatment is given five or six times a week for an average total course of fifty hours of coma. Although the number of treatment days may be somewhat smaller in acute cases and in those patients who have shown no benefit from treatment, the total number of hours should not be less than thirty. More than fifty coma days are given by some therapists to patients who are continuing to show beneficial results. If a relapse takes place, it usually occurs within a month after discontinuance of treatment. The patient should therefore continue under observation for nearly that period of time.

Complications of Treatment

Since dangerous, and even fatal, complications may readily occur, it is essential that both physician and nurse possess sufficient experience and skill to enable them to recognize and deal immediately with emergency situations. Even though both possess these qualities, the mortality rate will be from 0.5 to 1 per cent.

PROLONGED COMA. Ordinarily there is a coincident termination of hypoglycemia and of coma following the administration of carbohydrates. Sometimes, however, the termination of hypoglycemia is not accompanied by a return to consciousness. If there is no evidence of returning consciousness within five minutes after intravenous administration of glucose or within twenty minutes after administration by gavage one is confronted with a delayed awakening which may be the forerunner of prolonged or irreversible coma. Treatment of delayed awakening consists of the intravenous administration of 100 ml. of 33⅓ per cent of glucose and 100 mg. of thiamine chloride. The latter stimulates the utilization of available glucose. If the patient has not already received intragastric glucose he is given 500 ml. of warm 50 per cent glucose by gavage. If the patient does not respond within fifteen minutes, it must be considered that prolonged coma exists. This is an emergency condition and accounts for over one half of all deaths resulting from insulin coma. Persistent coma terminating in one to three hours is usually followed by complete recovery but longer periods are dangerous. While not definitely proven, prolonged or irreversible coma is presumably caused by the nerve cells having become exhausted or otherwise irreversibly altered so that they are no longer able to utilize glucose even though there is an ample supply present in the blood stream. In view of the marked diaphoresis which most patients manifest, there must be changes in water metabolism, also associated changes in electrolytic balance. The brain, following death from prolonged coma, shows either degenerative or hemorrhagic lesions together with cerebral edema. Even when prolonged coma is reversible, some patients are left with a permanent organic dementia. This mental deterioration is probably caused by the fact that in deep insulin shock the insulin depletes the cells of the cerebral cortex of their contained glycogen as well as excessively reducing any available free glucose. Under these circumstances the cells cannot utilize oxygen in their metabolic processes, with consequent damage to their structure. In other words, the hyperinsulism brings about a state of anoxia even in the presence of an abundance of oxygen. Histological examinations show that the cellular changes are identical with those alterations residual to severe degrees of cerebral anoxia in cases of carbon monoxide poisoning or mechanical strangulation.

If the patient is in Stage II or III and shows signs of cortical irritability, 50 ml. of 50 per cent sorbitol or sucrose are given intravenously as a dehydrating measure. If there is no response within fifteen minutes, or if the patient is in deep coma (Stage IV or V), 50 ml. of doubly concentrated human plasma are given intravenously. If the patient shows motor excitement, he should be restrained. Narcotics and sedatives should be avoided. Oxygen by nasal catheter, even in the absence of cyanosis, is usually advisable. If the patient's temperature is over 103°F. he should receive alcohol sponges or an ice water enema. Circulation and respiration should be supported by Coramine, 2 to 5 ml., given intravenously every three to four hours until the patient awakes. Epinephrine and caffeine are not recommended. If the patient has not responded within thirty minutes after having received plasma, the coma may continue for hours or days. Normal blood sugar level should be maintained by 10 per cent intravenous glucose drip. Blood sugar content should be checked every two to three hours. The administration of sucrose and of thiamine chloride should be repeated every two to three hours. Other measures previously described should be repeated as indicated. When the patient eventually recovers, insulin therapy should not be resumed for several days, the period of interruption depending upon the severity of the coma experienced. When treatment is begun again, it must be with a much smaller dose of insulin since the patient will now be found to be very sensitive to the drug. In those who recover from prolonged coma the episode is often followed by a dramatic improvement in the mental state.

A much less serious complication is the not infrequent and sometimes unavoidable secondary hypoglycemia or "*after-shock*." In this condition the patient has emerged from the coma in a normal manner but within twelve hours again develops signs and symptoms of hypoglycemia. It is usually prevented by giving an adequate amount of carbohydrates at the meal following emergence from coma with interval nourishment during the afternoon and evening. It is readily controlled by the intravenous injection of 50 ml. of 33⅓ per cent solution of glucose. This may be followed by sweetened fruit juice and other carbohydrates if the patient can be encouraged to cooperate.

Respiratory Complications. These are second in frequency as the cause of death in insulin therapy. A moderate degree of salivation is usual in insulin shock but may be so excessive that pneumonia may result from aspiration of saliva. It is therefore important that the patient's head be kept turned to the side during treatment and that secretions be aspirated or absorbed by a gauze wick. A lung abscess may follow regurgitation and aspiration of tube feeding or by a poorly given gavage. If symptoms suspected to be due either to pneumonia or to abscess appear, the patient should receive antibiotics. Pulmonary edema is usually of cardiac origin and should be treated accordingly. Laryngospasm may be helped by atropine. Edema of the glottis may require tracheotomy. Hiccough, usually due to disturbing changes in the medulla, should be regarded as a dangerous symptom. Here, as in other complications, the patient should receive intravenous glucose.

Cardiovascular Complications. Such minor complications as tachycardia, bradycardia, or arrhythmias usually respond to glucose alone. More serious complications, such as myocardial failure, cardiac dilation, aortic insufficiency or general vasomotor collapse, require intravenous glucose, Coramine, strophanthin and the usual supportive measures.

Convulsions. There are two types of convulsions, the early and the late. The former are of a grand mal type and usually occur in Stage II. These are not dangerous and are successfully controlled by intravenous injection of glucose and subsequent prophylactic use of anticonvulsants. Late convulsions occur in Stage IV and are dangerous. The late seizure is usually abortive or atypical with apnea and cyanosis. If not followed immediately by death it frequently eventuates in a prolonged or irreversible coma. The patient should receive intravenous glucose at once, also a similar injection of 2 to 4 ml. of Coramine. If there is respiratory embarrassment oxygen and artificial respiration should be employed. Following either type of convulsion there should be a rest period of one to several days, following which the dosage should be reduced 10 to 20 per cent.

Allergic Reactions. These may be either local or general. The former reaction is more common and is manifested by an itching, burning sensation at the point of injection which becomes indurated and painful. The erythema and induration disappear after a few days of local treatment. The generalized allergic reaction is exhibited in the form of urticaria with much itching. It is relieved by an injection of epinephrine or other antihistaminic agents.

Results of Treatment

As already implied, the use of insulin shock therapy is limited to the treatment of schizophrenia. There is complete agreement among therapists that there is an inverse ratio between the duration of illness and the recovery rate. The best results are obtained with patients who have not been ill for more than one year. After an illness of two years, the percentage of recovery or of improvement falls rapidly. The highest recovery or remission rate is among patients in their twenties who previously had well integrated personalities, who have had a stormy onset of the illness and have come to treatment within six months after its onset. Conversely, the results of treatment are poorer in the case of patients who have had limited personality resources, have long manifested schizoid traits, have had an insidious onset of their illness and become overtly psychotic before fifteen or after forty years of age. It is generally believed that patients showing tension or mixture of affective and of schizoid features have a more favorable outlook for recovery, also that patients who show a high resistance to insulin or fail to gain considerable weight during treatment do poorly. Much better results are secured with the paranoid and catatonic types of schizophrenia than with the simple and hebephrenic types, which respond very poorly.

There is admittedly a high rate of recurrence among schizophrenic patients treated with insulin therapy but the remission or recovery rate for those who have been adequately treated with insulin is significantly higher than for a similar group of untreated patients. With the possible exception of electric convulsion therapy in acute catatonia, insulin coma therapy is the most useful somatic treatment for schizophrenia. It has been said that over long periods of time recoveries are more stable in non-shock-treated patients than in those so treated. The use of insulin coma therapy is much less extensive than formerly.

Combined Insulin-Convulsive Therapy

Some psychiatrists prefer to combine insulin and convulsive therapies in the treatment of schizophrenia. The aim is to secure a summation of the therapeutic benefits of each procedure. Specific indications for the use of combined therapies are not precisely defined. However, these are commonly used: (1) when the patient fails to improve on either insulin coma therapy or electroshock therapy; (2) when the patient's improvement has failed to progress and further improvement is desired; (3) when he presents serious nursing problems, such as extremely overactive, unco-operative, assaultive, regressive behavior or suicidal tendencies; (4) if the patient is stuporous; or (5) if the patient shows definitely affective features.

Various techniques are followed in the application of combined insulin-convulsive therapy. In the "block" method, the therapist gives short series (two to four treatments) of electroconvulsive therapy widely spaced throughout a course of insulin coma therapy. In the "alternating" method, electroconvulsive therapy is given on the days when no insulin shocks are given. In a "crossing" of the methods, a course of electroconvulsive therapy is given before and/or after a course of insulin therapy. Commonly the most acute symptoms are relieved with electroconvulsive therapy prior to the use of insulin. If indications for its use arise during a course of insulin therapy, convulsive treatment is added. It is considered advisable to defer the induction of convulsions until the patient is smoothly obtaining coma hours each day since electroconvulsive therapy usually increases the insulin requirements and makes management difficult. It is therefore customary (except in the case of catatonic patients) for therapists to wait until the fifth or sixth week of an insulin shock course, or until a total of fifteen to thirty hours of coma has been reached before instituting both insulin and electric shock treatments. When the convulsive treatment is to be added, the patient receives 1/150 grains of atropine sulfate hypodermically and the convulsion is induced fifteen minutes later in Stage II of the insulin coma. At this point in the coma the convulsive threshold is relatively low, muscular rigidity is not prominent and the danger of fracture and of other complications is minimal. Despite the fact that at that time the dangers are greater and the response atypical, some therapists prefer to induce the convulsion during the deepest hypoglycemic coma in an attempt to intensify the therapeutic effects. The coma is terminated immediately following the convulsion by means of glucose given by vein, by stomach tube introduced before the convulsion or by both routes. To continue the coma beyond this point places undue physical strain on the patient. A course of electroconvulsive therapy during one of insulin shock is adapted to the needs of the individual patient and varies from one of a few treatments to one consisting of twenty to twenty-five treatments given three times a week. There is no evidence that risks are increased by combined treatment. It is a clinical impression that better results are secured in many cases by combined insulin-convulsive treatment but such has not yet been satistically proven.

Electric Convulsive Therapy

In 1938 Cerletti and Bini, after ensuring its safety by comprehensive animal experiments carried on in the former's laboratory in Rome, described a method of producing convulsions by electricity and began its use in the treatment of schizophrenia. It was first used in this country at the Pennsylvania Hospital in 1940.

The *apparatus* operates on 110-volt, 60-cycle, alternating current and contains mainly a variable transformer, ohm, volt, and ampere meters, and an automatic timer. The combined voltage and time settings constitute the "dose." Applications may range from 70 to 130 volts continuing from 0.1 to 0.5 second. Usually one starts with 80 volts for 0.2 second. If this fails to produce a convulsion, the voltage may be increased to 90 or 100 volts and the period of application increased. If this does not result in a seizure, no further application should be made until the following day. Only generalized seizures are productive of desired results. The operator will find that the dose must be determined by the convulsive threshold of the individual patient. This threshold is higher in female than in male patients, and higher in middle-aged than in younger persons. The threshold is raised after the first seizure.

The patient becomes unconscious immediately after the current is applied even if no seizure follows. He will have no memory of a "shock." The convulsion conforms closely to those of spontaneous origin with a tonic phase continuing for approximately ten seconds followed by a clonic phase of somewhat longer duration. The convulsion is accompanied by apnea.

Technique and Responses

In addition to the usual physical examination, including blood pressure, before receiving electric convulsive therapy, a roentgenogram should be made of the patient's chest and of the lateral aspect of the spine together with an electrocardiogram. An electroencephalogram is recommended by some therapists. If the patient is to be treated in the morning, he receives either no breakfast or a glass of fruit juice and one slice of toast two hours before treatment. The patient should void and dentures should be removed before treatment. If the patient suffers from nausea following the seizure, he may be given 50 mg. of Dramamine prior to treatment. He may receive the treatment either on a well padded table or on a bed the springs of which are supported by a board between spring and mattress. Compression fractures of vertebrae are occasional complications. Formerly it was believed that their frequency would be reduced if the spine were slightly overextended either by placing a firm pillow under the small of the back or by placing the patient on a Gatch bed during the treatment. This overextension is no longer generally recommended. The patient is placed in a comfortable dorsal position or the spine may be slightly flexed. The shoulders and arms are held lightly by a nurse to prevent extreme movements of the latter. Usually a restraint sheet is sufficient for the thighs but if they are held the control should not be too rigid lest fractures of an acetabulum or of a femur result. A padded tongue depressor or other resilient mouth gag is placed between the teeth to prevent biting the tongue or other injury. The assistant who holds the mouth gag in place will hold the patient's chin firmly upon the gag so that the jaw cannot open too far and become dislocated. Electrode paste is rubbed into the skin on both sides of the forehead and the electrodes, soaked in saturated salt solution, are applied to the prepared areas. The apparatus button is pressed and the patient becomes instantly unconscious. Following the clonic phase there is a phase of muscular relaxation with stertorous respiration. It is well to roll the patient on his side to prevent inhalation of saliva. The patient remains unconscious for about five minutes, then slowly rouses during the next five to ten minutes. After the treatment there is a period of confusion during which the patient should be watched lest he fall out of bed. He should usually be permitted to lie for one half to one hour after treatment. If left undisturbed he may sleep an hour or more. In most cases there is no postconvulsive excited state but a patient who is subject to this disturbance should receive 3 ¾ grains of Sodium Amytal intravenously just prior to application of the electricity.

There is insufficient evidence to show that unidirectional or brief stimuli techniques or the use of other types of currents or variant methods of application are superior to the ordinary form of treatment just described.

Frequency

Treatments are usually given three times a week. The period for which treatment should be continued depends largely upon the results of treatment and upon the nature of the disorder treated. In depressive reactions the patient may have received the maximum benefit after five to ten treatments. In disorders in which the patient is slowly but definitely improving, treatment may continue to twenty-five or thirty applications followed, if desirable, by maintenance treatments. Two treatments per day may be given for two or three successive days in the case of acutely disturbed patients who are threatened by psychotic exhaustion.

Indications

The greatest usefulness of electroconvulsive therapy is in depression. Its most frequent use, therefore, is in the treatment of involutional melancholia and of the depressive phase of manic-depressive psychosis. In case depression is an associated symptom in other disorders, this form of therapy may be followed by beneficial results. It is frequently used as a substitute for insulin shock therapy in acute and subacute schizophrenia reactions. Its use as a "maintenance" treatment in chronically disturbed schizophrenics and in the manic phase of manic-depressive psychosis will be discussed later.

Contraindications

As experience with electroconvulsive shock therapy has increased, conditions regarded as contraindications have decreased. *Age*, in itself, is not considered a contraindication. The aged patient should, of course, be very carefully examined for physical abnormalities. While the condition of the *cardiovascular system* should be carefully evaluated before giving electric convulsive therapy, the strain of the convulsion on that system has probably been exaggerated. Hypertension, abnormal electrocardiograms or a history of angina pectoris or of coronary thrombosis are not in themselves contraindications to treatment if the patient has a good cardiac reserve. Cardiac decompensation usually debars electroconvulsive therapy. The presence of aortic aneurysm also excludes the use of this treatment. If hypertension is largely caused by emotional factors, it need not be a cause for rejection of treatment but, on the contrary, may be an indication for its use. Vascular accidents as a result of electroconvulsive therapy are exceedingly rare. The use of electric convulsive therapy in the presence of myocardial disease depends upon its seriousness and the urgency of the need for treatment. If agitation is producing a constant strain on the heart, convulsive treatment may be used. Generally speaking, *tuberculosis,* if there is a history of recent hemorrhage or evidence of high activity, excludes treatment, but the patient who is a feeding problem is often benefited through the resulting gain of weight. Latent tuberculosis is rarely activated. Except for recent fractures *bone disease* is not a frequent contraindication to treatment. *Pregnancy* is not usually considered a contraindication. Electric shock is a safer form of therapy than insulin in the psychoses of pregnancy.

Complications

Impairment of Memory. Scarcely to be called a complication is the almost constant impairment of memory that accompanies electroconvulsive therapy. It may vary from a mild tendency to forget names to a severe confusion of the Korsakoff type. At first it tends to cover a long period prior to treatment, then gradually to diminish to events immediately before treatment. It is often distressing to the patient and may continue to some degree for several weeks or a few months following the termination of treatment. Full return of memory finally occurs. Psychological investigations indicate that electric convulsive therapy is not followed by any intellectual impairment.

Fractures and Dislocations. The most frequent complications in electroconvulsive therapy are fractures and dislocations caused by muscular contraction. The most frequent fracture is a *compression fracture of vertebrae* occurring between the second and eighth dorsal vertebrae, usually the third, fourth or fifth. Approximately 20 per cent of patients suffer this injury which occurs twice as frequently among men as among women. Apparently a majority of the fractures occur early in the course of treatment. They are not of major clinical importance and do not require special treatment. Many are found only on roentgenologic examination. Back pain may persist for a few days or weeks. Fractures of the femur, of the acetabulum and of the neck of the humerus may occur. Dislocation of the jaw is frequent unless pressure is applied to prevent the opening of the mouth at the onset of the tonic phase.

Apnea. Apnea occurs physiologically in any general convulsive seizure but in electroconvulsive therapy the respiratory arrest may be disturbingly prolonged. Some therapists use artificial respiration immediately after the convulsion as a safety measure. If apnea persists, artificial respiration should be continued. A metal airway should be available to prevent the tongue from falling back and to lead air through accumulations of saliva and mucus. Deaths as a result of electroconvulsive therapy are exceedingly uncommon.

"Softening" of Seizures

In order to avoid fractures or dislocations and to diminish the risk in elderly or infirm patients, convulsions may be modified or softened by means of curare. This inhibits the action of acetylcholine or neuromuscular junctions and softens the muscular contraction. It is used in the form of a concentrated aqueous extract known as Intocostrin which contains 10 mg. of active curare principle per cubic centimeter of the preparation. Not over 1 ml. per 40 pounds of body weight should be given. The maximum dose is therefore 4 to 5 ml. Bennett, who introduced curare as a means of softening the seizures, formerly injected Intocostrin (intravenously) at the slow rate of 1 ml. per minute. Later he recommended giving the entire amount within one minute. One to two minutes should be allowed after completing the injection before applying the electric current. D-tubocurarine chloride in the same amount is now often used. Prostigmine® is a reliable and quick antidote to curare and 1 ml. of a 1 to 2000 solution should be given intravenously after termination of the convulsion. In case of failing respiration, epinephrine should also be used.

In recent years succinylcholine dichloride (Anectine) has largely supplanted curare preparations as a muscle relaxant because of less risk of respiratory paralysis attending its use. From 10 to 40 mg. of succinylcholine dichloride may be mixed in the same syringe with 0.8 mg. of atropine and 2 ml. of Pentothal. At the end of the convulsion oxygen under positive pressure is administered until the patient breathes spontaneously.

Results of Treatment

In the depressions of involutional melancholia and of manic-depressive psychosis the improvement following electroconvulsive shock therapy is striking. In 80 per cent or more of these disorders five to ten treatments are followed by full or social recovery. Prior to the treatment of involutional melancholia by electric shock therapy protracted depression, sometimes lasting for years, was the rule. Early treatment of this disorder and of the depressions of manic-depressive psychosis by shock therapy will save many patients who would otherwise commit suicide. Electroconvulsive shock therapy has no influence on the recurrence of manic-depressive episodes. Guilt, self-punishing and self-accusatory trends are usually rapidly alleviated. In less than one half of the cases of the paranoid type of involutional psychosis is treatment followed by much improvement even though the maximum number of convulsions is induced. Senile depressions are usually relieved unless arteriosclerotic or senile brain changes have been important determinants. The results of treatment of the manic phase of manic-depressive psychosis are less favorable than of the depressive but have been greatly improved by the practice of giving treatments more frequently. Best results are secured by giving two treatments a day for the first two or three days. These are usually followed by much confusion but as this clears the patient is found to be definitely improved.

The effectiveness of electroconvulsive treatment of schizophrenia has been the subject of much discussion. It is generally agreed that this form of treatment is beneficial in a large percentage of schizophrenics with affective features. It is also helpful in hastening a remission in early, acute forms of the disorder. It is of little value in hebephrenia or when the onset has been of a prolonged, insidious nature. The best results are secured in catatonic excitement. Like other shock therapies this treatment is not followed by material improvement in the chronic, disorganized schizophrenic. The schizophrenic who has been ill less than a year and has not improved by a course of insulin should receive one of electroconvulsive shock. Similarly, such a patient who has not been helped by electroconvulsive therapy should receive insulin. Many schizophrenics treated by electric shock suffer relapses but it is doubtful if the percentage is any greater than after insulin shock therapy.

The relative value of electroconvulsive and of insulin shock therapies in early schizophrenia has been a controversial subject. Probably if the patient receives thirty to forty convulsive treatments the results of electroconvulsive therapy are not greatly inferior to those secured by insulin.

Electroconvulsive therapy is of little value in the treatment of psychoneuroses except in those manifesting depressive features. Its use should be accompanied by psychotherapy.

Maintenance Treatment

Formerly electroconvulsive therapy was extensively used as a "maintenance treatment" of chronically disturbed patients, especially those suffering from schizophrenia. While such treatment given once every week or ten days facilitated the care of these patients, it has been largely replaced by the use of tranquilizing drugs.

Ambulatory Treatment

For several years after the introduction of electroconvulsive therapy it was considered essential that its application be limited to patients resident in a hospital. In more recent years there has been considerable relaxation in this practice. Whether, however, electric convulsive treatments are administered to patients continuously confined to a hospital or to those who are not hospitalized they should be given only by a qualified psychiatrist well trained in the technique. Many patients, particularly those suffering from mild depressions, continue to reside at their homes but periodically visit a psychiatric or a general hospital to receive shock treatments. Later in the treatment day, after consciousness has become fully clear, the patient returns to his home. Some physicians, without untoward results, administer the treatment in their private offices.

More conservative physicians consider that the hazards, in the absence of trained nursing personnel and of all facilities for the meeting of emergencies, are too great to permit office treatment. In some instances ambulatory treatment is employed so that hospitalized patients who have sufficiently recovered to do so may return home and yet continue to receive treatments as required. In other cases patients who, after careful examination, are believed not to require an initial period of hospitalization visit hospital or office periodically for treatment. Prudence would seem to require, however, that there be a preliminary period of psychiatric hospital care so that the patient may become thoroughly known to the physician and the danger of suicide or other behavior disturbance be evaluated. The degree of knowledge, understanding and responsibility of relatives, and their ability to exercise constant supervision of the patient in his home, must be carefully determined. If treatment is undertaken in a general hospital or in a private office, provisions for dealing with postconvulsive confusion and excitement or with respiratory or other complications must be made. The patient should remain in the hospital or in the physician's office until there is no longer any danger of undesirable after effects. He should never be permitted to return home unaccompanied and there should be reliable and instructed persons there to supervise him during the entire course of treatment. Some psychiatrists doubt the advisability of the use of electroshock on an ambulatory basis except in an out-patient clinic connected with a psychiatric hospital.

Mode of Action

The use of electroconvulsive shock is entirely empirical. Many theories, both psychogenic and physiogenic, have been suggested as explanations for its therapeutic action but no one has offered a satisfactory explanation for the results obtained either by electroconvulsive or by insulin therapy. Some investigators suggest that cerebral anoxia, a result common to all the shock therapies, may somehow be the basis for the mental improvement. In both hypoglycemic and convulsive shock therapies, the brain is deprived of energy and oxidative metabolism to a degree that renders it inadequate to support cerebral function. The mechanisms producing these conditions are different however. With hypoglycemia the brain is deprived of glucose and cerebral metabolic rate is depressed. With electroshock, brain activity is raised to such a high pitch that cerebral function cannot be sustained by the oxygen and glucose coming to the brain in the blood.

Psychosurgery

The operation of lobotomy, a surgical procedure consisting of a severance of the connection between the thalamus and frontal lobe, was developed by a Portuguese neurologist, Egas Moniz, and first performed by the neurosurgeon, Almeida Lima, in 1935. Moniz published his monograph in 1936, immediately following which the operation was introduced into United States by Dr. Walter Freeman and Dr. James Watts. In 1949 Moniz received the Nobel Prize in Medicine for his work in prefrontal lobotomy.

It is generally accepted that the dorsomedial nucleus of the thalamus is the physical substratum of emotion. It is known that fibers run from this nucleus to the frontal poles and it is believed that the stimuli that pass along these radiations are concerned with the conscious experience of emotion. It is postulated that a cutting of these fibers so alters affective responses that tensions do not accumulate and that therefore regressive, reparative behavior is no longer necessary. Abundant experience has now shown that a severing of these fibers contributes greatly to the control of pathological emotional states. It is the aim of the neurosurgeon to sever the thalamofrontal radiation in such a manner that the emotional component of the neurosis or psychosis can be reduced to the point where the ideas no longer dominate the behavior of the patient, yet that the incisions leave sufficient quantities of the frontal lobes to permit the patient to retain the capacity for productive work and to make a satisfactory adaptation in a social environment. Following the section of the thalamocortical fibers, there is a retrograde degeneration of the dorsomedial nucleus.

Techniques

Several types of operation have been derived from the original prefrontal leukotomy developed by Moniz. One of the most widely used techniques is the modification developed by Freeman and Watts. This is a "blind" procedure performed through small lateral burr holes. The white matter in both frontal lobes is cut in the plane of the coronal suture. Unless the patient is disturbed, the operation is performed under local anesthesia. The burr holes are made in both sides of the skull at a point 6 cm. above the zygomatic process and 3 cm. behind the lateral rim of the orbit. A leukotome is introduced through the burr holes and section of the frontal white matter in both hemispheres is made. The cortex is not cut except in a small area for the introduction of the leukotome. The exact plane of the cortical incision is of great importance. If the incision is too far anteriorly the results of the operation are negligible; if it is made too far posteriorly apathy, inertia, and some degree of dementia may follow.

In order that he might operate with the advantage of clear vision Lyerly, in 1947, devised an "open" procedure permitted by the use of an osteoplastic flap. By a superior approach he separated the frontal lobe fibers and by means of a lighted speculum he worked under direct vision.

Another technique developed in 1948 by Scoville is known as *cortical undercutting*. In this operation a line of cleavage is made at the junction of the gray and white matter in the prefrontal cortex, thus severing the underlying long association fibers.

A few neurosurgeons have limited frontal lobe operations to a full sectioning of the white matter on either the right or the left side but not on both.

In 1948 Pool, Mettler and a group of workers from Columbia University and from the New Jersey State Hospital at Greystone Park developed an operation called "*topectomy*" consisting of the removal of symmetrical areas of the frontal cortex, especially of Brodmann's areas 9 and 10. In this study an attempt was made to evaluate the ablation of various selected areas. Apparently the therapeutic results are not determined so much by the excision of any one specific area as by the amount of brain substance removed. Topectomy does not seem to be followed by the unpleasant personality changes often seen in prefrontal lobotomy. It is, however, followed more frequently by convulsions than are other operative procedures. For this reason the operation is now rarely employed.

Spiegel and Wycis conceived the idea, not of interrupting the frontothalamic connections by cutting the radiations but by coagulating the dorsomedial nucleus of the thalamus. By elaborate technique they accurately locate this nucleus in which they then produce a lesion by electrolysis or by electrocoagulation. This procedure is known as *thalamotomy*.

In 1937 Fiamberti of Vareze, Italy, developed a different technique for severing the thalamofrontal radiations. In 1946 Freeman introduced this technique into the United States where it has become extensively employed. In this operation, known as *transorbital lobotomy*, the frontal lobes are entered through the bony cavity above the eye and the thalmofrontal radiations severed just lateral to the anterior horn of the lateral ventricle. The superior part of these radiations is supposed to underly areas 9 and 10 of Brodmann. The severance of the connections of these areas with the thalamus is, as in other forms of lobotomy, supposed to dissociate by surgical means the pathological thinking from its emotional reverberations and permit reorganization of more nearly normal patterns of cerebral activity. In carrying out the technique of transorbital lobotomy, a general anesthetic is not given. Anesthesia is secured by the administration of two electroshocks within one or two minutes of each other. The lobotomy is then performed in the postconvulsive coma. A slender, sharply pointed instrument is inserted in the conjunctival sac and driven through the skull at a point opposite the pupil and 2 cm. posterior to the frontal sinus. The base of the frontal lobe is penetrated about 3 cm. lateral to the midline and 2 cm. behind the frontal pole. The total depth of penetration from the tip of the instrument to the edge of the upper eyelid is 7 cm. Connections of this part of the frontal lobe with the thalamus are severed on an arc of 30 degrees by moving the handle of the instrument laterally about 15 degrees and medially the same distance. When the handle of the instrument, the leukotome, is in the lateral position at the 7 cm. mark, a deep frontal cut is made. The handle of the leukotome is strongly elevated until the shaft lies as nearly parallel as possible to the orbital plate. From this position the handle is then returned to the parasagittal plane and withdrawn. Following the completion of the operation on one side, the patient receives a third electroshock treatment, or, if he becomes restless, a fourth shock before the second side is done. There are no important structures such as vessels, nerves or glands in the path of the instrument. No preparation of the operative field is necessary since the conjunctival sac is normally sterile.

Advocates of transorbital lobotomy stress that complications are less frequent and mortality less than in other forms of psychosurgery. Among the advantages claimed are: (1) ease of performance; (2) economy of of time; (3) minimal hospitalization and nursing care; (4) minimal expense to patient and institution; (5) the apparent fact that undesirable personality traits following operation are less frequent; and (6) postoperative hemorrhage and seizures are less frequent.

Since the operation of transorbital leukotomy appears relatively simple and does not require the accouterments of major neurological surgery, there is a fear on the part of some psychiatrists that the operation may be used too indiscriminately and performed by physicians inadequately trained. Most neurosurgeons, too, hesitate about the blind passing of an instrument through the orbit into the brain with the possibility of damage to paranasal sinuses, and without full neurosurgical facilities for dealing with complications that may arise.

In 1951 Greenblatt, Solomon and Levine introduced what is known as the *bimedial* operation. This, too, is a bilateral prefrontal lobotomy carried out in the frontal or coronal plane. Instead, however, of cutting all the white matter in both frontal lobes, the bimedial operation is restricted to cutting only the medial half of the white matter in each frontal lobe. Reports suggest that this operation is followed by a greater relief of anxiety, tension, hostility and disorganization than are the full bilateral or unilateral operations.

Acute Effects of Operation

Immediately after either the open or blind type of prefrontal lobotomy the patient loses his nervous tension and may appear stuporous or confused for a few days to a week. He remains indifferent to his surroundings, pays no attention to excretory functions, has to be fed and moved about in bed, is somnolent and may vomit. He may confabulate and deny that he has had an operation. A few patients are noisy and manifest a repetitious, destructive overactivity. In many instances the success of the operation depends upon the supervision the patient receives for several weeks following. He must be forced out of bed, taken to the toilet at regular intervals, made to bathe, dress and feed himself. An excessive appetite is common and may result in a great gain in weight. In even the simplest matters the patient should be specifically instructed and guided for a considerable time. It is usually desirable that the patient go home as soon as possible after the operation in order that the constant social pressure of the home may stimulate more adequate social behavior. It is highly important that the operation be followed by an active rehabilitation program which should include retraining and re-educational measures and a system of graded privileges.

The chief complication of lobotomy is the development of convulsive seizures. These are usually of the grand mal type and can be controlled by anticonvulsive medication.

Indications

Prefrontal lobotomy is a radical procedure which will be undertaken only after other forms of treatment, including tranquilizing drugs and some form of shock therapy, have failed. Its use since the introduction of the tranquilizing drugs has greatly decreased. Patients are selected for operation on the basis of symptoms rather than of diagnosis. The best results are secured in patients who show tension, agitation and distress, depression, worry, emotional aggressiveness, hostility and excited, impulsive behavior. Such symptoms as phobias, obsessions, hallucinations and delusional experiences are relieved if they have not existed for extended periods, although the basic pathology of the thought process is not affected. Cruelty, avoidance of responsibility and excessive use of alcohol before the development of the psychosis are contraindications. In *schizophrenia* prefrontal lobotomy has no effect on the fundamental disease process but in well selected cases may be followed by a great improvement in adjustment. The better organized the prepsychotic personality the better the results, provided deteriorated, psychotic habits have not existed for several years. In general, lobotomy may be recommended after a year's illness provided the patient has in the meantime received active treatment with tranquilizing drugs, insulin and electroconvulsive therapy without beneficial results. If the patient is a chronically deteriorated, inactive hebephrenic whose affect has been "burned out," little benefit is to be expected from operation. On the other hand, the behavior of the overactive, resistive, excitable, destructive, restless, unmanageable schizophrenic may be greatly improved. Such a patient may become quiet, somewhat sociable, and perhaps later be able to leave the hospital and even become self-sustaining. Not a few patients become free, cheerful, relaxed, interested in events of the day and able to carry on a conversation on various topics. Sometimes activity may be so reduced that the patient sits about in a lethargic state. Lobotomy will rarely be undertaken in acute *manic-depressive* psychosis since most cases will yield either to electroconvulsive therapy or to tranquilizing drugs. It may be advisable in prolonged depressive states with tension that have not yielded to electric convulsive therapy. It has not usually been of value in chronic manic states. Since the recovery rate in *involutional melancholia* following convulsive therapy is high, lobotomy will rarely be used in this disease. There are, however, some cases of rut depression and rumination on abnormal ideas, or cases with schizophrenic features which do not respond to convulsive therapy. In such cases and in the paranoid type of involutional psychosis lobotomy may be a beneficial procedure. In severe obsessive-compulsive, obsessive-ruminative, and hypochondriacal types of *psychoneuroses* that have not been benefited by psychotherapy the disabling tension and anxiety states may be relieved by lobotomy. Obsessive ideas may continue but the relief from tension may permit the patient to pursue his normal activities. In general, previous conflicts remain but the quantity of emotional charge is reduced. Probably the best results in lobotomy are secured in agitated depressions and in severe obsessive-compulsive reactions accompanied by so much tension that the patient is incapacitated. One should, however, be conservative in recommending lobotomy for the treatment of psychoneuroses.

The success of prefrontal lobotomy in controlling emotional disturbance and overactivity arising from it as seen in some chronic manic and schizophrenic states suggested that the operation might be of benefit in the treatment of severe behavior disorders following acquired brain disease or in pathological personalities. The results, however, have been poor and the operation is not considered justifiable.

Any explanation for the beneficial effect produced by prefrontal lobotomy in relieving tension and anxiety remains speculative. It has been suggested that the operation may act in one of three ways: (1) a prevention of the relay to the frontohypothalamic mechanism of the nervous activities engendered by the mental conflict; (2) the intensity of the mental conflict loses its force when no longer stimulated by this mechanism; or (3) the mechanism of a mental conflict at a cortical level is highly complex and may be directly interfered with by the operation to such an extent that it can no longer develop the intensity required to stimulate the emotions.

Unpleasant Sequences

Observation of patients who have been subjected to prefrontal lobotomy suggests that the function of the "silent" regions of the frontal lobe is to elaborate and integrate affective responses with the other modes of response of the individual to the environment so as to secure an emotionally harmonious life. A change in personality with an accentuation of previous unpleasant traits is not uncommon but is by no means true in all cases. The patient's relatives must expect him to show an absence of self-consciousness, a facetiousness and childlike pleasure in simple things. Sarcastic remarks and undesirable behavior must be overlooked. Not for several months, if ever, should most patients be permitted to assume financial responsibilities or to attempt unusual social adjustments. Long and persistent re-educating and rehabilitating efforts should be continued. With the best results the patient loses his anxiety, becomes cheerful and friendly, takes an interest in matters about himself and even works regularly but without ambition. Even in cases where results are otherewise good the patient's sense of responsibility and his feeling for others may be impaired. Frequently there is a reduction in depth of feeling, in sensitivity and in richness of inner life. Affect is more shallow than before the illness and the patient usually lacks former sympathies and altruistic motives. There is an increase in self-esteem, tactlessness, lack of self-criticism and of restraint. Imaginative foresight is usually less than normal. "He doesn't care whether school keeps or not." With less desirable results the patient may be lazy, tactless, suggestible, childish and manifest a silly euphoria. He may be unrestrained in word and action, careless in eating habits and personal appearance and perhaps vulgar and profane. In the usual case the outstanding change is in affect and not in intellect. There is not a permanent impairment of the latter unless the incisions have been posterior to the usually accepted area. Some patients, particularly those schizophrenics who have led a purely vegetative existence without active mental conflict, may show no improvement and even exhibit an organic dementia also. Patients whose prepsychotic tendencies were characterized by active aggressiveness may, after operation, manifest an undesirable lack of restraint of these impulses.

Results of Operation

The percentage of improvement is highest in patients who are operated upon as soon as all other measures have been tried and failed. Not even a tentative evaluation of the results should be made for at least six months after the operation and usually a period of at least one year should be allowed for the attainment of the patient's best level. In the bilateral sectioning of all white matter in suitable patients on whom operation has not been unduly deferred, approximately one third will leave the hospital and make a tolerable or better adjustment. In some instances the degree of recovery is dramatic, the patient regaining a completely successful social, occupational and economic adjustment. Another third will show a significant improvement. Some of them can be cared for at home and the institutional adjustment of the remainder will be improved. A third of those operated upon will show no improvement. Paul, Fitzgerald and Greenblatt report that in a 5-year follow-up of patients who had received a bimedial operation 65 per cent showed a significant improvement.

BIBLIOGRAPHY

Alexander, Leo: Treatment of Mental Disorders. Philadelphia, W. B. Saunders Co., 1953.

Bond, E. D.: Results of treatment in psychoses—with a control series. Am. J. Psychiat., *110:*881–887, 1954.

Cerletti, V.: Old and new information about electroshock. Am. J. Psychiat., *107:*87–94, 1950.

———, and Bini, L.: L'Ellettroshock. Arch. Gen. di Neurol., Psichiat., e Psicoanal., *19:*266, 1938.

Committee on Public Health Relations, New York Acad. of Med.: Electroshock therapy. New York State J. Med., *51:*653, 1951.

Courville, C. B.: Late cerebral changes incident to severe hypoglycemia (insulin shock). Arch. Neurol. & Psychiat., *78:*1–14, 1957.

Ebaugh, F. E., et al.: Fatalities following electric convulsive therapy. Arch. Neurol. & Psychiat., *49:*107, 1943.

Ferraro, A., and Roizin, L.: Cerebral morphologic changes in monkeys subjected to a large number of electrically produced convulsions. Am. J. Psychiat., *106:*278–284, 1949.

Fiamberti, A. M.: Proposta di una tecnica operatoria modificata e simplificata per gli interventi alla Moniz sui lobi prefontali in malati de mente. Rassegna di Studi Psichiat., *26:*797, 1937.

Freeman, Walter, and Watts, J. W.: Psychosurgery in the Treatment of Mental Disorders and Intractable Pain, 2nd ed. Springfield, Illinois, Charles C Thomas, 1950.

Fulton, J. F.: Frontal Lobotomy and Affective Behavior. A Neurophysiological Analysis. New York, W. W. Norton, 1951.

———; Aring, C. D., and Wortis, S. B.: The Frontal Lobes. Proceedings of Assoc. for Research in Nerv. and Ment. Dis., Vol. XXVII. Baltimore, Williams & Wilkins Co., 1948.
Grassi, J. R.: Impairment of abstract behavior following bilateral prefrontal lobotomy. Psychiatric Quart., *24:*74, 1950.
Greenblatt, Milton, and Solomon, H. C.: Psychosurgery. New England J. Med., *248:* 19–25, 56–67, 1953.
Group for the Advancement of Psychiatry: Report No. 15, Revised Shock Therapy. Topeka, 1950.
Himwich, H. E.: Brain Metabolism and Cerebral Disorders. Baltimore, Williams & Wilkins Co., 1951.
Impastato, D. J., and Berg, S.: Methods of administration of succinylcholine dichloride in electroshock therapy with a description of a simple and modified technique and a succinylcholine dichloride test. Am. J. Psychiat., *112:*893–897, 1956.
Kalinowsky, L. B., and Hoch, P. H.: Shock Treatments, Psychosurgery and Other Somatic Treatments in Psychiatry, 2nd ed. New York, Grune & Stratton, 1952.
Landis, Carney: Psychological observations on psychosurgery patients. Psychiatric Quart., *25:*409, 1951.
Lennox, M. A., and Coolidge, J. C.: Electroencephalographic changes after prefrontal lobotomy. Arch. Neurol. & Psychiat., *62:*150–161, 1948.
Levine, J., Greenblatt, M., and Solomon, H. C.: Bimedial lobotomy. New England J. Med., *245:*888, 1951.
Moniz, Egas: Tentatives Opératoires dans le Traitement de Certaines Psychoses. Paris, Masson et Cie, 1936.
Overholser, Winfred: Proceedings of the Third Research Conference on Psychosurgery. Washington, Public Health Service Publications, No. 221, 1954.
Paul, N. L.; Fitzgerald, Edward, and Greenblatt, Milton: The long-term comparative results of three different lobotomy procedures. Am. J. Psychiat., *113:*808–814, 1957.
Pool, J. L.; Heath, R. G., and Weber, J. J.: Topectomy: Surgical techniques, psychiatric indications and postoperative management. J. Nerv. & Ment. Dis., *110:*464–477, 1949.
Prout, C. T., and Hamilton, D. M.: Results of electro-shock therapy in patients over 60 years of age. Bull. New York Acad. Med., *28:*454–461, 1952.
Regan, Peter F.: Effective utilization of electric convulsive treatment. Am. J. Psychiat., *114:*351–356, 1947.
Sakel, M.: The Pharmacological Shock Treatment of Schizophrenia. New York, Nervous and Mental Diseases Publishing Co., 1938.
Sargant, William, and Slater, Eliot: Physical Methods of Treatment in Psychiatry, 3rd ed. Baltimore, Williams and Wilkins Co., 1954.
Scheflen, A. E., Reiner, E. R., and Jetter, W. W.: Fatalities in insulin therapy of the psychoses. Arch. Neurol. & Psychiat., *67:*32–43, 1952.
Shurley, J. T., and Bond, E. D.: Insulin Shock Therapy in Schizophrenia. Washington, Veterans Administration Technical Bulletin, *10:*501, 1948.
Solomon, H. C., and Greenblatt, M.: Frontal Lobes and Schizophrenia. New York, Springer, 1953.
Spencer, A. M.: Posthypoglycemic encephalopathy in Sakel's insulin treatment. J. Ment. Sc., *94:*513–554, 1948.
Stengel, E.: The patient's attitudes to leucotomy and its effects. J. Ment. Sc., *98:*382–388, 1952.
Tyndel, M.: Hyaluronidase as an adjuvant in insulin shock therapy. J.A.M.A., *162:* 32–34, 1956.

CHAPTER XXXVI

Psychotherapy

Definition

Psychotherapy may be defined as the treatment of emotional and personality problems and disorders by psychological means. Although many different psychological techniques may be employed in an effort to relieve these problems and disorders and make the patient a happy, mature and independent person, an important therapeutic factor common to them all is the therapist-patient relationship with its interpersonal experiences. Through this relationship the patient knows that he can share his feelings, attitudes and experiences with the physician and that the latter with his warmth, understanding empathy, acceptance and support will not depreciate, censure or judge him no matter what he may reveal, but will respect his dignity and worth. This desired, positive, patient-therapist relationship with its psychotherapeutic value is often known as *transference*. Since the patient goes to the physician for help and the latter offers this to him, the patient usually brings this positive transference attitude to the therapeutic situation. It should not be confused with the patient's carry-over to the analyst of the emotional reactions directed in childhood to a meaningful person in the former's environmental, usually family, situation. This carry-over established in psychoanalytical procedure and formerly known as transference neurosis is also often referred to as transference although the term *transference situation* is preferable.

Types of Psychotherapy

Types of psychotherapy fall into two general groups. One may be described as genetic-dynamic, the other as supportive, suppressive, nonexploratory or nonspecific. In the former are included both Meyer's psychobiological therapy and Freudian psychoanalysis. No single psychotherapeutic method, approach, or technique is desirable for all patients or for all kinds of emotional difficulties. The pattern of psychotherapy must be determined by such factors as nature of the patient's problems, dynamic diagnosis, age of patient, intelligence, emotional maturity, family and social situation and the specialized training and skill of the therapist. The therapist, regardless of the type of therapy he employs, must have certain qualities. He should have a liking for people, possess a warm capacity for projecting himself into the situations and feelings of others and be able to understand human motivation. He should not possess too many personality characteristics that are defensive in nature. For psychotherapy to be successful, too, the patient must not only want to get well but he must give genuine and whole-hearted cooperation to the therapist. Both therapist and patient must relate meaningfully each to the other.

Genetic-Dynamic Therapies

While varying greatly in the techniques used, psychobiological therapy and psychoanalysis have in common the assumption that the patient's emotional or personality difficulty had its genesis in significant psychological experiences and developed in accordance with the dynamic processes of psychopathology, that the patient's present attitudes and specific modes of reaction to life experiences are largely determined by reactions and attitudes to experiences in the past. Both forms of psychotherapy should be based on a knowledge of personality development. Although both psychobiological therapy and psychoanalysis recognize the existence and operation of dynamic psychological processes, the latter alone assumes that infantile conflictual factors are the important genetic ones and explores the deep unconscious for their existence. While psychobiology acknowledges that reactions to experiences in early childhood greatly influences the development of the personality and the patterns of reactions in adult life, it maintains that reactions to experiences occurring in various phases and periods of development throughout the life of the individual may be nearly or equally as potent genetic factors. Although many other phases and differences characterize the techniques of the two therapies, it may be said that in psychoanalysis, problems and their genesis are ascertained by an exploration of the unconscious through free associations; and that in psychobiological therapy these problems are approached at a largely conscious level and discussed directly in the form of an ordinary conversation with attention directed toward definite situations and the patient's reactions to them. In both forms, the therapist seeks to modify the unhealthy attitudes that have prevented the patient from carrying on in his daily tasks without disturbing his relations with others or creating anxiety within himself. The therapist aims to assist the patient in establishing a more rational, more constructive and therefore healthier pattern of living.

Psychobiological Therapy

Because of the principles involved, Adolf Meyer characterized as *distributive analysis* and *synthesis* the technique of psychotherapy often known as psychobiological therapy. Briefly Meyer meant about as follows by this term: Guided by the therapist, the patient analyzes or critically examines one by one and in their relative importance the various factors, situations and his personality reactions thereto which in the light of his symptoms and complaints may have been of dynamic importance in producing his emotional problem or pattern of behavior. Then by inductive reasoning and by discussion with the therapist, the patient from the material secured through analysis reconstructs his difficulties and formulates how the understanding acquired thereby may be used constructively to modify emotional reactions and established patterns of behavior and a wholesome integration of the personality be thereby achieved.

This type of therapy without an exploration of subterranean mental processes, yet genetic-dynamic in its approach, begins with a study of the various fields which contribute to the personality formation. This study with its search for dynamic factors includes a history of the physical, physiological and psychological components of the personality and a knowledge of the present status of each. Its approach is one of biographical analysis and through the conscious mind rather than the unconscious. Quite early in his interview with the patient the therapist encourages the former to talk spontaneously about any feelings, troubles or problems with which he is now faced and with which, perhaps, he has long had to cope. This not only provides material for future analysis, critical examination and discussion but aids in an early establishment of the necessary patient-physician relationship. Among other subjects discussed will be the family history, not only with reference to hereditary background but as to beliefs and its interpersonal relationships, including any particular attachments or antagonisms. Early situations and experiences are analyzed for material that will shed light on the patient's personality development and make-up. Factors and situations which the patient's complaints and symptoms suggest may have been of importance in producing his present problems, including difficulties with himself and with others, are examined with careful scrutiny. The patient is encouraged to state the concrete circumstances under which his symptoms and unwholesome reactions first appeared.

One object of the dissection (distributive analysis) of the patient's past, his previous experiences, his modes of reaction and the various other lines suggested by his complaints or recognized by the therapist, is to make it apparent to the patient that his present mode of functioning with all its attendant distress and difficulties is to a very large extent the natural product of his past life. Discussions are held with the patient not only concerning his problems and complaints for which he seeks help but also varied problems and topics, some obviously related to his difficulties while others may have no apparent connection with them. The discussion will include both those life experiences of which the patient is more or less completely aware and those which he comes to recognize during the discussion of experiences and events. There will be various material of which the patient will wish to remain oblivious as well as experiences and situations which he will not discuss because he is not fully aware of them. Included in the study of the personality are emotionally colored thoughts, desires and strivings which may be only faintly recognized and not accepted by the patient. Occasionally the patient can be led to recognize that his behavior has been influenced by fear, resentment, hate, guilt, frustration, inferiority feeling or anxiety. In such cases a re-education of the abnormal attitude may be possible. In some cases the patient-physician relationship will help the patient to acquire insight or to work through material that has been repressed. Since it is difficult for the patient to study himself objectively, the therapist must often give him direction and careful guidance. The discussion, however, is limited to processes occurring at a conscious level and attention is directed more to actual situations and circumstances than to the discovery of unconscious attitudes and mechanisms. The therapist does not, as in psychoanalysis, attempt to have the patient relive early experiences but to have him understand the present meaning of them and his present attitude toward them. The physician's interested and receptive attitude and his noncritical acceptance of the patient's problems, feelings and fears help him to recognize his own emotions and to understand himself better. In psychobiological therapy, as in psychoanalysis, one must be careful not to overwhelm the patient with interpretations and thereby cause him to build up his defenses and resistances.

The discussions aim to help the patient trace genetically the origin of his complaint in past experience, both in that of which he is aware and in that which has been excluded from memory. Such a biographical analysis includes a study of somatic factors, of drives and activities and a survey of the patient's psychosexual development. It will emphasize human relationships in general, including difficulties with others and social successes and failures. Not rarely common factors will be found to have been operative in the production of seemingly unrelated symptoms and reactions.

Only those factors are discussed which seem to the patient to be intelligible in terms of human experience, and with particular reference to those facts which appear, both to the patient and the therapist, to have a meaningful place in the particular life experiences of the patient. The patient's life history is discussed with him in considerable detail and his life experiences and their implications are evaluated. The therapist asks questions frequently not so much for the purpose of securing an answer as for promoting a study by the patient himself of his modes of reaction to life experiences. Comments based on an understanding of the dynamic diagnosis may be made by the therapist. The patient is asked to analyze past experiences and to study them for factors involved. His conclusions are subjected to a critical review and made a topic for therapeutic discussion.

After various experiences, situations and symptoms have been discussed and analyzed, the patient is asked to reformulate them into a dynamic life story with its motivations in order that thereby he may as nearly as possible reproduce the origin and development of his problem and understand the means whereby he attempted to meet it. Great care must be exercised lest any interpretations to which an effort is made to guide the patient be not made too early, without fact, or in terms not acceptable to him. Usually the psychological therapist makes use also of other appropriate measures, such as reassurance, guidance, persuasion, desensitization and ventilation.

With a synthetic review and constructive use of the material obtained by an analysis of his life biography, the patient is aided in securing a helpful perspective of his behavior and of the factors that have determined it. To quite an extent the therapist becomes an educator and explainer of the patient's life experiences and reactions. Among his objectives is that of re-educating conscious attitudes which have been warped by resentment, guilt, hostility, frustration, overambition or depression. With the clarification of special problems and the acquisition of new insight and orientation and with synthesis of the facts that may contribute to the patient's security and social adaptation, it is hoped that there may be a certain reintegration of the personality with increased harmony and internal balance. Psychobiological psychotherapy assumes that the patient, having through the discussions, discovered and analyzed the factors that contributed to his difficulties, will be able to make the changes necessary for better adaptation. Frequently it is advisable to discuss the patient's assets and possibilities. Advice is often offered in the form of questions. Re-education, as may be determined by special needs, is frequently desirable.

Some physicians, although adhering to the principles of distributive analysis and synthesis, believe there should be more emphasis on unconscious processes and therefore also use word association tests, Rorschach's ink blot test, dreams and even Freudian free associations for securing material which may be used as topics for discussion. It is generally agreed that Meyer's psychobiological psychotherapy is more practical than orthodox psychoanalysis for the treatment of a majority of psychotic patients. If the patient has the intelligence and personality maturity to participate in analysis and synthesis it is often helpful in psychoneuroses, affective disturbances that are of reactive origin, immaturity reactions, mild paranoid reactions and psychosomatic or somatization reactions.

Reference was made in the previous paragraph to the use of word association tests. This is a method begun by Francis Galton but developed by Jung, having for its purpose the discovery of experiences and tendencies to which the patient is sensitive and therefore are of psychodynamic import. It is based on the observation that if a stimulus word arouses emotional conflict, the response is delayed, distorted or inhibited. In the use of this test a list of one hundred words designed to touch on all the common emotional problems is called and the patient is requested to respond after each word with the first thought that comes to him. Words that stimulate some sensitive topic are followed by a delay in answering or they evolve unusual or apparently irrelevant response words. After the list has been called the one hundred words are repeated with instructions to give after each word the same response as was first given. A failure to understand the word, or its repetition before giving a response, betrays the fact that a sensitive problem has been touched. The topics and tendencies thus betrayed may be used as subjects of discussion.

The unpleasant association may also be used as starting points for psychoanalytic free associations.

Psychoanalysis

It should be borne in mind that the term psychoanalysis is used in two very different senses. Freud originally applied the word to a particular therapeutic method but it is now employed also as the name of a system of theoretical psychology based on the assumption that there is a part of the mind of which one is not conscious. It is therefore a technique for both the investigation and the treatment of mental and emotional disorder. Some psychiatrists believe that the value of psychoanalysis with its emphasis on the unconscious background of conscious phenomena and as a method of investigating the workings of the mind has been greater than its value as a psychotherapeutic method. It has elucidated many aspects of human behavior that had baffled interpretation and has led to a deeper understanding of the factors that have determined personality development and patterns. Through psychoanalysis it has been learned that phenomena in adult life which are seemingly unintelligible take on meaning when understood in terms of chronologically earlier experiences. It has, too, been of immense value in bringing into awareness the unconscious roots of the problems of the mentally ill. The application of the increased knowledge of the mind secured through psychoanalysis has moreover been of great therapeutic value. As a system of psychotherapy, it aims to establish its methods on the general principles and knowledge of the dynamics of emotional life. Psychoanalysis makes possible a study of deep psychological forces and attempts to demonstrate how certain inner situations and roles persist and result in attitudes and motivating mechanisms that lie behind consciousness but may determine the whole course of life. It emphasizes, more than other psychological theories, the role of infantile experience in determining adult behavior. Probably many psychoanalysts underestimate the influence of later experiences in life. Often these are of more than precipitating significance.

It is an etiological, uncovering or insight type of therapy in contrast to the supportive, nonexploratory types to be described later. Doubtless the most important discoveries of Freud in relation to psychotherapy were those of *free association* as a means of exploration of the patient's mind, the study of *resistance* and the analysis of the *transference*. Psychoanalysis is a highly specialized procedure which should not be undertaken except by one who has had systematic training in its techniques. The goal of psychoanalytical therapy is the uncovering and modifying of unconscious psychological forces. Through the analysis the patient should discover the influences of these unconscious forces upon the pattern of his daily life and upon his relationship to other persons. Theoretically, at least, psychoanalysis is the choice of psychotherapy if a thoroughgoing modification of the personality is sought. The analyst seeks to bring about changes in personality structure by undoing the unfavorable patterns established in earlier years. Psychoanalysis aims to explore the deeper layers of the patient's mind with the hope that thereby he may acquire a maximum of self-knowledge and effect an alteration in the structure of his personality by undoing and reorganizing the unfavorable patterns that were established in an earlier period.

It is now generally agreed that an analytical psychotherapist should have a personal analysis as a basic preparation for analytical therapy. In this analysis the prospective therapist undertakes a penetrating psychological study of himself. With the aid of his analyst he is expected to explore thoroughly the unconscious realms of his mind, trace his personality development back to the formative experiences of his childhood and arrive at a fuller knowledge and a more realistic appaisal of himself. Such an analysis helps the therapist to recognize his own impulses, wishes, anxieties and defenses and reduces the danger that they interfere with the therapeutic relationship with the patient, or that the physician be rendered anxious by a hostile patient because of arousal of his own hostile or sadistic impulses. As in all patient-physician relationship types of psychotherapy, the therapist must avoid treating the patient as a projected part of himself. The personal analysis also enables the therapist to avoid many problems that may otherwise arise out of countertransference to be discussed later. A personal analysis, too, is extremely helpful in acquainting one's self with the technique of an experienced analyst. The future therapist should also receive a long period of supervised clinical work before undertaking psychoanalytical therapy without the guidace of a trained therapist.

Psychoanalysis finds its greatest therapeutic usefulness in the psychoneuroses, character disorders and some cases of incipient schizophrenia. The greatest success obtained in these disorders is with what Freud designated the transference neuroses in which he included hysteria, phobias and obsessive neurosis. These neuroses are characterized by a greater potentiality for transference (a relationship to be discussed later) than exists in other neuroses, and are therefore more amenable to therapy. In the psychoses the usefulness of psychoanalysis is definitely limited.

Even though the nature of his neurosis would indicate that a patient is a suitable subject for psychoanalysis, certain other elements may contraindicate any therapy of this nature. Unless the patient sincerely wishes for relief from the neurosis and is prepared to undertake the therapy seriously and resolutely, no attempt at psychoanalysis should be made. Since a person cannot profit by such therapy unless he has a well-developed capacity for introspective understanding, the analysis of a person of subnormal intelligence cannot be successfully undertaken. Rarely can much be accomplished by the analysis of persons over forty-five years of age although more depends upon the plasticity and receptivity of one's personality pattern than upon chronological age.

Psychoanalytical therapy involves, among other psychological principles, such important ones as *unconscious content*, *free association*, *resistance*, *transference*, *countertransference*, *interpretation* and *analysis of dreams*. These will be discussed briefly but no attempt will be made either to present them in detail or to examine the many problems that arise in the actual employment of the technique.

The analyst should be a graduate in medicine, have had considerable experience with both psychotic and neurotic patients and be well acquainted with the principles of dynamic psychology. He should be relatively free from conflicts and anxieties and from rigid convictions and other personality defenses. Interviews are held five or six days per week for periods extending from forty-five minutes to one hour. From one to three years are usually required for an analysis. It is generally considered desirable that the therapist and the patient should not have been previously acquainted, also that their relationship continue to be a strictly professional one free from social association. In order that free association may be facilitated, the patient reclines during the interview, relaxed on a couch, while the analyst is seated a little behind and to one side of him. The analyst can observe the patient but as the latter cannot see the analyst he is not constantly looking for signs of the therapist's response. One of the basic steps in psychoanalytical procedure in an exploration of the unconscious.

While dream analysis and other techniques are employed as supplementary means, the principal method is that of free association. To obtain such consciously unguided associations, the therapist asks the patient to say whatever comes to his mind, and warns him against changing the sequence of his undirected thoughts and against withholding anything because it seems irrelevant or distressing. There should be an uncensored, uninhibited verbalization of everything and anything that comes to mind. The permissive atmosphere of the therapeutic relationship facilitates free association. Opinions and feelings are expressed with a minimum or no guidance by inquiry. As material through the free association process emerges, often in symbolic form, from the consciously inaccessible portion of the mind it becomes conscious. That it may be used therapeutically, however, it is not only necessary that the patient's repressed material be made conscious but also that interrelations and implications of the material be recognized. It is essential that the therapist be exceedingly guarded and discrete in pointing out connections among the material produced by free association or of suggesting interpretations of it. The meaning of the material, as we shall see later, must be largely discovered by the patient himself. Through the free association process the patient explores early memories, recreates significant experiences and the feelings contingent on them, reactivates relations with parents, siblings or other persons and tries to bring into consciousness feelings and ideas about himself and his attitudes as they existed in childhood. The purpose of the analysis, however, is not in any way to secure a history but rather for the patient through free association and his interpretation of its products to discover the tendencies, motives, desires and other influences that have led to his personality problems, his defenses against anxiety and have constituted dynamic forces in his life. Gradually, as associations increase in number and in their richness of material from the unconscious, what has appeared irrelevant and meaningless to the patient begins to assume significance to him. As previously indicated, the therapist should bear in mind that interpretations of the material replete with symbolic disguises should scarcely be suggested, much less be forced on the patient who should be advised to discover for himself the meaning of his associative products. This does not mean that comment or carefully restrained aid in interpreting these products is not permissible but that the associations must be purely of an autogenous nature and that the patient must, in so far as possible, discover this significance for himself and come to appreciate that his symptoms bear a relation to some deep-seated personality problem. As will later be indicated more clearly, free association may be regarded as a method of recovering the history of a symptom and its defensive function. Because of the great degree of self-revelation that it makes possible, free association is perhaps the most valuable of all methods in disclosing psychodynamics. Although not employed by the orthodox psychoanalyst, some therapists use as a basis for analysis the unconscious material disclosed by the Rorschach or other projective test.

Free association does not, however, assure smooth and easy passage of all repressed memories and emotions into consciousness. Although the patient's trust in the analyst and the confidence that he is not being judged by the therapist aid him in facing emotional constellations with which he could not deal in the past, yet as certain repressed and forgotten experiences and emotions are about to be brought within the scope of immediate observation, an opposition to their complete awareness, an aversion to facing the unconscious basis of his motive appears. This opposition, known technically as *resistance*, may be manifested by sudden silences, denials, blockings, forgettings, evasions, embarrassments and strong emotional reactions. The dynamic significance of the repressed material may be estimated by the degree of resistance to its emergence, by the severity of the defensive reaction. By noting the occasion and the topics which evoke the patient's defensive resistances, the analyst secures clues as to the nature of the repressed material. Not rarely the patient's inflection or sudden change of subject indicates that the nucleus of a conflict is being approached or that he is unwittingly attempting to avoid recognition of an unconscious motivation. Again the resistance represents an unconscious effort to evade memories or insight. The analyst seeks to detect and bring to the patient's attention a recognition of his deep-rooted and repressed feelings and drives. This tends, however, to lead to an unconscious resistance to therapy. The resistance serves, of course, as a defense mechanism against the anxiety that would be aroused by a threatening self-knowledge of repudiated feelings and impulses. Care must be taken not to probe too deeply or too rapidly in the early stages of an analysis.

What is perhaps regarded as the most significant concept in psychoanalytical therapy, and one of the most important discoveries of Freud, is the emotional reaction of the patient toward the analysis known as the *transference* or *transference situation.* Transference is usually defined as a repetition in the patient's present life, and particularly in his relationship to the analyst, of unconscious emotional attitudes developed during childhood within the family group and especially toward the parents. It represents a carrying over, and attaching to the therapist, of the friendly, hostile or ambivalent attitudes and feelings which the patient formerly entertained in relation to the parent or other meaningful person of the past who played a significant role in his life. The patient reacts toward the therapist as if the latter were this person. The significance of the transfer is that it throws light upon the patient's relationship with the individual whom the therapist represents. The patient comes to react as if the therapist were actually the other person and therefore interprets the behavior of the analyst in conformance with his concept of the person toward whom he originally had the reaction. Important unconscious factors are therefore revealed not only by free associations and dreams but also by transference behavior. In the resulting reaction, often referred to as the transference neurosis, the original pathogenic conflicts of the early family relationships are repeated with lesser intensity in relationship to the analyst. This may lead to extreme anxiety, illogical hostility with paranoid implications, to clinging affecton or to serious acting out of impulses in order to invite the therapist's punishment. The therapist must not be surprised or disturbed by a hostile or critical attitude of the patient toward him. Rather does he objectively study those feelings with the patient, point them out to him and seek to trace them to their origin. An effort is made to make it clear to the patient how his feelings really arose out of earlier relationships. The patient's reliving of his original conflict in the transference situation is used by the therapist as an important therapeutic experience. By encouraging the patient to retrace his memories to early childhood, he may find the source of these feelings and make it possible to eliminate them or lessen their influence. The secret of the patient's illness may often be found in these transferred feelings. The discovery and understanding of the emotions originally felt toward other significant persons in the patient's past experience and transferred during therapy to the physician may have a definite therapeutic effect on him. This will be accomplished by the principle of interpretation to be discussed later. One aspect of the transference situation that may arise is the tendency of the patient to repeat in relation to the therapist a pattern of dependent emotional relationship such as hampered his emotional adjustment and personality development in the past.

A phenomenon that accounts for many mistakes and failures of psychotherapy is that known as *countertransference.* This consists of such negative attitudes of physician to patient as anger, impatience or resentment. These and similar attitudes are almost certain to interfere with the therapeutic effectiveness of the physician. For the most part the countertransference reactions arise in the therapist as a result of the patient's influence on the physician's unconscious feelings and have their origin in the latter's irrational projections and identifications. The therapist must not permit his own unconscious feelings and attitudes aroused during phases of treatment to intrude in his relations toward the patient.

As a rule the therapist himself should have received psychotherapy in order that his own problems may not blind him to similar ones in the patient.

It should be added, however, that just as countertransference can account for failure in therapy, so it can also in the hands of a skillful therapist be put to good use diagnostically and therapeutically. For instance, a patient, not intending to do so, may nevertheless arouse annoyance in the therapist. The latter perceives this as an index of the patient's hostility. The therapeutic task is then to find out, first, why the patient is afraid to express overt hostility, and second, what the patient's hostility represents.

Reference has been made to unconscious content, free associations, resistance, transference and countertransference as important psychoanalytical concepts. Another principle, especially important in its relation to therapy, is *interpretation*. This is the process whereby the therapist helps the patient to understand the meaning of his mental phenomena and behavior—usually mental phenomena the existence of which he is not even aware. In order that the patient may acquire an understanding insight into his difficulties and thereby improve his adjustment and reconstruct his personality to a desirable extent, there are many phases of his mental life of which he should have an understanding knowledge—an emotional, not merely an intellectual, knowledge. The impartment of such an understanding, however, is one of the most difficult tasks of psychotherapy and requires great skill and tact and discreet timing. The therapist attempts to penetrate the patient's personality defenses and bring the anxiety and underlying conflicts into consciousness so that they may be dealt with rationally. The acquiring of an insightful understanding by the patient is a slow process and must not be hurried. Newly gained insights may produce fright and terror. A premature interpretation mobilizes anxiety and alarms or antagonizes the patient. He must not be expected to tolerate the deeply disturbing experience and painful revelations which a self-knowledge of his motivations may bring until preparatory interpretations by the therapist have brought about a necessary stage of readiness. An interpretation of unconscious mental content as brought out by free association is a necessary part of any exploratory therapy. Before this is done, however, there should have been sufficient interpretation of the patient's defenses so that he is almost ready by himself to see the implications of what is brought forth through his free associations. A cautious interpretation will be necessary in order that the patient may acquire an understanding of the significance of transference phenomena. As is to be expected, the patient, through his need for protection against anxiety, will manifest a resistance to the therapist's interpretations. An added task for the therapist will be to assist the patient in interpreting his resistance. As has already been indicated, the therapist should never confront the patient with a blunt interpretation of the meaning of his symptoms. The more obvious their meaning the more cautious he should be in explaining them. It has been correctly said that whenever the patient cannot see the obvious it is because he needs his blindness. The therapist should not impose his own interpretations. The patient is likely to gain more insight into his problems and behavior through making his own associations, or at least in being merely guided and helped to draw his own conclusions and thereby meaningfully assimilate his interpretations into his psychology.

The efforts of the therapist and patient should lead to an undoing of repression in order that the repressed may be brought to consciousness and its critical judgments. Thus a rational decision can be made if all the facts are at hand instead of having only part of them available as was previously the case when some were unconscious. One aim of analysis is to bring about such a state that the conscious ego with its reason, logic and critical abilities, may assume control when it is confronted with unrealistic, pleasure-seeking, infantile demands that cannot be satisfied by reality. In other words, we can make a decision about our infantile demands when we see them and observe how inappropriate they are to present reality. Previously these infantile demands secured some gratification through neurotic symptoms. In every neurotic individual there is overt anxiety when the repressed approaches consciousness. This anxiety then causes the ego to renew its efforts to secure repression, often through the aid of other defense mechanisms. In the analytical transference situation, the patient will allow himself to experience the anxiety without renewed efforts at repression by the ego. This the patient can do since he identifies himself with the analyst who is there to help him and will, he is confident, protect him from danger. Thus, over a period of time, there is a fractionizing of the anxiety, a gradual exposure of the repressed, until finally the reasonable, judging portion of the ego recognizes that what was repressed is not appropriate in the present life of the patient.

Another important method employed by psychoanalysis for rendering contents of the unconscious available for conscious scrutiny is the examination of *dream material.* The dream is no longer regarded as an accident of our psychic life but as a phenomenon directly connected with it. Since presumably it represents a product of the patient's thinking that lacks the directing and inhibiting forces exercised by awareness, the material it presents for examination discloses more clearly than does consciously directed thinking the underlying strivings of the personality. Tendencies which may not be expressed in the presence of clear consciousness work freely in dreams. They serve as a convenient disguise for the patient's unacceptable, rejected emotions. In them the analyst finds a symbolic expression of the patient's inner tensions and clues to his repressed thoughts, feelings, childhood memories and experiences. When a dream persists in memory or is repeated it has special significance because it specifically fits and reveals something constant and basic in the forces that make the personality.

Freud divided the content of thought of dreams into two categories. One he called the *manifest content*—the content as it appears to and is recalled by the dreamer. The recollected or obvious content is not, however, the significant element which is contained in what is known as the *latent content*. The latent content, were it to appear in its naked form, would be too disturbing and painful and is therefore distorted and disguised so that its recollection will not disturb the dreamer. The disguise of mental material, the repression of which suffers a nocturnal relaxation, is brought about by the mechanisms of displacement, condensation, symbolization, dramatization and elaboration. The joint activity of these mechanisms is known as the *dream work*, a process by which the latent dream content is transformed into the manifest content. By condensation two or more ideas, wishes or persons are fused into one, emphasis on significant mental material is displaced and the content is dramatized and filled out by a deceptive secondary elaboration. As a result of the dream work the manifest content may appear to be merely an irrelevant, confused product, yet it really represents the symbolic expression of inner tensions and of other important psychic material the hidden meaning of which must be interpreted in terms of the total life situation of the individual. It will be noted that the mechanisms which in the dream work cause the latent content of the dream to assume the form presented in the manifest content are the same ones that are operative in producing many neurotic symptoms. Such symptoms are in their dynamics identical with dream processes. In both, one notes the operation of the psychological laws of the unconscious.

In psychoanalysis the dreamer is encouraged to report to the physician any recent or recurring dream. Starting from the manifest content of the dream, free associations are employed. The latent or underlying significance of the symbolic imagery in the manifest content is brought to light. There arises here, of course, the same problem of symbolization and interpretation as in free association, and the analyst must in the same way encourage the patient to discover the meaning concealed in the manifest content of the dream rather than impose the arbitrary acceptance of fixed symbols. It should be remembered, however, that the object in dream interpretation is not so much the translation of certain symbols as the discovery of the ideas and motives that are dynamic in determining the patient's reactions in his waking life. Jung speaks of the dream as essentially a rational and logical statement but one that appears illogical only because it is written in a language which cannot be understood without special study.

To be successful, psychoanalysis should so thoroughly reveal to the patient his underlying strivings and problems that with the assistance of the therapist he can reorganize the forces of his personality, redirect his affective energy into constructive channels and prevent its further dissipation in dissociation, substitution and other evasive, neurotic ways. It aims to give the patient freedom from disabling fears, distress and inhibitions and to enable him to achieve insight sufficient to handle ordinary conflicts and reasonable reality stress. In psychotic patients it is usually too difficult to overcome resistance or to establish transference to a degree that will permit successful analytic treatment.

Because of the time required for a standard Freudian analysis, and therefore the relatively few persons who can be treated thereby, attempts are being increasingly made to develop a brief interpretative psychotherapy based on psychoanalytical principles. Many psychiatrists combine selected features from psychobiological, supportive and psychoanalytical therapies. Franz Alexander, although making use of psychoanalytical principles, sought to make psychoanalysis less time-consuming. He believes that prolonged, uninterrupted, daily interviews may favor the development of a too dependent relationship and consequently postpone recovery. He therefore reduces the contact with the patient as much as possible, gives the patient more independence and discourages regressive tendencies. Even in those therapies, not extensively employed, which do not follow a classical Freudian analysis but nevertheless supplement their techniques with certain psychoanalytical principles, the therapist seeks to bring his patient to recognize the significance of his patterns of behavior and their relationship to early environmental and cultural influences or to interpersonal relationships and experiences. It is hoped that the insight acquired by the patient may enable him to modify these behavior patterns. It is also the hope of the therapist, whether he employs orthodox psychoanalysis or one of its modifications, that through his efforts the development of the personality which has been warped or stunted in its growth may resume its progress toward maturity.

Other Psychotherapeutic Techniques

In addition to the genetic-dynamic therapies, in which group, psychobiological therapy and psychoanalysis may be included, there are various other psychotherapeutic techniques. These may be classified in numerous ways. The following classification seems, however, to be a logical one: (1) Superficial Expressive Therapy; (2) Suppressive Therapy; and (3) Supportive Therapy. While classical psychoanalytic techniques are not employed in these forms, they are often to some degree psychoanalytically oriented.

SUPERFICIAL EXPRESSIVE THERAPY

In the discussion concerning psychoanalysis, attention was called to the fact that free association and an observation of its sequence of ideas, dreams and the associations to them, transference phenomena and defensive reactions, such as resistances, served both as a means of exploration and of expression of unconscious material. In the superficial expressive therapies, various techniques, sometimes with associated adjunctive devices (such as drugs which alter the level of consciousness), are employed for the purpose of exploring and securing expression of the preconscious and other relatively superficial mental content. Among the superficial expressive therapies would be included: (*a*) Narcosynthesis; (*b*) Ventilation; and (*c*) Abreaction.

Narcosynthesis

In this form of therapy, the patient is given an intravenous injection of Pentothal sodium or Sodium Amytal to the point of thorough relaxation but not of sleep. In this state censorship is less active and suppressed or repressed material emerges. Conscious control is obliterated and inhibitions removed. The patient's subconscious is revealed relatively rapidly and with the minimum of psychic trauma. Positive or negative feelings may be overtly expressed and trends disclosed. The technique is of considerable value when the patient has recently been subjected to severe traumatic experiences which stirred impulses and anxiety to a degree that they could not be handled without repression and symptom formation. Under these circumstances, abreaction often contributes to the therapeutic process. The greatest usefulness of narcosynthesis is in acute anxiety states, early traumatic neuroses and conversion hysterias. It is not satisfactory in obsessive-compulsive states or in chronic neuroses. The technique not only breaks down inhibitions but favors the establishment of rapport, puts the patient in a suggestible frame of mind and appeals to him because it uses a physical means of approach which he usually accepts more readily. Resistance, or an unconscious effort to evade memories and insight, is reduced by the narcosis and interpretation is thereby facilitated.

Ventilation

Ventilation is an expressive type of therapy in which the patient's anxiety is relieved to a greater or lesser degree by his being given an opportunity in a tolerant, empathic setting frankly to "talk out" and discuss with the therapist personal problems and "worries" which he ordinarily would not discuss with others. The physician, with an attitude of understanding and encouragement, interrupts the patient as little as possible although occasional questions may be necessary to keep the thread of the story in meaningful channels. Among topics that may require ventilation may be doubts, impulses, conscious anxieties, family problems and feelings of guilt. Some phases of the material expressed may be a sort of confession. Others may consist largely of "blowing off steam" regarding resentments. Frequently a joint discussion of present conflicts and past life situations as they seem to relate to emotional or psychosomatic symptoms may bring relief to troublesome aspects of the patient's life. Perhaps in this way the patient may discover a linkage of events and feelings with present reactions and symptoms. An occasional question may help the patient to find the meaning of his symptoms himself. A correction of misinformation regarding personal problems may result in some diminution of the patient's anxiety. The patient-physician relationship adds to the therapeutic effect of ventilation. Where "talking things out" has removed some of the anxiety and guilt from a crucial life situation, ventilation may at times be supplemented by a superficial psychotherapy based on a knowledge of psychodynamics.

Abreaction

This is a superficial expressive type of psychotherapy in which anxiety is lessened by an emotional re-living of the stress situation which produced the neurosis. A therapeutically beneficial discharge of dammed-up emotions associated with the recall of a repressed memory occurs. The existence of a high degree of emotional tension is the basic indication for abreaction. It often tends to produce a desensitization, *i.e.*, a reduction of emotional tension related to a repressed psychological conflict. The emotional reactions discharged are usually those of grief, rage or fear. Sometimes the abreaction may include an expression of hostility toward the therapist. Abreaction with its beneficial effect in bringing about a re-living and possible working out of the emotional aspects of a stressful experience may be spontaneous, suggested under hypnosis or facilitated with barbiturates.

SUPPRESSIVE THERAPY

Suppressive psychotherapy aims to strengthen repression and other usual defenses or to lessen the intensity of a disabling symptom by such means as dogmatic assurance, persuasion, suggestion and hypnosis. It makes no search for, or any effort to solve, the actual dynamic problem. If, therefore, it produces any relief the problem still remains and may readily return under any stress or strain.

Persuasion

Persuasion as a form of psychotherapy is particularly associated with the name of Paul Dubois of Berne. This therapy is based upon the principle of intellectual explanations and moralizing discussions. It is explained to the patient how faulty intellectual and emotional attitudes on his part were reactions to certain difficulties; also how such tendencies led to undesirable habits and unhealthy emotional and mental conditions. According to Dubois, an important method of therapeutic approach is through self-criticism and through reasoning as to the nature of the symptoms and as to the false ideas and bad mental habits which led to the symptoms. In persuasion the emphasis is on rationalism and on moral suasion, on an appeal to "reason" and to will rather than on an understanding of the personality and the dynamic factors in its formation. By means of persuasion, the therapist seeks to create, convert or strengthen certain impulses and to remove or diminish others, to create or strengthen some inhibitions and to free the patient from enslaving ones. It is the aim of the physician, through reasoned argument, to implant in the patient's mind the conviction that his symptoms will disappear. Persuasion probably overestimates the potency of rational processes in any attack upon the products of emotional factors.

Suggestion

In suggestion the therapist seeks to aid the patient by subtly, often indirectly, implanting or inducing the idea or belief that unpleasant or disabling symptoms are being relieved. The successful use of suggestion requires that the physician manifest an attitude of assurance, professional authority and sympathy. The patient, because of his respect for and confidence in the physician, tends to accept the idea presented. His critical ability is lessened and his mood is influenced. His attention becomes narrowed. In his state of expectancy he comes to believe that the results predicted will actually take place. The best results in suggestion therapy are secured when there is no deep-seated disturbance of the personality, as in hysterical conversion symptoms of recent and superficial origin, or in anxiety states following accidents. The employment of electricity, massage or manipulation in conjunction with suggestion is not advisable since the patient may atribute the recovery to external agencies. In such cases the recovery is frequently not permanent and at best is only the disappearance of a symptom and not a cure. In the event of a probable recurrence, the same agencies must be employed in exactly the same manner and frequently by the same person.

Suggestion does not, of course, give the patient any understanding of the cause or dynamics of his disability and in hysteria tends to fix even more firmly the usual propensity to receptivity so characteristic of that disorder. It tends to restrict rather than increase insight. Even though a symptom is relieved by suggestion, the problems and psychological needs that produced it remain unchanged and their evasion may soon be sought by some other symptom. For this reason the use of suggestion should be accompanied by some kind of re-education.

In spite of the limitations of suggestion, its use may be considered permissible in children, in persons of limited intelligence and in immature, hysterical personalities. Assuming, for example, that the symptom to be removed is a hysterical conversion symptom, such as a recent paralysis, the physician deals with it by direct suggestion accompanied by some explanation as to the nature of the paralysis. His attitude must be one of conviction and certainty and the patient must have confidence in him. The physician demonstrates that the capacity for passive movement still exists. He informs the patient that no organic disability that can interfere with function is present. In referring to the patient's disability, the physician comments as to what a nuisance the former's disability must be to him. At the same time he instructs the patient to move the extremity naturally and without forced effort. The patient is apt to make the mistake of attempting the movement by a strenuous effort that leads also to an innervation of the antagonist group of muscles resulting in a rigid immobility. The interview with its atmosphere of conviction must continue until voluntary exercise of the function is restored even though an hour or two be required. The physician, through the very full life story he has obtained from the patient and through a knowledge of the circumstances under which the disability occurred, must be able to convince the patient not only of the meaning and purpose of the symptom but also that the loss of function has persisted because he believed it to be a real loss. The restoration of function is not a matter of attempt to exercise it on the part of the patient, not a matter of "will," but a matter of belief that it is possible. The physician must be careful both in word and manner not to create the impression that he considers the patient to be either feigning or exaggerating his inability. Anything that will tend to offend the patient's self-respect must be avoided. Ross emphasizes that the atmosphere of the interview during which the physician attempts the removal of the symptom must be one of reasoned logic and of scrupulous avoidance of dramatic demonstration or of artful deception. The patient would prefer to believe that manipulation or some agency outside of himself removed the disability but he must be made to see that no external interference was instrumental. The patient must be convinced that the disability disappeared because he recognized its purpose and unreality.

The loss of the symptom is at first accompanied by a feeling of relief and pleasure, but unless he fully recognizes the sequence and relation of events and feelings the patient may suffer a relapse when again confronted with the same problem or unpleasant situation from which the symptom had unconsciously provided an escape. In that case the sense of relief is followed by anxiety, sleeplessness, mild depression, physical distress and perhaps by disability. A frank discussion of the situation with the patient may enable him to make an emotional adjustment to it; again, if the problem springs from the environment a removal from the source of the difficulty may be wise. Unfortunately the presenting symptom is often not an isolated affair but an expression of characterological tendencies which are apt to lead to difficulties of adjustment unless a thorough reconstruction of the personality occurs. Direct suggestion does not usually have as far-reaching an effect as does hypnotic suggestion which, therefore, is often preferable.

Hypnosis

Hypnosis may be defined as an induced dissociative state produced through suggestion. Although there is much prejudice against its use it nevertheless has a place as a form of therapy. Its greatest value is in hysteria. It also serves as a means of investigating behavior and the observation of hypnotized persons has contributed much to dynamic theories of mental activity. Freud's psychoanalytical theory and practice had their beginnings in hypnotism. Verbal suggestions are used in producing hypnosis. Through suggestion the patient's attention is diverted from all other stimuli and is directed to the therapist's procedure. His consciousness becomes progressively narrower, he becomes increasingly drowsy and passes into a trance-like sleep. In this state of semiconscious suggestibility inhibiting mechanisms may be by-passed, at least temporarily.

One of the most important characteristics of hypnosis is that of posthypnotic suggestion. Suggestions given during hypnosis may be acted upon after the termination of the hypnosis or even at a suggested period after its termination. This phenomenon may permit the physician to influence symptoms favorably. Hypnosis may be used as a means for commanding the disappearance of symptoms, particularly those produced through the use of repression as a defense mechanism. While a symptom may often be made to disappear dramatically through hypnosis, yet the factors which produced it are merely repressed and the fundamental personality problem is unchanged. Another reason why hypnosis is not a measure that is permanently successful when used alone is because suggestions lose their effect after a time. It also has the disadvantage that when the patient's symptoms are suggested away he may become dependent on the hypnotist instead of developing an ability to solve his problems independently. For these reasons hypnosis should be supplemented by an insight-producing and constructive form of psychotherapy. Any real cure requires a knowledge of the underlying factors which produced the symptoms.

Hypnosis may be of value when painful experiences have been repressed and given rise to symptoms. The memory of the traumatic experience may be revived by hypnosis and the symptom made to disappear with an accompanying abreaction in which the patient goes over and over the traumatic situation crying and sobbing or showing other expression of pent-up emotions.

Mention has already been made of the fact that hypnosis may be used as a means of investigating aspects of the patient's mental life beneath full awareness. Under hypnosis, forgotten experiences may be revived and the patient can discuss material about which he cannot or does not want to talk in the waking state. The use of intravenous barbiturates as a means of recovering repressed memories is more certain and requires less time than does hypnosis. It does not, either, involve the emotional dependence often prerequisite to successful hypnosis.

SUPPORTIVE PSYCHOTHERAPY

Supportive psychotherapy is not based on genetic and dynamic considerations but aims to reduce the tensions of anxiety or of other incapacitating tensions by supportive techniques. Care must be taken, however, not to disturb important and acceptable personality defenses. The techniques employed are of a simple type and the choice of selection will be determined by many factors, such as the personality characteristics, age, life situation and the nature of the patient's emotional problem or illness. Among the measures employed will be reassurance, use of authority, permissive attitudes that relieve guilt, reasoning, encouragement, counseling, explanation, advice and manipulation of environment including, perhaps, an attempted alteration of attitudes of key persons in the patient's life situation. Little attempt is made to bring about an adjustive personality change but rather to help the patient to maintain or improve his ability to face and handle his reality at his best integrative level.

It is often said that how the physician acts toward the patient, how he listens and speaks to him, is more important than what he tells the patient. While the therapist's attitude is important regardless of the type of psychotherapy employed, this is in itself a basic element in supportive therapy. The therapist must, in fact, be an understanding, thinking, feeling and responding person who recognizes the patient's individual problem. While supportive therapy consists essentially of strengthening old, but socially acceptable, defenses and the cultivation of new but related ones, the therapist should usually not be satisfied with the exclusive use of such mechanisms but as circumstances permit should try to work beyond the symptoms and aid the patient in acquiring at least some insight. In employing supportive therapy, the physician should bear in mind the danger that he may thereby encourage dependence and a regressive passivity in the patient. Support should be accompanied by efforts to promote maturity of personality. In both genetic-dynamic and in supportive therapy, only limited results can be expected if there are harsh environmental pressures from which the patient cannot escape.

Group Psychotherapy

A. *Rationale*

Following its introduction in this country by Pratt in 1905, group treatment in the practice of psychotherapy developed slowly until the last two decades. The application of group therapy, of the principles of dynamic psychiatry and the added impetus of the experiences of World War II have contributed to its rapid growth as a systematic treatment during recent years. Although it was first used for its morale effect upon physically ill patients whose activities were restricted, its scope has gradually been broadened through successive stages of experiment and evolution to embrace both hospital and out-patient treatment of psychoses, psychoneuroses, emotional disorders of children, situational reactions and behavior disorders. As a system of therapy, it was born of three considerations: (1) exigency; (2) specific indications; and (3) the sociodynamic nature of human maladjustment.

Its least recommending factor, perhaps, is that of exigency based on the fact that there are far more patients in need of therapy than there are therapists equipped to treat them on an individual basis. While the latter is certainly true, the proponents of group psychotherapy maintain that this mode of managing psychiatric illnesses neither supplants individual psychotherapy nor necessarily offers itself as a substitutive treatment for those to whom other psychotherapeutic doors are closed. On the contrary, it is claimed that specific indications are found among patients which recommend the use of group psychotherapy. Slavson notes that certain patients manifest aversion to the individual therapies because of fear, competitiveness, distrust, or antagonism toward all parental figures. Sometimes individual psychotherapy is too threatening and the patient finds in the group the acceptance and support necessary for the examination of his problems. For such persons, group psychotherapy alone may be successful, or it may serve as a preparation for individual treatment. Patients lacking sibling experiences, having antagonistic sibling attitudes, living in situations without opportunities for participation, experiencing destructive family relations, showing character disorders, presenting evidence of generalized social maladjustment or for whom the danger and fear of homosexual involvement with an individual therapist exist are often selected for group treatment. Patients with dull intelligence may benefit more from group than from individual therapy. Generally, all children gain from group association and it is believed that a large group of children is needed for this form of therapy to be successful. Exclusive group treatment is frequently considered successful when feelings of inadequacy, sibling rivalry, and social maladjustments are the presenting problems in children. Analytical group psychotherapy is considered the treatment of choice for adolescent girls with confused sexual identifications.

Perhaps the most significant consideration giving rise to the concept of group interaction as a method of psychotherapy is the sociodynamic pattern of human maturation. The development of the infant from helplessness and dependency to tempered autonomy and acculturation is a social event. The need to adjust and the unprofitable systems for avoiding discomfort are created by group life. This consideration has given rise to the hypothesis that if maladjustments are caused to develop by inadequate or unwholesome group situations during the formative periods of life, then it should be possible to undo and modify them by exposing the maladaptations to continuous, structured group action in a more adequate and more wholesome setting. The psychotherapeutic group recommends itself through its employment of the following factors: acceptance of the selected individuals, avoidance of unnecessary restrictions, permissiveness toward uninhibited verbal expression and critical evaluation of reactions to group interaction as opposed to platitudinous judgment.

In general the constituency of the group will be determined by the needs of the members, *i.e.*, the group is structured to meet their needs. The approach will be quite different in case of schizophrenics from that in "psychopaths."

B. Some Dynamisms Relating to Therapeutic Groups

The group is virtually an amalgamation of individual needs. Experience with therapy groups has revealed that the principles of treatment employed in individual psychotherapy are applicable to groups. The relationship between each member and the therapist possesses the qualities of individual therapy, and in addition all the patient-members become, in a sense, auxiliary therapists, thus increasing the emotional interplay. The group setting is a continuous reality factor which presents an ever-fresh stimulus and provocation to behavior. Although the group support diminishes individual anxiety, many group therapists feel that the amount and character of affective interactions may be increased and accelerated. The actual therapeutic benefits are realized by the participants rather than by the group as a whole.

A phenomenon of unmistakable significance is the factor of idea and affect contagion which permeates a group. Le Bon has likened the result with reference to group participants to the relationship between subject and hypnotist. The individual in a group behaves as though greatly influenced by a group will. Certain ego functions of integration, also of affective and conative censorship, are given over to the group and its leader. This factor makes group formation possible but it also highlights the degree of immaturity of the members. The suggestibility and unreasoning obedience found in group participants demonstrate their dependency. This may be used as a criterion in determining therapeutic improvement, for as maturation progresses some degree of individual independence develops and a more rational and more realistic relationship to the group ensues.

The group situation is such that mechanisms are mobilized for self-defense against real or imagined threats occasioned by the presence of others. In large part this is a result of *transference*, the avenue through which projections, displacements and other mechanisms operate. While the entrance of this attitudinal force into the group work presents a barrier, it becomes the very focal point toward which therapeutic interpretations and insight formations are directed.

C. Aims and Goals

Although employing many of the skills, techniques and psychological mechanisms of individual psychotherapy, group psychotherapy is more complex because of the additional factors inherent in the group process. The complexity may impair to some extent the depth of insights that can be gained. Group goals represent a summation of the members' motivations and the leader's aims. Generally, group leaders aim in their patients to relieve emotional stress, resolve some of their conflicts, help them to a clearer realization of the reasons for their difficulties and assist them in supplanting defensive reactions with more acceptable and satisfying modes of behavior.

D. Systems of Group Therapy

The large variety of conscious motivations entertained by patients usually gives way in the course of group work to the goal of insight formation. However, there are many people for whom the development of deep insight is impossible or even undesirable. Several schools of group treatment have therefore been evolved which range between extremes on a nondirective-directive therapeutic scale. At one end of the scale are the analytical or free association therapies. At the other end are inspirational approaches directed toward the suppression of symptomatic behavior. The following is not a comprehensive listing but sets forth a brief description of some representative group management systems. For the sake of psychiatric accuracy all of the methods listed cannot be called psychotherapy. The number of participants in each is a moot question. There is much overlapping and the classification scheme is entirely arbitrary. The number of systems of group organization does not reflect the psychotherapeutic validity of this mode of treatment but rather indicates the necessity for employing varying approaches to the manifold diagnostic categories group therapists undertake to treat.

I. Nondirective Methods (Psychoanalytical)

1. *Analytical Group Psychotherapy and Group Analysis (Slavson, Wolf, Foulkes and Others)*
   This system is applicable in psychoneurotic adults and adolescents. There may be four to twelve participants. Some homo-

geneity in respect to age, sex and type of problem is desirable. An analytically trained therapist is leader.

2. *Activity Group Psychotherapy (Slavson)*
This may be used with children from seven to fourteen years of age. There are usually seven to eight participants. It is especially indicated for children rejected by school and play companions. The atmosphere should be permissive and the therapist analytically trained.
3. *Activity-Interview Group Psychotherapy*
This is applicable in case of school-age children with serious problems or with deeply disturbed children who have need both to talk about their anxieties and to act out feelings. There may be eight to ten participants. The therapist should be analytically trained.
4. *Play Group Psychotherapy (Slavson)*
This is used for preschool age children who are not mature enough to gain from acting out. Children are supplied with play materials. Hidden resentments, feelings of frustration, fears and confusions are conveyed in play. An analytical therapist interprets the feelings expressed and the object in the family environment toward whom the feelings are directed. The number of participants varies from eight to sixteen.
5. *Group Interview Psychotherapy, Analytically Oriented (Wender and others)*
This technique is applicable in most age groups and may be employed with psychoneurotic patients, psycho-physiologic states, social maladjustments and mild psychoses. Six to ten members are desirable. There is spontaneous verbal participation by the group. Group interaction with interpretation leading to mutual support and relative insights is desired. This method may be combined with a didactic approach.

II. Clinical Methods with Didactic (Educational and Directive) Orientation

1. *Group Interview Psychotherapy (Hinckley and others)*
This may be employed with most age groups and in a wide variety of psychiatric conditions. There may be from eight to twenty members. The type of leadership depends on psychotherapeutic orientation.
2. *Interview-Inspirational Group Therapy (Hadden and others)*
This technique may be followed with most age groups and diagnostic categories. There may be a variable number of participants. Spontaneous lectures are given by the leader and free expression by participants is encouraged. Interpretations may be analytically oriented or may be directed toward conscious dynamisms and social mechanisms.
3. *Social Relationship Groups (F. Redl)*
This method is followed with seriously disturbed and aggres-

sive children who are usually denied other therapies. Camp activities, trips, tours and group projects are employed. Leaders may aid rapport in traditional social ways, *e. g.*, giving of gifts, treating, group playing, etc. Environmental manipulation is a part of the management.

III. Didactic Methods with Clinical Orientation

1. *Psychodrama (J. C. Moreno)*
   There are two to six or more participants and the method may be employed in many conditions. A special stage is required. A spontaneous acting out supplemented by discussion and interaction by audience ("auxiliary egos") is followed. A variation of this technique employs prepared scripts. Other therapeutic systems sometimes use the role-playing elements of psychodrama adjunctively.
2. *Group Orientative Therapy, "Affective Re-education" (Klapman)*
   There may be a variable number of participants. Many conditions are treated. The leader plays an authoritative role. The following types are employed:
   a. Planned Program. A series of lectures is given by the leader. It may be used effectively with combat emotional casualties and veterans.
   b. Assigned Reading. A classroom method is followed.
   c. Call Method. This is often effective with groups having difficulty in developing group identity, *e.g.*, seniles. Members are called upon by the leader.
   d. Rotation Method. A serial order of members agreed upon for recitation is established.
   e. Question System. In this method members submit problems or questions for group discussion or for leader-authority to answer.
3. *Nonclinical Group Management*
   a. Sociological Groups. Six to twelve members participate. Group tensions and group dynamics are observed and interpretations are directed toward group development.
   b. Social Group Work. Here there may be work and living project, recreational or socialized occupation therapy groups.
   c. Confessional-Inspirational Group Method (J. Pratt). Inpirational talks are given by leader in an attempt to stimulate admission of problems.
   d. Counseling. In this authoritative advice, guidance and direction are employed. There may be changing leadership and variable membership.
   e. Repressive-Inspirational Groups. (Anonymous organizations, *e.g.*, Alcoholics Anonymous). There may be any number of participants, up to 500 or more. Group unifi-

cation based upon group allegiance, mutual support and the deep acceptance of cultural, moral and religious values is developed. Appeals to reason and conscious elements of ambition are made. There may be changing leadership.

f. Revival Groups. There may be any number of participants. This well known "religious conversion" experience may in its casual application convert some behavior problems into full-fledged obsessional neuroses. A reaction approaching revival may occur among groups led by amateur or unskilled "therapists."

E. Organization of Group

When possible it is considered desirable to convene interview groups in round table formation in esthetically pleasant surroundings with an informal atmosphere predominating. Activity therapies may require work tables and a meeting room constructed of especially durable materials. Because of extra-therapeutic actings-out which may limit group work or fragment the group, it is usually desirable to separate the sexes. Groups may meet at any time of day or evening on a rigidly scheduled basis. Except for the intensive therapies the group convenes once a week for sixty- to ninety-minute periods. More frequent meetings are necessary for groups having deep insight goals.

The proponents of the analytical psychotherapies urge that the group leaders have had personal intensive psychotherapy and further training in psychopathology. It is believed that group psychotherapists should have special training in the therapies including a broad didactic educational background as well as a penchant for this form of treatment. The personality and motivations of the group leader are considered of importance and it is felt that therapists who normally experience discomfort in groups should not undertake group therapeutic leadership. A competent therapist of either sex may be a group leader. When both group and individual therapy are required for a patient, the therapist must be the same person.

Many groups maintain "open" membership, allowing participants to terminate therapy when they wish to do so and permitting others to join at any time. As a rule, the deeper the insight goal the less variable the group membership. Some groups set date limits while others go on indefinitely for several years. Goals, number of participants, and systems of therapy vary according to whether the groups are hospital or clinic patients. Group psychotherapy is used in mental hospitals, out-patient clinics, private practice, affiliate therapeutic agencies of educational institutions, family agencies, with relatives of hospitalized patients and with children. Certain groups employ a totally permissive atmosphere without rules. Some groups employ agreed-upon taboos relative to group work. Many leaders, for example, regard it desirable to inculcate ethical principles in the group relative to privileged communication and to forbid physical acting out during meetings.

Group homogeneity and the number of participants are still debated subjects. Too much unification of interest may present the therapist with a symptom wall used as a rallying point for group resistance in the form of monothematic ruminations. On the other hand, too little homogeneity causes scattered interest. Extreme heterogeneity, *e.g.*, alcoholic patients mingled with symptom-neurotic patients, or psychotic persons with transference-neurotic patients, may engender name-calling and mutual distrust. The groups should be large enough for an adequate amount of interaction yet not so large that members are neglected.

The criteria for denying patients admission to therapeutic groups depend largely upon the orientation of the therapy involved. Most groups suffer from the inclusion of acute psychotic, aggressive paranoid, regressed schizophrenic, and manic patients. Patients with psychoses tending toward depression, with potential or overt perversion, with suicidal behavior, psychopathic personality, involutional states with compulsive and obsessional drives, or with hallucinated thought life are generally excluded from analytical groups. Such patients tend to disrupt, dominate, and exploit the group. They may also stimulate pathological processes in a deleterious way in other patients. In general, it is the feeling among group therapists that patients must have some capacity to participate in groups and at least a minimal amount of social hunger to gain from a therapy group.

F. The Group Process

Group psychotherapy possesses a characteristic which contrasts it with individual therapy in that it more closely resembles actual life situations and ordinary social intercourse, thus endowing the process with continuous reality meanings. Whereas in individual psychotherapeutic situations all attitudes, conditionings, and transferences are isolated in the patient and channelled into the one participant-observer, in group interaction there exists a multiplicity of targets and a dilution of transference. These have both positive and negative values. On the one hand, these factors reduce anxiety and fear activated by hostile and aggressive feelings toward figures of authority, and they allow for redirection or deflection of the hostilities and resentments toward fellow members. On the other hand, these factors may add an almost insuperable complexity to the production of insights. This is due to the multiplicity of possible emotional interrelationships.

Probably all groups traverse phases of development roughly approximating three periods: (1) a stage of *group unification* with the emergence of group identity; (2) a stage of *group interaction* with the observation of dynamisms; and (3) a final stage of understanding and *resolution of dynamisms* with the production of insights.

Therapy takes place at different levels according to group goals. The factors of mutual support and reliance engendered by group sanction parallel the formation of group esprit and contribute toward the establishment of morale which may be all that is desired for some groups. Simple ventilation through the phenomenon of emotional release may relieve tensions in given situations. Popular superstitions and ignorance may respond to educative group reorientation with the consequent lessening of fears and anxieties.

Analytically oriented group psychotherapies make use of the classical factors of catharsis, resistance, analysis of transference, interpretation and insight formation. The leader plays an important role in interpretation when resistance must be overcome, also in the resolution of transference. The group setting offers opportunities for the manifestation of social mechanisms and dynamisms not ordinarily found in individual psychotherapy. In addition to those mentioned above, the following are a few commonly encountered: (1) *Displacement.* A variety of feelings toward the therapist which the patient may be afraid to express are displaced on less threatening group members or on persons not present. (2) *Escape.* This is achieved by selective silence or by a change of subject. (3) *Deflection.* This may be used for escape by redirecting attention to another group member. (4) *Catalysis.* This dynamism represents the manner in which each member activates all the others. Frequently it is valuable, especially in institutional group psychotherapy, to transplant a particularly alert or well indoctrinated member as a nuclear cadreman around whom new groups may be built. Such a catalyst accelerates early group work. (5) *Identification.* This primary mechanism in personality development is the insigne of civilization and enters importantly into the therapeutic process. (6) *Universalization.* This is the term given the dynamism occurring in patients when they discover that other people have problems similar to their own, that others entertain the same forbidden thoughts or experience similar unacceptable impulses. This mechanism alone is considered by some to be therapeutic. It reduces guilt, heightens self-esteem and diminishes emotional burdens.

Frequently small groups not only have supportive value but permit the expression of hidden anxieties and conflicts. Also members, by seeing their unconscious motives in action in the ways the members feel toward each other and to the therapist, may gradually gain insight into their difficulties.

Since anxiety is reduced and transference modified in group psychotherapy, the depth of insight may be less than in intensive individual psychotherapy although some therapists claim that a depth of insight comparable with that of individual psychoanalysis may be attained.

An important consideration of group therapy is the realization that in chronically aggressive children the very antagonisms and violent hostilities which constitute their antisocial tendencies are factors common to such groups and tend to promote unit formation, while the nonneurotic elements of the ego respond to the persevering interest and patience of the group leader.

The mobilization of certain defenses may be all that is desired in the treatment of many psychotic patients. The group process often encourages re-repression of unconscious fantasies which present themselves clinically as delusions. As the psychotic mechanisms are removed from consciousness, more normal ego elements resume their supremacy and the patient may become eligible for noninstitutional life or individual psychotherapy.

Mention should be made of the ever-increasing senile segment of the population with whom considerable group therapeutic work is now being done in some institutions. A significantly greater number of senile patients so treated is enabled to return to better levels of adjustment than is the case when group therapy is not employed. The group process appears to increase alertness, dispel confusion, bring affects toward normal and improve memory and orientation. Often the amount of incontinence is found to diminish in many patients on this program.

G. Results of Group Therapy

The statistical evaluation of therapeutic results of group work, as in all the therapies, is wanting in adequate objectivity. Unusually good results with analytical group therapy were secured by Schilder, who found 9 cured and 15 improved out of 31 neurotic patients treated. However, improvement was obtained with hypochondriacal patients. A high degree of cure or improvement was obtained with hysteric patients suffering from anxiety neurosis and obsessional and social neuroses. A recent study of twenty-two juvenile delinquents treated with interview and activity group therapy and of the same number of controls revealed statistically significant improvement in the experimental group as measured by psychometric test, school achievement and maturity tests as well as by Rorschach personality assessment technique. Also, neurotic depressions are said to respond well to group psychotherapy. Most therapists of well constituted groups report results which compare favorably with those of individual psychotherapy.

BIBLIOGRAPHY

Abraham, Karl: Collected Papers on Psychoanalysis. London, Hogarth Press, 1927.

Adler, Alfred: The Practice and Theory of Individual Psychology. New York, Harcourt, Brace & Co., 1927.

Alexander, Franz: Psychoanalysis and Psychotherapy. New York, W. W. Norton & Co., Inc., 1956.

———: Principles and techniques of briefer psychotherapeutic procedures. Proceedings of Assoc. for Research in Nervous and Mental Diseases, Vol. XXXI, pp. 16–20. Baltimore, The Williams & Wilkins Co., 1953.

———, and Ross, Helen, Eds.: Dynamic Psychiatry. Chicago, University of Chicago Press, 1952.

Appel, K. E.: Long term psychotherapy. Proceedings of Assoc. for Research in Nervous and Mental Diseases, Vol. XXXI, pp. 21–34. Baltimore, The Williams & Wilkins Co., 1953.

———: Principles and practice of psychotherapy. Am. J. Psychoanaly., *15*:99–106, 1955.

Balser, B. H.: Psychotherapy of the Adolescent. New York, International Universities Press, 1957.

Bartemeier, Leo: Presidential Address, American Psychiatric Association. Am. J. Psychiat., *109*:1–7, 1952.

Bernheim, H.: De la suggestion et ses applications à la thérapeutique. Paris, Octave Doin, 1886.

Blaine, Jr., G. B.: Short term psychotherapy with college students. New England J. Med., *256*:208–211, 1957.

Brenman, Margaret and Gill, M. M.: Hypnotherapy. New York, International Universities Press, 1947.
Brill, A. A.: Freud's Contributions to Psychiatry. New York, W. W. Norton & Co., 1944.
Cameron, D. E.: General Psychotherapy: Dynamics and Procedure. New York, Grune & Stratton, 1950.
Clark, D. H.: Functions of the mental hospital. Lancet, *271:*1005–1009, 1956.
Colby, K. M.: A Primer for Psychotherapists. New York, The Ronald Press Co., 1951.
Coleman, J. V.: Patient-physician relationship in psychotherapy. Am. J. Psychiat., *104:* 638–641, 1948.
Diethelm, Oskar: Treatment in Psychiatry, 2nd ed. Springfield, Illinois, Charles C Thomas, 1950.
Dorcus, A. M.: Hypnosis and Its Therapeutic Applications. New York, Blakiston, 1956.
Dubois, Paul: The Psychic Treatment of Mental Disorders, 6th ed. New York, Funk and Wagnalls, 1949.
Foulkes, S. H.: Introduction to Group-Analytic Psychotherapy. New York, Grune & Stratton, 1949.
Freud, S.: Collected Papers (5 Vols.). New York, International Psychoanalytical Press, 1924–1950.
———: The Interpretation of Dreams. New York, The Macmillan Co., 1933.
———: Group Psychology and the Analysis of the Ego. London, Hogarth Press, 1948.
Fromm-Reichmann, Frieda: Principles of Intensive Psychotherapy. Chicago, University of Chicago Press, 1950.
———: Notes on the personal and professional requirements of a psychotherapist. Psychiatry, *12:*361–378, 1949.
———: Psychoanalytic and general dynamic conceptions of theory and of therapy. J. Am. Psychoanalyt. Assoc., *2:*711–796, 1954.
———: Psychotherapy of schizophrenia. Am. J. Psychiat., *111:*410–419, 1954.
Galdston, Iago: Dynamics of the cure in psychiatry. Arch. Neurol. & Psychiat., *70:* 286–298, 1953.
Glover, Edward: The indications for psychoanalysis. J. Ment. Sc., *100:*393–401, 1954.
Greenacre, Phyllis: The role of transference. J. Am. Psychoanalyt. Assoc., *2:*671–684, 1954.
Hampshire, Alice: The use of groups in motivation for analytic group psychotherapy, *4:*95–102, 1954.
Hinckley, R. G., and Hermann, Lydia: Group Treatment in Psychotherapy. Minneapolis, University of Minnesota Press, 1951.
Hoch, P. H.: Aims and limitations of psychotherapy. Am. J. Psychiat., *112:*321–327, 1955.
Hordern, Anthony: The response of the neurotic personality to abreaction. J. Ment. Sc., *98:*630–639, 1952.
Janet, Pierre: Psychological Healing. New York, The Macmillan Co., 1925.
Jones, Ernest: Papers on Psychoanalysis, 4th ed. Baltimore, Wm. Wood & Co., 1938.
Jung, C. G.: Two Essays on Analytical Psychology. London, Ballière, Tindall and Cox, 1928.
Kelman, Harold, et al.: Goals in therapy. Am. J. Psychoanalysis, *16:*3–23, 1956.
Knight, R. P.: Evaluation of psychotherapeutic techniques. Bull. Menninger Clin., *16:* 113–124, 1952.
Kubie, L. S.: Practical and Theoretical Aspects of Psychoanalysis. New York, International Universities Press, 1950.
Muncie, Wendell: Psychiobiologic therapy. Am. J. Psychotherapy, *7:*225–240, 1953.
Nunberg, H.: Principles of Psychoanalysis; Their Application to the Neuroses. New York, International Universities Press, 1955.
Oberndorf, C. P.: A History of Psychoanalysis in America. New York, Grune & Stratton, Inc., 1953.
Orr, D. W.: Transference and Countertransference: A historical survey. J. Am. Psychoanalyt. Assoc., *2:*621–670, 1954.

Powdermaker, F. B., and Frank, J. D.: Group Psychotherapy. Cambridge, Harvard University Press, 1953.
Rickman, John: The role and future of psychotherapy within psychiatry. J. Ment. Sc., *96:*181–189, 1950.
Semrad, E. V., and Arsemian, J.: The use of group processes in teaching group dynamics. Am. J. Psychiat., *108:*358–363, 1951.
Slater, Ralph: Interpretations. Am. J. Psychoanalysis, *16:*118–124, 1956.
Slavson, S. R.: Analytic Group Psychotherapy with Children, Adolescents and Adults. New York, Columbia University Press, 1950.
Whitehorn, J. C.: Psychodynamic considerations with treatment of psychotic patients. West Ontario Med. J., *20:*27–41, 1950.
———: Understanding psychotherapy. Am. J. Psychiat., *112:*328–33, 1955.

CHAPTER XXXVII

Pharmacological Therapy

Phenothiazine Derivatives

Chlorpromazine Hydrochloride

This is a synthetic drug, one of the series of alkyl, amine derivatives of phenothiazine, its full chemical name being 10-(3-dimethylamino-propyl)-2-chlorphenothiazine hydrochloride. It was developed in the Rhone-Poulenc Specia Laboratories in France during research on potentiating agents in anesthesia. The first clinical investigations with the drug were carried out in that country in 1952 where, as in other European countries, it is marketed under the trade name Largactil. In this country it is marketed under the trade name of Thorazine.

Chlorpromazine is a white crystalline powder that is readily soluble in water. Since only a small part of the drug is eliminated by the kidneys, most of it is presumably metabolized in the body although the route is unknown.

PHYSIOLOGICAL EFFECTS. One of the early effects of the administration of chlorpromazine is a fall in blood pressure according to dose and individual reaction. Other effects are slowing of the pulse and of respiration, lowering of temperature and of basal metabolic rate and transient leukopenia. Also, it frequently causes dryness of the mucous membranes and nasal congestion. It has an antiemetic effect as well. In large doses chlorpromazine produces motor retardation, muscular hypotonia and an unsteady gait, and during the first two or three days of treatment, patients show a varying degree of somnolence but can be awakened without difficulty and are able to take food. However, as a rule, the increased need for sleep is reduced after a few days. Patients may complain of feeling faint, weak, cold and drowsy, but the sensorium remains clear. The action of the drug is maximal at one hour after administration and appreciable effects continue for six hours. It potentiates the effects of barbiturates and of narcotics.

ADMINISTRATION. Chlorpromazine is available in 10-, 25-, 50-, 100- and

200-mg. tablets, also in 25-mg. (1 ml.) and 50-mg. (2 ml.) ampouls. There is no standard dose of the drug; this must be individualized. Chlorpromazine may be administered by oral or by intramuscular routes; however, it is so irritant that it should not be administered subcutaneously. Intramuscular injections should be given deeply in the upper and outer quadrant of the buttock, and when injected the solution supplied by the manufacturer should be diluted with physiological salt solution or a 2 per cent procaine solution and administered very slowly. Massaging the site of the injection for three or four minutes will help to reduce local irritation. Some physicians add hyaluronidase in order to facilitate absorption and prevent abscess formation. If quick action is desired, the patient may receive 25 mg. by deep intramuscular injection, and if this amount is not effective an additional 25-mg. injection may be given within an hour unless contraindicated by marked hypotension. Subsequent intramuscular dosages may be increased gradually, even up to 400 mg. every six hours. The higher doses should be reached over a period of several days. If, as frequently occurs, the acutely disturbed patient becomes quiet within 48 hours, oral doses (mg. for mg. or higher) may gradually replace intramuscular doses. Injections should not be continued for more than three or four days without beginning to replace them with oral therapy. It will not usually be necessary to increase oral administration to more than 800 mg. a day but if sedation is not secured the dosage may gradually be increased up to as much as 1200 mg. a day. Usually this amount is sufficient for a maximum dose although some psychiatrists give a maximum of 2000 mg. in 24 hours. Amounts up to 4000 mg. have been given but large doses cause confusion and are not to be recommended. As the patient begins to grow quiet, the dose may gradually be reduced over a period of weeks or months. If signs of returning symptoms appear, the amount should be increased immediately and additional parenteral doses be given if necessary. When the patient is no longer disturbed, the dose may usually be reduced gradually and then continued for an indefinite period on the smallest amount that will control symptoms. Usually in the chronically disturbed patient this will be approximately 600 to 800 mg. daily. If there has been no improvement in symptoms after the patient has received these amounts daily for two months, the drug should be gradually discontinued.

In the less acutely agitated patient, treatment may be begun with 50 mg. given orally three times a day. This should be increased gradually until an effective and tolerable level is reached. Frequently doses of 100 to 400 mg. daily if continued over a long period will maintain sedation.

The most obvious response to chlorpromazine is a somnolent effect varying from slight drowsiness to deep sleep. The somnolence is most marked within fifteen to twenty minutes after an injection; however, even when the somnolence is deepest, it is possible to rouse the patient easily. He shows little or none of the residual clouding of consciousness which follows comparable barbiturate sedation. Acutely agitated, restless or excited patients show a greater response than do less disturbed patients. The tranquilizing effect does not seem in any way related to the underlying nature of the excitement, whether schizophrenic, manic or confusional. If the patient responds well to the drug, he develops an attitude of indifference both to his surroundings and to his symptoms. He shows decreased interest in and response to his hallucinatory experiences and a less assertive expression of his delusional ideas. Even though not somnolent, the patient may lie quietly in bed, unoccupied and staring ahead. He may answer questions readily and to the point but offer little or no spontaneous conversation; however, questioning shows that he is fully aware of his circumstances.

INDICATIONS FOR USE. Chlorpromazine usually exerts a tranquilizing effect in a wide variety of disturbed psychiatric states—tension, psychomotor overactivity, agitation, impulsiveness, aggressive outbursts, destructiveness and in overtly anxious, antagonistic, paranoid reactions. It, therefore, has a wide field of usefulness in schizophrenia, both in acute reactions and in overactive chronic patients. The more destructive and aggressive the patient the more likely is he to respond to chlorpromazine. In the acutely ill, schizophrenic hallucinations and delusional ideas frequently disappear within the first two weeks of treatment. Here, as elsewhere when rapid sedation is required, chlorpromazine is to be preferred to reserpine. The percentage of remissions or of improvements among schizophrenic patients who have been ill for less than six months is gratifyingly large and seems to be larger than in those who have received reserpine.

The longer the patient has been ill the less are his chances of attaining a moderate or marked improvement. Of schizophrenics who receive chlorpromazine (or reserpine) relatively early in their illness, more become able to leave the hospital and make adequate social adjustment than has been the case with any previous method of treatment. Among them will be many who despite electroconvulsive, insulin coma and other forms of treatment have shown no improvement. Chronic psychotic patients should be treated for extended periods (6 to 8 months) before assessing the result. Best results are secured with patients who have not been ill for more than two years. Among these the results will depend largely on the clinical manifestations of the disorder, the degree of improvement being much greater in the overactive, disturbed patients. Many patients previously so ill and preoccupied with the symptoms of their illness that they remained indifferent to or hostile to attempts to alter their behavior, thinking or emotional set become more amenable to therapy when taking chlorpromazine. While many schizophrenics who have been hospitalized for years show some improvement, not more than 5 per cent of those hospitalized for five continuous years become able to leave the hospital. It will later become necessary that an appreciable number of them return to the hospital. The number of chronic schizophrenics who will be able to leave the hospital and remain in the community will depend on the understanding and tolerance of the patient's family and the guidance and supervision of the social worker but it actually is not quite accurate to refer to the most favorable outcome of the chronic schizophrenic patient's illness as a cure.

From 30 to 35 per cent of chronic schizophrenics who have long been hospitalized will not be materially improved by administration of chlorpromazine, yet the care of the approximately 60 per cent who do improve but are not able to leave the hospital is greatly eased. Delusions and hallucinations may persist but are usually no longer disturbing to the patient. The sullen, sarcastic and antagonistic patient is less irritable and frequently becomes quiet, co-operative and accessible, and there is a remarkable improvement in the atmosphere of the ward for disturbed patients. Many who long occupied seclusion rooms because of their assaultive and destructive tendencies may mingle with other patients and participate in occupational and useful activities. Even in patients whose response is less favorable, there is usually a lessening of tension and perhaps an attitude of quiet indifference. While the withdrawn, inactive, unresponsive, regressed schizophrenic patient does not usually improve sufficiently to leave the hospital, he frequently is able to modify his behavior, discontinue soiling and no longer discard his clothing. Not the least desirable result of the use of chlorpromazine and of reserpine in the disturbed ward is the easing of the burden of the nurse and the aide, allowing them more time for creative activity with the patient. The relief from the anguish, bitterness, hostility and despair from which many patients suffer is of incalculable value. The chronic schizophrenic who improves, whether through use of chlorpromazine or through reserpine, and whether or not he is able to leave the hospital, should continue on a carefully determined maintenance dose for an extended period.

In manic-depressive psychosis, chlorpromazine is not a substitute for electroconvulsive therapy but in the early stages of the manic phase it is a useful adjunct if the patient is overactive and unmanageable and the period required for recovery is usually shortened. It is probably desirable to administer the drug by intramuscular injections for two or three days and then to continue it by mouth in 50 per cent larger doses. If the depressed patient is agitated, chlorpromazine will usually relieve, or perhaps more accurately, mask the agitation. However, reactive depressions do not respond particularly well to chlorpromazine and may be aggravated by reserpine. Electroconvulsive therapy still remains the most effective means of treating depression.

The usually difficult problem of the restless or agitated patient suffering from senile dementia is often rendered much easier by the use of chlorpromazine. Sedation by means of the barbiturates may confuse him still further. Under chlorpromazine, in amounts of 25 to 50 mg. three times a day, he often becomes calm and manageable and can be cared for at home. Memory loss and disorientation are, of course, unaffected.

Occasionally, especially in institutions for their care, epileptic patients who are subject to episodic or chronic disturbed states are observed. In these states the patient may be hyperactive, noisy, hostile, aggressive, resistive, assaultive, destructive and given to temper outbursts or furor states. A parenteral injection of 100 mg. of chlorpromazine is highly effective in quieting the acute, excited states. Most epileptic patients who exhibit chronic disturbed states are also quieted and relaxed by the drug.

This may at first be given in 300 mg. daily and later reduced to 150 mg. Since chlorpromazine tends to potentiate the activity of barbiturates, it is well to reduce the dose of the latter drug during the administration of the former.

In relatively large doses, chlorpromazine is extremely helpful in the management of acute alcoholic states. It produces prompt control of motor excitement and of nausea and vomiting, permits restful, relaxed sleep and contributes to the relief of tension and anxiety. Its sedative effect hastens recovery in delirium tremens. It is definitely beneficial in nearly all short-lived mental disturbances of a delirious type. The use of chlorpromazine should supplement and not replace the administration of glucose solution, of insulin and of vitamin B complex. It is not, of course, of value in the treatment of the Korsakoff syndrome or in the alleviation of chronic alcoholism.

As with reserpine, to be discussed later, the results to be obtained by chlorpromazine do not depend upon the specific psychiatric diagnosis but upon the type of behavioral disturbance.

Encouraging reports concerning the treatment of depression with chlorpromazine and promethazine have been published. The dose of promethazine is 12.5 mg. orally twice a day. The dose of chlorpromazine is individualized for each patient.

UNTOWARD EFFECTS. Mention has already been made of some of the physiological effects of chlorpromazine. At times these side effects are troublesome and may rarely lead to serious complications. Occasionally the somnolence may become excessive and require a reduction of dosage. Usually, however, it disappears after the first or second week of therapy. Not infrequently an unpleasant taste and a dryness of the mouth and "stuffiness" of the nose result in discomfort. Tachycardia, palpitation, persistent constipation even to the point of fecal impaction, headaches, pyrexia and pains in the legs or abdomen may occur. A pale and "pinched" facial appearance is common in patients receiving full intramuscular doses. Both chlorpromazine and reserpine cause hypotension of the orthostatic type. This may lead to sensations of faintness or to actual fainting, especially on changing from recumbent to standing position. Both drugs should be given with great caution to patients suffering from atherosclerosis, cardiovascular disease or other conditions in which a sudden drop in blood pressure may be undesirable. Photosensitivity confined to areas exposed to sunlight may be produced by chlorpromazine. Usually this will result merely in redness and itching but sometimes it will lead to edema and vesicle formation. Ordinarily interruption of the drug, the application of bland lotions and the administration of antihistamines are sufficient treatment of the dermatological reactions. About 8 per cent of patients receiving chlorpromazine develop allergic skin reactions. One of the most frequent forms is a maculopapular, erythematous, pruritic eruption involving the trunk and arms.

Jaundice, usually appearing from the second to eighth week after beginning the use of the drug, develops in approximately 4 per cent of cases and its duration is variable. Since there is no evidence of damage to the hepatic parenchyma, the jaundice is undoubtedly cholestatic in origin. The total bilirubin content of the blood is greatly elevated and the alkaline cholesterol is much increased as is the percentage of eosinophils. However, there is little or no disturbance of the cephalin flocculation and thymol turbidity. The obstruction is within the intralobular canaliculi and a result of a pericanalicular lymphocytic infiltration.

If the patient's mental state is such that he can note and report his observations, it is well to ask him if there has been any change in the color of his urine or stools, also if he has been aware of pruritus. As a precursory symptom of jaundice, this has been known to occur within two days after the administration of chlorpromazine. Since it is simple and can easily be done at the bedside as a screening measure, some internists advise doing a sodium bilirubinate test twice a week for three weeks after beginning the drug. If jaundice appears, the drug should be discontinued and glucose administered intravenously if indicated. Vitamins should be given, also a high carbohydrate, high protein and low fat diet. It is often difficult to determine whether the jaundice is caused by the drug or by extrahepatic obstruction. Surgery for supposed disease of the biliary tract should be avoided. Liver function tests should probably be continued until they show that normal function has been restored. To what extent, if any, the liver will suffer harmful effects as the result of long continued administration of chlorpromazine is as yet unknown. Although the jaundice is apparently related not so much to dosage as to a special sensitivity on the part of the patient, the drug may be resumed after normal function has been restored. The beginning dosage should not exceed 25 mg. given three times a day and increased slowly thereafter.

Chlorpromazine depresses the production of leukocytes. Agranulocytosis is fortunately of low incidence, probably less than 0.3 per cent and it occurs within three to six weeks after the beginning of treatment. It is more frequent in women, particularly in those between 40 and 60 years of age and its onset is sudden. Patients should be asked to report at once the sudden appearance of sore throat or of lesions in the mouth. Any rise in temperature should also suggest an immediate blood count. These cannot be relied upon as the sole criterion for agranulocytosis. A weekly blood count is in order but is of little value in detecting an impending agranulocytosis. In case blood dyscrasia develops, chlorpromazine should be stopped at once and penicillin and the broad-spectrum antibiotics be given immediately. Corticotropin (ACTH) is also usually employed and transfusion is often advisable. In spite of active treatment the outcome is often fatal.

Occasionally nurses who administer chlorpromazine develop a troublesome contact dermatitis which clears when further exposure is avoided. The irritant qualities of the drug were dramatically illustrated in the case of one patient who rubbed an eye with a tablet of chlorpromazine. An extensive and violent inflammatory process resulted in loss of vision. A few patients have attempted suicide with large doses of chlorpromazine but only one death has been reported.

Parkinsonism appears in about 10 per cent of patients receiving full doses of chlorpromazine. The clinical picture is the usual one of muscular rigidity, slowing of movement, festinating gait, sialorrhea and at times a pill-rolling tremor. The condition is always reversible and may be relieved with benztropine methane sulfonate (Cogentin), 1 mg., twice a day.

Miosis or blurring of vision is noted at times.

DISCONTINUANCE. It is not difficult to decide when the administration of chlorpromazine should be discontinued in the case of acute confusional excitement or in the case of acute manic episode of manic-depressive psychosis. In the former, its use may be terminated soon after the sensorium becomes fully clear. In the latter, the dose may be reduced as the symptoms subside and the drug may be discontinued after mood and motor activity have been entirely normal for two weeks. Experience thus far suggests that in chronic schizophrenia the drug should be continued indefinitely in optimal individual dosage. Although undesirable side effects of the drug usually appear within two months after beginning its use, yet the patient who continues on a maintenance dose after leaving the hospital should report frequently to a physician.

A number of phenothiazine derivatives are now available for clinical usage. The indications for their prescription are essentially similar to those for chlorpromazine. Some are suggested as less toxic in one respect or another:

Promazine

This drug, sold commercially as Sparine, is identical chemically with chlorpromazine except for the absence of a chlorine atom on the ring structure. The general pharmacological properties are similar, also. There is evidence that toxic manifestations such as jaundice and hypoplastic anemias are less likely to occur with its use although clinical experience with the drug remains limited. Transient leukopenia, agranulocytosis and convulsive seizures have been reported but are infrequent in occurrence. Promazine is available for both oral and parenteral administration. The tablets for oral use may be given in doses of 25 to 200 mg. every four to six hours, varied according to the response of the patient.

Perphenazine

This drug, known commercially as Trilafon, combines the phenothiazine and piperazine rings. It is said to have fewer side effects than chlorpromazine. Photosensitivity, has as yet to be reported nor have bone marrow suppression and narrowing of the visual fields been reported. Perphenazine is supplied in tablets of 2, 4 and 8 mg., and is recommended in oral doses of 6 to 16 mg. daily although as high as 64 mg. have been given. It is said to be useful for tension headaches, intractable pruritus and certain neurodermatoses as well as the psychotic states.

Prochlorperazine

This drug, sold as Compazine, has recently been recommended for use in the treatment of various neurotic conditions. It is given orally as 5-mg.

tablets three or four times daily. Since in large doses it produces extrapyramidal syndromes in a high percentage of individuals, it is not suggested for the disturbed psychotic.

N-Methylpiperidyl-(3)-methyl Phenothiazine

It is doubtful whether this drug, sold commercially as Pacatal, is superior to other phenothiazines. The indications for its use are the same, but reports on its toxicity are contradictory. It may be useful as a substitute for chlorpromazine in certain instances.

Urine Test for Phenothiazines. Recently a simple test for detection of chlorpromazine and other phenothiazines in urine has been described. To a small amount of urine (1 ml.) is added an equal volume of a solution containing equal parts of 10 per cent H_2SO_4 and 5 per cent $FeCl_3$. The mixture is gently shaken. The presence of phenothiazines is indicated by the development of a violet color.

Rauwolfia Derivatives

Reserpine

For centuries the root of the plant *Rauwolfia serpentina* Bentham, indigenous to India and known there as the "insanity herb," was used in that country for the treatment of a wide variety of diseases including mental disorders. In 1953 Dr. R. A. Hakim of Ahrnabad, India, was awarded a gold medal for the presentation of a paper on the cure of schizophrenia with a compound, the major ingredient of which was this drug. Reference to its sedative effect had, however, been previously made by many Indian writers. In 1943 note was made in the Indian Medical Gazette of its increasing popularity in the treatment of mental disease and report was made of improvement following use of the drug in manic-depressive psychosis, schizophrenia and other forms of mental disorder. In 1953, prompted by Hakim's report, Kline, at the Rockland (N. Y.) State Hospital, began the experimental use of reserpine, a colorless, crystalline, ester alkaloid, the chief active principle of *Rauwolfia*, and concluded it is an effective sedative for use in mental hospitals.

Pharmacologically, the Rauwolfia derivatives have an effect on the metabolism of serotonin (5-hydroxytryptamine). Serotonin, a product of tryptophan metabolism, is produced by the argentaffin cells which are dispensed throughout the body, particularly in the small intestine and nervous system tissues. The administration of Rauwolfia alkaloids liberates serotonin from the brain. This, it is believed, accounts for its tranquilizing effect. So far, no other tranquilizing drugs have shown this serotonin-releasing effect.

Administration and Dosage. Reserpine (Serpasil) may be given intramuscularly or orally and frequently in the early stages of treatment both methods are used simultaneously. However, the dosage must be individually adjusted in accordance with optimal results and tolerance of the patient. Many physicians recommend 5 mg. intramuscularly once a day for ten days and 1 mg. orally twice a day. If necessary, the oral dose may gradually be increased to 10 mg. and continued indefinitely. The maximum dose should not exceed 15 mg. in 24 hours. Sometimes the dose must be reduced to 2 mg. or 1 mg. because of side effects. Reserpine acts more slowly than does chlorpromazine. In its effect, 10 mg. of reserpine are equivalent to about 300 to 400 mg. of chlorpromazine. As with chlorpromazine, a confusional state may develop in case of overdosage; the optimal level of the dosage appearing to be proportional to the intensity of the emotional disturbance. If a patient shows no improvement after two months of treatment, it is probably useless to continue the drug but if improvement follows, treatment should be continued for at least three consecutive months. As is the case with chlorpromazine, it is usually desirable to continue reserpine indefinitely for the chronic psychotic patient who has improved with its use.

Clinical Effects. Even though the chemical structures of reserpine and of chlorpromazine are completely different, they are used for almost identical purposes and their clinical effects are strikingly similar. Although the psychological effects of these drugs are subject to quantitatively large individual variations, they both usually have a definitely relaxing and quieting influence. Typically the patient receiving reserpine is somnolent and lethargic but is readily aroused and then seems quite alert. Recent studies of the effects of reserpine upon pathological activity suggest that these are less than were originally assumed, and that the apparent results are a result largely of the increased somnolence during hours of the day when the patients would be normally awake. It is not certain that they are direct effects of the drug. Occasionally, from about two weeks to two months after beginning treatment, especially when receiving full doses of the drug, the patient may develop parkinsonism, usually of a more marked type than that produced by chlorpromazine. This syndrome may be quite complete even to the pill-rolling tremor, slow, shuffling gait and rigidity with cogwheel phenomena but the syndrome disappears with a reduction of the dosage. Some patients receiving reserpine rapidly increase their tissue water and this hydration may occasionally cause convulsions. Among other side effects occasionally observed are lactation in the nonpregnant woman and impotence in men. A serious drop in blood pressure occurs more frequently in the patient receiving reserpine than in the one receiving chlorpromazine. Reserpine also increases both the volume and acidity of gastric secretion and it is, therefore, contraindicated in patients with a known history of peptic ulcer. A rise of temperature occasionally occurs, as also does asthma. Clinical experience seems to show that in general the side effects of reserpine are less hazardous than those of chlorpromazine yet deaths have occurred because of sudden and excessive drop of blood pressure.

Clinical Use. While reserpine is of value in other disorders, its greatest use is in schizophrenia. In the acute schizophrenia with tension and anxiety or in milder chronic reactions, its use, as is true also of chlorpromazine, may shorten or prevent hospitalization. Perhaps one of its widest fields of use has been with the restless, combative, hostile, overactive, tense and threatening patient. It has been extensively used also for the untidy, regressed patient who refuses to wear clothing and usually requires seclusion. The longer the patient has been ill the less effective will be the treatment. Perhaps 10 per cent of restless, combative or destructive schizophrenics who have been hospitalized for less than five years, and 5 per cent of those who have been in a hospital for more than five years, will be able to return home under supervision. The ward adjustment of 70 per cent of chronic schizophrenics will be improved to varying degrees. The improvement in behavior in the overactive and aggressive patient is less marked than that observed following the use of chlorpromazine. There is usually an improvement in eating habits, toilet habits, and in social participation. In some patients the modified behavior following the administration of reserpine is maintained only as long as they are receiving the drug. In other cases there is a prolonged improvement.

Experience has shown that reserpine may have a sedative effect in the irritable, quarrelsome, demanding and hostile senile patient. Treatment may be begun with 0.5 mg. after each meal and 1.5 mg. at bedtime given in tablet form. This may be increased every third day up to a maximum of 40 mg. a day if the patient does not become somnolent. As improvement occurs, the dosage may be reduced to a maintenance amount of 6 to 10 mg. daily by mouth. It is believed that the use of reserpine will enable many ambulant seniles who would otherwise require institutional supervision to remain in the care of their families.

Both reserpine and chlorpromazine may exert a highly desirable sedative effect on the overactive, brain-injured child. It also often relieves the anxiety, fear and restlessness frequently seen in the chronic asthmatic.

The physician will not, whether using reserpine or chlorpromazine, be satisfied with a change in the chronic schizophrenic from a state of turbulence to one of quiet indifference. All other available therapeutic resources, including occupational and the many other therapies, should be employed. This is exceedingly important. A considerable number of patients will become sufficiently accessible so that they may participate in some form of psychotherapy.

Reserpine may aggravate depressions and, in fact, has produced depression eventuating in suicide in the hypertensive patient. Such depressions are occasionally of such a severity that electroshock therapy is required for their relief.

There have been a few reports indicating that a combination of reserpine or chlorpromazine with electroconvulsive therapy may be dangerous.

COMBINED USE OF RESERPINE AND CHLORPROMAZINE. Because of the observation that chlorpromazine potentiated the effects of hypnotics and sedatives, the effect of combining reserpine and chlorpromazine was investigated. Consequently, it was found that the combined use of the drugs is sometimes more effective in chronically disturbed patients than is either drug alone.

While the dosage scheduled in combined reserpine-chlorpromazine therapy may be varied, particularly with reference to the degree of the patient's disturbance, the following is recommended by Kline for the patient who is moderately disturbed. The patient is started on 3 mg. of reserpine and 25 mg. of chlorpromazine once a day. After ten days, the chlorpromazine is increased to 25 mg. twice a day. At the end of three weeks, if the patient is not showing satisfactory progress, the amount of chlorpromazine is increased to 50 mg. twice a day, the dose of reserpine remaining at 3 mg. daily. If, after another three to four weeks, the patient is not improving satisfactorily, 5 mg. of reserpine given by intramuscular injection should be added daily for ten days. If the patient still does not improve, the intramuscular dose may be increased to 10 mg. and continued until maximum results have been secured when the intramuscular injections are gradually withdrawn but oral medication is continued indefinitely. In many patients receiving combined therapy, it is not necessary to add intramuscular injections of reserpine.

Patients receiving reserpine alone do not develop either jaundice or agranulocytosis but those receiving combined reserpine-chlorpromazine therapy may develop either of these toxic reactions.

Both chlorpromazine and reserpine have been widely and, many believe, too indiscriminately used in private office and in clinic practice in the treatment of psychoneurotic and mildly psychotic patients. They are much less effective in these disorders than in the active, grossly psychotic patient. Both drugs, if accompanied by psychotherapy, may be helpful in treating the early schizophrenic patient, and they also may make psychotherapy easier in anxiety reactions. They usually have little value, however, in the treatment of obsessive-compulsive neuroses. Chlorpromazine sometimes seems to be helpful in phobic reactions, and psychosomatic disorders accompanied by tension are often made more comfortable by these tranquilizing drugs. Sometimes, especially in office or clinic practice, the patient may be so alarmed by a feeling of strangeness and even of depersonalization that these drugs must be discontinued.

After the disappearance of psychotic symptoms, some patients reject any suggestion that they receive psychotherpy while others express a wish for and should receive it. In the large public mental hospital psychotherapy is all too often not available for many who should receive it.

Because these drugs relieve tension, some patients may be reluctant to discontinue their use but since they have no euphorizing effect they do not lead to addiction in the true sense of the term. The improvement often produced by them is merely symptomatic and not etiological—a reduction in the quantity of the symptoms. The mechanism of their action is not yet certain. Somehow they seem to block autonomic response; perhaps they block impulses from the cortex to the reticular substance. It is not yet clearly determined whether their direct action is by influencing neurophysiological or chemical processes.

Diphenylmethane Derivatives

Several synthetic, tranquilizing drugs are now in an experimental stage in respect to their therapeutic usefulness. While apparently clinically useful, none has a sedative potentiality equal to chlorpromazine and reserpine. One of them is the chemical α-(4-piperidyl) benzhydrol hydrochloride, also known as azocyclonal, sold under the trade name Frenquel. It has been established that acute, exogenous, hallucinogenic psychoses analogous to those produced by cocaine, hashish and mescaline may be produced in normal subjects by D-lysergic acid diethylamide (LSD-25). It was discovered that the administration of Frenquel for a few days prior to the ingestion of LSD-25 prevented the dissociation reaction which otherwise occurred, and that the intravenous administration of 20 mg. of Frenquel during a LSD-25 psychosis will terminate the psychotic reaction in some persons. Similar results followed the use of Frenquel as a blocking or protective agent against mescaline psychosis and as a means of terminating it. Comparable action has been reported in the case of chlorpromazine.

Based on these observations, Fabing began the use of azocyclonal in the treatment of acute schizophrenic reactions, alcoholic hallucinosis and acute paranoid reactions. Treatment of these acute psychoses with azocyclonal met with considerable initial success especially when supplemented by chlorpromazine. Additional usage by others indicates that azocyclonal does not have therapeutic value in the chronic, disturbed schizophrenic, in psychotic depressive reactions or in obsessive-compulsive disorders. Brief experience suggests that it may be of therapeutic benefit in acute postoperative psychotic states and in delirium tremens.

The gamma isomer of azocyclonal, known as Meratran, has been suggested as a useful agent in treating depressed states and for chronic schizophrenics without delusions or marked anxiety. More recent clinical trials indicate that the expectations for this agent have not been extensively realized. Additional new derivatives of diphenylmethane, now under trial, are hydroxyzine (Atarax) and benactyzine (Suavitil).

Other Agents

Meprobamate

Meprobamate, 2-methyl-2-n propyl-1, 3-propanediol dicarbamate, commercially sold as Miltown or Equanil in the United States, is known to synchronize selectively interneuronal electrical activity in the thalamic nuclei and to act as an anticonvulsant and muscle relaxant. It is said, in contrast to the previously described drugs, not to affect activity of the autonomic nervous system.

It is reported of value in anxiety and tension states, phobias, tension headaches, psychosomatic disorders, insomnia, premenstrual tension and neurodermatitis. It often produces relief of headaches that are the result of constant, almost unremitting contraction of the posterior muscles of the neck.

Continued ingestion of large doses of meprobamate can create physical dependence, manifested on abrupt withdrawal of the drug by hyperirritability of the central nervous system and convulsions. The type of addiction caused by meprobamate resembles that caused by chronic intoxication with excessive amounts of barbiturates or alcohol. Especial care should be exercised in prescribing meprobamate for alcoholies or narcotic drug addicts.

A wide variety of side effects and untoward reactions has been reported. Among them have been dermal hypersensitivity reactions and acute nonthrombocytopenic purpura. Large doses taken with suicidal intent may produce complete respiratory and vasomotor collapse. The drug is not as effective in the treatment of the psychoses in the seriously disturbed as the phenothiazine derivatives.

It is available in tablets of 400 mg. which may be prescribed three to four times daily. Blood, urinary changes and local disturbances have not followed its prescription. In a few persons, allergic reactions have been noted with urticaria, erythematous rashes, and rarely fainting spells and bronchial spasm.

Effect of Tranquilizing Drugs in Public Mental Hospitals

The use of the tranquilizing drugs has made possible the discharge of many patients who seemed to be destined to permanent hospitalization. Even more striking is the fact that large segments of public mental hospitals now filled with orderly, quiet people were, before the introduction of these drugs, occupied by disturbed, noisy, destructive and hostile patients. The use of these drugs has brought many such patients to the point where other therapeutic techniques which formerly could not be employed because of their disturbed state are now applicable. As a result, the need for more personnel, especially for more professional personnel, has been increased. For example, more physicians are needed for the many patients who can now be helped by individual and group psychotherapy, and more nurses, occupational therapists and recreational workers are needed for the development of new activity, rehabilitation and resocialization programs.

BIBLIOGRAPHY

Annals N. Y. Academy of Sciences, *67:*671–894. Meprobamate and other agents used in mental disturbances. New York, 1957.

———, *61:*1–280. Reserpine in the treatment of neuropsychiatric, neurological and related clinical problems. New York, 1955.

Anton-Stephens, D.: Preliminary observations on the psychiatric uses of chlorpromazine (Largactil). J. Ment. Sc., *100:*543–557, 1954.

Ayd, F. J.: The treatment of anxiety, agitation and excitement in the aged. A preliminary report on Trilafon. J. Am. Geriatric Soc., *5:*1, 1957.

Baker, A. A.: Observations on the effect of Largactil in psychiatric illness. J. Ment. Sc., *101:*175–182, 1955.

Barsa, J. A., and Kline, N. S.: Combined reserpine-chlorpromazine in treatment of disturbed psychotics. Arch. Neurol. & Psychiat., *74:*280–286, 1955.

———: Treatment of two hundred disturbed psychotics with reserpine. J.A.M.A., *158:* 110–113, 1955.

Bird, E. G.; Gross, J. D., and Denber, H. C. B.: Chlorpromazine in the treatment of mental illness: a study of 750 patients. Am. J. Psychiat., *111:*930, 1955.

Bonafede, V. I.: Chlorpromazine (Thorazine) treatment of disturbed epileptic patients. Arch. Neurol. & Psychiat., *74:*158–162, 1955.

Borrus, J. C.: Meprobamate in psychiatric disorders. M. Clin. North America. W. B. Saunders Co., March, 1957.
Cutler, R. P., Monroe, J., and Anderson, T. E.: Effects of "tranquilizers" upon pathological activity in psychotic patients: I. chlorpromazine. Arch. Neurol. & Psychiat., *77*:616, 1957.
———: Effects of "tranquilizers" upon pathological activity in psychotic patients: II. reserpine. Arch. Neurol. & Psychiat., *78*:61–68, 1957.
Ewing, J. A., and Fullilove, R. E.: Addiction to meprobamate. New England J. Med., 257:76, 77, 1957.
Fabing, H. D.: Frenquel, a blocking agent against experimental LSD-25 and mescaline psychosis. Neurology, *5*:319–328, 1955.
Feldman, P. E.: A comparative study of various ataractic drugs. Am. J. Psychiat., *113*: 589–594, 1957.
Forest, F. M., and Forrest, J. S.: A simple test of chlorpromazine in urine. Am. J. Psychiat., *113*:931–932, 1957.
Goldman, Douglas: Comparison of clinical effects of chlorpromazine and reserpine in psychotic patients. Am. J. Med. Sc., *233*:439–441, 1954.
Hodges, H. H., and LaZerte, G. D.: Jaundice and agranulocytosis with fatality following chlorpromazine therapy. J.A.M.A., *158*:114–116, 1955.
Hollister, L. E.: Complications from the use of tranquilizing drugs. New England J. Med., *257*:170–177, 1957.
Kinross-Wright, Vernon: Chlorpromazine treatment of mental disorders. Am. J. Psychiat., *111*:907–912, 1955.
Kline, N. S.: Use of Rauwolfia Serpentina Bentham in neuropsychiatric conditions. Ann. New York Acad. Sc., *59*:107–132, 1954.
———, and Stanley, Alfred M.: Use of reserpine in a neuropsychiatric hospital. Ann. New York Acad. Sc., *61*:85–91, 1955.
Laborit, H.; Huguenard, P., and Alluaume, R.: Un nouveau stabilisateur végétatif (LE4560 RP). Presse méd., *60*:206–208, 1952.
Lehmann, H. E., and Hanrahan, G. E.: Chlorpromazine. Arch. Neurol. & Psychiat., *71*:227–231, 1954.
Lemere, Frederick: Combined chlorpromazine-reserpine therapy of psychiatric disorders. Arch. Neurol. & Psychiat., *74*:1–2, 1955.
Lesse, Stanley: An evaluation of promazine hydrochloride in psychiatric practice. Am. J. Psychiat., *113*:984–987, 1957.
New and Nonofficial Remedies: Promazine hydrochloride. J.A.M.A., *164*:171, 1957.
Noce, R. H.; Williams, D. B., and Rapaport, W.: Reserpine (Serpasil) in the management of the mentally ill. J.A.M.A., *158*:11–15, 1955.
Mitchell, P. H.: Effects of 'Pacatal' on symptoms of chronic psychotic female inpatients. Brit. M. J., *1*:204–207, 1957.
Osinki, W. A.: Withdrawal of meprobamate. J.A.M.A., *163*:489, 1957.
Perera, G. A.: Edema and congestive failure related to administration of *Rauwolfia Serpentina*. J.A.M.A., *159*:439, 1955.
Promazine Hydrochloride. J.A.M.A., *164*:171, 1957.
Rosner, B. S.; Fierman, L. B., and Kramer, J. F.: Clinical evaluation of Meratran and Frenquel on a chronic psychotic population. Am. J. Psychiat., *113*:993–996, 1957.
Rudy, L. H.; Himwich, H. E., and Tasher, D. C.: Clinical evaluation of two phenothiazine compounds, promazine and mepazine. Am. J. Psychiat., *113*:979–983, 1957.
Schultz, J. D.; Rea, E. L., Fazehas, J. F., and Shea, J. C.: Chlorpromazine in the management of acute alcoholic states. Quart. J. Stud. on Alcohol., *16*:245–250, 1955.
Sussman, R. M., and Sumner, P.: Jaundice following the administration of 50 mg. of chlorpromazine. New England J. Med., *253*:499–502, 1955.
Tourney, Garfield; Isberg, E. M., and Gottlieb, J. S.: The use of reserpine in an acute psychiatric treatment setting. Arch. Neurol. & Psychiat., *74*:325–328, 1955.
Vaughan, G. F.; Leiberman, D. M., and Cook, L. C.: Chlorpromazine in psychiatry. Lancet, *268*:1083–1086, 1955.
Woodson, Jr., R. E., et al.: Rauwolfia: Botany, Pharmacognosy, Chemistry and Pharmacology. Boston, Little, Brown & Co., 1957.

CHAPTER XXXVIII

Psychiatry and the Law

BOTH psychiatry and the law—the former to a large degree, the latter to an important but lesser extent—deal with human behavior. Psychiatry seeks to ascertain the forces that result in behavioral deviations and how they may be redirected to lead to greater intrapersonal serenity and to more constructive and socialized purposes. The law deals largely with the social control of behavior. Although these two disciplines deal with two quite different aspects of behavior they have many contacts, and since they approach problems of behavior from quite different points of view it is not surprising that differences of emphasis and of opinion sometimes exist.

Hospitalizing the Mentally Ill

One of the important differences between the psychiatrist and the lawyer is in their respective attitudes toward the admission of the mentally ill person to a hospital. The psychiatrist urges that the dignity of the patient be respected and that the obstacles to his admission be no greater than those experienced by the physically sick person. The laws of many states still contain much archaic legal phraseology carrying connotations of criminal prosecution and guilt in their provisions for the hospitalization of the mentally ill. Since in many instances the mental patient does not recognize that he is ill, he does not seek treatment and may even resist measures designed to provide it, and since the Constitution of the United States provides that a person may not be deprived of his liberty without adequate notice and a chance to be heard, the law insists on a punctilious observance of what it regards as human rights. A few years ago a special committee of the American Bar Association, in referring to the formal legal procedures of commitment of the mentally ill person, stated that these are "fundamental principles of justice which cannot be ignored. Without them, no citizen would be safe from the machinations of secret tribunals, and the most sane member of the community might be adjudged insane and landed in a madhouse." While it is perhaps theoretically possible that a sane person might be "railroaded" into an institution, it probably never occurs now in this country, certainly not in a public mental hospital. The lawyer should not be criticized too severely for his vigilant solicitude for the legal rights of the individual.

The physician believes, however, that one's medical rights are no less fundamental than his legal rights, and that the sick person should not be subjected to heartless and harmful mental torture incident to commitment. Until very recently one state in the United States required that a mentally sick person must, except for temporary commitment, have a "trial by jury." (A jury trial is now optional.) The laws governing commitment are, however, gradually becoming more liberal in respect to legal formality and its accompanying humiliating publicity. In England a special Royal Commission on Mental Health has recently (1957) recommended that the present laws dealing with the treatment and welfare of the mentally sick be repealed and replaced by an act founded on the general principles of putting mental patients, insofar as possible, on the same status as other patients. The commission recommended that the term "certification" (commitment) be dropped, also that when compulsory measures for the admission of a mental patient are necessary the authorization for admission should consist of the recommendation of two physicians, one of whom should be experienced in the treatment of mental disorders.

All but six states have laws that permit a mentally ill person to apply for treatment in a public mental hospital. Such laws frequently state that the applicant must be mentally competent to make application and must give a certain number of day's notice in writing if he desires to leave. The extent to which persons apply for admission under the provisions of such a statute varies greatly among the states. For many reasons the number who apply for admission is usually not large.

In addition to any laws providing for the voluntary admission of patients, every state has various laws governing the commitment of mentally ill persons. Frequently the patient with mental disorder caused by, or associated with, impairment of brain tissue function is not mentally competent to make application for his admission to a hospital. Among such persons may be those suffering from acute brain disorders associated with intoxication or infection, or from chronic brain disorder associated with cerebral arteriosclerosis or senile brain disease. The laws of four states wisely permit the legal guardian or close relative of such an incompetent person to arrange for his admission. "A person who is a fit subject for mental treatment should not be denied the easy method for admission merely because he may be too indecisive, weakminded or incompetent to sign his own papers." (Addendum, Law of Maryland, March 1944, page 63, 34A.)

Many states provide for the emergency commitment of a patient. These commitments are temporary and commitment for an indeterminate period must be completed before the expiration of the period for which the emergency commitment is permitted. The procedure to be followed in an emergency commitment varies greatly. In some states the law merely requires that a petition be filed with the hospital to which commitment is desired, together with a certification of one physician that the patient is in need of immediate hospital care.

In most states the law provides in general that when an involuntary commitment for an indeterminate period is contemplated, a petition for the patient's commitment must be filed with a judicial agency, that the patient be notified of the proposed judicial hearing on his mental state and that he be examined by two physicians who will certify that he is suffering from mental disease. The judge presiding at the hearing is the committing agent although in 21 states the hearing may be held before a jury if requested by the patient.

In a few states the law permits, without a judicial hearing or order, the superintendent of a mental hospital to receive a mentally sick person and detain him for an indeterminate period. Usually in such a case a relative or other responsible person submits to the superintendent a petition for the patient's admission. This petition contains a sworn statement setting forth reasons why the petitioner believes the patient is mentally ill. Accompanying the petition is a certification by two physicians that they have, within a prescribed period, examined the patient and that in their opinion he is mentally ill and in need of care and treatment in a hospital for the mentally sick. In one state most patients are admitted under the provisions of such a statute. It has been operative in practically the same form for over 70 years and has proven eminently satisfactory.

Model Act Governing Hospitalization of the Mentally Ill[1]

As previously indicated each state has its own laws governing the commitment of the mentally ill. For this reason there is great disparity among the states as to legal procedure in commitment. In many states, too, these procedures subject the patient to indignities and humiliations. For this reason the National Advisory Mental Health Council in 1949 requested the United States Public Health Service to develop what might be considered as a model act. Very few states have enacted a law patterned on this "Model Act" but presumably, as states gradually modify their commitment laws, there will be a tendency to incorporate into concrete legal procedure the modern thinking reflected in the provisions of this suggested act. The act will not be quoted but attention is called to some of its most important features.

Voluntary Hospitalization

The proposed act is so drawn as to facilitate voluntary admissions but provides that upon the patient's written request he shall be forthwith discharged. If, however, in the opinion of the head of the hospital the release of the patient would be dangerous to himself or others this official may notify the court and the patient's discharge be postponed for as long as the court deems necessary for the commencement of proceedings for judicial hospitalization, but in no event for more than five days.

Involuntary Hospitalization

The draft of the proposed act distinguishes between involuntary hospitalization and compulsory hospitalization. Commitment proceedings

[1] *A Draft Act Governing Hospitalization of the Mentally Ill*, U. S. Federal Security Agency, Public Health Service, Publication No. 51, U. S. Government Printing Office, 1951.

may be involuntary in the sense that they are initiated by someone other than the patient himself but the patient accepts the judgment of the physician and his family. In that case there is no judicial hearing and the commitment procedure consists merely of the filing of a request for the patient's admission and the certification of two qualified physicians that they have examined the individual and that in their opinion he should be hospitalized. It is presumed that most patients would be admitted on this medical certification were statutes based on the "Model Act" adopted.

Compulsory Hospitalization

If the patient refuses hospitalization, a judicial hearing is necessary before the commitment may be made compulsory. In such a case a petition for the patient's commitment may be filed with the court. This petition must be accompanied by a certificate of a physician stating that he has examined the patient and is of the opinion that he is mentally ill and should be hospitalized. Upon receipt of the application, the court gives notice thereof to the patient and appoints two physicians to examine him. If the examiners report that the patient is mentally ill, the court sets a date for a hearing at which the patient is afforded an opportunity to appear. If, upon completion of the hearing, the court finds that the patient is in need of custody and treatment, it orders his hospitalization for an indeterminate period or for a temporary observational period not to exceed six months.

The "Model Act" also has humane provisions for the emergency commitment of a patient pending opportunity to initiate proceedings for an indeterminate commitment.

The proposed draft contains various provisions designed to promote the welfare and protect the rights of the patient requiring hospitalization. Among these is one that pending his removal to a hospital a committed patient shall not, except because of and during an extreme emergency, be detained in a nonmedical facility used for the detention of individuals charged with or convicted of penal offenses. As is already provided in many states, the "Model Act" would, except under unusual circumstances, permit the patient to communicate with official agencies inside or outside the hospital; to receive visitors and confer with counsel; to exercise all civil rights, including the right to dispose of property, execute instruments, make purchases, enter contractual relationships, and vote, unless he has been adjudicated incompetent. The act also greatly restricts the information which may be divulged concerning a patient except with the permission of either himself or his guardian.

Observation Commitment

Several states have legal provision whereby a person charged with or under indictment for a criminal offense, or if having been found guilty is awaiting sentence, may be committed to a public mental hospital for a limited period of observation. Following the examination of the prisoner, the hospital submits a report to the court. The hospital does not, of course, express any opinion as to the guilt or innocence of the prisoner. If he is found to be psychotic, commitment will usually be recommended. Frequently the report may include a statement as to whether or not the prisoner's mental condition is such that he is capable of conferring with counsel and preparing his defense. Some courts, especially juvenile courts, may, if the hospital has thoroughly investigated the social situation of the patient, welcome suggestions as to disposition of the prisoner. A juvenile court is, however, more an administrative than a judicial tribunal. Courts are, to an increasing extent, committing prisoners for observation before trial or sentence. Many criminal courts in large cities now employ a full time or part time psychiatrist. Occasionally a prisoner, while serving a sentence, develops a psychosis under the stress of confinement. He will then be transferred to a mental hospital where he will remain until his recovery or until his sentence expires.

Commitment, Competency and Civil Rights

Commitment does not in itself automatically adjudicate incompetency; in most states, in fact, a mentally ill patient is not by his commitment adjudged incompetent or deprived of his "civil rights." If, at the time of his commitment, the patient is formally adjudged as "insane" by judicial action, he is thereby rendered incompetent and deprived of certain civil rights. He may not buy or sell property or sign legal papers; he may not vote or hold office; it suspends his driver's license; it usually vacates his license to practice medicine, law or other learned profession; takes away from him the right to consent to or refuse to consent to the adoption of a child; it casts doubt on his right to make a will; and it impairs his right to marry, although usually, if he does marry while psychotic, the marriage will be valid unless specifically set aside. In most states he cannot start a divorce action.

The methods of erasing the adjudication and of restoring legal competency vary from state to state. Generally speaking, if commitability and incompetency are determined by separate procedures, then discharge (not leave-of-absence or parole) will vacate the commitment order but have no effect on the finding of incompetency. Another court action will be necessary to declare the patient competent and to discharge a guardian.

Habeas Corpus

A right which the psychotic person preserves, even though he has been legally adjudicated as insane, is that of applying for a writ of *habeas corpus.* This writ has for its object the speedy release by judicial decree. Under American and English law this writ may be sued out on behalf of anyone who claims he is being restrained of his liberty illegally. Since a commitment may continue only so long as the patient needs care and custody, he may at any time petition for the issuance of such a writ on the ground that he is now sane and so entitled to release. At the hearing on the petition the sanity of the patient is inquired into and if the court finds him sane he may be discharged. In some jurisdictions the court impanels a jury to determine the issue of sanity. In only a few jurisdictions are there any restrictions imposed on the frequency with which application for a writ may be made.

Privileged Communications

In nearly all jurisdictions, a physician on the witness stand is not allowed, without the patient's consent, to disclose any information acquired in attending the patient in a professional capacity. It is generally held that the confidentiality of a patient's relations with his psychiatrist is peculiarly close, even more so than in ordinary medicine, and is not subject to violation even on a court summons. Usually courts have held that relations between a patient committed to a mental institution and a staff doctor are likewise of a privileged professional nature and are therefore protected from disclosure on a witness stand. The privilege has, in fact, been extended so far beyond the premise of protecting confidential communications that courts assume without argument that all statements of inmates to hospital doctors come within the rule.

Physicians in public mental hospitals receive so many requests for information about their patients that they frequently forget the extent to which the hospital records are really of a privileged nature. They should therefore be guarded lest they divulge more information concerning patients than is permissible.

Marriage

In most states the criterion of legal capacity to marry is the ability to understand the nature of the marriage contract and the duties and obligations such a contract entails. The statutes are of little help in defining the degree of mental unsoundness that will suffice to void a marriage. If it is clear that one party was so psychotic, drunk or defective at the time of marriage that he or she did not understand the obligations assumed by the marriage contract, an annulment will usually be decreed. In general, however, courts are reluctant to declare a marriage void. Many states have laws forbidding mentally ill persons to marry. The objective of such laws is presumably to prevent the procreation of defective children. If such is the case, the law is not based on any scientific proof of the inheritability of the disorder. Usually the courts will not annul a marriage on the grounds of fraud if a concealment of previous mental disease is the basis of the charge. Concealment of previous commitment to a mental hospital is not a ground for annulment on the basis of fraud unless the party concerned affirmatively stated that he never was in a mental hospital.

Divorce

In most states insanity is not a ground for divorce; however, in some states divorce will be granted if the insane spouse has been committed to a hospital for mental diseases for a period of years. The statutes in some states specify that the spouse must be "incurably insane." The psychiatrist is reluctant to testify that any mental illness is absolutely incurable. Perhaps he can say that in the light of present-day medical knowledge it is his opinion that the patient's disorder is incurable. He will remember that at the beginning of the present century he would have testified that general paresis, even in its early stage, was incurable. He certainly would not do so now.

Wills

A person's competency to make a will is known as testamentary capacity. This capacity must meet three criteria. The testator, or a person making a will, must (1) know that he is making a will, (2) know the nature and extent of his property and (3) know the natural objects of his bounty. Expressed a little more simply, the person signing a will must know clearly what he is doing when he signs it. While it is not necessary that he know the minutest details concerning his property he must have a substantially accurate knowledge of what he owns. By "natural objects of his bounty" is meant the members of the testator's family, his warm friends, others to whom he feels especially grateful, or institutions or organizations in which he has felt an interest. While he must know who are his living near relatives, the law does not require that he bequeath them anything. The failure of a testator to include a member of his family because of paranoid delusions of a psychotic intensity concerning the relative would probably render the will invalid since the delusion would affect his understanding of the natural objects of his bounty. Statutes sometimes state that the testator must be of "sound mind and memory." This phrase means, in effect, that the testator must possess the testamentary capacity just described. The fact that the testator was psychotic or was committed to a hospital for mental disorders when he made the will does not necessarily mean that he lacked mental capacity to make a will or renders it invalid. The psychiatrist must at all times bear in mind the three basic criteria as to testamentary capacity.

Since it is often difficult to draw a line between simple senility and senile dementia, the question of testamentary capacity of the elderly person may arise. Even though the testator's mental processes be slow, the courts will consider him competent if he can call to mind his property and the natural objects of his bounty. Senile persons may suffer not only impairment of mind and memory but also increased suggestibility and therefore be subject to undue influence. Many aged individuals are easy prey to the flattery of younger persons. The courts will hold invalid a will obtained by deception, threat or the persistent suggestion of a domineering relative or of a flattering confidant.

Occasionally the psychiatrist will be requested to testify in court concerning the testamentary capacity of a testator, now deceased, at the time he made his will. In such a case the attorney will ascertain from witnesses every possible fact concerning the testator's behavior which will be helpful to the psychiatrist in forming an honest opinion concerning the testator's capacity on the day he made his will. These facts will be assembled in the hypothetical question describing the testator's behavior. At times a lawyer will request that his client be examined as to his competency at the time a testator prepares his will. The psychiatrist's examination will then be directed with special reference to the three basic criteria of testamentary capacity. He will secure from the testator a description of his property and its estimated value. He will ask the patient to name the members of his family and indicate their relationships. As he secures a description of each relative the physician will note the nature of the emotional response evoked by the respective discussions concerning each. The physician's report to the lawyer should contain such verbatim statements made by the patient as will later suggest his testamentary capacity.

Competency and Contracts

Every person of legal age is presumed to be mentally competent, *i.e.*, to have the mental capacity to carry on his everyday affairs. The burden of proof is, therefore, on one who would declare the adult incompetent. To determine that a person is incompetent it must be shown that he has mental disorder, that this mental disorder causes a defect in judgment and that this defect in judgment renders him incapable of managing his property, the prudent making of contracts, or the taking of some other specific action.

The establishment of a mental disorder is not sufficient to warrant a finding of incompetency. It must also be shown that the mental disorder causes an impairment of judgment. No valid generalization can be made on the relationship of the various mental disorders to competency. The diagnostic label attached to the disorder is not as important as the degree to which judgment is impaired. Consideration must also be given as to whether the condition is static, progressive or improving. A progressive organic disease of the brain is typically a disorder that renders a patient incompetent but many patients suffering from psychogenic disorders such as manic-depressive psychosis, schizophrenia or paranoid disorders suffer from such seriously impaired judgment that they are rendered incompetent.

If a person is considered incompetent and he has business affairs which require attention, a petition for the appointment of a guardian will be filed with the appropriate court. The issue of incompetency is usually tried before either a probate or county court, without a jury. In several states a jury is still used. Usually a member of the patient's family is the petitioner but anyone who has an interest in preserving the patient's estate may petition the court for the appointment of a guardian. Notice of a hearing on the petition must be given to the person, and in many states to certain others, such as his next of kin. A few states provide not only that the person is entitled to be present if he desires but that his presence is required. It must be shown, usually by medical evidence, that there is danger that in the absence of a guardian for the person's estate he will dissipate his property or become the victim of designing persons. Some courts require personal testimony by a physician while others will accept a certificate of incompetency in lieu of personal testimony. If the person is declared incompetent, the court will decide whether his interests are best served by the appointment of a friend, relative, stranger or corporation as the guardian. In some states the fact of commitment automatically adjudges the patient as incompetent. In such a case the appointment of a guardian is merely an administrative matter and requires no judicial hearing. Usually a guardianship obtains only in respect to the patient's estate and does not, unless so specified, include guardianship of his person.

CONTRACTS. Courts will usually rule that a contract or other legal transaction will not be set aside on the grounds of mental incompetency if the person had sufficient mental capacity to understand the nature and effect of the particular transaction. A higher degree of mental capacity may be required to understand a complex instrument or transaction than a simple one. The degree of judgment needed may vary greatly. It is sometimes claimed that a contract was executed during a lucid interval of a person admittedly disordered. Psychiatrists are inclined to question whether in most cases the patient's lucidity during such intervals was not more apparent than real. It is the prevailing theory that where the incompetency of one party was not known to the other party, where no advantage was taken of the incompetent and where the contract has been executed and the parties cannot be put back *in statu quo*, the contract is binding and cannot be voided on the grounds of incompetency.

Criminal Responsibility

The concepts of mind held by psychiatry and by the law are so disparate that it is difficult for the two professions to agree as to responsibility for behavior, especially criminal behavior. According to the concept held by law, the mind is dominated by reason and full will, and behavior results from a consciously determined intent. The law does not recognize partial responsibility although to the psychiatrist responsibility does not have definable boundaries and degrees. Law confines its exploration of behavior to conscious data and assumes that a disorder of the cognitive faculty (knowledge) is the only basis for the determination of responsibility for behavior termed criminal. Psychiatry, on the other hand, assumes that mental processes are controlled by both conscious and unconscious factors, the latter playing a very important part; that behavior is an expression of the personality as a whole as determined by a multiplicity of complex factors including the unconscious effect of early experiences, and later pressures and emotional needs. To the psychiatrist the unlawful act may not be the result of a consciously determined "intent" but the surface manifestation of a more profound psychic disturbance, an indicator of breakdown in a system of psychic adaptive defenses erected to balance inner conflicts. The psychiatrist would go beyond the act itself and evaluate the total personality both in its conscious and unconscious aspects. He recognizes the role of the intellect, but would give to emotions and the unconscious a greater weight in the balance of forces in mental life.

The difference in these concepts is a logical result of the gradual development of psychological knowledge. In ancient times lunatics were not regarded as suffering from disease but were believed to be possessed of demons and were beaten, kept in chains, and not uncommonly sentenced to death by burning or hanging. Even if the alleged lunatic had committed some crime there was no consideration as to the offender's responsibility. Gradually, however, rules to determine criminal responsibility were formulated. Since American law is based largely on English law, it is of interest to note the early application of responsibility tests in the laws of England. In 1723 an English court declared that for an accused to escape punishment he must "not know what he is doing, no more than . . . a wild beast." This requirement that to qualify for immunity the accused shall know no more than a wild beast was altered and moderated somewhat about 1760 when the terms "right and wrong" were substituted for "good and evil." Slightly earlier, however, an accused person was executed after it had been determined that he had not shown a "*total* want of reason."

The American law generally prevalent at this time stems directly from the famous M'Naghten case. In 1843 Daniel M'Naghten was tried for the willful murder of Edward Drummond, the private secretary of Sir Robert Peel. For several years M'Naghten had suffered from delusions of persecution. He had attempted to escape from his persecutors by leaving Scotland and going to England or to France. On many occasions he had complained to his father and to various public authorities. He became increasingly embittered and finally determined to right his imaginary wrongs by killing Sir Robert Peel. With this object in mind he watched Peel's house. Seeing Drummond come out, he followed and shot him under the belief that he was shooting Peel. At M'Naghten's trial his counsel entered a plea of "partial insanity." He was declared of unsound mind and committed to an institution for the criminally insane.

This case caused a great sensation in England with the result that a few days after the trial a discussion took place in the House of Lords which proposed five questions to the fifteen Judges of England regarding the law of insanity. The answers of the Judges can be reduced to two rules to determine the responsibility of a person who pleads insanity as a defense to a crime:

(1) "To establish a defense on the ground of insanity it must be clearly proved that, at the time of committing the act, the party accused was laboring under such a defect of reason, from disease of the mind, as not to know the nature and quality of the act he was doing, or if he did know it, he did not know he was doing what was wrong."

As a rule the defendant "knows" the facts concerning the particular criminal act which he has committed, knows its harmfulness ("quality"), and its unlawfulness and consequences, but does not know the unconscious basis for it.

(2) "Where a person labors under partial delusions only and is not in other respects insane" and commits an offense in consequence thereof, "he must be considered in the same situation as to responsibility as if the facts with respect to which the delusion exists were real."

It should be borne in mind that the M'Naghten Rules are not a test of sanity and were not formulated as such. They are a test of responsibility in law for acts done. In 28 states the M'Naghten formula is the sole test of responsibility and in 17 others and in American Military Law it is still the main test supplemented by the "irresistible impulse test."

In 1922 the Lord Chancellor of England appointed a committee to consider and report upon what changes, if any, were desirable in the existing law, practice and procedure relating to criminal trials in which the plea of insanity as a defense was raised. The committee approved of the M'Naghten Rules and held they should be maintained. It recommended an addition to the effect that "a person charged criminally with an offense is irresponsible for his act when the act is committed under an impulse which the prisoner was by mental disease in substance deprived of any power to resist." As indicated, the laws in 17 states of the United States exempt from criminal responsibility persons suffering from irresistible or uncontrollable impulse. To most psychiatrists, however, the word "impulse" is unsatisfactory for it covers only a small and very special group of the mentally ill. It suggests some sudden episode, yet in many cases the sufferer acts, not suddenly or impulsively, but coolly and with ingenious calculation. This is characteristic of many who suffer from paranoid schizophrenia or paranoid psychosis. Although courts have hung tenaciously to the M'Naghten "right and wrong test" it has been severely criticized, and increasingly, not only by psychiatrists but also by many eminent lawyers. In 1953 Justice Felix Frankfurter stated in testifying before the British Royal Commission on Capital Punishment: "The M'Naghten Rules were rules which the Judges, in response to questions by the House of Lords, formulated in the light of the then existing psychological knowledge. . . . I do not see why the rules of law should be arrested at the state of psychological knowledge at the time when they were formulated."

The above statement, quoting the opinion of one of the most eminent American jurists, reflects the view of an increasing number of lawyers.

In 1869, influenced by Dr. Isaac Ray, doubtless the most enlightened American psychiatrist in the medical jurisprudence of insanity, the Supreme Court of New Hampshire handed down an opinion sweeping aside the M'Naghten Rules. The court recognized simply that an accused person is not criminally responsible if his unlawful act was the result of mental disease or mental defect. Under this decision, insanity is no longer defined as a matter of law; instead it is made a question of fact to be determined by the jury like any other fact. This determination rests upon testimony of the psychiatric expert respecting the latest knowledge of human behavior and his interpretation of such knowledge in terms of his observations of the accused. If the accused has a mental disease and if the criminal act is the product of it, he is found not guilty by reason of insanity.

In 1954, the case of Durham v. United States, the Court of Appeals for the District of Columbia Circuit handed down a decision adopting in substance the same rule as the New Hampshire one. This case involved a defendant, Durham, who had been convicted of housebreaking. He had previously been committed to a hospital for mental diseases. At Durham's trial the issue of responsibility was raised. A psychiatrist testified that he thought Durham was of unsound mind but that he might give the correct answer if a question of right or wrong were put to him. The appeal court ruled that the trial court was in error in declaring Durham sane on an obsolete test of responsibility. The essence of the decision is contained in the following passage:

"We find that as an exclusive criterion the right-wrong test is inadequate in that (a) it does not take sufficient account of psychic realities and scientific knowledge, and (b) it is based upon one symptom and so cannot validly be applied to all circumstances. We find that the 'irresistible impulse' test is also inadequate in that it gives no recognition to mental illness characterized by brooding and reflection and so relegates acts caused by such illness to the application of the inadequate right-wrong test. We conclude that a broader test should be adopted. . . .

"The rule we now hold must be applied on the retrial of this case and in future cases is not unlike that followed by the New Hampshire court since 1870. It is simply that an accused is not criminally responsible if his unlawful act was the product of mental disease or mental defect."[1]

In 1957 the Vermont legislature adopted the following test of insanity when this is used as a defense in criminal cases:

"1. A person is not responsible for criminal conduct if at the time of such conduct as a result of mental disease or defect he lacks adequate capacity either to appreciate the criminality of his conduct or to conform his conduct to the requirements of law.

2. The terms "mental disease or defect" do not include an abnormality manifested only by repeated criminal or otherwise anti-social conduct. The terms "mental disease or defect" shall include congenital and traumatic mental conditions as well as disease.

3. The M'Naghten test of insanity in criminal cases is hereby abolished."

This statute seems to reflect the increasing dissatisfaction with the M'Naghten Rules as a test of criminal responsibility.

When testifying at a trial the psychiatrist should remember that the determination of responsibility is a legal issue. The psychiatrist's function is to present the data; the application of the law to the facts is for the court and the jury. He will therefore not express any opinion as to whether or not the defendant can distinguish between right and wrong. Any testimony beyond professionally recognized medical data descriptive of the defendant's mental status, and informative to the court and jury, is therefore beyond the province of the psychiatric expert. All expert testimony should be free of moral and value statements. The psychiatrist will be wise not to attempt to scale degrees of responsibility in terms of symptoms.

If a person charged with crime is found not guilty by reason of insanity he may, in some states, at the discretion of the court be committed to a state hospital for mental diseases. In other states the law is mandatory that he be committed. In some states the patient may, upon recovery, be discharged by the court which ordered his commitment; in other states if regarded as no longer dangerous if allowed at large, may be dis-

[1] Durham v. United States: 59 App. D. C. 144 (1929).

charged by the governor. In one state the patient may be discharged only by act of legislature.

Patients are not tried or executed while insane. The issue in such a case is not the patient's ability, or lack of it, to distinguish between right and wrong, but his ability to confer with counsel, and prepare his defense.

In one state, Massachusetts, the law (the so-called Briggs Law) provides that a person who commits a capital offense or commits more than one felony, or who commits the same crime more than once must be referred for examination by experts appointed by the State Department of Mental Health. The examinations are usually made at the jail where the defendant is being held. The psychiatrist's report is filed with the clerk of the court and is accessible to the court, to the district attorney, and to the counsel for the accused. If the examiner reports that the prisoner is suffering from mental disease, he is not directly asked to say whether the patient is able to distinguish between right and wrong, or whether he is able to refrain from doing wrong because of an irresistible impulse, but he is asked whether the patient suffers from a mental illness sufficiently severe to affect his responsibility and to require treatment in a mental hospital. It is apparently assumed that the examiner bases his opinion on the right-wrong test and the irresistible impulse test but the reports submitted to the courts neither ask nor answer the question in these terms.

Under this law juries have shown a commendable tendency to take the word of the impartial examiner as against that of psychiatrists hired by either side. The "battle of experts" has become almost unknown in Massachusetts.

BIBLIOGRAPHY

Alexander, J. E.: Commentaries on the Law of Wills. San Francisco, Bender-Moss Co., 1918.

Barrow, R. L., and Fabing, H. D.: Epilepsy and the Law. New York, Paul B. Hoeber, Inc., 1956.

Davidson, Henry A.: Forensic Psychiatry. New York, Ronald Press Company, 1952.

Diamond, B. L.: Isaac Ray and the trial of Daniel M'Naghten. Am. J. Psychiat., *112:* 651–656, 1956.

G. A. P. Report No. 26: Criminal Responsibility and Psychiatric Expert Testimony. Topeka, Kansas, 1954.

Glueck, Sheldon: Mental Disorder and the Criminal Law. Boston, Little, Brown & Co., 1925.

Guttmacher, Manfred: The quest for a test of criminal responsibility. Am. J. Psychiat., *111:*428–433, 1954.

———, and Weihofen, Henry: Psychiatry and the Law. New York, W. W. Norton & Co., 1952.

Overholser, Winfred: The place of psychiatry in the criminal law. Psychiatric Quart., 10:197–223, 1936.

Ray, Isaac: The Medical Jurisprudence of Insanity. Boston, Charles C. Little, and James Brown, 1838.

Sobeloff, S. E.: From M'Naghten to Durham and beyond. Psychiatric Quart., 29: 357–371, 1955.

Tracey, J. E.: The Doctor as a Witness. Philadelphia, W. B. Saunders Co., 1957.

Usdin, G. L.: The physician and testamentary capacity. Am. J. Psychiat., *114:*249–255, 1957.

Weihofen, Henry: The Urge to Punish. New York, Farrar, Straus & Cudahy, Inc., 1956.

Index

R

S

T